W9-BVY-909

Behavioral Neurology

Behavioral Neurology: Practical Science of Mind and Brain

Second Edition

Howard S. Kirshner, MD
Professor and Vice Chair, Department of Neurology,
Vanderbilt University School of Medicine,
Nashville, Tennessee

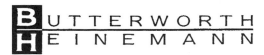

BUTTERWORTH
HEINEMANN

BOSTON   OXFORD   AUCKLAND   JOHANNESBURG   MELBOURNE   NEW DELHI

BS

Library of Congress Cataloging-in-Publication Data
A catalog record for this book is available from the Library of Congress

British Library Cataloguing-in-Publication Data
A catalogue record for this book is available from the British Library

ISBN 0-7506-7228-5

The publisher offers special discounts on bulk orders of this book.
For information, please contact:

Manager of Special Sales
Butterworth-Heinemann
225 Wildwood Avenue
Woburn, MA 01801-2041
Tel: 781-904-2500
Fax: 781-904-2620

For information on all Butterworth-Heinemann publications available, contact our World Wide Web home page at: http://www.bh.com

10 9 8 7 6 5 4 3 2 1

Printed in the United States of America

3/21/04

Contents

Preface   vii

PART I
INTRODUCTION TO BEHAVIORAL NEUROLOGY

1 Introduction and Historical Overview   3

2 The Science of Behavioral Neurology   9

3 Consciousness and the Brain   19

4 Bedside Mental Status Examination   25

PART II
FOCAL NEUROBEHAVIORAL SYNDROMES

5 Speech and Language Disorders   45

6 Alexias and Agraphias: Disorders of Reading and Writing   97

7 Apraxia   125

8 Agnosias   137

9 Disorders of the Right Hemisphere   159

10 Frontal Lobe Syndromes   179

11 Amnesias: Focal Syndromes of Memory Loss   207

12 Syndromes of the Corpus Callosum   233

PART III

GENERALIZED, DIFFUSE, MULTIFOCAL, AND "PSYCHIATRIC" DISORDERS

13 Dementia and Aging   247

14 Delirium and Acute Confusional States   307

15 Psychosis   325

16 Behavioral Aspects of Movement Disorders   341

17 Emotion and the Brain   359

PART IV

NEUROBEHAVIORAL ASPECTS OF SPECIFIC DISEASES

18 Cognitive Aspects of Multiple Sclerosis   377

19 Behavioral Aspects of Epilepsy   387

20 Behavioral Aspects of Traumatic Brain Injury   415

21 Neurorehabilitation and Recovery from Behavioral Effects of Stroke   427

Index   445

Preface

This monograph, like its first edition, *Behavioral Neurology: A Practical Approach*, represents my personal intellectual odyssey through the exploration of questions of mind and brain. At first, I was attracted to the subject by strictly philosophical interests: how can the intricacies of consciousness and behavior reside in the soft, gray, convoluted organ called the brain? Later, in pursuing a career in behavioral neurology and stroke, I felt a different motivation: the practical need to evaluate disorders of the higher functions and to diagnose the responsible lesion sites and disease processes. Most physicians and even neurologists devote attention to the "hard" neurological findings of the cranial nerve, motor, sensory, and cerebellar examinations, but pay little heed to the practical importance of the "higher functions" in neurological diagnosis. Patients suffer both from the failure to diagnose the underlying brain disorders and from the lack of recognition of the behavioral limitations they face. This book, like the first edition, represents the melding of these two themes in behavioral neurology: the relationship of mind and brain, and the practical diagnosis of disorders of the higher functions.

Fifteen years have passed since the publication of the earlier book. These years have been fruitful ones not only for behavioral neurology but also for the related fields of biological psychiatry, neuropsychiatry, and cognitive neuroscience. The influx of new information about the nervous system and behavior or cognition has been truly astounding. In updating the work, I have been struck by the fact that the evolution of behavioral neurology is much more dependent on other fields than was true 15 years ago. For example, our increased understanding of Alzheimer's disease is largely the result of advances in neurochemistry and neurobiology, which have led us closer to the pathogenesis of the condition and also to treatments. The Ph.D. cognitive neuroscientists who study behavior in animals now apply the techniques of functional neuroimaging (functional MRI, PET, and SPECT) to study behavior in individual human patients, much in the manner that behavioral neurologists have always done. Behavioral neurology is thus merging with neurobiology and with cognitive neuroscience in ways not considered possible a few years ago. If behavioral neurology is to continue to develop as a discipline, it must make increased use of the techniques and knowledge of these other specialties.

As in the first edition, I thank my mentors, including the late Drs. Norman Geschwind and D. Frank Benson, Drs. C. Miller Fisher, Raymond D. Adams, and J. P. Mohr, all of whom influenced my interest in this field. In more recent years my practical work has centered increasingly on stroke, and again I owe major debts to Drs. C. Miller Fisher and J. P. Mohr, who preceded me in this evolution. At Vanderbilt University, Dr. Robert T. Wertz has been a valuable collaborator and a source of inspiration in studies of language and the brain. Dr. Gerald Fenichel, my Chairman, has always been supportive of my work. Dr. Bassel Abou-Khalil has helped polish my effort on epilepsy. I thank Mark Kelly, Ph.D., for his major contribution to the chapter on frontal lobe disorders, now Chapter 10, in the first edition of this book. His contribution lives on in this edition. Dr. Herbert Meltzer and my brother, Dr. Lewis Kirshner, have provided advice on psychiatric disorders. Perhaps I shall some day convince Lew that neurology is not the specialty that answers only "how" questions about the mind and brain, whereas psychiatry attempts to answer the "why" questions. Susan Pioli of Butterworth-Heinemann has been as considerate and helpful an editor as any striving medical author could hope for.

No clinical monograph should omit mention of the patients, those unfortunate enough to develop neurological disorders involving the higher functions. These patients are indeed "patient" teachers, helping the physician to learn and, almost without exception, grateful for any understanding they can impart.

Finally, I thank my wife, Carol, and my children, Josh and Jodie (now grown and in careers themselves), for their forbearance in allowing me to spend long evenings retreating to my study, even after long hours of clinical work, instead of pursuing family matters. Without all of these individuals, this book would not have come to fruition.

Howard S. Kirshner, MD

PART I

Introduction to Behavioral Neurology

1

Introduction and Historical Overview

Some people say that the heart is the organ with which we think and that it feels pain and anxiety. But it is not so. Men ought to know that from the brain and from the brain only arise our pleasures, joys, laughter and tears. Through it, in particular, we think, see, hear and distinguish the ugly from the beautiful, the bad from the good, the pleasant from the unpleasant.... To consciousness the brain is messenger.

(Hippocrates)

Behavioral neurology is the study of the relationship of brain lesions and processes to human behavior and cognitive functions, much in the sense evoked by Hippocrates. Since the publication of the first edition of this book (Kirshner 1986), behavioral neurology has grown apace and has become a recognized subspecialty of neurology. In addition, considerable popular attention has been devoted to the relationship between the mind and the brain. How the brain subserves activities such as perception, consciousness, emotions, personality, language, and reasoning, to name but a few of the topics of behavioral neurology, has inherent fascination not only for physicians but also for philosophers, theologians, and the general public. In the words of the Nobel Laureate Francis Crick (1994), the codiscoverer with James Watson of the structure of DNA, the brain and its electrical and chemical processes make up the mind: 'You, your joys and your sorrows, your sense of personal identity and free will, are in fact no more than the behavior of a vast assembly of nerve cells and their associated molecules.'

Behavioral neurology must now be regrounded within the current explosion of knowledge in neuroscience. Tom Wolfe (2000), the popular journalist and novelist, wrote: "If I were a college student today, I don't think I could resist going into neuroscience. Here we have the two most fascinating riddles of the twenty-first century: the riddle of the human mind and the riddle of what happens to the

3

human mind when it comes to know itself absolutely." Closely related is the genetics revolution, which also has provided expanded knowledge of inherited patterns in behavior, temperament, and emotional states. The Human Genome Project promises to revolutionize our knowledge of inherited diseases. Wolfe (2000) quotes the biologist Edward O. Wilson as saying that the human newborn does not have a blank slate, or 'tabula rasa', for a brain, but rather a photographic film that just awaits being developed. On the other hand, we have just learned from the Human Genome Project that the human genome contains only twice as many genes as the fruitfly, and only a few hundred more than the mouse. Surely this small number of new, human genes suggests that human behavior is not solely determined by genes.

With the cognitive tools of behavioral neurology and neuropsychology, together with new technologies for brain imaging and electrophysiological analysis of brain activity, we can now begin to study how the firing patterns of brain neurons give rise to the phenomenon of consciousness, the sense of self, and the ability to process information and develop decisions and attitudes. The pattern of an individual's decisions and attitudes over time leads to a recognizable personality. In other words, recent advances in cognitive neuroscience, electrophysiology, and brain imaging have made mind–brain questions the subject of practical scientific and clinical study.

The purpose of the book is to show how cognitive neuroscience has advanced and to demonstrate how its subject matter has practical relevance for the diagnosis and treatment of patients. To medical students and residents, practicing physicians, and even some neurologists, the field of behavioral neurology comprises the most arcane, theoretical, and philosophical aspects of an already complex discipline – brain science. Behavioral neurology, however, is at its heart a practical discipline. The behavioral neurologist uses the mental status examination, just as the general neurologist uses the cranial nerve, motor, and sensory examinations, to localize lesions within the nervous system. As in all of neurology, the examination indicates where the lesion is, whereas the history indicates what the lesion is, or what specific disease process is active. Laboratory tests such as computed tomography (CT) and magnetic resonance imaging (MRI) scans are used for confirmation, but the diagnosis cannot be made without the traditional history and physical examination (Tanridag and Kirshner 1987). In behavioral neurology more than any other area of medicine, the bedside diagnosis is paramount. This book will emphasize the ways in which bedside diagnosis contributes to the diagnosis and treatment of patients with neurobehavioral syndromes.

In its development, behavioral neurology has increasingly overlapped with the disciplines of neuropsychology, cognitive neuroscience, biological psychiatry, and neuropsychiatry. Neuropsychology is a diagnostic subspecialty of psychology that deals with assessment of brain disease by standardized psychological tests. The clinical and experimental results of such tests will be discussed and compared with bedside clinical findings throughout this book. Neuropsychology may be seen as complementary to behavioral neurology in providing quantitative data for the disorders that the behavioral neurologist evaluates and treats.

Cognitive neuroscience is an investigational field in which neurobiologists study the basic mechanisms of cerebral processes including cognitive functions, behavior, and mood. This field is very closely related to behavioral neurology; until recently, however, cognitive neuroscientists tended to be basic scientists who investigated animal models or even computer models of brain function. In recent years, the advent of functional brain imaging has made it possible to study cerebral processes in a living, cognating human being, and the result is that the fields of behavioral neurology and cognitive neuroscience have effectively merged. In fact, the behavioral neurology section of the American Academy of Neurology decided during the 2000 meeting to change its name to include both behavioral and 'cognitive' neurology.

The field of biological psychiatry is the effort to discover biochemical or structural brain abnormalities underlying psychiatric diseases: mood changes, personality alterations, and thought disorders. These disorders were once thought to be purely in the realm of 'mental illnesses', but many, such as schizophrenia and bipolar affective disorder, have compelling evidence for a genetic or biochemical basis. Since psychiatrists rather than neurologists usually manage these diseases, the degree of overlap with behavioral neurology is limited, but patients with focal brain lesions occasionally manifest disorders resembling psychiatric diseases.

Finally, the field of neuropsychiatry also overlaps behavioral neurology. Its practitioners are again psychiatrists by training, rather than neurologists, but the subject matter is much the same: mood changes, thought disorders, personality changes, and the like, in the setting of neurological diseases such as Parkinson's disease, Alzheimer's disease or epilepsy. In recent years, practitioners of the two disciplines have sought to work together in unraveling some of the mysteries of the mind and brain. Unlike the first edition, this volume will consider key contributions of both biological psychiatry and neuropsychiatry to the clarification of brain–behavior relationships.

The history of behavioral neurology has had three somewhat distinct phases. The first phase, in the nineteenth and early twentieth centuries, involved the descriptions of classical syndromes of aphasia, apraxia, agnosia, and dementia, among other topics, by clinicians who studied their patients and often waited for them to die so that the brain could be examined. Physicians like Broca, Wernicke, Liepmann, and Alzheimer worked at about the same time that the modern classification of neurological diseases and neuropathology were developed by physicians such as Jackson, Gowers, and Charcot.

During the first half of the twentieth century, the interest in the behavioral sphere of neurology waned. Two prevalent patterns of thought accounted for the stagnation of behavioral neurology as an area of research. First, psychological theories considered personality and behavior to emanate from the brain as a whole, rather than from the activity of localized brain centers. The work of the psychologist Karl Lashley (1938) was especially influential in this regard. Second, religious beliefs held human psychological functions to be sacred and not amenable to medical or scientific understanding. During this period, many of the important discoveries and insights of nineteenth century behavioral neurology were forgotten.

The contemporary period of behavioral neurology, which began in the 1950s and 1960s, has been a golden era. The late Dr. Norman Geschwind deserves credit more than any other individual for rediscovering the descriptions of the nineteenth century clinicians and renewing the study of the higher cortical functions. Wilder Penfield, among others, stimulated similar interest in studies of patients with epilepsy. This second era of behavioral neurology has been aided immensely by the advent of new technologies for brain imaging. During this period a tremendous burgeoning of our knowledge of brain structure and function has occurred. Whereas the nineteenth century neurologist had to outlive his patient in order to correlate a brain lesion found at autopsy with a syndrome manifested during life, the contemporary neurologist can obtain immediate localization of a lesion by CT or MRI scanning. Geschwind himself went somewhat beyond the localizationist concepts of the nineteenth century to discuss 'disconnections' between brain centers, rather than destruction of cortical areas, as a source of behavioral symptomatology.

The third phase of behavioral neurology has involved the contributions of neuroscience and cognitive science to the understanding of brain–behavior relationships. The 1980s and 1990s witnessed the birth of a new type of technology, the imaging of functional activity in the brain. These technologies truly provide a 'window' into the brain, through which the examiner can observe the activation or inhibition of elements of the neuronal switchboard in response to stimuli. These functional imaging modalities of positron emission tomography (PET), single photon emission computed tomography (SPECT), and functional MRI (fMRI) permit visualization of language processing, thought, attention, self-monitoring, internal visualization or imagery, and perception of novelty in 'real time', during the performance of cognitive operations. In the words of Posner (1993), these imaging techniques amount to 'seeing the mind'. In addition, new techniques to map epileptic foci in the cerebral cortex have included direct electrical stimulation of the cortex or, more recently, transcranial magnetic stimulation. These techniques have provided another source of information about the loci in the brain involved in specific brain functions.

All of these techniques, taken together, have permitted new conceptions of brain organization and function. In place of localized 'centers' or even connections between centers, the cognitive neuroscientist speaks of 'networks' of brain regions in which individual 'modules' of cells carry out a specific function. The network approach to behavioral neurology, discussed further in the next chapter and throughout the book, is much more complex and sophisticated than earlier models. It is clear that holes in the brain, whether ascertained at autopsy or in imaging studies, do not reveal the richness of human behavioral disturbances brought about by brain disease. Lesions in specific different areas, however, may affect networks in ways that can be visualized by functional imaging techniques.

The book begins with a conceptual review of brain anatomy for behavior, followed by chapters on consciousness, the bedside mental status examination, aphasia and language disorders, reading and writing disorders, apraxia, agnosia, right hemisphere disorders, frontal lobe syndromes, memory and amnesias, the corpus callosum, dementia, delirium, psychosis, behavioral effects of movement disorders, emotion and the brain, behavioral effects of multiple sclerosis, traumatic brain injury, epilepsy, and neurorehabilitation, with an emphasis on stroke. These are the broad topics of behavioral neurology for adult patients. Subjects not covered in this book include developmental and pediatric syndromes such as mental retardation, autism, idiot savant syndromes, learning disorders, dyslexia, and attention deficit hyperactivity disorders.

Behavioral neurology, as a study of human behavior and especially of those most distinctly human 'higher cortical functions', has implications not only for medicine but also for the social sciences, philosophy, ethics, and religion. Because the functions studied are peculiarly human, animal models have been less useful than in other areas of neurology. Advances in behavioral neurology have depended, both traditionally and currently, on the careful study of patients with acquired brain lesions. Behavioral neurology is one of the few areas of medical science in which careful observation of a patient at the bedside can still provide important research information and can serve to prove or disprove new theories about cognitive function. The activities of the behavioral neurologist thus bridge the gap between medical care and research into the complex interrelationships of mind and brain, between brain science and social science or philosophy. It is hoped that this book, in expounding the principles of how brain disorders can be evaluated at the bedside, can bridge this gap for the reader.

REFERENCES

Crick F. The Astonishing Hypothesis: The Scientific Search for the Soul. New York: Charles Scribner's Sons, 1994;3.

Jones W, Withington E, eds. Hippocrates. The Loeb Classical Library, Vol. 2, The Sacred Disease. Cambridge: Harvard University Press, 1923;127–185.

Kirshner HS. Behavioral Neurology: A Practical Approach. New York: Churchill Livingstone, 1986.

Lashley KS. Factors limiting recovery after central nervous lesions. J Nerv Ment Dis 1938;88:733–755.

Posner MI. Seeing the mind. Science 1993;262:673–674.

Tanridag O, Kirshner HS. Magnetic resonance and CT scan imaging in neurobehavioral syndromes. Psychosomatics 1987;28:517–528.

Wolfe T. Hooking Up. New York: Farrar Straus Giroux, 2000;107.

2

The Science of Behavioral Neurology

The body was a cage, and inside that cage was something which looked, listened, feared, thought, and marveled; that something, the remainder left after the body had been accounted for, was the soul.

Ever since man has learned to give each part of the body a name, the body has given him less trouble. He has also learned that the soul is nothing more than the gray matter of the brain in action. The old duality of body and soul has become shrouded in scientific terminology, and we can laugh at it as merely an obsolete prejudice.

(Milan Kundera 1984)

Another problem is the overwhelming evidence that the mind is the activity of the brain. The supposedly immaterial soul, we now know, can be bisected with a knife, altered by chemicals, started or stopped by electricity, and extinguished by a sharp blow or by insufficient oxygen. Under a microscope, the brain has a breathtaking complexity of physical structure fully commensurate with the richness of the mind.

(Steven Pinker 1997)

CEREBRAL CORTEX

In Chapter 1, we referred to Crick's (1994) 'astonishing hypothesis' that all of human behavior, thinking, personality, aesthetics, and even ethics comes from the operations of the human brain. Even literary figures like Milan Kundera (1984) seem to have accepted this premise. Steven Pinker, a cognitive neuroscientist at MIT, refers in the quotation above to the physical evidence that damage to the brain affects mental processing – the litany of causes sounds almost like a summary of disease processes studied by the behavioral neurologist (Pinker

1997). Much of the rest of this book will be taken up by discussions of regional brain functions and of the disease processes that disrupt them. In order to study the brain origins of human behavior, it is necessary to give at least brief consideration to the organizational blueprint of the brain, known as gross and microscopic neuroanatomy. This brief discussion will emphasize the broad patterns of organization of the human cerebral cortex. Descriptions of the specific, functional neuroanatomy devoted to systems such as language, memory, praxis, and visuospatial function will be considered in the chapters on these functions. More detailed descriptions of the neuroanatomy can be found in textbooks of neuroanatomy (Carpenter 1978) or neuroscience (Kandel *et al.* 2000).

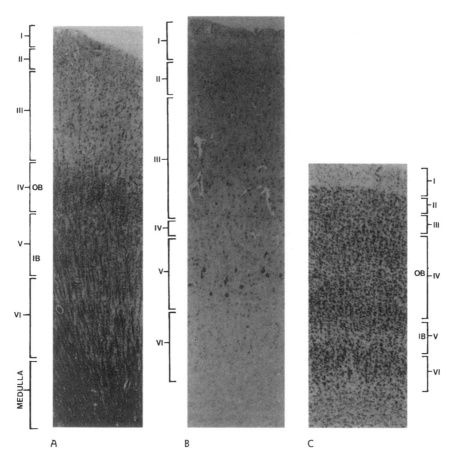

Figure 2.1 Microscopic sections of cerebral cortex from the precentral gyrus (A), another motor cortex (B), and visual cortex (C). Layer I is the molecular layer, II the external granular layer, III the external pyramidal layer, IV the internal granular layer, V the internal pyramidal layer, VI the multiform layer (see text). (Reprinted with permission from JL Wilkinson. Neuroanatomy for Medical Students (3rd edn). Oxford: Butterworth-Heinemann, 1998;176.)

The cognitive operations of the human brain take place among a large network of cortical cells and connections, which can be thought of as a neural switchboard. This network model of the brain provides the physical model for the subjective phenomena of mental activities. The cortical mantle of the human brain contains in excess of 20 billion nerve cells, arranged in a wrinkled pattern of gyri that allows a vast surface area of cortex to be enfolded into the relatively small space inside the human skull. The information stored in the human cerebral cortex rivals that of large computers or major libraries. As many as 70% of neurons in the human central nervous system reside in the cerebral cortex, and 75% of those are in the association cortex (Nauta and Feirtag 1986). Higher cortical functions, with few exceptions, take place in the association cortex.

In comparing the evolution of brain structure from animals to primates to man, the greatest increase in the number of neurons and size of brain elements is found in the association cortices of the brain, those regions that have no primary motor or sensory function but integrate the activities of primary motor and sensory areas of the brain. The greatest enlargement has come in the parietal and frontal association cortices.

The neuroanatomy of the cerebral cortex is well delineated. Cytoarchitectonic studies, including those of Brodmann (1909) and of the Vogts (1919), show that specific anatomic features distinguish the cortex in specific regions of the brain. Within each cortical area are columns of cells that have similar structure and, presumably, function. An experienced neuroanatomist can look at a slide of cortex from one region and immediately determine the type and function of cortex. Figure 2.1 shows the microscopic anatomy of the cerebral cortex. All areas of

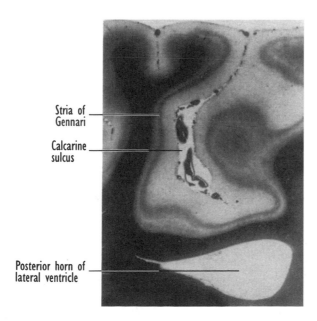

Stria of Gennari

Calcarine sulcus

Posterior horn of lateral ventricle

Figure 2.2 Section through the occipital cortex, showing the line of Gennari in the calcarine cortex (primary visual cortex). (Reprinted with permission from JL Wilkinson. Neuroanatomy for Medical Students (3rd edn). Oxford: Butterworth-Heinemann, 1998;178.)

the neocortex contain six layers: I, the outer molecular layer; II, the external granule cell layer; III, the external pyramidal cell layer; IV, the internal granular layer; V, the internal pyramidal cell layer; and VI, the multiform layer. There are, however, important variations. For example, the primary motor cortex of the precentral gyrus of the frontal lobe contains large pyramidal neurons but virtually no internal granular layer, layer IV; hence the motor cortex is sometimes referred to as 'agranular cortex'. Sensory cortices do not have large, pyramidal cells but have large internal granular layers and are hence called 'granular cortex'. The visual

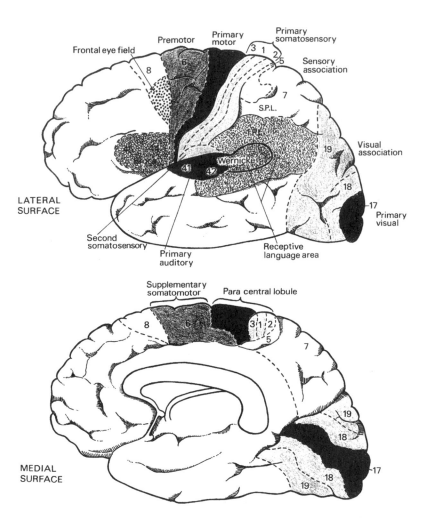

Figure 2.3 Drawings of the lateral and medial surfaces of the brain, with Brodmann cortical areas drawn in for the most important areas. SPL = superior parietal lobule, IPL = inferior parietal lobule. (Reprinted with permission from JL Wilkinson. Neuroanatomy for Medical Students (3rd edn). Oxford: Butterworth-Heinemann, 1998;181.)

cortex has an identifying white matter bundle layer called the line (or stria) of Gennari, visible even to the naked eye (see Figure 2.2). Areas of the cortex with the same cytoarchitectonic structure carry Brodmann numbers that are still in widespread use today (see Figure 2.3). Columns of cells with one structure and function are called 'modules', as proposed by Fodor in his 1983 monograph, *The Modularity of Mind*. Each module carries out a specific function, such as motor innervation, sensory perception, or a myriad of other activities. These modules communicate with other modules through cortical–cortical connections. Figure 2.4 shows the major white matter bundles that interconnect areas of the cerebral cortex.

The motor system has been understood for centuries, because of the obvious paralysis on the contralateral side of the body that follows a stroke or traumatic injury to the posterior frontal cortex. The primary motor area lies in the precentral gyrus, though many motor cells are also found by electrophysiological testing in the postcentral gyrus as well. A supplementary motor area in the medial frontal cortex also helps to program movements, and the prefrontal areas seem necessary to plan and initiate movement.

Primary cortical sensory areas include the visual cortex in the occipital lobes, the auditory cortex in the temporal lobes, the somatosensory cortex in the parietal lobes, and likely gustatory and olfactory cortices in the parietal and temporal lobes, respectively. Each of these primary cortices processes stimuli from only one sensory modality (vision, hearing, somatosensory function, taste, and smell) and has cortical–cortical connections only to adjacent portions of the

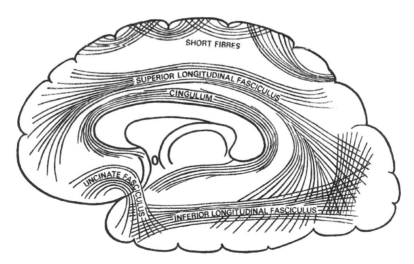

Figure 2.4 Drawing of the principal white matter bundles connecting areas of the cortex. Not shown on this figure is the 'arcuate fasciculus' connecting the temporal and frontal lobes (see Chapter 5). (Reprinted with permission from JL Wilkinson. Neuroanatomy for Medical Students (3rd edn). Oxford: Butterworth-Heinemann, 1998;178.)

association cortex also dedicated to this modality, called 'unimodal association cortex'. Sensory information is sequentially processed in increasingly complex fashion, leading from raw sensory data to a unified 'percept'.

The Visual Cortex

The organization of a primary sensory and unimodal association cortex has been especially well studied in the visual system, through the Nobel Prize-winning research of David Hubel, Torsten Wiesel and others. Retinal ganglion cells are activated by light within a bright area of the visual field, called a 'center', inhibited by light in the 'surround'. These cells project through the optic nerve to the lateral geniculate body of the thalamus, and then via the optic radiations to the primary visual cortex in each medial occipital lobe. In the primary visual cortex, a vertical column of neurons may detect an edge or bar of light rather than a spot; such a cell likely integrates the responses of several retinal ganglion cells. This vertical column of neurons in the primary visual cortex is a good example of a 'module' devoted to visual perception. The 'simple' cells of the visual cortex respond to bright central bars with dark surrounds. Several such cells in turn project to 'complex' cells, which may detect an edge or line with a specific orientation, or with a specific direction of movement, but without specifying the exact location of the line within the visual field. The firing of complex cells makes possible the perception of visual shapes and motion. Complex cells, in turn, project to cells in the visual unimodal association cortex (Brodmann areas 18 and 19), where cells may detect not only shapes but also patterns and movements; such cells may respond to movement anywhere in the visual field, an important characteristic in terms of the organism's need to maintain visual attention for possible dangers in the environment. In the visual association cortex, columns may respond to specific shapes, colors, or qualities such as novelty. In this fashion, the functions of cell columns or modules become more sophisticated as one moves from the primary cortex to the association cortex. By Fodor's model, the modules of primary visual perception project to 'central systems', by which we mean the higher levels of visual association cortex, then on to more complex systems of the brain. Examples of aspects of visual perception requiring higher levels of brain activation include the appreciation of beauty in a starry sky, or the adaptation of a ballet to a specific musical accompaniment.

Heteromodal Association Cortices

Unimodal association cortices communicate with each other via still more complex connections to the 'heteromodal association cortex', of which there are two main areas (Fuster 1989). The posterior heteromodal association cortex involves the posterior inferior parietal lobe, especially the angular gyrus. The posterior heteromodal cortex enables human beings to perceive an analogy between an association in one modality, for example a picture of a dog and the printed word 'dog' in the visual modality, with a percept in a different modality, for example the sound of the spoken word 'dog' or the sound of the dog's bark. Such intermodality associations are reportedly difficult for animals to learn, even chimpanzees, but easy for human beings. Cross-sensory associations involve the functioning of networks of multitudes of neurons, again rivaling the networks of the most sophisticated computers. The cognitive impression of perceptions in more than one modality can be called a 'concept' (Benson and Ardila 1996).

We will see in Chapter 5 how the parietal heteromodal cortex is crucial for language functioning. When we learn to read, we associate visual symbols with previously learned auditory word images, stored predominantly in the temporal lobe. The processes of reading and writing are disrupted by damage in the left parietal area. The parietal cortex is important for recognition of objects via sensation (stereognosis), as well as for the functions of calculation (originally learned from numbers in the body image of fingers and toes?), right and left discrimination, the body image of the contralateral half of the body, and spatial reasoning. Learned patterns of movement also appear to require the left parietal lobe for their planning and execution; lesions in this region produce apraxia (Chapter 6). Mesulam (1990) discusses the parietal cortex as part of a large network for attention, language, and memory.

The second heteromodal association cortex involves the lateralprefrontal region (Goldman-Rakic 1996). This region is thought to be involved with attention or 'working memory' (Baddeley 1992), and with sequential processes such as the registration and retrieval of stimuli in order of presentation, or the planning of motor activities. A related concept of cognitive neuropsychology is 'executive function', by which is meant the determination of which of the many sensory stimuli reaching the brain merit attention, and which motor outputs should be activated at a given time. The frontal lobes initiate behavior, and correspond to what might be referred to in philosophy or religion as 'free will'.

Supramodal Cortex

Another frontal cortical area, the orbitofrontal and anterior frontal portion of the prefrontal cortex, is thought to be involved in emotional states and in appetites and drives, or in the integration of internal bodily states and sensations with the external world. This part of the frontal cortex is referred to as 'supramodal cortex' (Benson and Ardila 1996), because it determines which of the many unimodal and heteromodal inputs from other brain regions should be attended to at a specific time, and how these exteroceptive inputs should be dealt with in reference to interoceptive inputs. The orbitofrontal cortex has close connections with the more primitive, emotional structures of the brain involved in drive-related behavior. These structures were referred to as the 'limbic system' by Paul MacLean (1958), though the term 'limbus' was used by Broca to designate the gray matter areas bordering the corpus callosum and upper brainstem, including the cingulate gyrus and parahippocampal region. These brain areas receive projections from the body's interoceptive functions, including autonomic and visceral processes. MacLean's 'triune brain' (1973) included the 'reptile brain', involving mainly the brainstem, responsible for elementary biological functions such as feeding, fighting, and mating; the 'limbic system', responsible for emotions and their role in drives and rewards; and the cortex, involved in memory and cognitive functions. MacLean developed the concept that the internal and emotional centers of the limbic system must be tied into the newer, neocortical areas responsible for intellectual function. The linking of these two systems may underlie the phenomenon of consciousness (see Chapter 3).

Although the model of Benson and Ardila (1996) speaks of the orbitofrontal cortex as an association cortex, it is more primitive in its structure. Only the neocortex of the human brain contains the classical six-layered organization discussed above. The 'allocortex', containing a simpler, layered structure, includes the hippocampus and related structures such as the dentate gyrus, called 'archicortex', and the pyriform or primary olfactory cortex, called 'paleocortex'. Basal forebrain areas included in the limbic system comprise the septal region, amygdala, and substantia innominata, which occupy mainly subcortical locations. These two more primitive regions, the allocortex and basal forebrain structures, form the limbic cortex. The 'paralimbic' cortex or mesocortex includes the orbitofrontal cortex, the insula, parts of the temporal pole, the parahippocampal areas, and the cingulate cortex (Carpenter 1978).

CORTICAL AND ORTICAL–SUBCORTICAL NETWORKS

This somewhat simplified model of the nervous system provides an idea of how the modular arrangement of cortical cells can give rise to networks that subserve complex functions. The discussion thus far is mainly centered on the cerebral neocortex. In order to remember an association, memory storage must occur via the hippocampus and its projections called 'Papez's circuit' to the septal region, mammillary bodies, and thalamus, thence to the frontal lobes and back to the hippocampus. The brain systems for memory storage and retrieval will be discussed in detail in Chapter 10. When emotional reactions such as pleasure and fear are involved in making the memory more vivid, the amygdala is involved. Other types of memory, such as motor learning and conditioning, may involve the basal ganglia and cerebellum (see Chapter 11). In motor functioning, the firing of prefrontal neurons that plan actions must be combined not only with the activation of the cortical motor cells but also of descending axonal pathways towards the spinal cord motor neurons, which in turn activate nerves and muscles, the basal ganglia circuits that integrate movement patterns, and connections to the cerebellum that coordinate the individual movements into smooth performances. Motor planning also involves prefrontal regions involved in attention and sequential executive function. On the sensory side, we must consider the role of the thalamus in relaying some sensory inputs in a way that reaches conscious attention, or alternatively serves as a gate that keeps them out of consciousness.

Mesulam (1998) divides the higher cortical functions into five principal 'neurocognitive networks':

1. A spatial awareness network, involving the right parietal cortex, the right frontal cortex, and the cingulate cortex (see Chapter 9)
2. A language network, involving principally Wernicke's area in the left temporal lobe, Broca's area in the left frontal lobe, and the circuitry between them (see Chapter 4)
3. The memory circuit, involving primarily the medial temporal structures and connections via Papez's circuit, as outlined above and in Chapter 11
4. A working-memory and executive function network, involving mainly the prefrontal cortex, with connections to the parietal cortex (see Chapter 10)
5. A network for face and object identification, centering on the temporal cortices of both hemispheres (see Chapter 8).

These networks are interconnected, and components of more than one network may be activated in specific cognitive tasks.

The brain is a complex organ that will likely continue to resist our explorations and attempts at full understanding, despite the technological advances that have made cognitive neuroscience possible. Some authorities even question whether a human brain can ever achieve understanding of its own intricate processes. The journalist Tom Wolfe (2000) discusses the new generation of neuroscientists whose attitude is 'Why wrestle with Kant's God, Freedom, and Immortality when it is only a matter of time before neuroscience, probably through brain imaging, reveals the actual physical mechanism that fabricates these mental constructs, these illusions?'. Wolfe, however, feels that such self-examinations are bound to fail: "Being finite, hardwired, it will probably never have the power to comprehend human existence in any complete way. It would be as if a group of dogs were to call a conference to try to understand The Dog. They could try as hard as they wanted, but they wouldn't get very far. Dogs can communicate only about forty notions, all of them primitive, and they can't record anything. The project would be doomed from the start. The human brain is far superior to the dog's, but it is limited nonetheless. So any hope of human beings arriving at some final, complete, self-enclosed theory of human existence is doomed, too."

The organizational model of the human brain briefly summarized in this chapter, however, gives us a good basis for examining the practical aspects of our knowledge of brain and behavior. We will continue to examine knowledge of specific brain functions and behavior in the succeeding chapters.

REFERENCES

Baddeley A. Working memory. Science 1992;255:556–559.
Benson DF, Ardila A. Aphasia: A Clinical Perspective. New York: Oxford University Press, 1996;262–277.
Brodmann K. Vergleichende Lokalisation-lehre der Grosshirnrinde in ihren Prinzipien dargestellt auf Grund des Zellenbaues. 1909. Leipzig:Barth, 1-324.
Carpenter MB. Core Text of Neuroanatomy. Baltimore: Williams & Wilkins, 1978.

Crick F. The Astonishing Hypothesis. The Scientific Search for the Soul. New York: Charles Scribner's Sons, 1994;3.

Fuster JM. The Prefrontal Cortex: Anatomy, Physiology, and Neuropsychology of the Frontal Lobe. New York: Raven, 1989.

Goldman-Rakic PS. The prefrontal landscape: implications of functional architecture for understanding human mentation and the central executive. Phil Trans R Soc Lond B 1996;351:1445–1453.

Kandel ER, Schwartz JH, Jessell TM. Principles of Neural Science (4th edn). New York: McGraw-Hill, 2000.

Kundera M. The Unbearable Lightness of Being. New York: Harper & Row, 1984;40.

MacLean PD. Contrasting functions of limbic and neocortical systems of the brain and their relevance to psychophysiological aspects of medicine. Am J Med 1958; 25: 611–635.

MacLean PD. A Triune Concept of the Brain and Behaviour. Toronto: University of Toronto Press, 1973.

Mesulam M-M. Large scale neurocognitive networks and distributed processing for attention, language, and memory. Ann Neurol 1990;28:597–613.

Mesulam M-M. From sensation to cognition. Brain 1998;121:1013–1052.

Nauta WJH, Feirtag M. Fundamental Neuroanatomy. New York: W.H. Freeman, 1986.

Pinker S. How The Mind Works. New York: WW Norton & Co, 1997;64.

Vogt C, Vogt O. Allgemeine Ergebnisse unserer Hirnforschung. Vierte Mitteilung: Die physiologische Bedeutung der architektonischen Rindenreizungen. J Psychol u Neurol 1919;25:279–462.

Wilkinson JL. Neuroanatomy for Medical Students (3rd edn). Oxford: Butterworth-Heinemann, 1998.

Wolfe T. Hooking Up. New York: Farrar Strauss Giroux, 2000;98:108.

3

Consciousness and the Brain

My soul knows my meat is doing bad things, and is embarrassed. But my meat just keeps right on doing bad, dumb things. 'Your what and your what?' he said. 'My soul and my meat,' I said. 'They're separate?' he said. 'I sure hope they are,' I said. 'I would hate to be responsible for what my meat does.' I told him, only half joking, about how I imagined the soul of each person, myself included, as being a sort of flexible neon tube inside. All the tube could do was receive news about what was happening with the meat, over which it had no control.

(Vonnegut 1987)

All human beings feel a sense of self-awareness, which we refer to as 'consciousness'. Despite this universal understanding of what consciousness is, the neural basis for conscious awareness and the related sense of self is poorly understood. Consciousness, the self, and the soul were traditionally the province of philosophers or theologians rather than scientists. Neuroscience has begun to unravel the phenomena of consciousness. Neuroscientists such as John Eccles (1973; 1992), J. Z. Young (1988), and Wilder Penfield (1975) have written philosophical treatises on the mind–brain relationship, dealing with the phenomenon of consciousness, late in their careers. Clinical neurologists have long been familiar with brain disorders that affect consciousness. The neurological understanding of consciousness begins with this knowledge. Generations of neurologists have learned about the neurology of unconsciousness from a monograph by Plum and Posner (1982). This volume teaches the reader how to examine a comatose patient to determine the level of the nervous system at which a lesion has interrupted consciousness.

Lesions involving both sides of the brainstem at the level of the midbrain or pons regularly produce coma, especially acute lesions such as brainstem strokes. The ascending neuronal pathways of the reticular activating system are necessary to keep the brain awake. The reticular activating system projects up the brainstem, though the thalamus, and then to distributed areas of the cerebral cortex. Bilateral thalamic lesions can also cause coma. Above the level of the thalamus, focal lesions do not usually impair consciousness. The exceptions are: (1) lesions with mass effect sufficient to cause pressure downwards on the brainstem (herniation syndromes); (2) large, bilateral lesions (as in massive, bilateral strokes or head injuries); or (3) diffuse or multifocal lesions, as in states of hypoxic encephalopathy or hypoglycemia. Diffuse, bilateral lesions of the hemispheres produce prolonged states of lack of responsiveness to environmental stimuli. These diffuse lesions can be structural, as in hypoxic damage, or functional, as in drug overdoses, metabolic comas, and the like.

A series of other states of depressed consciousness have been recognized in patients recovering from coma or patients with lesions that produce partial reduction of consciousness. Patients may regain an alternation between periods of apparent sleep, with the eyes closed, and 'awake' periods, with the eyes open, staring in one direction or roving, but without any meaningful response to environmental stimuli. This state of consciousness is called 'persistent vegetative state', or 'coma vigile'. Vegetative state can occur as a temporary or lasting state, in which case it is called 'permanent vegetative state'. Much controversy exists as to the time after a brain injury when a vegetative state can be considered permanent, with all of the ethical consequences that derive from this decision (American Neurological Association Committee 1993; Childs *et al.* 1993; Multi-Society Task Force 1994). Legal cases such as the Karen Ann Quinlan case and the Nancy Cruzan case have dealt with the issue of whether patients in persistent vegetative state are living or dead, and whether they must be kept alive by all medical and nutritional means.

Lesser states of diffuse damage may produce an encephalopathy or delirium (see Chapter 14). Brainstem lesions that do not produce coma may produce inability to speak or move the facial muscles, a state called 'locked-in syndrome'. These patients are totally awake, but unable to move the limbs, facial muscles, or speech apparatus; such 'locked-in' patients may be able to communicate only by blinking or looking up and down. A fictional locked-in syndrome can be found in *The Count of Montecristo*. Another state of altered conscious resembling the persistent vegetative state is akinetic mutism or abulia, in which a patient looks awake but does not respond to stimuli, though occasionally complex motor behaviors and even speech emerge. Akinetic mutism is best documented with bilateral lesions of the prefrontal cortex. A second type of akinetic mutism, in which the patient looks less awake, has been described with lesions in the upper midbrain (Segarra 1970).

These pathological states of consciousness teach us that there must be activating stimuli for consciousness (the reticular activating system), and also a cortical mantle that is awake and carries the content of consciousness. In a conscious organism, only a small number of incoming sensory stimuli reach consciousness, and only a small amount of the external world is chosen on which to focus attention, or the 'spotlight' of consciousness. Neuroscience is helping us to understand these processes.

For Crick (1994), the best model for the study of consciousness is visual awareness, since the anatomy and physiology of the visual system are so well understood. Crick points out that neurons in the primary visual cortex likely do not have access to conscious awareness. Stated another way, we do not pay attention to much of what our eyes see. A perceived object, however, excites neurons in several different areas of the visual association cortex, each eliciting associations that can lead to conscious awareness or memory storage of the items perceived. Rees and colleagues (2000) have shown that patients with neglect of the left visual field show activation of the right occipital cortex in response to stimuli of which they have no conscious awareness. Crick and Koch (1995) argue that activation of the frontal cortex is necessary for these visual percepts to enter consciousness, though subconscious awareness in the form of 'blindsight' may exist at the level of the occipital cortex. Conscious visual perception seems to involve interactions between the visual parts of the brain and the frontal lobe systems for attention and working memory (Ungerleider *et al.* 1998).

There are many clinical examples of 'unconscious' mental processing, and a number of these involve vision. Patients with cortical blindness can sometimes show evidence of knowledge of items they cannot see, a phenomenon called 'blindsight' (see Chapter 8). Patients with right hemisphere lesions who 'extinguish' objects in their left visual field when presented with bilateral stimuli nonetheless show activation of the right visual cortex by functional magnetic resonance imaging, indicating that the objects are 'seen' in some sense, though not consciously (Rees *et al.* 2000). Libet (1999) demonstrated experimentally that visual and other sensory stimuli have to persist at least 500 milliseconds to reach conscious awareness, yet stimuli of shorter duration can elicit reactions. Motor responses to sensory stimuli can occur before conscious awareness, as in the ability to pull one's hand away from a hot stove before feeling the heat. Racers begin running before they are aware of having heard the starting gun (Crick and Koch 1998). A familiar example of unconscious visual processing is the drive home from work; most individuals can remember very little that they saw on the trip, yet they drove without accidents. A more arcane example from the visual system comes from the experiments of Gur and Snodderly (1997) on color vision in monkeys. When two colors are projected at a frequency of over 10 hertz, the monkey perceives a fused color, yet recordings from cells in the visual cortex clearly demonstrate that information about the two separate colors is coded in the monkey's visual cortex. Crick and Koch (1998) refer to the unconscious visual processing as an 'online visual system'. They suggest that the 'dorsal visual stream', an occipitoparietal system for perception of location and movement direction of objects, is largely conscious, whereas the 'ventral visual stream', an occipitotemporal system for identification of objects, is largely unconscious. Other examples of unconscious mental processing include 'implicit memory', including unconscious memories for how to perform tasks ('procedural memory'), priming memory, and classical conditioning; these types of memory can function normally in patients with severe short-term memory loss, who have no conscious awareness of possessing these memories (see Chapter 11).

In language syndromes, patients can match spoken to written words without knowledge of their meaning, suggesting that there are internal rules of language equivalence that are unconscious (Albert *et al.* 1973; Brust 2000). Brust (2000) refers to all of these varieties of unconscious mental processes as the 'non-Freudian unconscious'.

The frontal lobes, as stated in Chapter 2, are heavily involved in the phenomenon of consciousness. As conceived by Paul MacLean (1958), the orbitofrontal cortex contains neurons that integrate exteroceptive sensory inputs like vision with interoceptive stimuli related to drives, appetites, and emotional states as well as changes in the internal milieu. This integration of attention to external and internal stimuli may underlie conscious awareness. For Benson and Ardila (1996), the supramodal cortex in the orbitofrontal lobes represents the brain system that 'anticipates, conjectures, ruminates, plans for the future, and fantasizes'. In other words, it is this part of the brain that brings specific cognitive processes to conscious awareness and that may be responsible for the phenomenon of consciousness itself.

A recent study (Keenan *et al.* 2001) provided evidence that the right frontal lobe might be the part of the brain that recognizes the self. These investigators studied patients undergoing Wada tests, in which a barbiturate is injected into the carotid artery to determine cortical dominance for language. They presented subjects with a self-photograph and a photograph of a famous person, followed by a 'morphed' photograph of a famous person and the patient. When the left hemisphere was anesthetized, the subjects said that the morphed photograph represented the famous person, whereas with right hemisphere anesthesia the subject selected the self-face.

Clinically, extensive bilateral lesions of the orbitofrontal cortex may leave the individual awake but staring, unable to respond to the environment, a state already referred to as 'akinetic mutism'. Such patients have their eyes open, appearing awake, but they have very limited responses to stimuli, often after a delay. A question requiring a sentence answer is usually met with silence, but sometimes a question with a one-word answer will be responded to in a whisper, many seconds or even minutes after the initial query. Such patients are 'conscious' at least in a partial way. With lesser lesions, patients with frontal lobe damage may lose their ability to form appropriate or mature judgments, reacting impulsively to incoming stimuli in a manner reminiscent of animal behavior.

The frontal lobe contains the supramodal cortex, which, along with the heteromodal frontal cortex, is responsible for the 'executive functions', the cognitive processes that decide which of the myriad of incoming stimuli to attend to, which responses to activate, in which priority, and in which order. This area of the brain is also involved in 'working memory', the ability of the brain to maintain attention to a string of items. The prefrontal regions are thus involved in the focusing of attention and the 'stream of consciousness'. Once attention is lost, the items fade rapidly and are forgotten, unless a smaller set are deliberately 'memorized', or transferred into the short-term memory store, involving the limbic structures of the brain and especially the hippocampal regions (see Chapter 11). Executive function clearly defines what portions of our experience are allowed into conscious awareness. The sense of self emerges from the ongoing experience of self-consciousness, over time.

Mesulam (1998) builds on these anatomical facts with his concepts of brain networks, as outlined in Chapter 2. Consciousness is not embodied in any one brain network, but in interactions of all of them. In lower animals, consciousness is driven by simple reactions to immediate sensations, drives, and needs. In the human, the working memory function of the frontal lobes and the more complex systems for reasoning and analysis allow a more complex consciousness to develop. Mesulam summarizes human consciousness this way: "A more complex form of consciousness would be expected to emerge if some critical mass of neurons, freed from the household chores of sensation and action, could afford to form alternative and annotated representations of ambient events. One consequence of this process could be the emergence of an observing self who becomes differentiated from the sensory flux and who can therefore intentionally comment (introspect) on experience."

Another clinical window into the phenomena of consciousness comes from surgery to separate the hemispheres by cutting the corpus callosum. In 'split-brain' or commissurotomized patients, each hemisphere seems to have its own separate consciousness. The left hemisphere, which has the capacity for speech and language, can express this consciousness in words. For example, a split-brain patient can report words or pictures that appear in the right visual field. The right hemisphere cannot produce verbal accounts of items seen in the left visual field, but the subject can choose the correct item by pointing with the left hand, at the same time the subject claims to have no conscious knowledge of the item. In terms of the speaking left hemisphere, the right hemisphere has 'unconscious' visual knowledge, also called 'blindsight'. At times, the left hand of the patient may seem to operate under a different agenda from the right hand; a split-brain patient may select a dress from a rack with the right hand, while the left hand puts it back or selects a more daring fashion. This rivalry of the left hand with the right is called the 'alien hand syndrome', a phenomenon seen also in patients with strokes involving the corpus callosum (Chan and Ross 1997). This topic is discussed further in Chapter 12, on syndromes of the corpus callosum. The alien hand syndrome is a striking example of the separate consciousnesses of the two divided hemispheres.

Young and Pigott (1999), in a recent review of the neurology of consciousness, urged neurologists to forego vague diagnoses such as 'impaired consciousness' in favor of more specific analysis of the precise components of consciousness that are affected. For example, reticular activating system lesions may prevent consciousness from arising at all; frontal lesions may impair the focusing of attention; parietal or occipital lesions may affect the ability to perceive sensory experiences; limbic lesions may prevent association of new perceptions with past memories or with motivation to satisfy drives or build self-esteem. When specific components of consciousness are evaluated, much of behavioral neurology can be thought of in a context of alteration of the state or content of consciousness.

REFERENCES

Albert ML, Yamadori A, Gardner H, Howes D. Comprehension in alexia. Brain 1973;96:317–328.

American Neurological Association Committee on Ethical Affairs. Persistent vegetative state: report of the American Neurological Association Committee on Ethical Affairs. Ann Neurol 1993;33:386–390.

Benson DF, Ardila A. Aphasia. A Clinical Perspective. New York: Oxford University Press, 1996.

Brust JCM. The non-Freudian unconscious. Neurologist 2000;6:224–231.

Chan J-L, Ross ED. Alien hand syndrome: influence of neglect on the clinical presentation of frontal and callosal variants. Cortex 1997;33:287–299.

Childs NL, Mercer WN, Childs HW. Accuracy of diagnosis of persistent vegetative state. Neurology 1993;43:1465–1467.

Crick F. The Astonishing Hypothesis. The Scientific Search for the Soul. New York: Charles Scribner's Sons, 1994;3.

Crick F, Koch C. Are we aware of neural activity in primary visual cortex? Nature 1995;375:121–123.

Crick F, Koch C. Consciousness and neuroscience. Cerebral Cortex 1998;8:97–107.

Eccles JC. The Understanding of the Brain. New York: McGraw-Hill, 1973.

Eccles JC. Evolution of consciousness. Proc Natl Acad Sci 1992;89:7320–7324.

Goldman-Rakic PS. The prefrontal landscape: implications of functional architecture for understanding human mentation and the central executive. Phil Trans R Soc Lond B (1996);351:1445–1453.

Gur M, Snodderly DM. A dissociation between brain activity and perception: chromatically opponent cortical neurons signal chromatic flicker that is not perceived. Vision Res 1997;37:377–382.

Keenan JP, Nelson A, O'Connor M, PascualLeone A. Self-recognition and the right hemisphere. Nature 2001;409:305–306.

Libet B. How does conscious experience arise? The neural time factor. Brain Res Bull 1999;50:339–340.

MacLean PD. Contrasting functions of limbic and neocortical systems of the brain and their relevance to psychophysiological aspects of medicine. Am J Med 1958; 25:611–635.

Mesulam M-M. From sensation to cognition. Brain 1998;121:1013–1052.

Multi-Society Task Force on PVS. Medical aspects of the persistent vegetative state. N Engl J Med 1994;330:1499–1508.

Penfield W. The Mystery of the Mind. Princeton: Princeton University Press, 1975.

Plum F, Posner JB. The Diagnosis of Stupor and Coma (3rd edn). Philadelphia: FA Davis Co., 1982.

Rees G, Wojciulik E, Clarke K et al. Unconscious activation of visual cortex in the damaged right hemisphere of a parietal patient with extinction. Brain 2000; 123:1624–1633.

Segarra JM. Cerebral vascular disease and behavior. I. The syndrome of the mesencephalic artery (basilar artery bifurcation). Arch Neurol 1970;22:408–418.

Vonnegut, K. Bluebeard. New York: Delacorte Press, 1987;238.

Young CB, Pigott SE. Neurobiological basis of consciousness. Arch Neurol 1999; 56:153–157.

Young JZ. Philosophy and the Brain. Oxford: Oxford University Press, 1988.

4

Bedside Mental Status Examination

There is a widespread, usually tacit but often openly expressed, view that mental examination is a long and arduous task. Most physicians have learned that although a 'complete' survey of the heart, lungs, abdomen and other structures can take hours, intimate knowledge of the examination and repeated practice enable them to obtain essential information in a very brief time. Those who have learned the mental examination and have practiced it often can equally well obtain vital information rapidly and efficiently when necessary.

(Norman Geschwind 1977)

The bedside mental status examination is an integral part of the neurological examination, the tool by which neurologists localize lesions in the brain that affect the higher cortical functions. The mental status examination is just as important to lesion localization and neurological diagnosis as the examinations of the cranial nerves, motor, sensory, and cerebellar systems. Though the mental status evaluation is the most neglected area of the neurological examination, it generally takes only a few minutes, and its cost effectiveness compares well to brain imaging studies such as magnetic resonance imaging or positron emission tomography.

The most important aspect of the mental status examination is the necessity of performing it. One of the most common errors made by neurologists is to omit a systematic evaluation of mental function in patients who appear alert and oriented. Focal cognitive deficits affecting memory, knowledge, praxis, visual object recognition, calculation, or visual-constructional function may not impair the patient's ability to speak coherently; unless these functions are tested, the deficit will be missed. A patient who suffered a posterior cerebral artery stroke was discharged home without any recognition that he could not read, or that his memory was impaired, until he tried to function at home. Likewise, demented patients often develop a 'cocktail party' demeanor in which appropriate social phrases and comments belie widespread cognitive losses. Others may become so adept at

25

deferring questions to a spouse or family member that their own inability to answer goes unnoticed. The neurologist must decide which patients need formal cognitive testing, and whether to use an individual, informal test routine or whether to apply one of the standard tests. Again, it is more important to do the examination than to follow any specific format.

STANDARDIZED BEDSIDE ASSESSMENTS
The Mini Mental State Examination

Several bedside mental status assessments have been published. Perhaps the most widely used is the Folstein Mini Mental State examination (MMSE) (Folstein *et al.* 1975). The MMSE consists of 30 points: 5 for orientation to time, 5 for orientation to place, 5 for attention, 3 for registration of three items, 3 for recall of the three items after 5 minutes, 2 for naming objects, 1 for repeating a phrase, 3 for following a three-stage command, 1 for following a printed command, 1 for writing a sentence, and 1 for copying a diagram. The details of

Table 4.1 The Mini Mental State Examination (Folstein *et al.* 1975)

Specific Item	Points
Orientation – time	
Year	1
Season	1
Month	1
Date	1
Day	1
Orientation – place	
State	1
County	1
Town	1
Hospital	1
Floor	1
Attention	5
Choice of serial 7s, or	
Spell 'world' backwards	
Memory	
Register three items	3
Recall three items at 5 minutes	3
Naming (pencil, watch)	2
Repetition (no ifs, ands, or buts)	1
Following three-step command	3
Following printed command	1
('close your eyes')	
Write a sentence	1
Copy intersecting pentagons	1

the items are presented in Table 4.1. The advantages of the MMSE are that it is brief, easy to administer, and quantitative. The numerical score may help in documenting deficits and their progression over time; this may help to justify speech or cognitive therapy, drug treatments such as cholinesterase inhibitors for Alzheimer's disease, and disability status for insurance companies and governmental agencies.

The MMSE has several limitations. First, the normal range of scores depends on education; the low-normal cut-off is estimated by Crum *et al.* (1993) to be 19 for uneducated persons, 23 for elementary or junior high-school educated persons, 27 for high-school graduates, and 29 for college graduates. Age is also a factor; in a recent study, at age 75 MMSE scores ranged from 21 to 29 in community-dwelling people (tenth to ninetieth percentiles, respectively), but at age 95 the values were 10 to 27 (Dufouil *et al.* 2000). In addition, the test is weighted towards orientation and language; the only 'right hemisphere' test is the copying of intersecting pentagons, a relatively easy task. Others have suggested using the clock-drawing test (see below). The MMSE can be normal in patients with lesions in the right hemisphere or frontal lobes. The test may thus be insensitive to focal neurological disorders (Dick *et al.* 1984). Finally, even an abnormal score does not distinguish a focal lesion from a more diffuse disorder such as an encephalopathy or dementia. Although the test is useful in separating normal patients from those with brain damage, or psychiatric from neurological patients, the test score does not help the neurologist determine what sort of disorder is present, or where it is located in the brain.

The authors of the MMSE have recently presented an even shorter version of the test, called the 'Micro Mental State Examination'. The test is not yet well standardized or tested. It uses the clock drawing test rather than the intersecting pentagons test.

The Modified Mini Mental State Examination

Many behavioral neurologists use the MMSE as a screening test and supplement it with more focused tasks. Teng and Chui (1987) suggested adding four items to the test to make it more sensitive in both the 'ceiling' and 'floor' regions of the score. They added the patient's place or state of birth, in order to gauge recall of personal information. In the short-term memory task, they suggested using three specific words (shirt, brown, honesty; alternative versions, shoes, black, modesty; socks, blue, charity), in order to keep the difficulty of the memory words constant. On the recall portion, they included three multiple-choice alternatives. For the reverse registration task, they omitted serial sevens and suggested counting backwards from five, a task easy for even more impaired persons. They also added to the spatial orientation question, 'Are we in a hospital or office building or home?'. An additional category of naming up to ten four-legged animals in 30 seconds probes generative naming, not tested in the original MMSE. The Modified Mini Mental State Examination (3MS), as the authors call it, has definite advantages over the standard MMSE, but this version of the test has not gained wide acceptance.

Dementia Screening Tests

A series of bedside screening tests for dementia in elderly patients have been published, and several are used in research on dementia and Alzheimer's disease. It should be noted from the outset that the goal of these batteries is to distinguish demented individuals from elderly normals and elderly depressed patients, and there is no effort to detect or distinguish patients with focal brain lesions. Appelgate *et al.* (1990) and Ferris and Kluger (1997) have provided reviews of the available screening tests for dementia.

Blessed Rating Instruments

Blessed and colleagues developed the first brief, standardized tests for dementia in England in the 1960s. Initially four tests were developed: the Blessed Dementia Rating Scale (BLS-D), the Blessed Information Scale, the Blessed Memory Scale, and the Blessed Concentration Scale (Blessed *et al.* 1968; newer version, Blessed *et al.* 1988). In the pioneering work of these authors, deficits on the BLS-D late in life correlated with the degree of pathological change related to Alzheimer's disease at autopsy. More recently, a shortened version of the Blessed Dementia Scale, along with six items of the Information Scale, have been incorporated into the battery used by the Consortium to Establish a Registry for Alzheimer's Disease (CERAD; Morris *et al.* 1988).

Mattis Dementia Rating Scale

The Mattis Dementia Rating Scale, published in 1976, is a more detailed cognitive test that can take as long as 45 minutes to administer, though subjects who correctly answer the first of each series of questions can be presumed to know the easier items to follow, shortening the test considerably. This test is used mainly in research studies on Alzheimer's disease.

Alzheimer's Disease Assessment Scale

The Alzheimer's Disease Assessment Scale (ADAS; Mohs and Cohen 1988) is another research test scale that has been used extensively in clinical trials related to Alzheimer's disease. It has two parts: a non-cognitive battery, which is not frequently used, and the ADAS cognitive battery (ADAS-cog), which includes a word recall task, naming of objects and fingers, ability to follow commands, copying of geometric forms, folding a letter and writing the address, orientation, reading words aloud, a language rating scale for speech, comprehension of tasks, word-finding, and remembering test instructions. The test has proved useful in staging Alzheimer's disease and documenting response to treatment, but it is generally too involved for routine office use in diagnosis.

The 7-Minute Screen

Solomon and Pendlebury (1999) have developed a 7-minute screen for dementia, which is available free to physicians. The test includes orientation to month, date, year, day, and time; a naming test for four separate cards containing four pictures; a delayed recall test for the four items of each card, cued by class of item; a clock-drawing test; and a generative naming test for animals. The authors have presented evidence that their screening test is more sensitive and more specific than the MMSE in the diagnosis of dementia.

The Neuropsychiatric Inventory

The Neuropsychiatric Inventory is a measure of psychopathology in demented patients. Kaufer and colleagues (2000) have validated a two-page questionnaire version called the NPI-Q. This test is useful in testing effects of drugs designed to diminish psychiatric symptoms in patients with Alzheimer's disease.

INDIVIDUALIZED MENTAL STATUS EXAMINATIONS

Most behavioral neurologists use their own individualized mental status examinations, either alone or in combination with a standardized battery such as the MMSE. Several texts provide detailed mental status assessments (Strub and Black 1977; Weintraub and Mesulam 1985; Kirshner 1986). The following is the author's own approach to bedside mental status testing.

Assessment of Mental Status During History Taking

An experienced examiner can learn much about the subject's mental status by careful observation during the history. Considerable insight can be gained into the subject's recent memory, orientation, language function, affect or mood, insight and judgment. This technique, however, requires deliberate observation of the patient and carefully chosen questions that probe not only the history itself but also the patient's knowledge and memory of it. This information emerges without added time for the examiner and without the restraints of a formal test situation. The elements of this, informal mental status examination are listed in Table 4.2. Also included in the history should be a mention of handedness,

---

Table 4.2 Mental status assessment during history taking

Sensorium
  Level of alertness
  Hallucinations
  Attention span
Dress, grooming, and hygiene
Motor activity
Affect and mood
Insight and judgment
Reasoning, thought process
Language
Memory

---

because of its correlation with cerebral dominance for language and other functions, and of the patient's educational level.

Sensorium

The first observation to be made during the history is the patient's sensorium, or level of alertness. Level of alertness can be graded as normal, lethargic (the patient is slow to respond or requires repeated questions), or obtunded (the patient requires special alerting stimuli to respond, e.g. shouting, jostling, or noxious stimuli). Stupor and coma represent extremes of obtundation; the stuporous patient responds only to alerting stimuli, and the comatose patient does not respond at all. The specific stimuli needed to alert the patient should be documented; for example 'the patient awoke to calling his name' or 'the patient fended off the examiner's hand with his left hand in response to sternal rub'. Spontaneous hallucinations can also be noted under the category of sensorium. Attention span, or the subject's ability to stick to the subject of the examiner's serial questions, is also noted, as is distractibility.

Dress, Grooming, and Hygiene

Dress and grooming are noted as indicators of the patient's attention to personal hygiene and appearance. Patients may be unkempt, reflecting inattentiveness to personal hygiene, or so fastidiously groomed as to suggest undue attention to personal appearance. Occasionally half of the body reflects more attention than the other; a patient with unilateral neglect may shave only one side of his face, or leave food dribbling out of one side of the mouth. The patient's meal plate may also reveal inattention to one side of space; the patient may eat all of the food from only one side of the plate, then ask for more.

Motor Activity

The patient's level of motor activity is also an important indicator of mental state. Restlessness and agitation, as opposed to calmness and immobility, are the two poles of the dimension of spontaneous motor activity. The examiner should note spontaneous gestures or mannerisms, as well as tics, tremors, and involuntary movements.

Affect and Mood

Affect and mood reflect the patient's emotional state: affect is the examiner's judgment of the patient's mood, whereas mood is the patient's own subjective report.

Elation, sadness, anger, fear, anxiety, and apathy are examples of affective state. Facial expressions, vocal intonations, and gestures all indicate emotional states in ways obvious to any observant human being.

If there is doubt about the patient's mood state, the examiner should consider how the patient makes him or her feel. A depressed patient often makes the examiner feel depressed, while a manic patient makes the examiner feel happy and amused.

Moods may be fleeting emotions or sustained, pervasive personality traits. The examiner attempts to judge whether or not a patient's affect and mood are appropriate in quality and degree to the situation. For example, a right hemisphere stroke patient may be aware that he cannot move his left arm or leg, yet seem totally unconcerned. Finally, the examiner should ask during the history about bodily symptoms related to mood states. In the familiar example of depression, the examiner asks about the 'vegetative signs' of weight loss, anorexia, and insomnia. The anxious patient may complain of sweating, palpitations, or tremor.

Insight and Judgment

Insight and judgment are important to both psychiatric and neurological diagnosis. These functions are best evaluated by assessing the patient's understanding of his or her own illness. Most interviews begin with questions about why the patient has sought help. A patient demonstrates reduced insight, for example, if he states that he has come to the office because his wife thought he needed to, but he feels fine, or if he refers to a minor, incidental complaint such as ankle swelling. Further questions can probe the patient's understanding of the tests or consultations ordered, the diagnostic possibilities that have been discussed, the treatments prescribed, and the impact of the illness on the patient's ability to work or function.

Reasoning or Thought Process

As the patient tells his or her history, the examiner gains insight into the patient's mental processes, including thought and reasoning. Are the patient's thoughts logically connected? Are appropriate steps being planned between a goal and its execution? The patient may describe hallucinations or illusions (misperceptions of sensory stimuli, such as mistaking an intravenous line for a snake, or a dropped cup for a gunshot). Also included under this category are delusional thought processes and suspicious or paranoid ideation. These types of symptoms provide a window into the deranged thought processes of a psychotic or delirious patient. The breakdown of logical thinking and associations is called 'confusion', probably the most difficult word to define in behavioral neurology (see Chapter 14).

Language and Memory

The last two mental functions assessed during history taking – language and memory – are also the subjects of more detailed, formal testing. History taking is verbal communication, and the examiner should form at least a preliminary impression about the patient's fluency of speech and comprehension of spoken language. Word-finding pauses, circumlocutions, and word errors can be noted informally before the deliberate bedside testing of language function begins. Memory for personal events, both recent and remote, is also demonstrated by the patient's ability to recall elements of the history. Remote memory can be assessed by questions about the patient's background, hometown, education, employment, and medical and family history. Family members may need to verify the correct answers to these questions. Recent memory is reflected in the recall of recent symptoms, visits to physicians, tests, and treatments. A patient with short-term memory loss may, for example, not recall a spinal tap or operation performed earlier the same day.

All of the preceding functions can be assessed in a preliminary way through history taking. Reporting can be brief. A single sentence, such as 'this cheerful, well-dressed, articulate lady relates a detailed chronological history of progressive weakness of her left leg', can document or imply normal functioning in orientation, recent memory, language, insight, judgment, and mood, all in a few words. In selected cases, the bedside mental status examination can stop there, or perhaps after formal testing of orientation and memory. For patients in whom the results are not clear, the formal mental status examination should follow.

THE FORMAL MENTAL STATUS EXAMINATION

The formal mental status examination should include orientation, memory, language, praxis, gnosis or object recognition, calculations, visual–spatial–constructional functions, affect/mood, and insight and judgment. The categories of the examination are listed in Table 4.3.

Orientation

Orientation should always be tested explicitly for the date, place, personal identity, and situation. The awareness of the situation denotes the patient's understanding of why he or she is at the doctor's office or hospital. In some demented patients, an apparently lucid history may conceal the fact that the patient is confabulating information, and the patient may fail on the most simple of orientation questions. Failure on this test always requires a more detailed mental status examination.

Table 4.3   The formal mental status examination

Orientation
Memory
  Immediate memory (attention span)
  Short-term (recent) memory
  Long-term (remote) memory
Language
Praxis
Gnosis, object recognition
Calculations
Visual–constructional abilities
Frontal lobe functions
Insight and judgment, abstract reasoning

Table 4.4 Bedside memory tests

Immediate memory
    Digit span, or 'spell world backwards'

Recent memory
    Three words at 5 minutes (purple, baseball, Virginia)
    Three locations of hidden coins at 5 minutes
    Recent news, personal events

Remote memory
    Last five US Presidents
    State Governor
    Dates of World War II, Kennedy assassination
    Names of grandchildren

Memory

Memory has three stages, at least for the purposes of bedside testing: (1) immediate; (2) short-term (recent); and (3) long-term (remote). Tests of these three stages of memory are listed in Table 4.4.

Immediate memory refers to the ability to keep a series of items under immediate attention, such that they can be recited back. This function reflects attention and concentration, not memorization. The most popular immediate attention tests are forward digit span, serial 7 subtractions from 100, or the MMSE test 'spell world backwards'. As above, serial subtractions of 3s from 20 or even 1s from 5 can be done in patients who fail the more difficult tests. In the digit span test, numbers are called out one per second, after which the subject repeats them. Normal subjects can remember seven digits forward, which perhaps by coincidence is the number of digits in a local telephone number. Young people can hear a telephone number once, walk across the room, and dial the number without having to memorize it. Older individuals have more difficulty with this task. The backwards digit span, sometimes chosen as a more difficult test, may require some memorization for longer items. Spans of numbers greater than seven ('supraspan memory') definitely require memorization, and are tests of both concentration and short-term memory.

Short-term memory is the storage of information by memorization, for recall some minutes or hours later. It should be noted that some experimental psychologists use the term 'short-term' to mean what was just described as 'immediate' memory; by this nomenclature, long-term memory would be the recall of events for a few minutes. As used in clinical neurology, however, short-term memory refers both to the anterograde learning of new information over minutes to hours and to the retrograde recall of what happened a few minutes ago. Testing should include recall of three unrelated words at 5 minutes. The subject should always be asked to repeat the words after presentation, to make sure that the three items have been registered. Items should be from distinct semantic categories, such as 'purple', 'baseball', and 'Virginia', to discourage the subject from creating a mnemonic aid to recall the items. If the subject fails one or more items, semantic cues can be tried, such as 'it was a color'. Nonverbal short-term memory can also be tested by hiding three coins in different locations in the room and then asking the patient to find them, or by asking the patient to reproduce a drawing after a delay. These non-verbal memory tests can be useful in patients with verbal memory deficits related to left hemisphere lesions, but in whom non-verbal memory may be normal.

We test remote memory by asking the subject the names of children, grandchildren, or siblings, provided that a relative is available to confirm the answers. Fund of information can be tested with recent Presidents or other political figures, the dates of World War II or the Revolutionary War, the years of major events such as the assassination of John F. Kennedy, the Challenger disaster, the prolonged presidential election of 2000, or the terrorist attacks of September 11, 2001. For patients who do not pay attention to politics, use of athletic stars or television celebrities may be more appropriate. Even better are familiar tasks from the patient's work, such as the times of planting crops for a farmer, or the common drugs for hypertension for a physician.

Language

Language testing should include the seven items listed in Table 4.5: spontaneous speech, automatic sequences, naming, repetition, auditory comprehension, reading, and writing.

Spontaneous speech is characterized for its fluency and for the presence of articulation errors, hesitancy, word-finding pauses and circumlocutions (use of a phrase where one word would do), and 'paraphasic' errors. Paraphasic errors are called 'semantic' or 'verbal' if they involve the substitution of an incorrect word, such as 'fork' for 'spoon' or 'pencil' for 'pen'. Paraphasic errors are termed 'literal' or 'phonemic' if an incorrect sound is given, such as 'poon' for 'spoon' or 'ben' for 'pen'. If the words cannot be recognized at all, they are called 'neologisms', and the aphasic production is called 'jargon'.

Automatic sequences are familiar series items, such as counting to ten, or reciting the days of the week or the months of the year. Some patients can

Table 4.5 Bedside language tests

Spontaneous speech
Fluency
Articulation
Prosody
Content (literal, verbal paraphasias, neologisms)
Automatic sequences
Naming
Repetition
Auditory comprehension
Reading
Writing

produce these series utterances while remaining nearly mute in spontaneous conversation.

Naming is usually tested to confrontation, by showing the patient an item and asking for its name. Naming can also be tested by a 'fill in the blanks' format, or by asking the subject to produce as many animals as possible in 1 minute (generative naming). Items to be named should include objects (watch, ring, pen), object parts (watchband, winding stem), body parts (thumb, palm of the hand, elbow, wrist), and colors, since some patients have anomia that is relatively specific for classes of items.

Repetition should always be tested explicitly, as its involvement is pivotal for diagnosis of the classical aphasia syndromes. Repetition is tested for single words, polysyllabic words and phrases, and complex grammatical phrases. Polysyllabic words such as 'Methodist Episcopal' and 'British Constitution' are very difficult for patients with dysarthria and apraxia of speech, whereas complex grammatical phrases such as 'no ifs, ands, or buts' or 'the spy fled to Greece' are difficult for aphasic patients.

Comprehension has already been assessed informally during the history. In formal testing, the gauge of comprehension is the subject's ability to follow commands of one, two, and three steps (see Table 4.6). If the subject fails to carry out such commands, there are several possibilities in addition to language comprehension failure: deafness, inability to understand English, and apraxia, a failure to carry out motor acts in spite of intact comprehension. If apraxia is in question, the examiner can either ask yes/no questions or give commands with very simple motor requirements, such as 'point to the receptacle for trash'.

Reading should be tested both aloud and for meaning. Reading comprehension can be tested by use of printed commands similar to those used for testing of auditory comprehension. For patients with mild deficits, reading comprehension for paragraph-length material should also be tested.

Writing can include copying, writing phrases to dictation, and spontaneous writing of phrases or sentences. Many examiners have the patient sign his or her name, but this overlearned task may be preserved even in aphasic patients. Asking the subject to write a sentence explaining why he or she is presently in the hospital or office may tell much about the subject's awareness of the situation.

Table 4.6 Commands for testing of auditory comprehension

1. Close your eyes
2. Stick out your tongue
3. Point to the ceiling
4. Raise your left arm
5. Touch your right ear
6. Touch your left thumb to your chin
7. Hold up two fingers on your left hand
8. Close your right eye and touch your left thumb to your nose

Praxis

Apraxias are disorders of learned movement. Three types of movement are tested, each using one hand at a time. First, the subject is asked to demonstrate in pantomime the use of an imaginary object, such as a pencil, hammer, or comb. Second, the examiner demonstrates a similar, learned movement and asks the subject to imitate it. Third, the patient is given an actual object and asked to show how it is used. In addition to these motor patterns involving the extremities, commands should be chosen that require movement of the mouth, lips, and tongue (see Table 4.7). Finally, praxis should be tested for the execution of a multi-stage activity, such as taking out a pipe, filling it with tobacco, lighting, and smoking it; or filling a coffee maker with coffee and water, placing the filter properly, and turning it on to make coffee.

Gnosis

Testing of gnosis, or recognition of objects, is important in selected patients. This testing is usually carried out for specific sensory modalities, usually vision, hearing, and touch. For example, a patient with visual agnosia may be unable to identify a visual object, but able to identify the object by feel or by sound. Other patients may fail to identify the same item by touch (tactile agnosia) or by sound (auditory agnosia). These topics will be considered further in Chapter 8. A screening battery would include a series of pictures of objects and famous people for visual identification, a group of coins and small objects for tactile identification (e.g. a key, a paper clip, a safety pin), and a series of sounds (a bell, a whistle, and a series of animal noises such as an imitated dog bark, pig oink, and cat meow).

Calculations

We have already alluded to the serial sevens test, which is in actuality a test of both concentration and subtraction ability (Manning 1982). If the subject

---

Table 4.7 Praxis testing

Extremity praxis
  Items: hammer, saw, scissors, comb, toothbrush
  Pantomime the use of items ('show me how to use a ___')
  Imitation of the use of items ('do this after me')
  Demonstration of the use of actual items ('show me how to use this')

Orofacial praxis
  Show me how to:
    Stick out your tongue
    Blow a kiss
    Lick your upper lip
    Blow a smoke ring
    Cough

Series praxis
  Demonstrate use of coffee pot, including use of coffee powder, water, filter

performs this task accurately, calculation ability is likely intact. If the subject fails, simpler arithmetic problems such as change-making examples should be tested. For example, the patient may be asked to calculate the change from $1.00 for a drink costing 55 cents, or from $5.00 for a lunch costing $3.42. Written arithmetic tests may also be useful, especially in patients with visuospatial deficits related to right hemisphere lesions.

Visual-Constructional Ability

Visual, spatial, and constructional abilities are considered together, as these functions are all frequently affected by right hemisphere, and especially right parietal, lesions. Table 4.8 lists a brief battery of such tests. These tests are the most frequently omitted of all of the mental status examination categories, yet in a matter of 2 or 3 minutes and at no cost they can differentiate a right parietal lesion from a brainstem or spinal cord lesion. Bisection of a line is probably the easiest test to gauge neglect of one side of space. Drawing a clock and placing the numbers and hands tests both constructional ability and neglect, as long as digital watch designs are forbidden. The subject can be asked to draw from memory a bilaterally symmetric structure such as a Greek cross, a house, or a daisy; frequently, a subject with neglect will leave out details on one side of the drawing (see Figure 8.1). Copying a cube or a complex geometric figure tests constructional ability at a higher level; the intersecting pentagons figure from the MMSE can also be used. These tests should each be carried out on a blank, unlined piece of paper. We test topographical ability by asking the patient to draw a map of the state or country, with the locations of major cities. In the hospital, the patient can be asked to draw the ward or demonstrate the locations of the nurses' station and the elevators.

Frontal Lobe Function (Affect/Mood)

The frontal lobes are critical to behavior and personality, yet they are very difficult to test on a bedside mental status examination. An artificial test sometimes used to test frontal lobe processing is the copying and continuation of

Table 4.8 Visual–constructional tests

Draw a clock, place the hands at 20 minutes to 3
Draw (or copy) two-dimensional figures
  Daisy
  Greek cross
  House
Copy a cube
Copy a complex figure
Locate cities on a map
Demonstrate the location of hospital room, nurses' station
Repeating sequences (see Figure 4.1)

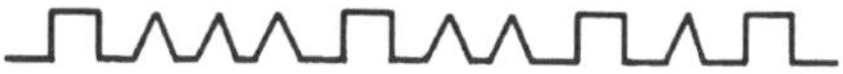

_Лᒀᐱᐱ_Лᐱᐱ_Лᐱᒀ

Figure 4.1 Alternating sequence test. The patient is asked to continue the visual pattern of alternating sequences on a blank sheet of paper. (Modified from RL Strub, RW Black. The Mental Status Examination in Neurology. Philadelphia: Davis, 1977; and AR Luria. Frontal lobe syndromes. In PJ Vinken, GW Bruyn (eds). Handbook of Clinical Neurology, Vol. 2. New York: American Elsevier, 1969.)

Luria's test of sequential squares and triangles (Strub and Black 1977; Figure 4.1). As will be seen in Chapter 10, frontal lesions may affect a patient's personality in ways very obvious to family members and friends, yet the entire neurological examination may be normal, even including the standard mental status examination. A tendency to perseverate or to have difficulty in shifting cognitive sets can be seen in the Luria test. Insight and judgment also reflect frontal lobe functioning (see below). Neuropsychological testing may be required to provide further, localizing information.

Recently, Dubois and colleagues (2000) have presented a frontal assessment battery called the 'FAB'. The test includes two similarity questions, a series naming test of words beginning with 's', a motor imitation task, a 'conflicting instructions' task ('tap once when I tap twice'), a 'go–no go' task ('tap once when I tap once'), and a screening test for utilization behavior or the environmental dependency syndrome (see Chapter 10): the examiner places his hands near those of the patient and says 'do not take my hands'. This test reportedly takes about 10 minutes to perform at the bedside and is sensitive to frontal lobe disorders.

Insight and Judgment, Abstract Reasoning

Insight and judgment have already been tested in the observational portion of the mental status examination. As stated earlier, the subject's understanding of his or her own illness is the most important test of insight. To some extent, these functions can also be tested by artificial problems. We can best assess the patient's capacity for abstract reasoning by formal testing. A commonly used test is the interpretation of proverbs such as 'people who live in glass houses should not throw stones', or 'absence makes the heart grow fonder'. These interpretations test insight and judgment, but they are culturally biased; patients who are mentally retarded or neurologically normal but uneducated often give concrete interpretations. Patients with psychiatric illness or delirium may give bizarre, idiosyncratic responses. Another way of testing abstract reasoning is to test similarities, for example, 'why is an apple like an orange?'. Finally, artificial judgment situations have been utilized, e.g. 'what would you do if you saw a fire in a movie theater?', or 'what would you do if you found a stamped addressed envelope on the sidewalk?'. Again, these artificial judgment situations may be more difficult to interpret than the patient's understanding of why he or she is visiting the doctor.

DETERMINATION OF MENTAL COMPETENCY

Neurologists, as well as psychologists and psychiatrists, are often asked to give an opinion on the mental competency of patients with neurobehavioral disorders. These determinations must be made not only for patients' financial decisions, but also for consent to receive treatments or to participate in research trials. Michael Alexander (1988) presented a framework for determination of competency, which is shown in Table 4.9. Chief among the criteria are deficits in attention, memory, and language. Alexander emphasized that patients with focal brain lesions, such as strokes, may fail to comprehend issues presented in one language modality, such as printed language or arithmetic calculations, but may understand the same issues presented orally. Another patient could read business reports but not understand the same information presented in spoken form. Such patients may be deemed competent, provided that a representative is present to be sure that the patient receives the information through the appropriate channel. Other patients should be declared incompetent, and decisions should be made by court-appointed legal guardians or representatives with power of attorney. Judgment of competency in a patient with a focal brain injury can be very challenging, and a behavioral neurologist may be the specialist most able to decide. Though other, more standardized batteries have been introduced (Kim *et al.* 2001), Alexander's clinical model has considerable usefulness for practicing neurologists.

In generalized dementias such as Alzheimer's disease, the determination of competency is usually more straightforward. As in patients with focal brain lesions, semantic ability and language comprehension are important in determining the competency of demented patients. In addition, demented patients may

Table 4.9 Neurological criteria for determination of mental incompetency (adapted from Alexander 1988)

Cognitive domain	Clinical threshold for likely incompetency
Attention	Digit span <5, distractibility, perseveration
Memory	Frank disorientation, inability to recall four words for 3 minutes, inability to provide recent history
Language	Impaired ability to express decisions; Poor comprehension of spoken or written language
Spatial/perceptual	Hemispatial neglect; major constructional deficits, agnosia
Reasoning	Concrete, autistic, or tangential thinking, or distortion of reasoning by delusional or paranoid thinking
Emotion	Anosognosia or unconcern about deficits, irritability, mania, euphoria, severe depression sufficient to disrupt judgment
Miscellaneous	Acalculia preventing comprehension of quantitative concepts

lack sufficient memory to consider the issues involved in a decision. With more complex issues, reasoning ability also comes into play. Two recent studies have shown that physicians not only showed good consensus in judging the mental competency of patients with Alzheimer's disease shown discussing treatment decisions in videotaped vignettes (Marson *et al.* 2000), but that these the physicians' judgments also correlated with neuropsychological testing, particularly in the areas of naming, language comprehension, and reasoning (Earnst *et al.* 2000). Bassett (1999) presented evidence that attention span, as measured by the Trails A test of the Halstead-Reitan battery, was highly correlated with mental competency in patients with Alzheimer's disease.

CONCLUSION

Like any part of the neurological examination, the formal mental status examination must be tailored to the individual patient. It is unrealistic to expect an internist or family practitioner to perform a detailed mental status examination on a patient with chest pain or gastrointestinal bleeding, but at least orientation and memory should be tested. It should be equally obvious that a patient with difficulty expressing him- or herself requires a detailed examination of language for proper diagnosis. Delineation of a specific type of aphasia aids in the localization of the lesion and in the diagnosis of the disease process. Similarly, a patient with left arm and leg weakness should be tested for visual–spatial–constructional ability, since a deficit may lead to the diagnosis of a right parietal lesion rather than a spinal cord disorder. Neurodiagnostic testing can then proceed directly to brain imaging, skipping the spinal cord MR imaging or myelography that would otherwise be considered. Patients with memory loss or dementia clearly require a detailed exploration of cognitive functions. More problematic are patients with complaints such as headache, in whom a screening mental status examination is as important as the motor and sensory examinations to exclude a focal, space-occupying lesion.

Succeeding chapters of this book explicate how specific mental status findings are used, together with findings of the rest of the neurological examination, to localize disease processes in the nervous system. The history of the onset of the current symptoms, together with the medical history and risk factors, then guides the examiner to the specific etiologic diagnosis.

REFERENCES

Alexander MP. Clinical determination of mental competence. A theory and a retrospective study. Arch Neurol 1988;45:23–26.

Applegate WB, Blass JP, Williams TF. Instruments for the functional assessment of older patients. New Engl J Med 1990;322:1207–1214.

Bassett SS. Attention: neuropsychological predictor of competency in Alzheimer's disease. J Geriatr Psychiatry Neurol 1999;12:200–205.

Blessed G, Tomlinson BE, Roth M. The association between quantitative measures of dementia and senile change in the cerebral gray matter of elderly subjects. Br J Psychiatry 1968;114:797–811.

Blessed G, Tomlinson BE, Roth M. Blessed–Roth dementia scale (DS). Psychopharmacol Bull 1988;24:705–708.

Crum RM, Anthony JC, Bassett SS, Folstein MF. Population-based norms for the mini mental state examination by age and educational level. JAMA 1993;269:2386–2391.

Dick JPR, Stewart A, Blackstock J *et al.* Mini-mental state examination in neurological patients. J Neurol Neurosurg Psychiat 1984;47:496–499.

Dubois B, Slachevsky A, Litvan I, Pillon B. The FAB: A frontal assessment battery at bedside. Neurology 2000;55:1621–1626.

Dufouil C, Clayton D, Brayne C *et al.* Population norms for the MMSE in the very old. Estimates based on longitudinal data. Neurology 2000;55:1609–1613.

Earnst KS, Marson DC, Harrell LE. Cognitive models of physicians' legal standard and personal judgments of competency in patients with Alzheimer's disease. J Am Geriatr Soc 2000;48:919–927.

Ferris SH, Kluger A. Assessing cognition in Alzheimer's disease research. Alzheimer's disease and associated disorders 1997;11(suppl. 6):45–49.

Folstein MF, Folstein SE, McHugh PR. 'Mini-mental state': a practical method for grading the cognitive state of patients for the clinician. J Psychiatr Res 1975;12:189–198.

Geschwind N. Foreword to Strub RL, Black FW. The Mental Status Examination in Neurology. Philadelphia: FA Davis Company, 1977;v–vi.

Kaufer DI, Cummings JL, Ketchel P *et al.* Validation of the NPI-Q, a brief clinical form of the Neuropsychiatric Inventory. J Neuropsychiatry Clin Neurosci 2000;12: 233–235.

Kim SY, Caine ED, Currier GW, Leibovici A, Ryan JM. Assessing the competence of persons with Alzheimer's disease in providing informed consent for participation in research. Am J Psychiatry 2001;158:712–717.

Kirshner HS. Bedside mental status examination. In HS Kirshner (ed.), Behavioral Neurology: A Practical Approach. New York: Churchill Livingstone, 1986;3–13.

Manning RT. The serial sevens test. Arch Intern Med 1982;142:1192.

Marson DC, Earnst KS, Jamil F, Bartolucci A, Harrell LE. Consistency of physicians' legal standard and personal judgments of competency in patients with Alzheimer's disease. J Am geriatr Soc 2000;48:911–918.

Mattis S. Mental status examination for organic mental syndrome in the elderly patient. In R Bellack, B Karasu (eds), Geriatric Psychiatry. New York: Grune & Stratton, 1976;77–121.

Mohs RC, Cohen L. Alzheimer's Disease Assessment Scale (ADAS). Psychopharmacol Bull 1988;24:627–628.

Morris JC, Mohs RC, Rogers H *et al.* Consortium to Establish a Registry for Alzheimer's Disease (CERAD). Clinical and neuropsychological assessment of Alzheimer's disease. Psychopharmacol Bull 1988;24:641–652.

Solomon PR, Pendlebury WW. The seven-minute screen. Available from Janssen Pharmaceutica/Research Foundation, 1999.

Strub RL, Black FW. The Mental Status Examination in Neurology. Philadelphia: FA Davis Co., 1977;1–182.

Teng EL, Chui HC. The modified mini-mental state (3MS) examination. J Clin Psychiat 1987;48:314–318.

Weintraub S, Mesulam M-M. Mental state assessment of young and elderly adults in behavioral neurology. In M-M Mesulam (ed.), Principles of Behavioral Neurology. Philadelphia: FA Davis Co., 1985;71–123.

PART II

Focal Neurobehavioral Syndromes

5

Speech and Language Disorders

Language is so tightly woven into human experience that it is scarcely possible to imagine life without it. Chances are that if you find two or more people together anywhere on earth, they will soon be exchanging words. When there is no one to talk with, people talk to themselves, to their dogs, even to their plants. In our social relations, the race is not to the swift but to the verbal–the spellbinding orator, the silver-tongued seducer, the persuasive child who wins the battle of wills against a brawnier parent. Aphasia, the loss of language following brain injury, is devastating, and in severe cases family members may feel that the whole person is lost forever.

(Pinker 1994)

Speech and language are perhaps the most 'human' of all attributes, the ability to communicate verbally with other people. Speech is defined as the articulation of language sounds by the vocal apparatus, whereas language refers to the manipulation of symbols in the production and comprehension of communicative symbols. The organization of the human brain for expressive speech may be under the control of a gene; patients with an autosomal dominant disorder of speech and language has recently been reported to have an abnormal gene on Chromosome 7 (Lai *et al.* 2001). Aphasias are acquired disorders of language secondary to brain disease (Alexander and Benson 1998). The aphasias represent a family of syndromes in which specific language functions are affected by focal lesions usually of the left hemisphere. The syndromes can be defined by the bedside examination of speech and language presented in Chapter 4.

Historically, speech and language were the first of the higher cortical functions to be correlated with specific focal lesions of the brain. Even now, they remain the clearest example of how careful analysis of human behavior at the bedside can lead to localization of brain functions. References to speech and articulation problems in persons with left hemisphere damage can be traced to ancient times, as in the Edwin Smith Papyrus, which spoke of a man with 'a wound in his temple'; 'he speaks not to thee...copious tears fall from both his eyes' (McHenry 1969). This Egyptian papyrus, written in approximately 3500 BC,

45

not only contains the first mention of acquired speech and language disorder, but also hints of depression associated with aphasia. The modern analysis of language disorders began with the 1861 publication of Paul Broca, who described a severe articulatory disorder in two patients who had relatively intact comprehension. Both patients died and had focal lesions of the left frontal lobe. This was the first demonstration that a higher function as complex as spoken language resided in a focal area of the brain, which could be damaged in a stroke.

During the later nineteenth and early twentieth centuries, physicians studied the speech and language of patients, and then examined the brain to see the location of the damage. In this painstaking and slow fashion, knowledge about the organization of language in the brain accrued. As in other areas of behavioral neurology, knowledge of brain–behavior relationships advanced largely through the study of patients with stroke, an 'experiment of nature' that damages one area of the brain, leaving other areas completely intact. In aphasia, moreover, animal models were unavailable to supplement this information, since the capacity of other species for articulate language is so limited.

During the second half of the twentieth century, clinical observations were greatly augmented by new technologies. First, standardized test batteries, administered by speech/language pathologists or neuropsychologists, have made the behavioral assessment of the aphasic patient more quantitative and comparable from one patient to another. Researchers in neurolinguistics have devised specific linguistic tests to study language and the brain. Second, new methods of brain imaging have permitted the correlation of behavior and brain pathology in the living patient. The computerized tomographic (CT) scan and magnetic resonance imaging (MRI) scan permit precise imaging of brain anatomy and pathology in the living patient. MRI provides views of the brain in sagittal and coronal planes in addition to the transaxial plane of the CT scan. MRI also avoids artifacts in the tissues adjacent to bone. Single photon emission computed tomography (SPECT), positron emission tomography (PET), and functional MRI (fMRI), so called functional imaging methods, permit the visualization of areas of isotope uptake or blood flow increase corresponding to areas of active brain metabolism. These techniques provide a functional map of brain activity for the study of language activation in normals during activities such as speaking, reading, and thinking, and they provide sensitive measures of decreased activity of the language cortex in disease states. These methods are especially useful in diffuse brain diseases such as Alzheimer's disease or primary progressive aphasia, in which no focal lesion may be evident on a static brain image such as a CT or MRI brain scan.

Another area in which new techniques have advanced the study of language is the electrical mapping of the brain in patients with epilepsy. Stimulation of brain areas can indicate which cortical areas are involved in language, and which can safely be removed in epilepsy surgery. The mapping of language zones by this technique has given a quite different view of language organization in the brain from studies of stroke patients, indicating that the traditional language areas may be smaller and less consistent in location than the experience with strokes suggested. Surgical ablations of epileptogenic cortex have served to confirm these impressions.

Speech and language disorders, like the other functions studied by behavioral neurologists, have fascination not only for physicians but also for psychologists, linguists, and philosophers. The analysis of aphasia is also of practical usefulness in the localization of lesions in the brain and in the diagnosis of neurological disorders. Brain imaging modalities confirm these clinical localizations and diagnoses, aiding both research and clinical medicine. New treatments in many of the brain diseases, including stroke, promise much more to offer aphasic patients.

APPROACH TO THE PATIENT WITH SPEECH AND LANGUAGE DISORDERS

The first task of the behavioral neurologist when evaluating a speech or language problem is to determine if the patient is aphasic. The definition of aphasia, an acquired disorder of language, is carefully constructed to exclude three other causes of abnormal communication. The examiner must first ensure in the history that the deficit is acquired, i.e., that premorbid speech and language skills were normally developed. Congenital or developmental language problems are referred to as 'dysphasias'. The reader should be aware of a conflicting terminology, used mainly in the UK and Europe, in which 'dysphasia' refers to a partial loss of language, whereas 'aphasia' denotes a total loss of language. Developmental language disorders are less well correlated with focal brain lesions than acquired aphasias; in most cases, the brain appears grossly normal by CT scan or *post-mortem* examination. Minor developmental anomalies may be seen in some cases. Acquired aphasias in children can be analyzed in the same manner as adult aphasias, with smaller differences than previously believed.

Second, the definition of aphasia excludes motor speech disorders, which disturb only spoken language output. The bedside examination presented in Chapter 2 should help in making this distinction. In motor speech disorders, written language expression and receptive language skills remain intact. We shall discuss motor speech disorders below.

Third, the definition excludes disorders of language content secondary to psychiatric disorders. In psychosis, the mechanics of speech and language are normal, but the underlying thought process, or manipulation of concepts, is abnormal. A psychotic patient may thus formulate and articulate perfectly normal sentences, using normal nouns, verbs, and other parts of speech, but the content is bizarre or nonsensical. In general, elementary language functions like those tested in the bedside assessment are normal in psychotic patients, as long as cooperation can be obtained (DiSimon *et al.* 1977). Paraphasic errors and neologisms are rare in psychosis, except in some very chronic, untreated schizophrenic patients who speak a jargon called 'word salad speech' (Gerson *et al.* 1977). Patients with bipolar affective disorder may occasionally have their speech derailed by 'clang associations', which represent punning or wordplay. The communicative errors in psychotic patients are often related to vague or confused references, unspecified or ambiguous meanings rather than true language errors

(Docherty *et al.* 1996). A key difference between psychosis and aphasia is in the patient's non-linguistic behavior. The psychotic patient manifests abnormal behavior as well as language, whereas an aphasic patient usually behaves appropriately, though unable to communicate. The presence of other focal left hemisphere signs in many aphasic patients also helps to indicate a neurological rather than psychiatric disorder. Psychosis will be considered further in Chapter 15.

MOTOR SPEECH DISORDERS

Motor speech disorders refer to abnormalities of speech articulation, in the absence of language dysfunction. On the bedside mental status examination, spontaneous speech, repetition, naming, and reading aloud may be abnormal, but auditory comprehension, reading comprehension, and writing should all be normal. In general, if the examiner transcribes the speech output of a dysarthric patient and then reads it aloud, it should sound normal. Motor speech disorders are generally divided into dysarthria and apraxia of speech.

Dysarthria

Dysarthria refers to a consistent misarticulation of phonemes. Darley and colleagues, of the Mayo Clinic, defined dysarthria as: "a group of speech disorders resulting from disturbances of muscular control over the speech mechanism due to damage of the central or peripheral nervous system, {creating} problems in oral communication due to paralysis, weakness, or incoordination of the speech musculature." (Darley *et al.* 1969, p. 246). By this definition, dysarthria is a neurological disorder and does not refer to local, structural disorders such as cleft lip or palate and laryngectomy. Dysarthria can aid in the diagnosis of disorders of the central and peripheral nervous system, based on the specific auditory–perceptual features of the dysarthria.

Classification of Dysarthria

Dysarthria has been divided into six subtypes (Darley *et al.* 1969) based on neuroanatomic lesions but distinguishable by auditory–perceptual characteristics that a physician can learn to recognize at the bedside. Table 5.1 lists a summary of the Mayo Clinic classification of dysarthria. The six types of dysarthria are: flaccid, spastic, ataxic, hypokinetic, hyperkinetic, and mixed. Subsequently, the Mayo Clinic group (Duffy 1995) has added a subtype of spastic dysarthria called 'unilateral upper motor neuron dysarthria'.

Flaccid dysarthria results from bilateral, lower motor neuron lesions, or bulbar palsy. The auditory characteristics include: (1) breathy voice quality; (2) hypernasality; and (3) imprecise consonants (errors or distortions of consonant sounds). Flaccid dysarthria may result from a brainstem stroke, traumatic

Table 5.1 Classification of the dysarthrias (adapted from FL Darley, AE Aronson, JR Brown. Differential diagnostic patterns of dysarthria. J Speech Hear Res 1969;12: 246–249; JR Duffy. Motor Speech Disorders. Substrates, Differential Diagnosis, and Management. St Louis: Mosby, 1995)

Type	Localization	Auditory signs	Diagnoses
Flaccid	Lower motor neuron	Breathy, nasal voice	Stroke, myasthenia gravis
Spastic	Bilateral upper motor neuron	Strain-strangle, harsh voice; slow rate; imprecise consonants	Bilateral strokes, tumors, primary lateral sclerosis
Unilateral upper motor neuron	Unilateral upper motor neuron	Consonant imprecision, slow rate, harsh voice quality	Stroke, tumor
Ataxic	Cerebellum	Irregular articulatory breakdowns, excessive and equal stress	Stroke, degenerative disease
Hypokinetic	Extrapyramidal	Rapid rate, reduced loudness, monopitch and monoloudness	Parkinson's disease
Hyperkinetic	Extrapyramidal	Prolonged phonemes, variable rate, inappropriate silences, voice stoppages	Dystonia, Huntington's disease
Spastic–flaccid	Upper and lower motor neuron	Hypernasality; strain-strangle, harsh voice, slow rate, imprecise consonants	Amyotrophic lateral sclerosis, multiple strokes

brain injury, or neuromuscular disorders such as myasthenia gravis, acute polio, or Guillain–Barré syndrome.

Spastic dysarthria results from bilateral upper motor neuron lesions, also referred to as 'pseudobulbar palsy'. The auditory characteristics are: (1) a strain-strangle, harsh voice; (2) slow rate; and (3) imprecise consonants, often with hypernasality. Causes of spastic dysarthria include bilateral strokes, tumors, and degenerative diseases such as primary lateral sclerosis.

Unilateral upper motor neuron (UUMN) dysarthria results from a unilateral upper motor neuron lesion. The auditory signs are similar to the spastic type, but less severe: (1) harsh voice; (2) slow rate; and (3) imprecise consonants. Common causes of UUMN are a unilateral hemisphere stroke or brain tumor.

Ataxic dysarthria results from damage in the cerebellum or its connections. The auditory signs are: (1) irregular articulatory breakdowns; and (2) excessive and equal stress on every syllable, also referred to as 'scanning speech'. Possible causes include cerebellar degenerations, strokes, and tumors. Multiple sclerosis frequently produces ataxic dysarthria, but it may be mixed with elements of flaccid, spastic, or unilateral upper motor neuron dysarthria.

Hypokinetic dysarthria is associated with extrapyramidal or basal ganglia diseases. The auditory characteristics are: (1) rapid rate; (2) reduced loudness; (3) monopitch (unvarying pitch level); and (4) monoloudness (unvarying loudness level). The most common cause of hypokinetic dysarthria is Parkinson's disease. Occasionally, strokes involving the basal ganglia can mimic this pattern.

Hyperkinetic dysarthria is also associated with extrapyramidal disorders, but those with increased rather than decreased movement. The auditory signs include: (1) prolonged phonemes (individual speech sounds are stretched out); (2) variable rate (sometimes too fast and sometimes too slow); (3) harsh voice quality; (4) inappropriate silences (abnormal pauses in the flow of speech); and (5) voice stoppages (inappropriate absence of phonation). Common causes of hyperkinetic dysarthria are dystonia (e.g. dystonia musculorum deformans), Joseph's disease, and Huntington's disease.

Mixed dysarthria has several subtypes. The auditory perceptual characteristics vary, depending on which neurological systems are involved.

Spastic–flaccid dysarthria results from involvement of both the upper and lower motor neuron systems. The auditory characteristics are: (1) hypernasality; (2) strain-strangle, liquid-sounding voice quality (phonation is accompanied by a gurgle); (3) extremely slow rate; and (4) severe consonant imprecision. Spastic–flaccid dysarthria is typically caused by amyotrophic lateral sclerosis (ALS), but may be seen in multiple strokes.

Multiple sclerosis may produce a mixed ataxic–spastic–flaccid dysarthria resulting from cerebellar, upper motor neuron, and lower motor neuron involvement. The ataxic features (excessive and equal stress, slow rate) may be most prominent. Similarly, Wilson's disease may produce auditory characteristics of hypokinetic, ataxic, and spastic dysarthrias.

Apraxia of Speech

Apraxia of speech is a disorder that can be thought of as intermediate between the dysarthrias and the aphasias. It is not completely accepted as an entity by all neurologists, though speech–language pathologists diagnose it routinely. Wertz *et al.* (1984, p. 48) define apraxia of speech as: "...an articulatory disorder resulting from impairment, as a result of brain damage, of the capacity to program the positioning of speech musculature and the sequencing of muscle movements for the volitional production of phonemes. The speech musculature does not show significant weakness, slowness, or incoordination in reflex and automatic acts."

This definition closely follows the more general definition of apraxia provided by Norman Geschwind (see Chapter 7). It implies that apraxia of speech is a motor speech disorder, not a language disorder or aphasia. In simpler terms,

Table 5.2 Auditory features of apraxia of speech

Effortful, groping, trial-and-error articulation, with attempts at self-correction
Difficulty with initiation of utterances
Difficulty most evident on initial phonemes of multisyllabic utterances
Dysprosody
Inconsistency on repeated productions of the same word

apraxia of speech is a disorder of the programming of rapid sequences of phonemes.

Apraxia of speech is distinguished from dysarthria because it results from defective patterns of phoneme utterances, and not from weakness, slowness, or incoordination of the articulators. In practical terms, speech apraxia causes articulatory errors that, in contrast to dysarthric mispronunciations, are inconsistent; the subject may pronounce the same word differently, and sometimes normally, in different utterances. Apraxia of speech is distinguished from aphasia by the lack of language disorder. In fact, however, apraxia of speech is rarely an isolated deficit and is often mixed with aphasia, and sometimes with dysarthria.

Table 5.2 lists the key features of apraxia of speech. First, the patient displays effortful, trial and error, groping articulatory movements, in an apparent attempt to produce the right sound sequences. Errors are often accompanied by several attempts at self-correction. Second, the speech is dysprosodic, or marred by disruptions in the rhythm, stress (emphasis), and intonation of speech. Third, apraxic speech is inconsistent. For example, a patient may make different errors in pronouncing the same word several times; this is especially evident with polysyllabic words with multiple consonant sounds, such as 'impossibility', 'artillery', or 'catastrophe'. A patient trying to say 'catastrophe' five times might produce 'capastrophy, catastroophy, catastrophe, caphastromy, calastrothy'. Fourth, the apraxic speaker has special difficulty initiating speech, with more errors at the beginning than at the end of a phrase.

Localization of Apraxia of Speech

The motor programming of speech sequences is not well localized in the nervous system. It may well relate to Broca's area in the left inferior frontal gyrus, since patients with Broca's aphasia (see below) frequently have an associated apraxia of speech. In fact, Broca emphasized the articulatory disorder in his original descriptions of two patients with left frontal lesions. Recently, Dronkers (1996) associated apraxia of speech with lesions of the insula. Twenty-five stroke patients who displayed apraxia of speech all had lesions involving the left insula, whereas none of the 19 patients without apraxia of speech had lesions in this area. Dronkers concluded that the insula appears to be specialized for the motor planning of speech.

Etiology of Apraxia of Speech

Duffy (1995) reported a large series of patients with apraxia of speech. The great majority of cases, 58%, had either single or multiple strokes, all of which involved the left hemisphere. Less common causes of apraxia of speech included degenerative diseases of the nervous system disease, traumatic brain injury, tumors, and multiple or unknown causes.

MUTENESS

A special problem in the diagnosis of speech and language problems is the mute patient. The mute patient may have dysarthria of severe degree, apraxia of speech, a non-neurologic disorder such as a laryngeal obstruction, a frontal lobe syndrome with akinetic mutism (see Chapter 10), an extrapyramidal disorder such as severe Parkinson's disease, a psychogenic state such as catatonia, simple uncooperativeness, or stupor. In general, some language output must be present before the examiner can confidently diagnose aphasia. Normal performance in writing and in language comprehension makes aphasia unlikely. Muteness and inability to follow commands in a patient who is seemingly alert may signify severe aphasia, but care must be taken in this diagnosis. Of course, other 'neighborhood signs' of left hemisphere injury such as right hemiparesis, right-sided sensory loss, and right hemianopsia aid in the diagnosis of aphasia. In general, the aphasic patient tries to communicate by gesturing, grunting, or pointing; he is mute in speech but not in other behaviors (Geschwind 1964).

APHASIAS

Aphasia is a common clinical problem, occurring in at least 20% of stroke patients (Pedersen *et al.* 1995). Aphasias can be divided behaviorally and neuroanatomically into syndromes involving the primary language cortex and those involving other cortical and subcortical centers. The primary language cortex is arranged as a circuit of centers around the left sylvian fissure, involving the operculum (or roof of the sylvian fissure) in the frontal, parietal, and temporal lobes. Since aphasia was first described in the nineteenth century, a number of clinical investigators have devised classifications of aphasia. The Boston classification of Benson and Geschwind, recently updated by Alexander and Benson (1998), offers the most practical system for clinical neurologists, because it utilizes the classical syndromes described in the nineteenth century but incorporates new knowledge of neuroanatomy and clinical findings. In addition, this classification scheme relates directly to both the bedside language examination and to test scores obtained on the Boston Diagnostic Aphasia Examination (BDAE). A preliminary classification is made from the bedside examination, but more reliable syndrome diagnosis is obtained from either the BDAE or its shortened adaptation, the Western Aphasia Battery (WAB).

In the past, there has been a tendency to classify aphasias by a dichotomous approach. Examples of dichotomous classifications that are familiar to neurologists are: expressive versus receptive, motor versus sensory, fluent versus non-fluent, and anterior versus posterior aphasias. The problem with the expressive–receptive and motor–sensory dichotomies is that aphasias are rarely purely expressive or receptive, motor or sensory. Virtually all aphasics have abnormal language expression; it is the type of the expressive deficit that is important. This classification scheme is often misleading, since naïve clinicians frequently term even the fluent, paraphasic speech of a Wernicke's aphasic as 'expressive aphasia', though this is not what the term originally meant. If a dichotomy is to be used, the author prefers the fluent–non-fluent scheme, since it is descriptive and less likely to be misleading.

The Boston classification divides the aphasias into eight classical syndromes: Broca's, Wernicke's, global, conduction, anomic, and transcortical motor, transcortical sensory, and mixed transcortical aphasia, also called the syndrome of the isolation of the speech area. In addition, we shall consider the syndromes of aphemia, pure word deafness, and the subcortical aphasia syndromes. Disorders of reading and writing (alexias and agraphias) will be considered in Chapter 6. For each aphasia classification, we shall consider the typical clinical findings, the associated neurological signs, and the localizations of the underlying brain lesions. Finally, at the end of the chapter, we shall consider the topics of aphasia in left-handers, 'crossed aphasia' associated with right hemisphere lesions in right-handers, and aphasia in bilinguals, or speakers of more than one language.

Broca's Aphasia

Paul Broca, a French surgeon, described two patients in 1861 who had a difficulty in articulation, producing only stereotyped utterances such as 'Tan tan'. These patients could comprehend spoken language. Broca chose the term 'aphemia' for this articulatory disorder, but the name 'aphasia', proposed by Trousseau, won out. Broca gets much of the credit for localizing the articulation of speech to the inferior left frontal region that now bears the name 'Broca's area'. As Carl Sagan (1974) stated in his essay *Broca's Brain*: "Articulate speech, it turns out, as Broca inferred on only fragmentary evidence, is to an important extent localized in and controlled by Broca's area. It was one of the first discoveries of a separation of function between the left and right hemispheres of the brain. But most important, it was one of the first indications that specific brain functions exist in particular locales in the brain, that there is a connection between the anatomy of the brain and what the brain does, an activity sometimes described as 'mind'."

In modern descriptions, the typical Broca's aphasic speaks little, or non-fluently. The deficit can range from complete muteness, to single word utterances, to phrases and short sentences produced hesitantly. The disorder is an aphasia rather than just a motor speech disorder, because grammatical constructions are disturbed. Expressive speech is agrammatic; it reads like a telegram. For example, a Broca's aphasic who wanted to express that his wife would be coming to the hospital at 4 pm might produce 'wife...come...hospital...today'. Table 5.3 displays the major clinical features of Broca's aphasia.

Table 5.3 Features of Broca's aphasia

Feature	Characteristic
Spontaneous speech	Non-fluent, hesitant, from mute to agrammatic, often dysarthric
Naming	Impaired ('tip-of-the-tongue')
Auditory comprehension	Intact for simple material; impaired for complex syntactic constructions
Repetition	Impaired, hesitant
Reading	Difficulty reading aloud, often poorer reading than auditory comprehension
Writing	Difficulty writing, even with left hand
Associated signs	Right hemiparesis, right hemisensory loss, apraxia of left limbs
Behavior	Frustrated, depressed, but appropriate

Naming in Broca's aphasia is usually impaired. Frequently the patient will have an idea of the name, for example he can produce the initial letter or phoneme or can correctly state the number of syllables in the word. This type of anomia is called the 'tip of the tongue phenomenon'. In some patients, naming of actions (verbs) is worse than naming of objects (nouns).

Repetition in Broca's aphasia is usually only slightly better than spontaneous speech, marred by similar articulatory difficulty and hesitancy. Auditory comprehension often seems normal, but sentences with complex grammatical structure reveal deficits in syntactic decoding. The patient with Broca's aphasia may not, for example, be able to comprehend sentences with embedded clauses – the sentence 'the book which Bill gave to Betty was long' may cause major difficulty; the patient may have difficulty answering questions regarding who received the book and who gave it. Complex syntax causes difficulty for patients with Broca's aphasia in comprehension, just as it does in expressive speech (Heilman and Scholes 1976; Goodglass *et al.* 1979). A recent study using functional activation of the brain with positron emission tomography (Caplan *et al.* 1997) showed that the left frontal Broca's area lights up during both expression and comprehension of sentences with embedded clauses. This modern evidence confirms what aphasiologists have known for 140 years, namely that Broca's area is involved in the production and comprehension of syntactic relationships.

Reading is often more affected than auditory comprehension in Broca's aphasia. Benson (1977) referred to this reading difficulty as the 'third alexia'. Writing is also deficient in Broca's aphasia. Most patients with this disorder have partial or total paralysis of the right arm and leg, making it difficult for the right-handed patient to write with the dominant hand. The patient may refuse to write, but if he or she attempts to do so only a few awkward letters emerge. Persons with injuries to the right arm, but with normal brain function, can learn to write awkwardly but intelligibly with the left hand. The agraphia of Broca's aphasia is thus not simply a motor disorder, but a central language disorder affecting the written language modality. Experimentally, some patients with Broca's aphasia and right hemiparesis have been taught to write with the right hand, by placing the arm in a device resembling a roller skate, with pen attached. Patients with some proximal movement of the arm can direct the writing instrument, and such patients often write better with the paralyzed right arm than with the non-paralyzed left arm (Brown *et al.* 1983; Whurr and Lorch 1991). This discrepancy in performance may reflect apraxia for use of the right limbs, or perhaps disconnection from input of language signals across the corpus callosum to the right hemisphere motor area.

Associated deficits with Broca's aphasia include weakness of the right face, arm, and leg, and often some sensory loss on the right side of the body. The visual fields are usually spared. Some studies on post-stroke depression have found an association between depression and infarctions of the anterior left hemisphere, though some recent surveys with a longer time period after the stroke have not found as much difference between the hemispheres (see Chapters 17 and 21). Behaviorally, Broca's aphasics seem appropriately concerned about their stroke deficits, often frustrated but fully aware (Robinson and Benson 1981). Some

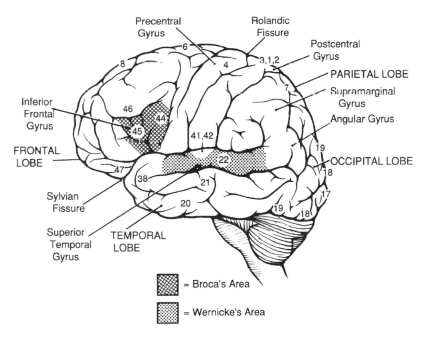

Figure 5.1 Simplified diagram of the lateral surface of the left hemisphere, showing the relationship of Broca's and Wernicke's language areas to the motor and sensory cortices, the angular and supramarginal gyri, and the lobar architecture of the brain. (Reprinted with permission from WG Bradley, RB Daroff, GM Fenichel, CD Marsden (eds). Neurology in Clinical Practice, Vol. I (3rd edn). Boston: Butterworth Heinemann, 2000.)

patients with Broca's aphasia may show apraxia of the left limbs, failing to follow commands for use of the left limbs that they can readily comprehend. It is important to recognize this apraxia and not mistake it for failure to comprehend.

The lesions of Broca's aphasia classically involve the posterior two-thirds of the inferior frontal convolution, pars triangularis and pars opercularis, Brodmann areas 44 and 45 (Figure 5.1). Figure 5.2 shows the relationship of the Broca's and Wernicke's language areas to the divisions of the middle cerebral artery; strokes in these territories are the most common cause of aphasia. Mohr and colleagues (1978) showed that lesions restricted to the cortical Broca's area are generally associated with virtually complete recovery, such that Broca's aphasia is present only during the initial days or weeks. Alexander and colleagues (1990) found that patients with lesions of areas 44 and 45 had mainly a deficit in initiation of speech, without true aphasia. Patients with lesions only of the lower motor cortex had only dysarthria and speech hesitancy. Both areas 44 and 45 and the lower motor cortex had to be damaged to produce the full picture of Broca's aphasia. Figure 5.3 shows an MRI scan from a patient with a transitory Broca's aphasia and apraxia of speech. Patients with lasting Broca's aphasia

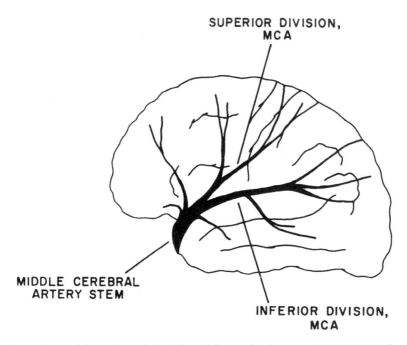

SUPERIOR DIVISION,
MCA

MIDDLE CEREBRAL
ARTERY STEM

INFERIOR DIVISION,
MCA

Figure 5.2 Cortical branches of the left middle cerebral artery (MCA). MCA branches, though more variable than depicted, are arranged into a superior division supplying the frontal and parietal lobes and an inferior division supplying the temporal lobe. Broca's area, along with the primary motor and sensory cortices, lies within the superior division territory. Wernicke's area lies within the inferior division territory.

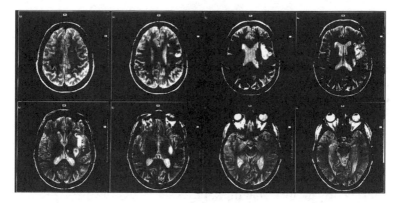

Figure 5.3 Magnetic resonance imaging scan from a patient with Broca's aphasia. The cortical Broca's area, the subcortical white matter, and the insula were all involved in the infarction. The patient had very hesitant speech, with dysarthria, apraxia of speech, and mild non-fluent aphasia. The patient recovered language function within 6 weeks. (Reprinted with permission from WG Bradley, RB Daroff, GM Fenichel, CD Marsden (eds). Neurology in Clinical Practice, Vol. I (3rd edn). Boston: Butterworth-Heinemann, 2000.)

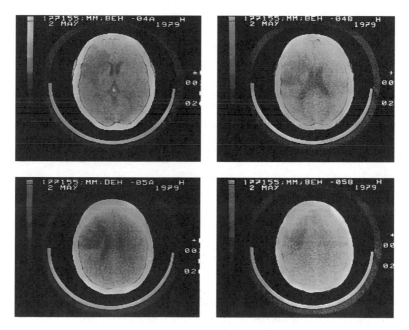

Figure 5.4 CT scan from a patient with persistent, severe Broca's aphasia. The large area of infarction on the four cuts includes most of the territory of the superior division of the left middle cerebral artery. Note that on this first generation CT scan, the left side of the brain is on the left side of the picture.

usually have much larger lesions, involving not only Broca's area but also much of the frontoparietal operculum (Figure 5.4). Broca's two original cases had such lesions, as have most reported cases over the ensuing century. Most such patients have global aphasia immediately after their stroke, which involves much of the left middle cerebral artery territory, and recovery towards Broca's aphasia occurs over a period of weeks to months. Mohr and colleagues (1978) referred to the transitory and permanent forms of Broca's aphasia as 'Baby Broca' and 'Big Broca' syndromes, respectively.

The prognosis for recovery in Broca's aphasia thus depends on the time after the stroke that the patient is examined. Naeser and colleagues (1989) reported that lesions associated with poor recovery of fluent speech always include two subcortical areas: (1) the subcallosal fasciculus deep to Broca's area; and (2) the periventricular white matter along the body of the left lateral ventricle. The combined cortical–subcortical frontal lesion appears to be required for lasting non-fluency.

Aphemia

In contrast to Broca's original use of the term 'aphemie' to describe the articulatory disorder of his two 1861 cases of Broca's aphasia, 'aphemia' is now used to designate a more restricted syndrome of non-fluent speech, with normal comprehension and writing (Schiff *et al.* 1983). Patients with aphemia are often mute initially, with hesitant speech emerging over the next few days, often with prominent phonemic errors.

Patients with aphemia often have right facial weakness but no major motor deficits, and their comprehension, reading, and writing are largely normal. The lesions may involve the face area of the motor cortex (Alexander *et al.* 1990). Alexander and colleagues (1989a) suggested that the deficits in aphemia are not distinguishable from those of isolated apraxia of speech. Both aphemia and isolated apraxia of speech are rare syndromes, often associated with nearly complete recovery over a few weeks. In strict terms, aphemia is not a true language disorder, but a motor speech disorder.

Wernicke's Aphasia

The second major aphasia syndrome, Wernicke's aphasia, appeared on the scene in 1874, in a monograph by the German physician Karl Wernicke. Wernicke's aphasia can in many ways be thought of as the opposite of Broca's aphasia. Whereas the speech of a Broca's aphasic is non-fluent and effortful, the patient with Wernicke's aphasia speaks effortlessly, often with a normal or even increased number of words per unit time ('logorrhea'). The content of the speech, however, is empty, containing stock phrases but few meaningful nouns and verbs. There are many paraphasic errors of both literal (phonemic) and verbal (semantic) type. If the speech is so filled with non-words that the meaning cannot be discerned, we speak of 'jargon aphasia'. In milder cases, sentences may begin appropriately, but the word order then goes awry and the meaning becomes lost.

A listener not familiar with the native language of a Wernicke's aphasic might not notice anything wrong, as the patient speaks fluently and effortlessly, in a pattern that sounds like the speaker's native language. A native listener, however, hears few meaningful phrases and many speech errors. Whereas Broca's aphasics comprehend semantic material fairly well, Wernicke's aphasics may comprehend almost nothing said to them. Patients sometimes seem to understand family members, but extralinguistic cues such as facial expressions and gestures facilitate communication. An unbiased examiner, testing comprehension by non-repetitive commands or by yes/no questions, finds deficits easily. Sometimes a nonsense question such as 'Do you vomit every day?' rapidly establishes that comprehension is lacking.

The features of Wernicke's aphasia are listed in Table 5.4. Naming is often bizarre and paraphasic, with utterances not resembling the target word and often not words at all. Repetition is usually impaired, with paraphasic substitutions. If the patient has difficulty understanding the request to repeat, whispering a phrase in the patient's ear, as in a hearing test, may provoke an attempt at repetition. Reading comprehension is often severely impaired, resembling auditory comprehension, but occasional patients may comprehend better auditorily than visually, or *vice versa* (Kirshner *et al.* 1989). These differences may be functionally important, as the use of a spared modality may greatly facilitate comprehension. Sign language, a visual modality, may have a place in communication therapy of patients with spared reading (Heilman *et al.* 1979; Kirshner and Webb 1981). Cases of Wernicke's aphasia with intact reading resemble the classical syndrome of pure word deafness (see below), whereas those with relatively spared auditory comprehension resemble the deficit of pure alexia with agraphia (see Chapter 6). Writing in Wernicke's aphasia is different from that of Broca's aphasia, in that the patient usually has no weakness or paralysis and can write well-formed letters easily. Written productions, however, are filled with empty phrases and erroneous words, like the speech of these patients. In addition, writing allows the analysis of spelling, which is usually full of errors. Abnormal

Table 5.4 Characteristics of Wernicke's aphasia

Feature	Characteristic
Spontaneous speech	Fluent, with paraphasic errors of both phonemic and verbal type
Naming	Impaired, often paraphasic
Auditory comprehension	Impaired, often for even simple questions
Repetition	Impaired
Reading	Usually impaired, with exceptions
Writing	Well-formed but paragraphic
Associated signs	±R hemianopia, usually no motor or sensory abnormalities
Behavior	Often unaware of deficits, may be inappropriately happy, later sometimes angry, suspicious

spelling can be a tip-off to the disorder in mild cases (see the classical 1972 paper by MacDonald Critchley, *The Detection of Minimal Dysphasia*, in Critchley 1979). As in the case of reading, a few atypical cases have been described in which writing is superior to verbal expression (Lhermitte and Derouesné 1974, Hier and Mohr 1977).

The associated deficits of Wernicke's aphasia are often minimal. Patients may have right visual field deficits, but these are inconsistent. Usually there is no significant paralysis or sensory loss. Patients with Wernicke's aphasia may be mistaken for psychotic or confused persons. Indeed, some Wernicke's aphasics seem confused at presentation. They often seem unaware of their deficits, and they do not appear depressed initially. Later, they may become angry at not being understood, and cases of agitation and even paranoid ideation and behavior have been reported in Wernicke's aphasia. Patients who recover from Wernicke's aphasia rarely recall having difficulty with comprehension. One patient with a vascular malformation of the left temporal lobe recalled brief episodes, likely seizures, during which she could not understand the speech of others; she recalled that it sounded like a foreign language. Lazar and colleagues (2000) recently reported a patient with an arteriovenous malformation who became aphasic during selective amobarbital injections into the inferior division of the left middle cerebral artery. This patient recalled the episodes well, and he appeared to understand questions better than the examiners had thought: 'In general, my mind seemed to work except that words could not be found or had turned into other words. I also perceived throughout this procedure what a terrible disorder that would be if it were not reversible due to local anesthetics'.

The lesions of Wernicke's aphasia classically involve the left superior temporal gyrus. Modern studies utilizing CT and MRI scans have largely confirmed this localization, though some authors include the inferior parietal lobule (supramarginal and angular gyri, Brodmann areas 39 and 40) as part of Wernicke's area. Kirshner and colleagues (1989) found differences in the deficit profile of Wernicke's aphasia, depending on whether the lesion was predominantly temporal or predominantly parietal. The temporal lesions were associated with more severe impairment of auditory comprehension than of reading, whereas the parietal lesions disturbed reading more than auditory comprehension. Figure 5.5 shows a CT scan from a patient with a left temporal lesion and Wernicke's aphasia but intact reading comprehension. Figure 5.6 shows a patient with a left parietal lesion and superior reading to auditory comprehension. MRI and PET studies of a patient with Wernicke's aphasia are shown in Figure 5.7. As Bogen and Bogen (1976) have pointed out, the appropriate question to ask of Wernicke's area is 'Where is it?', whereas the appropriate question to ask of Broca's area is 'What good is it?', since destruction of Broca's area appears to cause only temporary loss of the faculty of speech. Electrical stimulation studies have confirmed that activation of the posterior left superior temporal gyrus by surface electrodes interferes temporarily with language comprehension (Lesser *et al.* 1986; Boatman *et al.* 2000). Patients reported hearing sounds, but were unable to comprehend them.

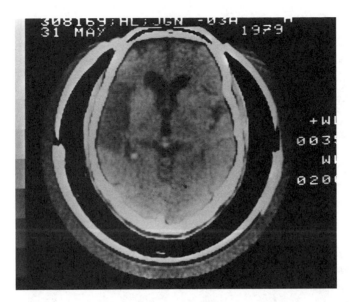

Figure 5.5 CT scan from a patient with Wernicke's aphasia but spared reading ability. Note that the lesion, though very large, is predominantly temporal.

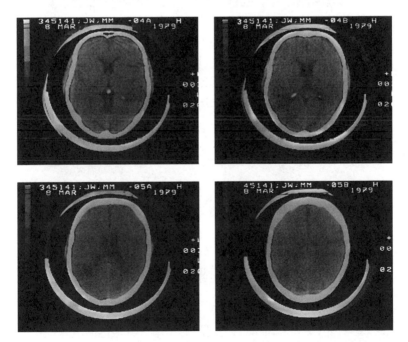

Figure 5.6 CT scan from another patient with Wernicke's aphasia. This elderly man suffered an acute confusional state with cortical blindness after cerebral angiography. After the confusion cleared, he was left with a mild, fluent aphasia and severe loss of comprehension, worse for reading than for auditory language.

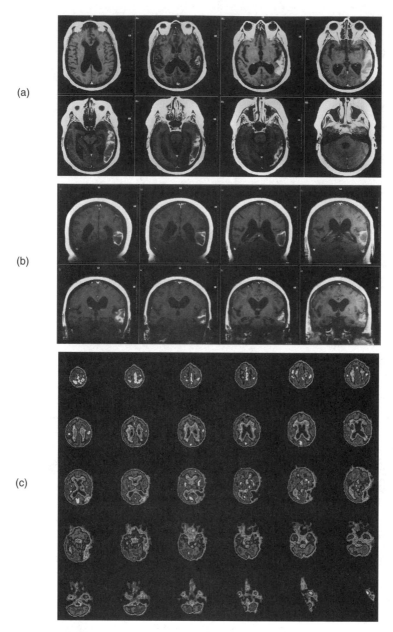

Figure 5.7 Axial and coronal magnetic resonance imaging slices (a and b), and PET scan images (c) of an elderly woman with Wernicke's aphasia. Note the large left superior temporal lobe lesion. The onset of the deficit was not clear, and the PET scan was useful in determining that the lesion had reduced glucose metabolism. This finding confirmed that the lesion was a stroke, rather than a brain tumor. (Reprinted with permission from WG Bradley, RB Daroff, GM Fenichel, CD Marsden (eds). Neurology in Clinical Practice, Vol. I (3rd edn). Boston: Butterworth-Heinemann, 2000.)

In Naeser and colleagues' studies (1987), lasting loss of single word comprehension is closely correlated with destruction of Wernicke's area. In the studies of Selnes *et al.* (1984) and Kertesz *et al.* (1993), on the other hand, lasting Wernicke's aphasia is usually associated with lesions much larger than just Wernicke's area, involving additional areas of the left temporal and parietal lobes. Lesions not totally destroying Wernicke's area might be compatible with recovery towards deficit profiles of conduction or anomic aphasia (see below), as comprehension improves.

Pure Word Deafness

Pure word deafness is a selective deafness for auditory language. It may be thought of as a more restrictive version of Wernicke's aphasia in which speech, writing, naming, and reading are normal, but there is an isolated auditory deficit affecting comprehension and repetition. The patient is deaf only to words; normal pure-tone hearing is a prerequisite for the diagnosis. The word-deaf patient can hear and interpret meaningful non-verbal sounds, such as the characteristic ring of a bell or telephone or the customary cries of animals. Most reported patients with pure word deafness have had some associated aphasic deficits, especially paraphasic speech and naming (Goldstein 1974).

Most patients with pure word deafness have no other neurological abnormalities, in terms of motor, sensory, or visual deficits. Neuroanatomically, pure word deafness has been classically explained as a disconnection of the intact Wernicke's area from both auditory cortices, located in 'Heschl's gyrus', a portion of the superior temporal gyrus on the superior surface of each temporal lobe, within the sylvian fissure (Geschwind 1964; Coslett *et al.* 1984). Cases of pure word deafness have been reported with bilateral temporal lobe pathology such as Herpes simplex encephalitis and bilateral strokes. Destructive lesions of both temporal lobes, involving the Heschl's gyrus bilaterally, cause the syndrome of 'cortical deafness', comprising loss of both word comprehension and also identification of other meaningful sounds, though patients with bilateral cortical lesions are not totally deaf. In some cases, initial cortical deafness has given way to more selective syndromes affecting language more than non-verbal auditory sounds (Kanshepolsky *et al.* 1973; Kirshner and Webb 1981; Mendez and Geehan 1988), or involving temporal sequencing of stimuli (Tanaka *et al.* 1987).

Geschwind (1970) pointed out that a unilateral left temporal lesion could cut off the left temporal Wernicke's area from input from both primary auditory cortices. Other more recent such cases have been reported (Takahashi *et al.* 1992). This would explain the clear overlap with Wernicke's aphasia, related to unilateral lesions of the left temporal lobe. As stated earlier, some patients with Wernicke's aphasia may have superior reading to auditory comprehension (Kirshner *et al.* 1989). Wernicke himself mentioned that some highly educated persons might be able to read without need for the auditory language centers. It is thus possible that some patients may retain reading ability to some extent even with destruction of much of Wernicke's area.

Global Aphasia

The third major aphasia syndrome, global aphasia, can be thought of as the sum of Broca's plus Wernicke's aphasia. The aphasia profile is quite simply the loss of all of the elementary language functions (Table 5.5); the patient speaks like a Broca's aphasic but comprehends like a Wernicke's aphasic – the worst of both worlds. Some patients speak only a verbal stereotyped phrase or 'stereotypy', such as 'wawawa'. The syndrome is also called 'total aphasia' or 'mixed aphasia' if not all of the deficits are severe.

Most global aphasics have severe associated deficits of right hemianopia, right hemiparesis, and right hemisensory loss, though there are exceptions. The syndrome of global aphasia without hemiparesis has been reported several times, with lesions that generally involve both Broca's and Wernicke's areas, but spare the motor and sensory cortices (Legatt *et al.* 1987; Tranel *et al.* 1987). In general, patients with global aphasia have extensive damage involving the left frontal, temporal, and parietal lobes. The most common causes would be strokes caused by embolism to the middle cerebral artery or occlusion of the internal carotid artery. The syndrome also results from large tumors, hemorrhages in the left basal ganglia and subcortical white matter, and other lesions. The patient with global aphasia often appears depressed and withdrawn, a phenomenon described by Kurt Goldstein (1948) as the 'catastrophic reaction' and by C. Miller Fisher (personal communication) as the 'ignoring aphasic'.

Global aphasia often improves over time, with the deficit evolving into another aphasia category. The evolution from global to Broca's aphasia is the most common path for these patients, as comprehension gradually improves over weeks and months (Mohr *et al.* 1978). In the study of Naeser and colleagues (1990), sparing of the cortical Wernicke's area in the superior temporal lobe was associated with recovery of comprehension. Occasional patients evolve towards Wernicke's or even anomic aphasia.

Table 5.5 Characteristics of global aphasia

Feature	Characteristic
Spontaneous speech	Non-fluent, mute, or restricted to a stereotyped phrase
Naming	Impaired
Auditory comprehension	Impaired
Repetition	Impaired
Reading	Impaired
Writing	Impaired
Associated deficits	Most have right hemianopia, right hemiparesis, right hemisensory loss, often apraxia
Behavior	Often depressed

Conduction Aphasia

Conduction aphasia is a much less common syndrome than Broca's, Wernicke's, or global aphasia, comprising about 10% of aphasia cases. It is important, however, both because of the striking nature of the deficits, and for its implications regarding theories of language function. Conduction aphasia can be thought of primarily as a disorder of repetition, as this function is impaired out of proportion to other language deficits. The patient with conduction aphasia may not be able to repeat even single words or phrases, despite the ability to explain these failures in well-constructed sentences. One patient could not repeat the word 'boy', but spontaneously said, 'I like girls better'. Asked to repeat 'hospital', he said, 'Hother... my hotheral... you know, this damned place where we are'. Speech in conduction aphasia is typically fluent, though many patients make frequent literal paraphasic errors. Some attempt to correct themselves, giving the speech pattern a choppy, hesitant quality, but still more fluent than seen in Broca's or global aphasia. Occasionally, speech output is more severely paraphasic. Naming varies from normal to very paraphasic. Auditory comprehension must be intact for conduction aphasia to be diagnosed, a key point in distinguishing conduction aphasia from Wernicke's aphasia. Reading for meaning is generally good, but reading aloud may produce errors resembling the repetition errors. Writing is usually preserved. These features are summarized in Table 5.6.

Associated deficits in conduction aphasia are more variable than in the other aphasia syndromes. Many patients have combinations of right-sided motor and sensory deficits, usually not severe, and many have apraxia.

The lesions of conduction aphasia may involve the superior temporal lobe, but without severe damage to Wernicke's area, or may involve the inferior parietal region (Figures 5.8, 5.9). As originally postulated by Wernicke, the lesions leave Broca's and Wernicke's areas intact but disrupt the connections between them. Geschwind later revived this hypothesis as one of the principal examples of a 'disconnection syndrome', in which a behavioral syndrome results not from damage to a cortical area, but from disconnection between two areas. The

Table 5.6 Characteristics of conduction aphasia

Feature	Characteristic
Spontaneous speech	Fluent, with literal paraphasic errors
Naming	Variably intact
Auditory comprehension	Intact
Repetition	Poor
Reading	Variable aloud, comprehension intact
Writing	Variably intact
Associated deficits	Right hemiparesis, right hemisensory loss, visual field defect, apraxia all variable
Behavior	No characteristic picture

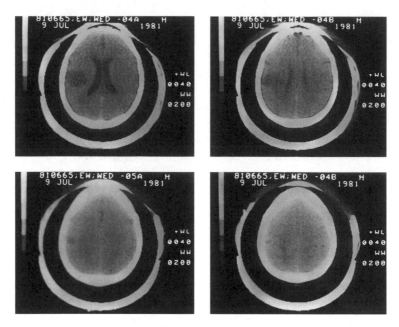

Figure 5.8 CT scan from a patient with conduction aphasia. The lesion predominantly involves the left inferior parietal cortex.

disconnection theory of conduction aphasia is shown diagrammatically in Figure 5.10, which has the arcuate fasciculus drawn schematically. This theory is useful as a convenient way of remembering the syndrome, but it is likely an oversimplification. Most cases of conduction aphasia involve cortical areas, and the syndrome should be understood in the light of current models of brain function, which consider networks and systems rather than isolated cortical centers. Jason Brown (1975) pointed out that conduction aphasia is almost never seen with white matter lesions disrupting the arcuate fasciculus, nor is it common in white matter diseases such as multiple sclerosis. Deep brain hemorrhages, which may also disrupt the arcuate fasciculus, again do not typically cause conduction aphasia (Hier *et al.* 1977). According to Benson and colleagues (1973) and Damasio and Damasio (1980), patients with conduction aphasia and parietal lesions have associated ideomotor apraxia, whereas those with temporal lesions do not. Levine and Calvanio (1982) postulated that damage to the inferior parietal cortex, rather than anatomic disconnection of the temporal and frontal cortices, might be the cause of some of the linguistic features of conduction aphasia. Recent literature concerning the inferior parietal lobule and especially the supramarginal gyrus indicates that damage to this area results in incorrect elicitation of phonemes and 'literal paraphasic errors' (Demonet *et al.* 1992; Kirshner *et al.* 1999). This is often a prominent problem in conduction aphasia, and it is another

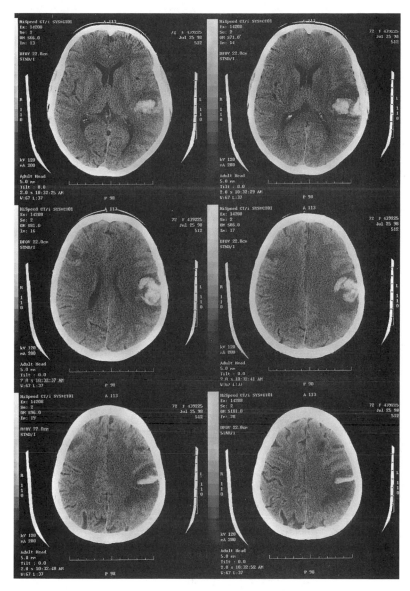

Figure 5.9 CT scan from a patient with conduction aphasia. This patient presented with aphasia and moderate right hemiparesis; she was given intravenous tissue plasminogen activator (tPA) and suffered a hemorrhage into the left inferior parietal lobe. Her aphasia, on examination 2 weeks later, was fluent and paraphasic, with poor naming and virtually no ability to repeat, but relatively preserved comprehension.

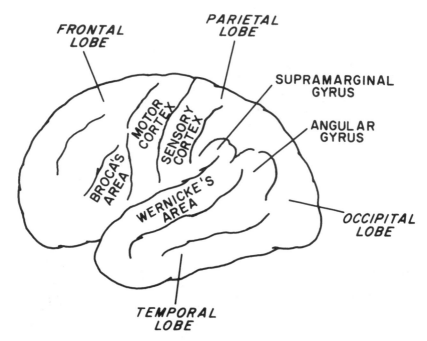

Figure 5.10 Diagram of the lateral view of the left hemisphere, outlining the path of the arcuate fasciculus, a white matter bundle connecting Wernicke's and Broca's areas. The disconnection theory of conduction aphasia, proposed first by Wernicke but later popularized by Geschwind, holds that a lesion interrupting the arcuate fasciculus is the anatomical cause of conduction aphasia.

piece of evidence that conduction aphasia is a cortical aphasia, and not just a disconnection of white matter fiber systems.

Other cognitive scientists have explained conduction aphasia as a loss of auditory–verbal immediate memory (Strubb 1974; Tzortzis and Albert 1974; Heilman *et al.* 1976b; Shallice and Warrington 1977). If a subject cannot keep a string of words in the immediate attention span for long enough to activate the articulatory system, a deficit pattern like conduction aphasia would result. In this regard, it is interesting that delayed feedback of the words to be repeated helps patients with conduction aphasia repeat better, while it seems to confuse normal subjects (Boller and Marcie 1978; Chapin *et al.* 1981). Finally, conduction aphasia has been conceptualized as a loss of 'inner speech' (Feinberg *et al.* 1986). These competing theories of conduction aphasia are difficult to separate, in terms of the key behavioral features of conduction aphasia.

Anomic Aphasia

Anomic aphasia, as the name implies, is a syndrome in which naming difficulty is the primary abnormality. The syndrome is also called 'amnestic aphasia',

Table 5.7 Characteristics of anomic aphasia

Feature	Characteristic
Spontaneous speech	Fluent, with word-finding pauses and circumlocutions
Naming	Impaired
Auditory comprehension	Intact
Repetition	Intact
Reading	Intact
Writing	Intact except for word-finding difficulty
Associated signs	Variable, often absent
Behavior	No characteristic features

meaning that there is a loss of memory for words and names (Benson, 1979). Spontaneous speech in anomic aphasia is fluent, with spontaneous word-searching pauses and circumlocutions. Naming is impaired out of proportion to all other language functions. Auditory comprehension, repetition, reading, and writing are all relatively preserved (Table 5.7). Note that this is the first syndrome we have discussed that is associated with normal repetition; Broca's, Wernicke's, global, and conduction aphasia all have defective repetition. Associated deficits are extremely variable; in many cases, no other obvious neurological deficits are present.

Naming, or elicitation of words, is the most fundamental language function, and as such it is deranged in virtually all of the aphasic syndromes (Henderson 1995). Even normal people, and especially elderly people, have occasional word-finding difficulty. Almost all aphasic patients have some degree of anomia, and in many recovering aphasics the mildest stage is a form of anomic aphasia.

Benson and Ardila (1996) divide anomia into four separate types: word production anomia, word selection anomia, semantic anomia, and disconnection anomia. Word production anomia is a difficulty with elicitation of words, seen particularly with left frontal lesions involving Broca's area, the prefrontal region, or the supplementary motor area. Patients with word production anomia recognize the correct word and benefit from cues of the first phoneme of the word. Patients with prefrontal damage may produce words very slowly, and they do particularly poorly on serial naming tasks such as the 'animal naming' subtest of the BDAE, in which the subject has to produce as many animal names as possible in 1 minute. Patients with prefrontal lesions also have perseverations on naming tasks. Patients with supplementary motor cortex lesions or lesions disconnecting the SMA and Broca's area have difficulty initiating articulation. In Broca's aphasia, and also conduction aphasia, phonemic errors occur, whereas in Wernicke's aphasia both phonemic and semantic errors are common.

Patients with word selection anomia cannot produce the word or benefit from cues, but they can always point to the object if given the name. This deficit may correlate with temporal lesions, usually not involving Wernicke's area, and more related to the memory system (see Chapter 11). The problem arises at the level of selecting a phonemic representation for a word meaning.

Patients with semantic anomia fail to produce the name or benefit from cues, and they cannot point to the object when given the name; they have simply lost the meaning of the word. This third type of anomia may arise from the angular gyrus region. Semantic anomia has also been described in dementias (Semantic dementia, see Chapter 13).

Disconnection anomia refers to anomia for selective classes of items, in which a disconnection prevents semantic information from reaching the left hemisphere 'naming center', by which we mean the posterior temporal and angular gyrus areas. Examples include category specific anomias, such as the color anomia associated with alexia without agraphia (see Chapter 6), or modality-specific anomias such as 'optic aphasia' in which specifically visual information does not reach the naming center. For example, an optic aphasic will not be able to name an object by sight, but will do so by touch or sound. This sort of deficit will be discussed in Chapter 8, with the agnosias. Finally, lesions of the corpus callosum prevent information from crossing from one hemisphere to the other. A patient with callosotomy surgery, for example, may be unable to name an object palpated with the left hand or shown visually by a tachistiscope into the left visual field, because the right hemisphere cannot transfer the information to the left hemisphere language centers for naming. Callosal syndromes are discussed in Chapter 12.

The lesions of anomic aphasia correspond to these separate types of anomia, and are extremely variable. The sparing of repetition suggests that the perisylvian language circuit, from Heschl's gyri to Wernicke's area to Broca's area, is all functioning well. The lesions, therefore, should be outside this circuit. Geschwind (1970) associated anomic aphasia with lesions of the left angular gyrus, in line with Benson and Ardila's (1996) localization of semantic anomia. Lesions of the angular gyrus produce a series of neurobehavioral deficits, including alexia, agraphia, acalculia, right–left confusion, 'finger agnosia' or loss of body image for fingers, and even constructional apraxia, all of which make the lesion localization rather obvious. The classic Gerstmann syndrome, thought to be localizing for a left parietal lesion, comprises four of these deficits: agraphia, right–left confusion, acalculia, and finger agnosia. Tumors of the deep left temporal white matter may produce isolated anomia. Anomic aphasia may also be the last stage in recovery in a variety of aphasic syndromes, including conduction, Wernicke's, and even Broca's aphasia. Anomia can be a sign of a subdural hematoma, it can be the principal language deficit at early stages of Alzheimer's (Appell et al. 1982; Kirshner et al. 1987) and Pick's diseases, and it also occurs in acute confusional states. Anomia is thus the least localizing of the aphasic syndromes. The more pure the deficit of anomia, however, the more likely it is to be associated with structural pathology of the left hemisphere. Some literature suggests that anomia for verbs is more associated with left frontal lesions, whereas anomia for nouns is more associated with lesions of the left temporal lobe (Damasio 1992). Common nouns and proper nouns may even have separate localizations, and either one may be disturbed selectively in some syndromes of anomia.

Transcortical Aphasias

Lichtheim used the term 'transcortical aphasias' to designate the anatomic sparing of the perisylvian language circuit; instead, the damage resided in the adjacent cortex, which Lichtheim called the 'area of concepts' (Lichtheim 1885). The term was also used by Goldstein in 1917. The practical consequence of the sparing of the perisylvian language cortex is the preservation of repetition, which these patients can perform normally, or even excessively, as in echolalia. While modern neuroanatomists do not speak of an area of concepts, the principle remains that damage to the association cortex outside the perisylvian language cortex underlies the transcortical aphasia syndromes. Characteristics of the three transcortical aphasia syndromes are presented in Table 5.8.

Transcortical Motor Aphasia

Transcortical motor aphasia (TCMA) is a Broca-like aphasia with preserved repetition (Rubens 1976). The patient speaks little, often responding after a long delay, or in a whisper, or with just a word or two to answer a question. In contrast to the paucity of spontaneous speech, the patient can repeat long sentences fluently. Naming performance may vary, but auditory comprehension and reading are usually preserved. Writing may share some of the same hesitancy as speaking. Most patients have at least a partial right hemiparesis. The Russian neuropsychiatrist Luria called the same aphasia syndrome 'dynamic aphasia', referring to the lack of initiation of speech (Luria and Tsvetkova 1968).

TCMA represents a frontal lobe syndrome affecting language. Frontal lobe disorders generally involve a lack of movement or a difficulty with the initiation of movement; in this case, a localized left frontal lesion causes the patient to have reduced initiation of speech. Lesions causing transcortical motor aphasia virtually always involve the left frontal lobe, often within the territory of the anterior cerebral artery. The site of damage may be anterior to Broca's area, deep in the subcortical frontal white matter, or on the medial surface of the

Table 5.8 Characteristics of transcortical aphasias

Feature	Transcortical motor aphasia	Transcortical sensory aphasia	Mixed transcortical aphasia
Speech	Non-fluent	Fluent	Non-fluent
Naming	Impaired	Impaired	Impaired
Repetition	Preserved	Echolalic	Echolalic
Comprehension	Preserved	Impaired	Impaired
Reading	Preserved	Impaired	Impaired
Writing	Reduced	Paragraphic	Poor
Associated signs	Right leg > arm weakness, abulia	Variable, often none	Right or bilateral hemiparesis

frontal lobe, in the vicinity of the supplementary motor area (Alexander and Schmitt 1980; Masdeu *et al.* 1982; Freedman *et al.* 1984). In the anterior cerebral artery stroke syndrome, the right hemiparesis differs from that associated with middle cerebral artery strokes in that the leg is affected more than the arm, and the shoulder is affected more than the hand (middle cerebral artery strokes tend to affect the hand most). Some patients demonstrate an involuntary grasp response in the affected hand. Since TCMA involves a separate vascular territory and a separate lobar anatomy from the aphasia syndromes of the middle cerebral artery, it tends to be relatively pure, with little overlap with other aphasia syndromes.

Albert and colleagues (1988) analogized TCMA to the motor akinesia of Parkinson's disease, and tried the dopaminergic drug, bromocriptine. While this approach to the pharmacotherapy of aphasia has remained of doubtful benefit, it has opened a new field of language rehabilitation (see Chapter 21).

Transcortical Sensory Aphasia

The syndrome of transcortical sensory aphasia (TCSA) resembles Wernicke's aphasia, except that repetition is spared. Speech is fluent and paraphasic, naming is also paraphasic, and auditory and reading comprehension are severely impaired. Associated signs may be absent. TCSA is uncommon as a stroke syndrome, though a few cases have been reported with lesions near the temporo-occipital junction, classically sparing Wernicke's area itself (Kertesz *et al.* 1982). Boatman and colleagues (2000), in studies of electrical stimulation of the superior temporal region, found areas in each subject that would produce Wernicke's aphasia (fluent speech, poor comprehension, and poor repetition), and areas in which stimulation produced the deficit profile of transcortical sensory aphasia (fluent speech, poor comprehension, intact repetition). At a few sites, the deficit profile of TCSA involved intact naming. TCSA with spared naming has also rarely been reported in stroke cases (Heilman *et al.* 1981). The authors proposed a dissociation between phonology and semantics. The syndrome has also been described as a stage in the language deterioration of Alzheimer's disease (Appell *et al.* 1982).

Mixed Transcortical Aphasia (Isolation of the Speech Area)

The syndrome of mixed transcortical aphasia (mixed TCA) can be thought of as the transcortical analog of global aphasia. Patients are nearly mute, cannot name, cannot follow commands or comprehend yes/no questions, and cannot read or write. The only language function they can perform is repetition, and they often repeat excessively, or echolalically.

One of the best-described cases of this syndrome was a 13-year-old girl, described by Geschwind *et al.* (1968), who suffered carbon monoxide poisoning, with large infarctions in the watershed distribution of both hemispheres. The patient repeated echolalically and sang songs. She completed familiar phrases begun by the examiner, and she could even learn the lyrics of new songs that had not been on the radio before her illness. By contrast, she could not speak propositionally or respond to questions or commands. In Lichtheim's model, this patient had no 'area of concepts' at all, just a circuit from temporal lobe to frontal lobe that could subserve repetition, and also connections to the limbic system for memory storage. The authors therefore termed the syndrome the 'syndrome of the isolation of the speech area'. Patients with less severe impairment of language modalities are better classified as 'mixed transcortical aphasia' (Heilman *et al.* 1976b; Ross 1980; Grossi *et al.* 1991). Mixed TCA can be thought of as the sum of the deficits of transcortical motor and sensory aphasia, just as global aphasia can be thought of as the sum of Broca's and Wernicke's aphasia. This syndrome, like TCSA, has been described as a late stage in the language deterioration of Alzheimer's disease (Whitaker 1976).

Summary of the Eight Cortical Aphasia Syndromes

The eight traditional cortical aphasia syndromes (Broca's, Wernicke's, conduction, global, anomic, and the three transcortical aphasias) can be classified based on three decision points: fluent versus non-fluent, repetition preserved or impaired, and comprehension preserved or impaired. For example, there are four non-fluent aphasias (Broca's, global, transcortical motor, and mixed transcortical aphasias), and four fluent aphasias (Wernicke's, conduction, anomic, and transcortical sensory aphasias). We can then separate the four non-fluent aphasias by two with impaired repetition (Broca's and global), and two with preserved repetition (TCMA and MTCA). We can distinguish these in turn by preserved or impaired comprehension. Figure 5.11 is a flow chart for the classification of the cortical aphasias.

The neuroanatomy of the classical aphasia syndromes, as summarized in the preceding sections, has generally been confirmed by brain imaging studies. Kreisler and colleagues (2000), in a study of 107 aphasic stroke patients from Lille, France, reported strikingly classical aphasia localizations: nonfluent aphasia was associated with frontal or putaminal lesions, whereas comprehension deficits correlated with posterior temporal lesions. Analysis of lesion site predicted a correct aphasia classification in over 2/3 of the patients. Other authors (Willmes and Poeck 1993) have reported much less accurate correlation between lesion location and aphasia syndrome, and others (Basso *et al.* 1985b) have pointed to 'exceptions' or anomalous cases. Every expert in aphasia has seen patients in whom the lesion localization is unexpected or surprising. The neuroscientific reasons for the variability in language organization in the brain are incompletely understood and should be the subject of future research (Kirshner 2000). Recent studies have suggested that patients with aphasia in the acute phase of a stroke, before any compensation or reorganization can occur, may have more predictable areas of brain dysfunction (see Chapter 21).

This eight-part classification is an oversimplification, since it does not account for intermediate cases, such as semifluent expression or mildly impaired comprehension. Some aphasia cases appear atypical for any of the classical syndromes. This classification system, however, remains the best starting point in the

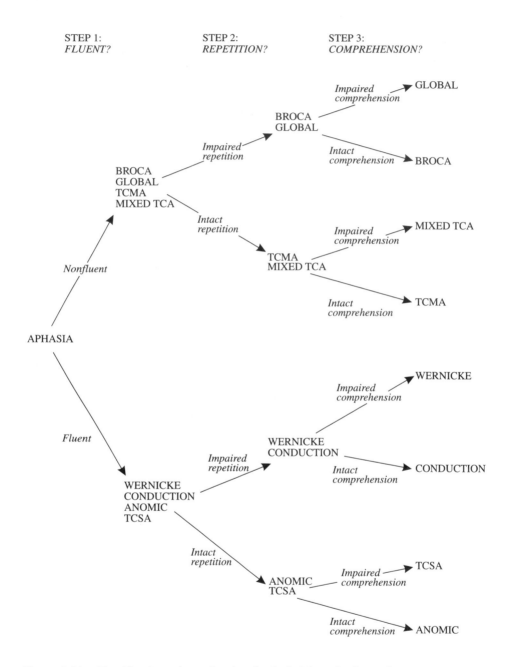

Figure 5.11 Classification scheme for the classical eight aphasia syndromes.

diagnosis of aphasia. The eight syndromes correlate not only with easily observed language behavior, but also with well-established localizations of brain pathology, of importance to the neurologist.

Subcortical Aphasias

Classically, aphasia has been assumed to represent damage to the left hemisphere language cortex. In recent years, many cases of aphasia from subcortical lesions have been reported, and a new category of 'subcortical aphasia' has been added to the aphasia classification. It should not be surprising that subcortical sites that project up or down from portions of the language cortex might themselves produce aphasic symptomatology when damaged. As the name implies, subcortical aphasias are defined more by the anatomy of the brain lesion than by specific language characteristics. Several patterns of language disorder have been defined in patients with subcortical lesions.

Thalamic Aphasia

The first type of subcortical aphasia is 'thalamic aphasia', first described in patients with thalamic hemorrhage (Fisher 1959; Mohr *et al.* 1975; Reynolds *et al.* 1979). The aphasia pattern usually associated with thalamic damage is fluent, often with paraphasic errors, but with better comprehension and repetition than Wernicke's aphasia. As with most subcortical aphasias, the syndrome does not match any of the classical cortical aphasia syndromes. Mohr and colleagues (1975) described a 'dichotomous' state in which patients fluctuate between a coherent speech pattern while alert and an unintelligible, paraphasic mumble when somnolent. Luria (1977) called thalamic aphasia a 'quasiaphasic disturbance of vigilance', meaning that the thalamus plays a role in keeping the language cortex awake. In fact, the posterior thalamus has extensive projections to Wernicke's area, and the anterior and paramedian thalamic nuclei connect to structures involved in memory and attention (Crosson 1984).

More precise anatomic localization in thalamic aphasia has come from cases of ischemic infarction of the thalamus, since ischemic strokes have less swelling and mass effect than hemorrhages, and therefore the structure–function correlation is more accurate. Bogousslavsky and colleagues (1988) divided their 40 cases of thalamic infarction into four separate vascular territories. Aphasia correlated best with infarctions within the territory of the tuberothalamic artery, which supplies the anterior thalamus, including the ventral anterior and part of the ventral lateral nuclei. Common features were hypophonia, verbal paraphasias, impaired comprehension, and intact repetition. Similar aphasic deficits were seen in patients with paramedian thalamic infarcts, within the territory of the thalamoperforating artery, though most patients had an initially depressed level of consciousness. The other two thalamic syndromes – posterior choroidal artery infarcts with infarction of the lateral geniculate body, and ventroposterolateral infarcts in the territory of the inferolateral arteries – had hemianopia and hemisensory loss, respectively, without language disturbance. Graff-Radford and colleagues (1984, 1985) also described fluent aphasia, anomia, perseveration, reduced comprehension, preserved reading, and intact repetition in cases of thalamic infarction. Deficits in short-term memory and attention have also been reported in cases of paramedian thalamic infarction (Fensore *et al.* 1988; Stuss *et al.* 1988).

Thalamic aphasia has also been reported in association with surgical thalamotomy (Bell 1968; Samra *et al.* 1969), thalamic tumors (Smythe and Stern 1938), arteriovenous malformation of the thalamus (Luria 1977), and thalamic abscess (Megens *et al.* 1992). Electrical stimulation of the thalamus can disrupt naming and memory (Ojemann *et al.* 1968; Ojemann 1975). Thalamic aphasia also has implications for cerebral dominance. Hemorrhages in the right thalamus have produced aphasia in left-handed patients, indicating that language dominance in one hemisphere extends down to the level of the thalamus (Kirshner and Kistler 1982; Chesson 1983). Figure 5.12 shows a CT scan from a patient with thalamic aphasia secondary to a right thalamic hemorrhage.

Anterior Subcortical Aphasia Syndromes

Lesions of the caudate nucleus, putamen, and adjacent white matter have also been associated with aphasia. As in thalamic aphasia, the first cases of anterior basal ganglia lesions with aphasia were patients with hemorrhages. The lateral basal ganglia region, including the putamen, globus pallidus, and internal capsule, is the most frequent site of hypertensive intracerebral hemorrhage. Hier

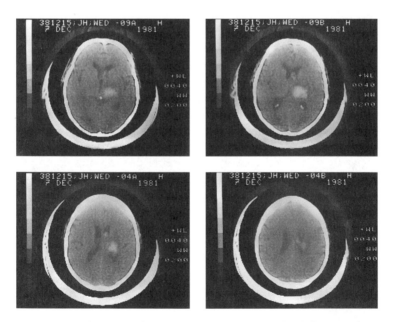

Figure 5.12 CT scan, showing a dense hemorrhage in the right thalamus. The patient was left-handed and had mild, fluent aphasia (Reprinted with permission from HS Kirshner, KH Kistler. Aphasia after right thalamic hemorrhage. Arch Neurol 1982;39:667–669).

and colleagues (1977) and Alexander and LoVerme (1980) reported patients with aphasia secondary to putamenal hemorrhages. These patients were often mute initially, but later fluent, with some paraphasias and relatively preserved comprchension and repetition. The aphasia characteristics in lateral basal ganglia hemorrhage vary with the exact location and size of the bleed, varying from dysarthria and minimal aphasia to severe global aphasia.

As in thalamic aphasia, better definition of the subcortical aphasia syndromes has come with study of patients with basal ganglia infarctions. The most common is the 'anterior subcortical aphasia syndrome' secondary to infarction of the head of the caudate nucleus, anterior limb of internal capsule, and anterior putamen, in the territory of lenticulostriate branches of the middle cerebral artery. Features of this syndrome include dysarthria and decreased fluency, but with longer phrase length than Broca's aphasia, and with associated paraphasias. Comprehension is usually only mildly affected, and repetition is spared (Damasio *et al.* 1982; Naeser *et al.* 1982; Cappa *et al.* 1983; Alexander *et al.* 1987). Many patients have an associated right hemiparesis and impaired attention and short-term memory. Recovery is typically quite good. The neuroanatomy of this syndrome likely involves disruption in the caudate nucleus or anterior limb of fibers projecting to the caudate from the auditory cortex, and from the caudate to the globus pallidus, ventrolateral thalamus, and premotor cortex. Figure 5.13 shows an MRI scan from a patient with the anterior subcortical aphasia syndrome. This patient walked into the outpatient clinic the day after her stroke. She had virtually no hemiparesis, but a non-fluent aphasia with anomia and mild dysarthria.

Subcortical aphasia syndromes are quite complex and probably not completely classified. Reported cases of subcortical aphasia have had a variety of aphasic characteristics. The correlations of aphasia symptomatology with subcortical anatomic structures have been based on small numbers of cases, inconsistent from one series to another. Damasio and colleagues (1982) stated that lesions of the white matter anterior to the caudate and putamen produced a picture similar to transcortical motor aphasia, while lesions of the posterior caudate, posterior limb of internal capsule, and posterior putamen generally produced only dysarthria. Naeser and colleagues (1982) delineated three syndromes: (1) the anterior syndrome described above; (2) a Wernicke-like syndrome with more posterior lesions (see below); and (3) a global aphasia syndrome with lesions involving both sites. Some of the larger infarcts described in Naeser's patients involved the temporal isthmus, a confluence of white matter fibers projecting to Wernicke's area, and therefore associated with comprehension deficit. Fromm and colleagues (1985) stressed the variability in their series of subcortical aphasia cases. Alexander and colleagues (1987) found that lesions restricted to the putamen or head of the caudate nucleus did not produce language disturbance – or at worst mild word-finding difficulty. Lesions involving the more posterior putamen were associated with hypophonia. There was still no language disturbance with involvement of the anterior limb of the internal capsule, except when this involved extensive injury to the caudate, putamen, and anterior limb of internal capsule, in which case the patients had the full anterior subcortical

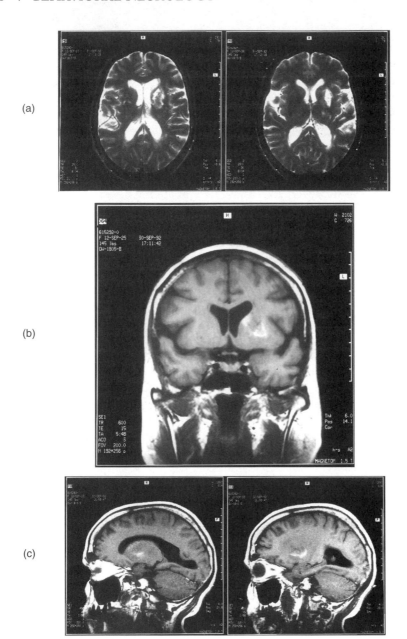

Figure 5.13 MRI scan in the axial (a), coronal (b), and sagittal (c) planes from a patient with the anterior subcortical aphasia syndrome. The lesion is an infarction involving the anterior caudate, putamen, and anterior limb of the left internal capsule. The patient presented with dysarthria and mild, non-fluent aphasia with anomia, with good comprehension. The advantage of MRI in permitting visualization of the lesion in all three planes is apparent. (Reprinted with permission from WG Bradley, RB Daroff, GM Fenichel, CD Marsden (eds). Neurology in Clinical Practice, Vol. I (3rd edn). Boston: Butterworth-Heinemann, 2000.)

aphasia syndrome. Dysarthria was also associated if the damage extended to the white matter of the periventricular region or the genu of the internal capsule. Lesions located more posteriorly, converging on the temporal isthmus, produced fluent aphasia, neologisms, and impaired comprehension. Lesions involving both areas, including the anterior caudate and putamen, internal capsule, periventricular white matter, and temporal isthmus, produced global aphasia. Finally, lesions more laterally placed, involving the insular cortex, extreme capsule, claustrum, and internal capsule, were associated with fluent aphasia, mild word-finding difficulty, and phonemic paraphasias that increased on repetition and reading aloud. This last syndrome is a subcortical version of conduction aphasia. Hence, nearly the full spectrum of cortical aphasia types can be seen with subcortical lesions. These syndromes, however, are uncommon, and for the most part it remains true that aphasia usually signifies cortical pathology.

Other authors have pointed out different features of aphasias secondary to subcortical lesions. Two reports have found disproportionate impairment of writing (Tanridag and Kirshner 1985; Basso *et al.* 1987). Selective lesions of the caudate nucleus have also been reported to produce 'frontal lobe' syndromes involving impaired attention, sequencing, and planning (Mendez *et al.* 1989). The study of subcortical lesions and their correlation with language and other cognitive functions is an area in which the astute clinician, armed only with bedside testing techniques and a CT or MRI scanner, can contribute new information to brain–behavior relationships.

The basis of subcortical aphasia likely involves connections between the basal ganglia and the cortex. Motor speech is likely similar in its organization to the general motor control system, involving a feedback loop from the cerebral cortex to the striatum (putamen and caudate) to the globus pallidus, then via projections to the lateral thalamus, via the anterior limb of internal capsule, back to the cerebral cortex. This loop is familiar to neurologists from discussion of movement disorders and Parkinson's disease. There are clear analogies between extremity movements and the speech. Hesitancy, initiation difficulty, and disturbed motor control can be seen in the dysarthrias and aphasias, just as limb movements and gait are deranged in basal ganglia disorders (Crosson 1985).

Aphasia in Left-Handers

In view of the intense interest in language dominance, surprisingly few studies have investigated language function in left-handed patients with acquired aphasia. A few general statements can be made. More left-handers than right-handers become aphasic after a stroke, regardless of the side of the stroke, suggesting that left-handed patients have some language representation in both cerebral hemispheres. Though aphasia is more common in left-handers, recovery may be better, suggesting that hemisphere dominance may be less rigid in left-handers, and either hemisphere can subserve recovery of language (Goodglass and Quadfasel 1954; Brown and Hecaen 1976). Naeser and Borod (1986) reported a series of 31 left-handed aphasic patients, of whom 27 had left and 4 right hemisphere lesions. Most patients with aphasia and left hemisphere lesions had similar aphasia syndromes to those of a matched group of right-handed aphasics with left hemisphere lesions. Two patients, however, had destruction of the right frontal, temporal, and parietal cortices with non-fluent speech output but preserved comprehension, suggesting a left hemisphere Wernicke's area but a right hemisphere Broca's area. Most left-handers, like right-handers, have left hemisphere dominance for speech and language, but some patients may have separate loci of dominance for handedness, motor speech, and auditory comprehension. Basso and colleagues (1990) also found only minor differences between matched right-handed and non-right-handed patients with aphasia; the one exception was a left-handed patient with conduction aphasia, whose matched right-handed patient with a similar lesion had global aphasia. In this study, recovery also differed little between left- and right-handed aphasic patients.

In summary, patients with aphasia confirm the results of Wada testing that most left-handed patients have relative left hemisphere dominance for language, though they may have a higher percentage of mixed hemispheric dominance for language or pure right hemisphere dominance than right-handed patients.

Crossed Aphasia in Dextrals

Although more than 99% of right-handed patients with aphasia have left hemisphere lesions (Gloning et al. 1969), occasional right-handed patients have been reported with aphasia secondary to right hemisphere lesions. Bramwell first called the phenomenon 'crossed aphasia' in 1899. Some early reports (Brown and Hecaen 1976) found non-fluent aphasia in all crossed aphasics, but later papers have documented a variety of types of aphasia, including Wernicke's aphasia (Henderson 1983; Sweet et al. 1984). As in left-handed people, the majority of crossed aphasia cases resemble those of left hemisphere strokes in the analogous areas. Language functions may be similarly located within a hemisphere, regardless of which hemisphere is dominant for language. Basso and colleagues (1985a) found expected language deficits for similar left hemisphere lesions in their seven crossed aphasics. Alexander and colleagues (1989b) distinguished 'mirror image' syndromes, paralleling left hemisphere lesions, from 'anomalous' cases. In their literature review, 22 of 34 cases had mirror image syndromes, whereas 12 cases had anomalous deficits. A common 'anomalous' aphasia syndrome was the preservation of fluent speech despite large suprasylvian, perirolandic lesions, which would be expected to produce non-fluent aphasia in the left hemisphere. Interestingly, 11 of these 12 cases had greater impairment of written expression than of speech, a finding also present in four of seven cases reported by Basso and colleagues (1985a). Overall, the 'anomalous' cases suggest that dominance for specific language functions may lie in separate hemispheres. For example, the left hemisphere may be necessary for fluent speech production, whereas the right hemisphere might subserve language comprehension. Semantics and syntax may also be localized to different hemispheres in occasional patients (Basso et al. 1985a). In addition to anomalous language, these patients also have other atypical findings. For example, many fail to show the ideomotor apraxia usually associated with aphasia, and many have neglect or visuospatial deficits, usually associated with right hemisphere damage but not with aphasia (Sweet *et al.* 1984; Basso *et al.* 1985a).

New techniques such as Wada testing, SPECT, and PET functional brain imaging are beginning to be applied to crossed aphasia. Wada testing, in which sodium amytal is injected into the left carotid artery, has not worsened the language performance of right-handed 'crossed aphasia' patients (Alexander *et al.* 1989b; Zangwill 1979), confirming the complete lateralization of language to the right hemisphere. Studies with SPECT or PET imaging have confirmed the atypical finding of reduced cerebral blood flow in the right hemisphere (Schweiger *et al.* 1987; Perani *et al.* 1988; Walker-Batson *et al.* 1988; Cappa *et al.* 1993; Gomez-Tortosa *et al.* 1994; Bakar *et al.* 1996), but some studies have found reduced blood flow or metabolism in the left hemisphere as well, not corresponding to structural lesions on CT or MRI scans. These left hemisphere metabolic or blood flow reductions may represent diaschisis, a reduced pattern of cerebral blood flow and metabolism in the opposite hemisphere after a stroke. Diaschisis could be one explanation for crossed aphasia. In one recent case, however, the left hemisphere metabolic activity recovered at a time when the aphasia remained severe (Bakar *et al.* 1996). Figure 5.14 shows a PET scan from a patient with a right hemisphere stroke and 'crossed aphasia'. Crossed aphasia likely results not from diaschisis, but from atypical cerebral dominance for language.

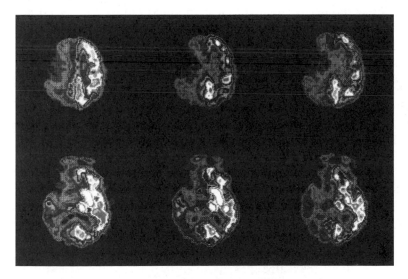

Figure 5.14 PET image from a patient with a right middle cerebral artery territory stroke and 'crossed aphasia'. After recovery, only the right hemisphere showed hypometabolism. (Reprinted with permission from M Bakar, HS Kirshner, RT Wertz. Crossed aphasia. Functional brain imaging with PET or SPECT. Arch Neurol 1996;53:1026–1032.)

Aphasia in Polyglots

The effect of acquired aphasia on different languages has been an area of interest to aphasiologists for generations. Early theories stated that the patient's original native language would fare better after a stroke than a newly acquired language (Ribot's Law, 1906), but a rival theory stated that the language used most before the stroke would recover better (Pitres' Law 1895). Minkowski (1927) followed Pitres in believing that the language in which the subject had the most emotional investment and the most motivation to recover would be better preserved, usually the language in which the patient speaks and works every day, also the language spoken by doctors and speech pathologists. In recent literature, neither theory has held up consistently. Obler and Albert (1977) reviewed 106 cases from the literature and three of their own with polyglot aphasia. They found that Ribot's law applied no more than half of the time, while Pitres' rule appeared to apply more regularly in younger aphasic patients. No rule had consistent predictive value in the recovery of different languages. Studies from Canada, where many people speak both English and French, have shown that subjects who learn both languages simultaneously in childhood (compound bilinguals) have similar patterns of aphasia in both languages, while subjects who learn one language and then the other (coordinate bilinguals) show greater differences between languages (Lambert and Fillenbaum 1959). Similarly, Mastronardi *et al.* (1991) reported a patient who learned English, French, and Italian simultaneously in childhood and showed a similar degree and pattern of aphasia in all three languages, whereas a second patient who grew up speaking Croatian but later learned Italian was more aphasic in Italian than in her native tongue. These authors postulated that compound bilinguals have similar neuroanatomic representations for each language, whereas coordinate bilinguals have different representations.

In a few studies, the aphasia type in bilingual patients was different in one language versus another; for example, a Russian immigrant to Israel developed global aphasia in the newly learned Hebrew language, but only a mild anomic aphasia in Russian (Obler and Albert 1977). Silverberg and Gordon (1979) studied two Israeli aphasics who both learned Hebrew much later than a native language. The first had a moderately severe non-fluent aphasia in Spanish and a milder fluent aphasia in Hebrew. She recovered completely in Hebrew, incompletely in Spanish. The second patient, whose Hebrew was very limited, was globally aphasic in Hebrew, while he had only a mild anomia in Russian.

Recently, PET imaging has been applied to the study of bilingual patients. Perani *et al.* (1998) found that subjects with very high proficiency for two languages showed similar patterns of brain activation in response to language tasks, but those with different levels of proficiency showed differences in activation patterns. These authors concluded that the level of proficiency, and not the time of acquisition, determines the cerebral organization of a second language.

Ojemann and Whitaker (1978) reported that electrical stimulation in two bilingual patients showed differential interference with the two languages; naming in the more newly learned language could be disrupted by stimulation in a larger area than naming in the primary language. A second language in the process of acquisition appears to require more widespread neural systems, and is therefore more susceptible to damage.

SPEECH THERAPY

Speech/language pathologists perform rehabilitative therapy for patients with both motor speech disorders and aphasia. It is helpful for the neurologist to have an understanding of what speech pathologists do, and knowledge of the evidence that it helps patients. This discussion will center on aphasia therapy (Wertz 1995). According to Byng and Black (1995), speech therapy techniques incorporate eight general principles; the therapist attempts to:

1. Delineate the subject's prior use of language
2. Facilitate accommodation to changes in communication
3. Investigate the specific aphasic deficits
4. Remediate the language deficits
5. Increase all possible communication modes
6. Enhance the use of remaining language skills
7. Provide opportunities to use new language skills
8. Modify the communication habits of family members and friends.

These efforts seek to aid the aphasic patient's deficit, the functional disability that results from it, and the handicap it imposes in daily life.

In general, there are three theories of speech therapy: stimulation–facilitation, cognitive neuropsychological and/or psycholinguistic treatment, and functional communication.

Stimulation–Facilitation Therapy

The most traditional and widely used speech therapy technique is stimulation–facilitation. The stimulation–facilitation approach (Schuell *et al.* 1964) targets four areas: auditory comprehension, reading, oral-expressive language, and writing, with emphasis on auditory processing. The treatment tasks employ intensive auditory drills in a stimulus–response format. The tasks begin with simple one-step commands and then become progressively more complex ('treatment hierarchies'). The theoretical premise is that an aphasic patient's use of language can be 'stimulated' or facilitated by repeated practice.

Stimulation–facilitation methods for treating different types of aphasia include visual action therapy (VAT) for treating global aphasia, voluntary control of involuntary utterances (VICU) for improving oral-expressive language, the Helm elicited program for syntax stimulation (HELPSS) for improving syntax, and treatment of Wernicke's aphasia (TWA) for improving auditory comprehension (Helm-Estabrooks and Albert 1991). An example of the stimulation-facilitation approach, employed in a hierarchical method, is melodic intonation therapy (MIT). Repetition of verbal stimuli, using exaggerated rhythm, pitch, and hand gestures, is employed to improve oral-expressive language in Broca's aphasics. The program begins with words and short phrases, then progresses to sentences, with the items first intoned musically, then spoken with exaggerated prosody, and finally spoken normally.

Cognitive Neuropsychological and/or Psycholinguistic Treatment

The cognitive neuropsychological and/or psycholinguistic approach to treatment views aphasia as disruption of specific steps in language processing. The treatment attempts to restore or bypass the impaired module or step in language or cognitive processing. The therapist must design single-case treatment programs to facilite access to intact information when the problem is impaired access, to reorganize processing through intact components, or to help the subject relearn lost information or linguistic rules.

An example of the psycholinguistic approach to treatment is 'mapping therapy', developed by Saffran and colleagues (1993) for treating agrammatic aphasic patients. The focus is on improving sentence comprehension and expression by helping the patient 'map' the relationships between nouns and verbs in both active and passive sentences, and thereby to overcome the problems with syntax that are a major part of Broca's aphasia. These methods can be employed to treat deficits in auditory comprehension, reading, oral-expressive language, and writing.

Functional Communication Treatment

A functional communication approach to aphasia treatment posits that communication reflects pragmatic rules, and aphasia in this context is simply ineffective use of language communication. The goal of treatment is to facilitate more normal communication by emphasizing pragmatic function, regardless of linguistic form, with flexible strategies for circumventing communication breakdowns (Holland 1991). Several functional communication therapy systems have been advanced. The most widely used is PACE (Promoting Aphasic's Communicative Effectiveness, Davis and Wilcox 1985). This approach emphasizes use of residual communicative strengths rather than attempting to overcome linguistic deficits. While verbal communication is encouraged, PACE promotes the use of other modalities – gesture, writing, drawing – to compensate for what the patient cannot say. For example, the patient might be asked to communicate information contained in pictures however he or she can. PACE simulates what people do when they communicate.

Efficacy of Aphasia Therapy

The efficacy of treatment for aphasia has remained controversial. The available data result from three designs: single treatment group, comparison of treatments, and treatment versus no-treatment comparisons. Single treatment group studies measure the severity of aphasia in patients before and after treatment. At least ten single treatment group aphasia treatment studies have reported improvement in 50–96% of patients. These studies, however, do not prove that the improvement resulted from the treatment rather than from spontaneous recovery. A comparison of treatments design involves comparison of specific treatment techniques in matched groups, with administration of a pre- and post-treatment outcome measure. Of five such studies, only one (Wertz *et al.* 1981) indicated a specific treatment effect, namely better improvement with individual versus group therapy. These studies do not include a no-treatment group, and hence do not establish the efficacy of treatment. A treatment versus no-treatment design can indicate that the treatment was efficacious, provided that the patients were randomly assigned. At least seven comparison of treatment with no-treatment investigations have been conducted with aphasic patients, but only three assigned patients randomly. The four investigations that did not assign patients randomly used self-selected no-treatment groups: patients who elected not to receive treatment, who could not afford treatment, who resided where treatment was not available, or who were placed on a waiting list. These studies are difficult to interpret, because variables that may influence response to treatment were not controlled. Nevertheless, three of the four investigations had positive results.

Two of the three investigations that employed random assignment of patients to treatment and no-treatment groups (Wertz *et al.* 1986; Katz and Wertz 1997) reported positive results of treatment. Wertz *et al.* (1986) assigned aphasic stroke patients randomly to treatment by speech pathologists for 8–10 hours each week for 12 weeks, or no-treatment for 12 weeks. At the end of 12 weeks, treated patients made significantly more improvement than those without treatment. After the crossover at 12 weeks, the group that switched to active treatment caught up most of the way with the previously treated group. This study probably provides the best and most direct evidence that speech therapy actually brings about improvement in aphasic patients. Katz and Wertz (1997) assigned aphasic patients at least 6 months post-onset randomly to three groups: computer language treatment, computer stimulation with no manipulation of language deficits, and no treatment. Patients received 3 hours of treatment each week for 6 months. At the end of the trial, the computer language treatment group did better than the computer stimulation and no-treatment groups, which did not differ from each other. The only negative study was that of Lincoln *et al.* (1984), who assigned aphasic patients randomly to treatment and no-treatment groups at 4 weeks post-onset. They prescribed 2 hours of treatment each week for 24 weeks, but few of the patients actually received the full 48 hours of treatment. The treated and untreated patients did not differ from each other at 24 weeks, but most authorities would say that the treatment was not adequate.

Three meta-analyses of aphasia treatment studies have been reported. Whurr *et al.* (1992) analyzed 45 aphasia treatment studies. The results indicated a medium-sized effect; 73% of treated patients showed improvement. Robey has reported two meta-analyses of aphasia treatment studies. The first (Robey 1994) included 21 studies, and indicated that treated patients improved nearly twice as much as untreated patients. In a more recent meta-analysis of 55 studies (Robey 1998), Robey concluded that outcomes for treated patients were superior to those for untreated individuals in all stages of recovery, but outcomes were best when treatment was begun in the acute stage of recovery.

In summary, aphasia therapy appears to benefit most patients. Patients most likely to improve include those with single strokes, treated soon after onset, in good general health, and receiving at least 3 hours of therapy weekly for a period of months. There is no evidence to support one type of treatment over another. A few studies have compared therapy by trained speech/language pathologists with that by lightly trained volunteers (Hartman and Landau 1987). Differences have been small or non-existent. Much research into specific methods of speech therapy is therefore needed. Aphasia therapy, however, has become a standard practice in rehabilitation. Were aphasia therapy a drug, the treatment would likely meet FDA approval. Neurologists should keep this in mind in comparing speech therapy for aphasia with other widely prescribed treatments.

Pharmacotherapy of Aphasia

A recent and potentially exciting area of aphasia research involves the use of drugs to stimulate recovery of language functions. Albert and colleagues (1988) began this research with a report that the anti-parkinson drug bromocriptine appeared to improve speech output in patients with transcortical motor aphasia. The authors pointed to the known effects of dopamine agonist drugs in stimulating initiation of movement in Parkinson's disease; transcortical motor aphasia shares with Parkinson's disease a difficulty in initiation of motor behavior, in this case speech. The drug has also been tried in other non-fluent aphasias, though two randomized trials did not find definite benefit (Gupta et al. 1995; Sabe et al. 1995).

Preliminary use of stimulant drugs such as methylphenidate has also shown promise in promoting speech output. This area of research is still in its infancy, but there is considerable hope that pharmacotherapy may be an adjunct to behavioral therapies for aphasia. In addition, the effects of stimulant and dopamine agonist drugs raise the concern that sedative and tranquilizing drugs may actually impede language rehabilitation. One study found that patients treated with the anticonvulsant drugs phenytoin and carbamazepine, benzodiazepines used for sleep or anxiety, and some antihypertensive drugs seemed to retard stroke rehabilitation. While a prospective study has not been reported, physicians caring for aphasic patients should avoid these drugs if possible.

Future Areas of Aphasia Research

The study of language in the new millenium will draw upon recent advances in brain technology, especially the imaging of functional brain activity (Kirshner 2000). These techniques (PET, SPECT, and functional MRI) provide a 'window' into the brain, through which an investigator can observe the neuronal switchboard turning on and off in response to stimuli. As stated by Posner (1993), PET is to neuroscience what the telescope was to astronomy or the microscope to pathology; it permits 'seeing the mind', visualizing language processes, thought, attention, self-monitoring, and perception of novelty. As we saw in Chapter 1, our concepts of brain organization are changing. In place of localized brain centers, we now speak of 'networks' connecting a series of cortical 'modules'. Another technique, the localization of language cortex by electrical stimulation in epileptic patients, has shown much greater variability than *post-mortem* studies in the precise cortical sites that represent the Broca's or Wernicke's areas. Rare patients have only a frontal or only a temporal language center (Ojemann *et al.* 1989). Such variability in functional brain anatomy may explain the discrepancies in aphasia localization, the 'atypical' cases referred to in this chapter. Functional imaging has also identified new language areas, in particular the 'inferior temporal language area' (Luders *et al.* 1986). This area has not been important in stroke cases, but cases of spontaneous seizures arising from this area have been reported (Kirshner *et al.* 1995). Figure 5.15 shows an MRI scan and PET scan from a patient with focal seizures originating from the left inferior temporal lobe. The PET scan was hypermetabolic, indicating increased glucose uptake in the region of the seizure. After control of the seizures, the aphasia resolved completely.

Functional imaging can now address questions long unanswered: Why can some 'atypical' patients have Broca's area destruction but not be aphasic? Why

(a)

(b)

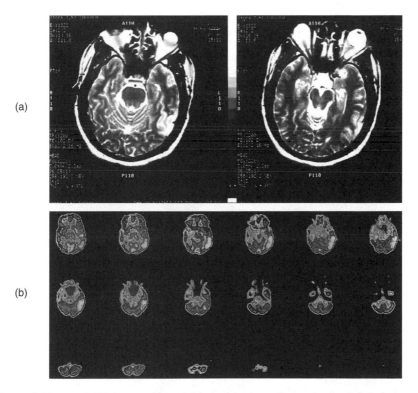

Figure 5.15 (a) MRI image, t2-weighted, showing a lesion in the left inferior temporal lobe. (b) The PET scan from the same patient showed hypermetabolism in the same area.

do occasional cases with temporal lesions manifest conduction or anomic aphasia, rather than the expected Wernicke's aphasia? Where is language comprehension mediated in these atypical patients? Is there a difference in how reading comprehension takes place in those Wernicke's aphasics with spared reading but impaired auditory language versus normal readers? Is 'inner thought' different in an aphasic patient versus a normal speaker?

The recovery of aphasia is among the topics of future studies (see Chapter 21). Functional imaging studies have found conflicting evidence regarding how the brain reorganizes to regain language function. Some studies have suggested right hemisphere participation in language recovery, based on resting increases in blood flow or glucose metabolism (Cappa *et al.* 1997), or from right hemisphere activation during language tasks (Weiller *et al.* 1995). Heiss and colleagues (1999), on the other hand, found evidence of recovery in the left hemisphere. In their studies, right hemisphere activation was a 'second best' attempt at recovery, always incomplete, whereas the left superior temporal gyrus activated in those destined for full language recovery.

In the future, functional brain imaging may permit prediction of spontaneous recovery and thereby help in planning the most effective course of behavioral and pharmacologic therapies. For example, Naeser and colleagues found that patients with destruction of Broca's area and the subcortical areas of the subcallosal fasciculus and periventricular white matter will not regain fluent speech (1989), and that patients with destruction of all of Wernicke's area will not regain language comprehension (1987). In such cases, traditional speech therapy will not be successful. Naeser and Palumbo (1995) have suggested that speech–language pathologists not bother with traditional therapy, but instead proceed directly to computer-based communication techniques such as Cvic, a computer therapy program marketed under the trade-name Lingraphica. Heiss and colleagues (1999) similarly reported that if the left superior temporal gyrus is not capable of functional activity, the prognosis for recovery of language function is poor. These conclusions require confirmation with larger series of patients. In addition, drug therapy with agents such as bromocriptine or amphetamine could be carried out in such patients, ideally with monitoring of functional imaging. Drug therapies are in their infancy, and we have little idea how they work. Estrogens have recently been shown to change PET patterns of activation in older women (Shaywitz *et al.* 1999). If drugs can influence the reorganization of language function after stroke, and if the 'best' therapies can be directed to the right patients from the beginning, improved outcomes are likely. Such studies promise new insights into the relationships of brain structure, brain function, and behavior.

REFERENCES

Albert ML, Bachman DL, Morgan A, Helm-Estabrooks N. Pharmacotherapy for aphasia. Neurology 1988;38:877–879.

Alexander MP, Benson DF. The aphasias and related disturbances. In RJ Joynt (ed.), Clinical Neurology. Philadelphia: Lippincott, 1998:1–58.

Alexander MP, LoVerme SR. Aphasia after left hemispheric intracerebral hemorrhage. Neurology 1980;30:1193–1202.

Alexander MP, Schmitt MA. The aphasia syndrome of stroke in the left anterior cerebral artery territory. Arch Neurol 1980;37:97–100.

Alexander MP, Naeser MA, Palumbo CL. Correlations of sub-cortical CT lesion sites and aphasia profiles. Brain 1987;110:961–991.

Alexander MP, Benson DF, Stuss D. Frontal lobes and language. Brain Lang 1989a;37:656–691.

Alexander MP, Fischette MR, Fischer RS. Crossed aphasias can be mirror image or anomalous. Brain 1989b;112:953–973.

Alexander MP, Naeser MA, Palumbo C. Broca's area aphasias: aphasia after lesions including the frontal operculum. Neurology 1990;40:353–362.

Appell J, Kertesz A, Fisman M. A study of language functioning in Alzheimer's patients. Brain Lang 1982;22:23–30.

Bakar M, Kirshner HS, Wertz RT. Crossed aphasia. Functional brain imaging with PET or SPECT. Arch Neurol 1996;53:1026–1032.

Basso A, Capitani E, Laiacona M, Zanobio ME. Crossed aphasia:one or more syndromes? Cortex 1985a;21:25–45.

Basso A, Lecours AR, Moraschini S, Vanier M. Anatomoclinical correlations of the aphasias as defined through computerized tomography: exceptions. Brain Lang 1985b;26:201–229.

Basso A, Della Sala S, Farabola M. Aphasia arising from purely deep lesions. Cortex 1987;23:29–44.

Basso A, Farabola M, Pia Grassi M *et al*. Aphasia in left handers. Comparison of aphasia profiles and language recovery in non-right-handed and matched right-handed patients. Brain Lang 1990;38:233–252.

Bell DS. Speech functions of the thalamus inferred from the effects of thalamotomy. Brain 1968;91:619–638.

Benson DF. The third alexia. Arch Neurol 1977;34:327–331.

Benson DF. Neurologic correlates of anomia. In H Whitaker, HA Whitaker (eds), Studies in Neurolinguistics, Vol 4. New York: Academic Press, 1979;293–328.

Benson DR, Sheremata WA, Bouchard R *et al*. Conduction aphasia: a clinicopathological study. Arch Neurol 1973;28:339–346.

Benson DF, Ardila A. Aphasia. A Clinical Perspective. New York, Oxford University Press, 1996.

Boatman D, Gordon B, Hart J *et al*. Transcortical sensory aphasia: revisited and revised. Brain 2000;123:1634–1642.

Bogen J, Bogen G. Wernicke's region – where is it? Ann NY Acad Sci 1976;280:834–843.

Bogousslavsky J, Regli F, Uske A. Thalamic infarcts: clinical syndromes, etiology, and prognosis. Neurology 1988;38:837–848.

Boller F, Marcie P. Possible role of abnormal auditory feedback in conduction aphasia. Neuropsychologia 1978;16:521–524.

Bramwell B. On 'crossed' aphasia and the factors which go to determine whether the 'leading' or 'driving' speech-centres shall be located in the left or in the right hemisphere of the brain, with notes of a case of 'crossed' aphasia (aphasia with right-sided hemiplegia) in a left-handed man. Lancet 1899;1:1473–1479.

Brown JW. The problem of repetition: a study of 'conduction' aphasia and the 'isolation' syndrome. Cortex 1975;11:37–52.

Brown JW, Hecaen H. Lateralization and language representation. Observations on aphasia in children, left-handers, and 'anomalous' dextrals. Neurology 1976;26:183–189.

Brown JW, Leader BJ, Blum CS. Hemiplegic writing in severe aphasia. Brain Lang 1983;19:204–215.

Byng S, Black M. What makes a therapy? Some parameters of therapeutic intervention in aphasia. Eur J Disord Commun 1995;30:303–316.

Caplan D, Alpert N, Waters G. Effects of syntactic structure and number of propositions on patterns of regional cerebral blood flow. Brain Lang 1997;60:66–69.

Cappa SF, Cavallotti G, Guidotti M *et al.* Subcortical aphasia: two clinical–CT scan correlation studies. Cortex 1983;19:227–241.

Cappa SF, Perani D, Bressi S *et al.* Crossed aphasia: a PET follow-up study of two cases. J Neurol Neurosurg Psychiatry 1993;56:665–671.

Cappa SF, Perani D, Grassi F *et al.* A PET follow-up study of recovery after stroke in acute aphasics. Brain Lang 1997;56:55–67.

Chapin C, Blumstein SE, Meissner B, Boller F. Speech production mechanisms in aphasia: a delayed auditory feedback study. Brain Lang 1981;14:106–113.

Chesson AL. Aphasia following a right thalamic hemorrhage. Brain Lang 1983;19:306–316.

Coslett HB, Brashear HR, Heilman KM. Pure word deafness after bilateral primary auditory cortex infarcts. Neurology 1984;34:347–352.

Critchley M. The detection of minimal dysphasia. In M Critchley, JL O'Leary, B Jennett (eds), Scientific Foundations of Neurology. London: Heinemann Medical Books, 1972. Reprinted in Critchley M. The Divine Banquet of the Brain. New York: Raven Press, 1979;63–71.

Crosson B. Role of the dominant thalamus in language: a review. Psychol Bull 1984;96:491–517.

Crosson B. Subcortical functions in language: a working model. Brain Lang 1985;25:257–292.

Damasio AR. Aphasia. New Engl J Med 1992;326:531–539.

Damasio H, Damasio AR. The anatomical basis of conduction aphasia. Brain 1980; 103:337–350.

Damasio AR, Damasio H, Rizzo M *et al.* Aphasia with non-hemorrhagic lesions in the basal ganglia and internal capsule. Arch Neurol 1982;39:15–20.

Darley FL, Aronson AE, Brown JR. Differential diagnostic patterns of dysarthria. J Speech Hear Res 1969;12:246–269.

Davis GA, Wilcox MJ. Adult Aphasia Rehabilitation: Applied Pragmatics. San Diego: College-Hill Press, 1985.

Demonet J-F, Chollet F, Ramsay S *et al.* The anatomy of phonological and semantic processing in normal subjects. Brain 1992;115:1753–1768.

DiSimon FG, Darley FL, Aronson AE. Patterns of dysfunction in schizophrenic patients on an aphasia test battery. J Speech Hear Disord 1977;62:498–513.

Docherty NM, DeRosa M, Andreasen NC. Communication disturbances in schizophrenia and mania. Arch Gen Psychiatry 1996;53:358–364.

Dronkers NF. A new brain region for coordinating speech articulation. Nature 1996;384:159–161.

Duffy JR. Motor speech disorders. Substrates, differential diagnosis, and management. St. Louis: Mosby, 1995.

Feinberg TE, Gonzalez Rothi LJ, Heilman KM. 'Inner speech' in conduction aphasia. Arch Neurol 1986;43:591–593.

Fensore C, Lazzarino LG, Nappo A, Nicolai A. Language and memory disturbances from mesencephalothalamic infarcts. A clinical and computed tomographic study. Eur Neurol 1988;28:51–56.

Fisher CM. The pathological and clinical aspects of thalamic hemorrhage. Trans Am Neurol Assoc 1959;84:56–59.

Freedman M, Alexander MP, Naeser MA. Anatomic basis of transcortical motor aphasia. Neurology 1984;34:409–417.

Fromm D, Holland AL, Swindell CS, Reinmuth OM. Various consequences of subcortical stroke. Prospective study of 16 consecutive cases. Arch Neurol 1985;42:943–950.

Gerson SN, Benson DF, Frazier SH. Diagnosis: schizophrenia versus posterior aphasia. Am J Psychiatry 1977;134:966–969.

Geschwind N. Non-aphasic disorders of speech. Int J Neurol 1964;4:207–214.

Geschwind N. The organization of language and the brain. Science 1970;170:940–944.

Gloning I, Gloning K, Haub G, Quatember R. Comparison of verbal behavior in right-handed and non-right-handed patients with anatomically verified lesion of one hemisphere. Cortex 1969;5:43–52.

Goldstein K. Die transcorticalen Aphasien. Ergebn Neurol Psychiat 1917;2:349–629.

Goldstein K. Language and Language Disturbances. Aphasic Symptom Complexes and their Significance for Medicine and the Theory of Language. New York: Grune & Stratton, 1948;10–16.

Goldstein MN. Auditory agnosia for speech ('pure word deafness'). A historical review with current implications. Brain Lang 1974;1:195–204.

Gomez-Tortosa E, Martin EM, Sychra JJ, Dujovny M. Language-activated single-photon emission tomography imaging in the evaluation of language lateralization: evidence from a case of crossed aphasia: case report. Neurosurgery 1994;35:515–519.

Goodglass H, Quadfasel F. Language laterality in left-handed aphasics. Brain 1954;77:521–548.

Goodglass H, Blumstein SE, Gleason JB *et al*. The effect of syntactic encoding on sentence comprehension in aphasia. Brain Lang 1979;7:201–209.

Graff-Radford NR, Eslinger PJ, Damasio AR, Yamada T. Non-hemorrhagic infarction of the thalamus: behavioral, anatomic, and physiologic correlates. Neurology 1984;34:14–23.

Graff-Radford NR, Damasio H, Yamada T *et al*. Non-hemorrhagic thalamic infarction. Clinical, neuropsychological and electrophysiological findings in four anatomical groups defined by computerized tomography. Brain 1985;108:485–516.

Grossi D, Trojano L, Chiacchio L *et al*. Mixed transcortical aphasia: clinical features and neuroanatomical correlates. A possible role of the right hemisphere. Eur Neurol 1991;31:204–211.

Gupta SR, Mlcoch AG, Scolaro C, Mortiz T. Bromocriptine treatment of non-fluent aphasia. Neurology 1995;45:2170–2173.

Hartman J, Landau W. Comparison of formal language therapy with supportive counseling for aphasia due to acute vascular accident. Arch Neurol 1987;24:646–649.

Heilman KM, Scholes RJ. The nature of comprehension errors in Broca's, conduction, and Wernicke's aphasics. Cortex 1976;12:258–265.

Heilman KM, Tucker DM, Valenstein E. A case of mixed transcortical aphasia with intact naming. Brain 1976a;99:415–426.

Heilman KM, Scholes R, Watson RT. Defects of immediate memory in Broca's and conduction aphasia. Brain Lang 1976b;3:201–208.

Heilman K, Rothi L, Campanella D, Wolfson S. Wernicke's and global aphasia without alexia. Arch Neurol 1979;36:129–133.

Heilman KM, Rothi L, McFarling D, Rottmann AL. Transcortical sensory aphasia with relatively spared spontaneous speech and naming. Arch Neurol 1981;38:236–239.

Heiss W-D, Kessler J, Thiel A *et al*. Differential capacity of left and right hemispheric areas for compensation of poststroke aphasia. Ann Neurol 1999;45:430–438; see also Heiss W-D, Luxenburger G *et al*. Speech-induced cerebral metabolic activation reflects recovery from aphasia. J Neurol Sci 1997;145:213–217.

Helm-Estabrooks N, Albert ML. Manual of Aphasia Therapy. Austin, TX: Pro-ed, 1991.

Henderson VW. Speech fluency in crossed aphasia. Brain 1983;106:837–857.

Henderson VW. Naming and naming disorders. In HS Kirshner, Handbook of Neurological Speech and Language Disorders. New York: Marcel Dekker, 1995;165–185.

Hier D, Mohr JP. Incongruous oral and written naming: evidence for a subdivision of the syndrome of Wernicke's aphasia. Brain Lang 1977;4:115–126.

Hier DB, David KR, Richardson EP, Mohr JP. Hypertensive putaminal hemorrhage. Ann Neurol 1977;1:152–159.

Holland AL. Pragmatic aspects of intervention in aphasia. J Neuroling 1991;6:197–211.

Kanshepolsky J, Kelley JJ, Waggener JD. A cortical auditory disorder. Clinical, audiological and pathologic aspects. Neurology 1973;23:699–705.

Katz RC, Wertz RT. The efficacy of computer-provided reading treatment for chronic aphasic adults. J Speech Hear Res 1997;40:493–507.

Kertesz A, Sheppard A, MacKenzie R. Localization in transcortical sensory aphasia. Arch Neurol 1982;39:475–478.

Kertesz A, Lau WK, Polk M. The structural determinants of recovery in Wernicke's aphasia. Brain Lang 1993;44:153–164.

Kessler J, Karbe H et al. Cerebral glucose metabolism as a predictor of recovery from aphasia in ischemic stroke. Arch Neurol 1993;50:958–964; and Heiss W-D, Karbe H, Weber-

Kirshner HS. Language studies in the third millennium. Brain Lang 2000;71:124–128.

Kirshner HS, Kistler KH. Aphasia after right thalamic hemorrhage. Arch Neurol 1982;39:667–669.

Kirshner H, Webb W. Selective involvement of the auditory–verbal modality in an acquired communication disorder: benefit from sign language therapy. Brain Lang 1981;13:161–170.

Kreisler A, Godefroy O, Delmaire et al. The anatomy of aphasia revisited. Neurology 2000; 54:1117–1123.

Kirshner HS, Casey PF, Kelly MP et al. Anomia in cerebral diseases. Neuropsychologia 1987;25:701–705.

Kirshner HS, Casey PF, Henson J et al. Behavioural features and lesion localization in Wernicke's aphasia. Aphasiology 1989;3:169–176.

Kirshner HS, Hughes T, Fakhoury T, Abou-Khalil B. Aphasia secondary to partial status epilepticus of the basal temporal language area. Neurology 1995;45:1616–1618.

Kirshner HS, Alexander M, Lorch MP, Wertz RT. Disorders of speech and language. Continuum 1999;5:61–79.

Lai CSL, Fisher SE, Hurst JA et al. A forkhead-domain gene is mutated in a severe speech and language disorder. Nature 2001;413:519–523.

Lambert WE, Fillenbaum S. A pilot study of aphasia among bilinguals. Can J Psychol 1959;13:28–34.

Lazar RM, Marshall RS, Prell GD, Pile-Spellman J. The experience of Wernicke's aphasia. Neurology 2000;55:1222–1224.

Legatt AD, Rubin MJ, Kaplan LR et al. Global aphasia without hemiparesis: multiple etiologies. Neurology 1987;37:201–205.

Lesser RP, Luders H, Morris HH et al. Electrical stimulation of Wernicke's area interferes with comprehension. Neurology 1986;36:658–663.

Levine DN, Calvanio R. Conduction aphasia. In HS Kirshner, FR Freemon (eds), The Neurology of Aphasia. Amsterdam: Swets & Zeitlinger, 1982;79–112.

Lhermitte F, Derouesné J. Paraphasies et jargonaphasie dans le langage oral avec conservation du langage ecrit: genese des neologismes. Rev Neurol (Paris) 1974;130:21–38.

Lichtheim L. On aphasia. Brain 1885;7:433–484.

Lincoln NB, Mulley GP, Jones AC et al. Effectiveness of speech therapy for aphasic stroke patients. A randomized controlled trial. Lancet 1984;1:1197–1200.

Luders H, Lesser RP, Hahn J et al. Basal temporal language area demonstrated by electrical stimulation. Neurology 1986;36:505–510.

Luria AR. On quasi-aphasic speech disturbances in lesions of the deep structures of the brain. Brain Lang 1977;4:432–459.

Luria AR, Tsvetkova LS. The mechanism of 'dynamic aphasia'. Foundations of language 1968;4:296–307.

Masdeu JC, Schoene WC, Funkenstein H. Aphasia following infarction of the left supplementary motor area. A clinicopathologic study. Neurology 1978;28:1220–1223.

Mastronardi L, Ferrante L, Celli P et al. Aphasia in polyglots: report of two cases and analysis of the literature. Neurosurgery 1991;29:621–623.

McHenry LC. Garrison's History of Neurology. Illinois: Springfield, 1969;3–4.

Megens J, van Loon J, Goffin J, Gybels J. Subcortical aphasia from a thalamic abscess. J Neurol Neurosurg Psychiatry 1992;55:319–321.

Mendez M, Geehan GR. Cortical auditory disorder: Clinical and psychoacoustic features. J Neurol Neurosurg Psychiatry 1988;51:1–9.

Mendez MF, Adams NL, Lewandowski KS. Neurobehavioral changes associated with caudate lesions. Neurology 1989;39:349–354.

Metter EJ, Wasterlain CG, Kuhl DE et al. [18]FDG positron emission computed tomography in a study of aphasia. Ann Neurol 1981;10:173–183; see also Metter EJ, Kempler D, Jackson C et al. Cerebral glucose metabolism in Wernicke's, Broca's, and conduction aphasia. Arch Neurol 1989;46:27–34.

Minkowski M. Klinischer beitrag zur Aphasie bei Polyglotten, speziell im Hinblick aufs Schweizerdeutsche. Schweiz Arch Neurol Psychiatr 1927;21:43–72.

Mohr JP, Watters WC, Duncan GW. Thalamic hemorrhage and aphasia. Brain Lang 1975;2:3–17.

Mohr JP, Pessin MS, Finklestein S et al. Broca aphasia: pathologic and clinical. Neurology 1978;28:311–324.

Naeser MA, Borod JC. Aphasia in left-handers: lesion site, lesion side, and hemispheric asymmetries on CT. Neurology 1986;36:471–488.

Naeser MA, Palumbo CL. How to analyze CT/MRI scan lesion sites to predict potential for long-term recovery in aphasia. In HS Kirshner (ed.), Handbook of Neurological Speech and Language Disorders. New York: Marcel Dekker, Inc., 1995; 91–148.

Naeser MA, Alexander MP, Helm-Estabrooks N et al. Aphasia with predominantly sub-cortical lesion sites. Arch Neurol 1982;39:2–14.

Naeser MA, Helm-Estabrooks N, Haas G et al. Relationship between lesion extent in 'Wernicke's area' on CT scan and predicting recovery of comprehension in Wernicke's aphasia. Arch Neurol 1987;44:73–82.

Naeser MA, Palumbo CL, Helm-Estabrooks N et al. Role of the medial subcallosal fasciculus and other white matter pathways in recovery of spontaneous speech. Brain 1989;112:1–38.

Naeser MA, Gaddie A, Palumbo CL et al. Late recovery of auditory comprehension in global aphasia. Improved recovery observed with subcortical temporal isthmus lesion vs Wernicke's cortical area lesion. Arch Neurol 1990;47:425–432.

Obler LK, Albert ML. Influence of aging on recovery from aphasia in polyglots. Brain Lang 1977;4:460–463.

Ojemann G. Language and the thalamus: object naming and recall during and after thalamic stimulation. Brain Lang 1975;2:101–120.

Ojemann GA, Whitaker HA. The bilingual brain. Arch Neurol 1978;35:409–412.

Ojemann G, Fedio P, Van Buren J. Anomia from pulvinar and sub-cortical parietal stimulation. Brain 1968;91:99–116.

Ojemann G, Ojemann J, Lettich E, Berger M. Cortical language localization in left, dominant hemisphere. An electrical stimulation mapping investigation in 117 patients. J Neurosurg 1989;71:316–326.

Pedersen PM, Jorgensen HS, Nakayama H et al. Aphasia in acute stroke: incidence, determinants, and recovery. Ann Neurol 1995;38:659–666.

Perani D, Papagno C, Cappa S et al. Crossed aphasia: functional studies with single photon emission computerized tomography. Cortex 1988;24:171–178.

Perani D, Paulesu E, Galles NS et al. The bilingual brain. Proficiency and age of acquisition of the second language. Brain 1998;121:1841–1852.

Pinker S. The Language Instinct. New York: William Morrow and Co., Inc, 1994;17.

Pitres A. Étude sur l'aphasie chez les polyglottes. Rev Med 1895;15:873–899.

Poeck K, Huber W, Willmes K. Outcome of intensive language treatment in aphasia. J Speech Hear Dis 1989;54:471–479.

Posner MI. Seeing the mind. Science 1993;262:673–674.

Reynolds AF, Turner PT, Harris AB et al. Left thalamic hemorrhage with dysphasia: a report of five cases. Brain Lang 1979;7:62–73.

Ribot T. Diseases of Memory, an Essay in the Positive Psychology. London: Kegan Paul, 1906:122.

Robey RR. The efficacy of treatment for aphasic persons: a meta-analysis. Brain Lang 1994;47:585–608.

Robey RR. A meta–analysis of clinical outcomes in the treatment of aphasia. J Speech Lang Hear Res 1998;41:172–187.

Robinson RG, Benson DF. Depression in aphasic patients: frequency, severity, and clinical–pathological correlations. Brain Lang 1981;14:282–291.

Ross ED. Left medial parietal lobe and receptive language functions: mixed transcortical aphasia after left anterior cerebral artery infarction. Neurology 1980;30:144–151.

Rubens AB. Transcortical motor aphasia. Studies in Neurolinguistics 1976;1:293–306.

Sabe L, Salvarezza F, Cuerva AG et al. A randomized, double-blind, placebo-controlled study of bromocriptine in nonfluent aphasia. Neurology 1995;45:2272–2274.

Saffran E, Schwartz M, Fink R et al. Mapping therapy: an approach to remediating agrammatic sentence comprehension and production. In J Cooper (ed.), Aphasia Treatment: Current Approaches and Research Opportunities, NIDCD Monograph 2. Bethesda, MD: National Institutes of Health 1993:77–90.

Sagan C. 'Broca's brain'. New York: Random House, 1974;8.

Samra K, Riklan M, Levita E et al. Language and speech correlates of anatomically verified lesions in thalamic surgery for parkinsonism. J Speech Hear Res 1969;12:510–540.

Sarno MT. Acquired Aphasia (2nd edn). San Diego: Academic Press, 1991.

Schiff HB, Alexander MR, Naeser MA et al. Aphemia: clinical–anatomic correlations. Arch Neurol 1983;40:720–27.

Schuell H, Jenkins JJ, Jimenez-Pabon E. Aphasia in Adults: Diagnosis, Prognosis, and Treatment. New York: Hoeber Medical Division, Harper & Row Publishers, 1964.

Schweiger A, Wechsler AF, Mazziota JC. Metabolic correlates of linguistic functions in a patient with crossed aphasia. Aphasiology 1987;5:415–421.

Selnes OA, Niccum N, Knopman DS, Rubens AB. Recovery of single word comprehension: CT-scan correlates. Brain Lang 1984; 21:72–84.

Shallice T, Warrington EK. Auditory–verbal short-term memory impairment and conduction aphasia. Brain Lang 1977;4:479–491.

Shaywitz SE, Shaywitz BA, Pugh KR et al. Effect of estrogen on brain activation patterns in postmenopausal women during working memory tasks. JAMA 1999;281:1197.

Silverberg R, Gordon HW. Differential aphasia in two bilingual individuals. Neurology 1979;29:51–55.

Smythe GE, Stern K. Tumors of the thalamus: a clinico-pathological study. Brain 1938;61:339–360.

Strub RL. The repetition defect in conduction aphasia: mnestic or linguistic? Brain Lang 1974;1:241–255.

Stuss DT, Guberman A, Nelson R, Larochelle S. The neuropsychology of paramedian thalamic infarction. Brain Lang 1988;8:348–378.

Sweet EWS, Panis W, Levine DN. Crossed Wernicke's aphasia. Neurology 1984;34:475–479.

Takahasi N, Kawamura M, Shinotou H et al. Pure word deafness due to left hemisphere damage. Cortex 1992;28:295–303.

Tanaka Y, Yamadori A, Mori E. Pure word deafness following bilateral lesions. A psychophysical analysis. Brain 1987;110:381–403.

Tanridag O, Kirshner HS. Aphasia and agraphia in lesions of the posterior internal capsule and putamen. Neurology 1985; 35:1797–1801.

Tranel D, Biller J, Damasio H et al. Global aphasia without hemiparesis. Arch Neurol 1987;44:304–308.

Tzortzis C, Albert ML. Impairment of memory for sequences in conduction aphasia. Neuropsychologia 1974;12:355–366.

Walker-Batson D, Wendt JS, Devous M *et al*. A long-term follow-up case study of crossed aphasia assessed by single-photon emission tomography (SPECT), language, and neuropsychological testing. Brain Lang 1988;33:311–322.

Weiller C, Isensee C, Rijntjes M *et al*. Recovery from Wernicke's aphasia: a positron emission tomographic study. Ann Neurol 1995;37:723–732.

Wertz RT. Efficacy. In C Code, D Muller (eds), The Treatment of Aphasia: From Theory to Practice. London: Whurr Publishers Ltd, 1995;309–339.

Wertz RT, Collins MJ, Weiss D *et al*. Veterans Administration cooperative study on aphasia: a comparison of individual and group treatment. J Speech Hear Res 1981;24:580–594.

Wertz RT, LaPointe LL, Rosenbek JC. Apraxia of speech in adults: the disorder and its management. San Diego:Singular Publishing Group, Inc., 1984.

Wertz RT, Weiss DG, Aten J *et al*. Comparison of clinic, home, and deferred language treatment for aphasia: A Veterans Administration cooperative study. Arch Neurol 1986;43:653–658.

Whitaker H. A case of the isolation of the language function. In H Whitaker, HA Whitaker (eds), Studies in Neurolinguistics, Vol. 2. New York: Academic Press, 1976;1–58.

Whurr M, Lorch M. The use of a prosthesis to facilitate writing in aphasia and right hemiplegia. Aphasiology 1991;5:411–418.

Whurr R, Lorch MP, Nye C. A meta-analysis of studies carried out between 1946 and 1988 concerned with the efficacy of speech and language therapy treatment for aphasic patients. Eur J Dis Commun 1992;27:1–17.

Willmes K, Poeck K. To what extent can aphasic syndromes be localized? Brain 1993;116:1527–1540.

Zangwill OL. Two cases of crossed aphasia in dextrals. Neuropsychologia 1979;17:167–172.

6

Alexias and Agraphias: Disorders of Reading and Writing

Reading maketh a full man, conference a ready man, and writing an exact man.

(Francis Bacon, *Essays* 1626)

Reading is to the mind, what exercise is to the body.

(Addison, *The Tatler*, No. 147 1709–1711)

Alexias and agraphias are acquired disorders of reading secondary to brain damage (Alexander and Benson 1998). Reading and writing are language modalities; alexias and agraphias therefore qualify as syndromes of aphasia, but ones in which the comprehension and production of written language are affected more than spoken language modalities. The term 'alexia' signifies an acquired reading disorder, just as 'aphasia' means an acquired language disorder. Developmental or congenital reading disorders are referred to as 'dyslexias'. The reader should be aware, however, that in Europe and in some neuropsychological and neurolinguistic writings, 'dyslexia' is used to denote partial as opposed to complete loss of reading.

Like the aphasias, the alexias and agraphias are categorized according to the patient's performance during the bedside language examination, presented in Chapter 4. Without the deliberate testing of reading and writing, this important and interesting group of disorders cannot be diagnosed or even detected. A history of intact premorbid reading and writing skills is also required. Deficits in reading and writing in association with other neurological signs serve the same practical usefulness as deficits in spoken language in the localization of brain lesions and the diagnosis of neurological disorders. In addition, neurolinguistic studies of the alexias and agraphias have been used to establish models of the component behavioral steps in normal reading and writing. The testing of these models has led to new understanding of the organization of reading and writing in the brain, and also to new classifications of alexia and agraphia, based on the specific neurolinguistic step in the reading or writing process which is disturbed.

ALEXIAS

Traditionally, the alexias are divided into three categories: pure alexia with agraphia, pure alexia without agraphia, and alexia associated with the aphasias ('aphasic alexia'). Several functions contribute to the ability to read written language. Reading may be compromised by attentional impairments, problems with sequencing, or speech or language disorders that make it impossible to read aloud. Reading involves several distinct steps in cognitive processing: the visuospatial perception of individual letters and word shapes, the learned correspondence between letters and sounds, the recognition of groups of letters to the spoken form of words, and the association of meaning to these letter strings.

In this chapter, we shall first discuss the classical syndromes, then consider the newer, neurolinguistic classification of alexias. Like the aphasic syndromes, the alexias have characteristic findings on bedside examination, associated neurological signs, and anatomically distinct lesion localizations.

Alexia with Agraphia (Parietal-Temporal Alexia)

The syndrome of alexia with agraphia, first described by the French physician Dejerine in 1891 as letter-blindness, is in effect an acquired illiteracy. Reading and writing are both disrupted without significant aphasia in other language modalities. Features of the bedside examination are presented in Table 6.1. Most cases of pure alexia with agraphia are not truly 'pure', in the sense that a mild fluent aphasia with paraphasias is usually present. Other terms for the same syndrome include: parietal-temporal alexia, angular alexia, central alexia, and semantic alexia.

Table 6.1 Characteristics of pure alexia with agraphia

Feature	Characteristic
Spontaneous speech	Fluent, often paraphasic
Naming	Often impaired
Auditory comprehension	Intact
Repetition	Intact
Reading	Impaired
Writing	Impaired
Associated signs	Gerstmann syndrome, right visual field defect
Localization	Left inferior parietal

The loss of reading and writing may be total, but is more often partial. Both reading words aloud and reading comprehension are affected. The understanding of words spelled orally is also typically impaired. The difficulty with letters is generally mirrored in number tasks (acalculia), and may also be seen in other symbolic forms of writing such as musical notation. Occasional cases may have some preserved ability to spell words, or to comprehend words spelled orally (Albert *et al.* 1973; Mohr 1976; Rothi and Heilman 1981). Writing is usually affected totally, such that the patient cannot write or spell even single words. Some patients can copy in a 'slavish' manner, but cannot write sentences spontaneously or to dictation.

Alexia with agraphia is frequently associated with other language deficits. Most patients have some paraphasias in running speech, and naming errors are also common. Repetition and auditory comprehension are preserved. Occasional cases of alexia with agraphia evolve from an initial deficit of Wernicke's aphasia, with some impairment of auditory comprehension as well as reading.

Other, associated neurological deficits are variable and may be completely absent. A right visual-field defect or right inferior quadrant defect is often present. Right-sided sensory and motor signs are usually mild if present at all. Other features of the Gerstmann syndrome (acalculia, finger agnosia, and right–left confusion) may also be present.

The anatomical basis of alexia with agraphia usually involves the left inferior parietal lobule, and in particular the left angular gyrus. The syndrome may be seen in strokes involving the inferior division of the left middle cerebral artery or a 'watershed' infarct between the left middle and posterior cerebral arteries. In stroke cases, however, alexia with agraphia is usually mixed with aphasia. Isolated left parietal lesions such as tumors, traumatic injuries, hemorrhages, and arteriovenous malformations can produce this syndrome. Figure 6.1 shows a cerebral hemorrhage in a patient with acute leukemia and thrombocytopenia, resulting in alexia with agraphia.

Gerstmann and Angular Gyrus Syndromes
In 1930, Gerstmann described four deficits associated with left parietal lesions: agraphia, right–left confusion, disorientation, acalculia, and finger agnosia.

Agraphia Agraphia will be discussed in the second part of this chapter. It is associated not only with the syndrome of alexia with agraphia, but also with the Gerstmann and angular gyrus syndromes.

Right–Left Disorientation Right–left discrimination is tested when a patient is given two- and three-step commands, usually involving both sides of the body. Right–left disorientation, detected by errors in right–left discrimination, is also associated with both the Gerstmann and angular gyrus syndromes.

Acalculia Acalculia is the loss of ability to perform calculations, either mentally or with paper and pencil. Hecaen and Angelergues (1961) divided acalculia

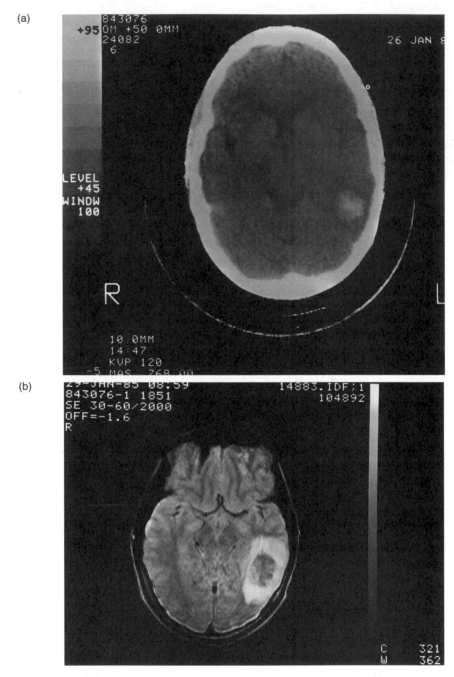

Figure 6.1 (a) CT scan from a young patient with acute lymphocytic leukemia. There is a localized hemorrhage in the left inferior parietal lobe, in the vicinity of the angular gyrus. The patient manifested a mild aphasia with anomia but complete inability to read or write (the syndrome of alexia with agraphia); (b) MRI scan, axial section, from the same patient, showing an area of hemorrhage with surrounding edema.

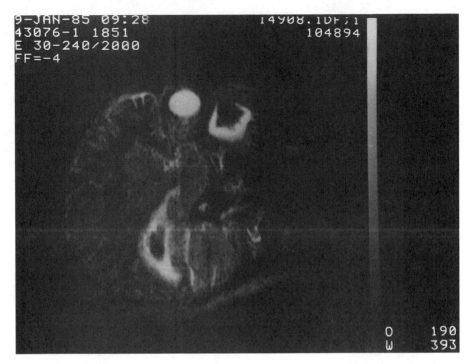

Figure 6.1 (c) MRI scan, sagittal section, showing the location of the hemorrhage in the left posterior, inferior parietal region. The advantage of the MRI for viewing of the lesion in different planes is evident.

into three types: (1) inability to read and write numbers; (2) spatial acalculia, or difficulty lining up the numbers correctly or keeping them in columns; and (3) anarithmetia, or true loss of ability to perform mental arithmetic, not explained by writing or spatial difficulties. The first and third types correlate with left parietal lesions (Jackson and Warrington 1986), whereas spatial acalculia correlates more with right hemisphere lesions. Patients with aphasia may be unable to verbalize calculations, yet some can perform silent calculations and indicate the correct answer by multiple choice (Benson and Denckla 1969). Occasional patients with severe aphasic deficits can play bridge or look at business ledgers and spreadsheets with apparent comprehension. Isolated left parietal lesions can impair calculations without producing any notable language disorder, the true syndrome of anarithmetia or loss of the concept of numbers (Grafman *et al.* 1982). Other studies have confirmed that calculation disorders are most common in posterior left hemisphere lesions, though they occur with lesions in other, varied sites (Boller and Grafman 1983).

Finger Agnosia The fourth element, finger agnosia, refers to a topographical and lateral difficulty with body parts, of which identification of fingers on the patient's own or the examiner's hand is perhaps the most sensitive index. The disorder may be related to the more severe body image deficits found with right parietal lesions (see Chapter 9).

The four elements of the Gerstmann syndrome do not necessarily all occur together; any combination of three items would indicate a left inferior parietal lesion, and other related deficits, including alexia and mild aphasia, may be combined. The syndrome lost adherents in the 1960s and 1970s because of this variability (Benton 1961; Critchley 1966). Benton went so far as to call the Gerstmann syndrome a 'fiction'. More recently, however, patients with focal left parietal lesions have manifested the classical Gerstmann tetrad (Roeltgen *et al.* 1983; Varney 1984; Mazzoni *et al.* 1990). In addition, Morris and colleagues (1984) documented that the four deficits could be produced by electrical stimulation in the left angular and supramarginal gyrus of an adolescent with epilepsy. Based on this new evidence, even Benton (1992) publicly accepted the Gerstmann tetrad as a valid syndrome.

Benson and colleagues (1982) described the angular gyrus syndrome as a variant of Gerstmann's syndrome and a mimicker of dementia. This vital confluence of the temporal and parietal lobes involves multiple cortical functions within a small anatomical territory. A patient with a single lesion in the left angular gyrus, documented by PET scan but not by CT, had combined deficits of anomia, fluent aphasia, alexia, agraphia, acalculia, right–left disorientation, finger agnosia, and constructional apraxia. The sheer multiplicity of these deficits resembled a dementia syndrome such as Alzheimer's disease. The features of the angular gyrus syndrome are shown in Table 6.2.

The role of the angular gyrus in alexia with agraphia, Gerstmann's syndrome, and the angular gyrus syndrome relates to larger, theoretical issues concerning the functions of this important brain region. Dejerine (1891) conceived of the angular gyrus as a visual word center, analogous to Wernicke's area as an auditory word center. Geschwind (1965) considered the area as a center for intermodality transfers, including the translation of visual into auditory language symbols, which is so important to reading. Geschwind also pointed out that this ability to translate from visual to auditory or tactile stimuli, which is so easy for

Table 6.2   Features of the angular gyrus syndrome

Anomia
Alexia
Agraphia
Acalculia
Right–left disorientation
Finger agnosia
Constructional apraxia
±mild, fluent aphasia
Right visual field defects

human subjects, is extremely difficult for experimental animals, including primates. The temporoparietal cortex is one of the areas that has enlarged the most in the evolution from animal to human brains, and perhaps this development was important to the emergence of language. As stated in Chapter 2, the angular gyrus and adjacent areas of the parietal cortex are now referred to as one of two 'heteromodal association cortices'. The principal role of this brain region is the coordination of information transfer among different sensory modalities.

Alexia Without Agraphia (Occipital Alexia)

Dejerine described the second acquired alexia syndrome, pure alexia without agraphia, in 1892, a year after pure alexia with agraphia. The syndrome has been referred to as occipital alexia, pure alexia, posterior alexia, pure word blindness, and letter-by-letter alexia. Not only are these patients not grossly aphasic, but they can also write, both spontaneously and to dictation. The hallmark of this syndrome is the paradoxical inability of the patients to read words they have just written. Pure alexia is a true 'word blindness', in which printed words have lost their meaning, though the patient is not blind. In other words, the patient has acquired not a total illiteracy as in alexia with agraphia, but rather a linguistic blindfold.

The features of alexia without agraphia are shown in Table 6.3. Spontaneous speech is usually normal, without paraphasias. Naming may be mildly impaired, especially for colors (see below). Auditory comprehension and repetition are typically intact, and most patients can spell words orally and comprehend words dictated in spelled form. Oral spelling and comprehension of orally spelled words is impaired in almost all other alexic syndromes, and is therefore useful in the diagnosis of pure alexia without agraphia. Reading may be completely absent at first. As recovery occurs, the patient may gain the ability

Table 6.3   Characteristics of pure alexia without agraphia

Feature	Characteristic
Spontaneous speech	Normal
Naming	Color naming difficulty
Auditory comprehension	Intact
Repetition	Intact
Reading	Impaired
Writing	Intact
Associated signs	Right hemianopsia; short-term memory loss; occasionally, motor, sensory signs
Localization	Left occipital lobe, splenium, medial temporal lobe

to recognize and name letters. The patient can then laboriously spell words out letter-by-letter, first aloud and then silently. Even at this stage, however, reading is slow and effortful, and reading for pleasure is impossible. Reading takes longer, or the error rates increase, as word length increases, presumably because of difficulty holding the letters in sequential memory. Such length-dependence of word reading is not seen in normal readers (Staller *et al.* 1978). Sometimes the patient will make errors in reading aloud; the beginnings of words are typically correct, but the endings may be guessed – for example, the patient may read 'medical' as 'medicine'. Writing remains intact, except that the patient cannot read his or her own written productions.

Associated symptoms and signs are quite different from those of alexia with agraphia. Primary motor and sensory deficits are usually absent. Occasional patients have partial right hemiparesis or hemisensory loss. Most patients, on the other hand, have a visual field deficit, either a hemianopia or a right upper quadrant defect. Rare patients have intact visual fields (Greenblatt 1973, 1977); some of these lose color vision in the right visual field ('hemiachromatopsia'; Damasio and Damasio 1983). These visual deficits are important to test for, since they may be the only elementary neurological deficits to aid in the detection of this syndrome.

Associated behavioral deficits in pure alexia include color anomia, visual agnosia, and memory loss. Geschwind and Fusillo (1966) analyzed the color naming difficulty in two patients with pure alexia. These patients could match and sort colors normally, indicating that the deficit is not a problem of visual perception. They could also name colors in the abstract, such as the typical color of a banana or the inside of a watermelon, so the problem is not an anomia (Damasio *et al.* 1979). These patients cannot associate a perceived color with its name. By Milner and Teuber's (1968) definition of an agnosia as a 'percept without a meaning', the name 'color agnosia' is a more correct designation for the syndrome than 'color anomia'. Occasionally the deficit in naming colors may extend even to pictures and objects, in which case the patient has a visual agnosia (see Chapter 8). Deficits in memory may manifest initially as confusion, but the sensorium then clears, and a pure short-term memory impairment remains. Immediate memory and memory for remote events are preserved. This memory loss can persist for weeks or months (see Chapter 11). Cases of pure alexia typically have no parietal lobe signs such as calculation difficulty or the other elements of the Gerstmann and angular gyrus syndromes.

Alexia without agraphia is specific for a consistent lesion site, the left posterior cerebral artery distribution in the medial occipital and medial temporal lobes, often including the splenium of the corpus callosum. A case example is shown in Figure 6.2. The left occipital lobe lesion produces a right homonymous hemianopia, while the lesion in the corpus callosum prevents visual information from the right occipital lobe from reaching left hemisphere language centers (see Figure 6.3, which is adapted from a similar figure in Dejerine's 1892 article). Alexia without agraphia, by this model, is a classic example of a 'disconnection syndrome'; that is, the symptoms result not from damage to a cortical center, but rather by interruption of connections between two centers.

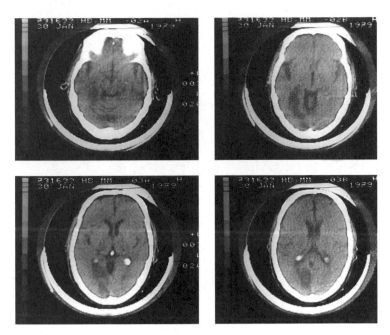

Figure 6.2 CT scan from a patient with pure alexia without agraphia. Note the infarction in the left medial occipital and medial temporal lobes, within the territory of the left posterior cerebral artery.

The complete syndrome of pure alexia without agraphia (alexia, color naming disorder, short-term memory loss, and right hemianopsia) results from occlusion of the posterior cerebral artery, with infarction of the occipitotemporal cortex, medial occipital cortex, splenium of the corpus callosum, and medial temporal cortex. If branches to the thalamus and cerebral peduncle are involved, right-sided motor and sensory deficits are associated. Those patients with more lateral occipital infarctions, sparing the splenium and medial occipital and temporal regions, have a more partial or transient alexia, sparing letters, and often sparing memory, color-naming, and visual field deficits (Johansson and Fahlgren 1979; Damasio and Damasio 1983).

A subgroup of patients with alexia without agraphia does not have a detectable right hemianopsia or quadrant defect. This syndrome has been termed 'subangular alexia' by Greenblatt (1973, 1977); the lesion does not affect the left occipital cortex or splenium, but rather the subcortical white matter in the parietal lobe, involving the connecting fibers from the occipital lobes to the left angular gyrus, where decoding of visual symbols into language is thought to take place.

Some patients with pure alexia, especially those without hemianopia, have been noted to have hemiachromatopsia, a color vision deficit in the affected visual field of patients who do not have a complete hemianopsia (Damasio and Damasio 1983). This deficit was present in Dejerine's original 1892 patient.

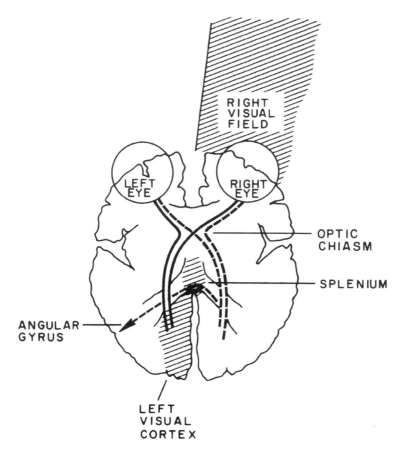

Figure 6.3 Disconnection model of alexia without agraphia, based on Dejerine's 1892 schema. Damage to the left visual cortex produces right hemianopsia. Visual information from the left visual field, perceived in the intact right occipital cortex, cannot reach the left angular gyrus because of damage to the splenium of the corpus callosum.

One last deficit often associated with alexia without agraphia is short-term memory loss, thought to result from involvement of the left hippocampus in the posterior medial temporal lobe. Despite the usual teaching that bilateral temporal lesions are required to produce lasting amnesia, unilateral left temporal lesions have been reported to cause clinically significant amnesia, especially for words (Benson *et al.* 1974; see Chapter 11). This deficit may contribute to the inability of a patient with pure alexia to read a sentence he or she has just written. Acutely, patients with left posterior cerebral artery territory strokes may seem confused or delirious (Devinsky *et al.* 1988); after the delirium clears, short-term memory loss remains.

Not all cases of pure alexia are caused by strokes. Other reported causes of pure alexia without agraphia, either on a transient or permanent basis, have included: a left occipital lesion including compression of the posterior cerebral artery in the course of transtentorial herniation from a frontal lobe tumor (Kirshner *et al.* 1982); occipital tumors (Greenblatt 1973; Vincent *et al.* 1977; Turgman *et al.* 1979); surgical resection of the left occipital lobe (Ajuriaguerra and Hecaen 1951); occipital lobe hemorrhage (Levine and Calvanio 1978); and traumatic brain injury (Lhermitte *et al.* 1929; Heilman *et al.* 1971). These conditions all affect the left occipital lobe, but not the splenium of the corpus callosum, raising further question about the necessity of anatomical disconnection as the cause of the disorder.

There are four simple bedside tests that distinguish between the syndromes of alexia with and without agraphia. First, test the patient's ability to recognize words spelled aloud. Patients with alexia without agraphia succeed, whereas those with alexia and agraphia fail. Second, have the patient copy written material, versus writing to dictation. Patients with alexia without agraphia write better to dictation than copying, while those with alexia with agraphia copy better than they write to dictation. Third, patients with alexia without agraphia can spell words orally and comprehend words spelled aloud to them, whereas patients with alexia and agraphia are usually impaired on both tasks. Calculations are also much more likely to be affected by lesions producing alexia with agraphia. Performance on these four bedside tasks indicates whether the lesion involves the occipital or parietal lobe.

Aphasic Alexia

Many patients with aphasia have associated alexia. Wernicke's aphasia, for example, frequently involves reading, though some patients have auditory comprehension impairment out of proportion to alexia, whereas others understand spoken language better than they can read. Patients with Wernicke's aphasia but relatively preserved auditory comprehension closely resemble the syndrome of alexia with agraphia.

In common usage, however, the term 'aphasic alexia' refers to the alexia associated with left frontal lesions and global or Broca's aphasia. Benson (1977) termed this the 'third alexia', following the two classical syndromes of alexia with and without agraphia. Aphasic alexia is also referred to as anterior or frontal alexia. Most patients with Broca's aphasia have difficulty in reading, usually out of proportion to auditory comprehension. Of Benson's series of 61 Broca's aphasics, all but 10 had significant reading deficits. As in both the expressive speech and auditory comprehension modalities, patients with Broca's aphasia often have difficulty with syntactic relationships. Broca's aphasics tend to comprehend familiar, meaningful words, such as nouns and verbs, but they become mixed up by phrases in which grammatical words or word endings determine the meaning. Phrases such as 'the book which Bill gave to Betty was boring' cause special difficulty for both reading and auditory comprehension; the patient may know that the sentence is about a gift book, but he cannot say whether Bill gave or received the book. Although these patients can read individual words, they cannot read texts for meaning.

In some patients the reading disorder affects even more elementary aspects of ability to derive meaning from printed symbols. In such severely impaired patients, naming individual letters may be difficult, a phenomenon first described in 1900 by Hinshelwood as 'letter blindness'. Benson *et al.* (1971) pointed out that the letter blindness of frontal lesions is different from the 'word blindness' seen in occipital lesions and the syndrome of alexia without agraphia. Patients can recognize and read short, familiar nouns and verbs, but not grammatical words or single letters. One famous patient could read 'be' but not 'b' (Gardner and Zurif 1975). This syndrome is sometimes referred to as 'literal alexia'. A long noun such as 'ambulance' may be read better than a connector word such as 'am'. In addition, these patients cannot read phonetically pronounceable non-words such as 'fod' or 'mip' (Kirshner and Webb 1982). The residual reading in such patients thus involves the recognition of whole, familiar words; processing of printed words into phonemes or letters is impossible. Most such patients also have severe agraphia. We shall return to this pattern of reading disorder later, under the term 'deep dyslexia'. It is important to recognize, however, that the one spared reading function in aphasic alexia, recognition of familiar words, is the precise function that is destroyed in the syndrome of pure alexia without agraphia.

The syndrome of aphasic alexia suggests that there are at least two ways in which an individual can read. The usual way is by visual perception of letters, translation of graphemes into phonemes, and then access to meaning. This is presumably the way we learn to read. The second way, seen in patients with acquired frontal lesions, is the direct access of familiar words to meaning. Figure 6.4 shows these two routes to reading. In this simple example, we have taken evidence from two acquired alexic syndromes to delineate the psycholinguistic processes

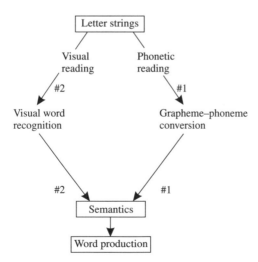

Figure 6.4 Two-part model of the reading system. Route 1 involves decoding of letter strings or graphemes into phonemes, then into semantics (meaning), and finally into oral production of the word. Route 2 involves direct recognition of words, with direct access to their meanings.

involved in reading. This type of analysis has been greatly expanded, as will be seen in the next section.

THE PSYCHOLINGUISTIC ANALYSIS OF ACQUIRED READING DISORDERS

Psycholinguists approach reading by defining the sequential cognitive operations required for reading, which they dissect out by testing individual patients with acquired reading disorders (Newcombe and Marshall 1981; Patterson 1981). These investigators have created models of the reading process, with component steps that are disrupted in specific cases. Part of this analysis involves the classification of reading errors (Marshall and Newcombe 1973; see Table 6.4).

In addition to hearing the patient's reading of a word, it is important to ascertain whether the patient has understood its meaning. For example, a patient who reads 'cat' as 'dog' (semantic error) or 'great' as 'greet (regularization or visual error) may perceive the correct meaning, or the meaning of the word chosen in error.

Psycholinguistic analysis of reading ability also makes use of specific classes of words that bring out differences in patients with different mechanisms of reading difficulty. Words vary in length, in frequency of occurrence, in concreteness or 'imageability', in part of speech (nouns, verbs, adjectives, function words), in regularity or phonetic character of spelling (for example, 'boat' is a regular word, 'yacht' is an irregular word), and in whether the word is a true word or a pronounceable non-word (e.g. 'hup'). All of these variables of words may influence the difficulty patients have in reading them.

Psycholinguistic Syndromes of Alexia
Letter-by-Letter Reading

'Letter-by letter alexia' (or 'dyslexia', as it is often called in psycholinguistic parlance), is the same syndrome as the traditional alexia without agraphia

Table 6.4   Classification of reading errors

Class of error	Description	Example
Visual error	Response looks like target	'canary' for 'carry'
Phonological error	Response sounds like target	'parody' for 'parrot'
Morphological error	Response shares word stem but different prefix/suffix	'edit' for 'edition'
Semantic error	Response related in meaning	'canary' for 'parrot'
Regularization error	Irregularly spelled word pronounced like regular one	'shoe' as 'show'
Homophone error	Meaning of homophone chosen in error	'billed' instead of 'build'

(Patterson and Kay 1982). Patients read aloud, letter by letter, rather than sounding out the whole word, and they then attempt to interpret the word based on the letter sequence they have named. As patients improve, they learn to do the letter-by-letter reading silently, but their latency to the identification of a printed word remains length-dependent, a phenomenon not seen in normal readers (Staller *et al.* 1978). Reading in these patients is always effortful and slow; they may scan the newspaper for headlines or sports scores of interest, but they rarely read for pleasure.

Whereas neurologists have emphasized the disconnection theory as the reason for alexia in this syndrome (see above), psycholinguists have emphasized that pure alexia or 'letter-by-letter reading' is a failure of one reading function, the ability to take in a word or visual word form at a glance. Warrington and Shallice (1980) referred to this type of alexia as 'visual word-form dyslexia'. The ability to take in a word at a glance appears to be a left occipital function; some investigators have related this deficit to an inability to perceive more than one stimulus at a time, called 'simultanagnosia' (Kinsbourne and Warrington 1962; Warrington and Rabin 1971). Levine and Calvanio (1978) interpreted the deficit as one of visual immediate memory; note the similarity to the discussion of conduction aphasia as either a disconnection of heard words from the structures that subserve repetition, versus an immediate auditory–verbal memory deficit (see Chapter 5). It is clear that normal, rapid reading requires perception of whole words; laborious, letter-by-letter or grapheme–phoneme reading is too slow and effortful to enable us to read novels or even the daily newspaper.

Deep Alexia (Dyslexia)

Deep dyslexia is similar to aphasic alexia, as defined above with regard to frontal lobe lesions and Broca's or global aphasia. Patients read mainly familiar words by recognition of the words and knowledge of their meaning (Saffran and Marin 1977; Kapur and Perl 1978). They cannot read phonetically, as in nonsense syllables, and sometimes they cannot name letters. Both letter naming and grapheme–phoneme reading appear to require the left hemisphere language cortex, especially the frontal lobe. Errors in deep alexia tend to be semantic ('jail' for 'prison') or visual ('perform for perfume'). Words seem to be directly recognized by access to their meaning. The ability of the subject to read a word is directly related to how common the word is, how concrete as opposed to abstract (or imageable versus nonimageable), and also whether the word is a noun or verb, as compared to adjective or adverb. Word length is not an important variable; as mentioned earlier, one famous patient could read 'ambulance' but not 'am'. Most patients with deep dyslexia have large left hemisphere lesions and significant nonfluent aphasia (Coltheart *et al.* 1980).

The ability to read familiar words by direct recognition of their meaning implies a separate mechanism of reading from the usual technique taught in elementary school, namely the ability to transform a printed letter string ('grapheme') into a sound (or 'phoneme'), and then to interpret its meaning. This is a rapid reading technique, but in deep dyslexia the words the subject can read are so limited that reading as a practical mode of communication is not possible.

The pathology involved in the deep alexia syndrome is incompletely known. Benson and Ardila (1996) point to involvement of the inferior frontal gyrus with extension into the anterior insula. Severe non-fluent aphasia may occur without associated alexia when the lesions do not involve the perisylvian region (Benson and Ardila 1996). Theories of the residual recognition or reading of familiar words have involved either spared areas of the left hemisphere, or perhaps the right hemisphere (Coltheart *et al.* 1980). Experiments on split-brain patients, reviewed in Chapter 12, suggest that the right hemisphere can read familiar words. A recent study utilizing PET scanning, however, has shown activation predominantly in adjacent left hemisphere cortical areas during reading of familiar words in two patients with deep alexia (Price *et al.* 1998).

Phonological Alexia (Dyslexia)

Phonological dyslexia is similar to deep dyslexia, with a loss of ability to read phonetically or to read non-words (Friedman 1995). In phonological dyslexia, however, single words are read relatively normally, and semantic errors are rare. The syndrome seems milder than deep dyslexia, since phonological dyslexics can read most words, and they can read aloud. They appear to read real words by a direct conversion of printed word to phonemes, without necessary access to meaning. This is called the lexical–phonological path to reading. Phonological dyslexia thus provides evidence of a third route to reading (see below).

Surface Alexia (Dyslexia)

Surface dyslexia is opposite to deep dyslexia, in that subjects can read only phonetically. They read nonsense syllables normally, but cannot read irregularly spelled words such as 'colonel', 'yacht', or 'wrench'. They may read 'pint' and 'lint' as if they rhyme, or they may read 'lout' and 'rough' with the same vowel sound. If they mispronounce a word, they interpret the meaning of the word pronounced in error; for example, a patient shown the word 'listen' pronounced it as 'Liston' and interpreted it as the famous boxer (Marshall and Newcombe 1973; Deloche *et al.* 1982). Other than such errors, however, patients with surface alexia can read words and recognize their meanings. They cannot, however, recognize words at a glance, and their reading is effortful, like that of elementary school children newly learning to read.

Psycholinguistic Model of Reading

The syndromes of deep, phonological, and surface dyslexia suggest that there are three separate pathways available in normal reading: a grapheme–phoneme route, a grapheme–semantics–phonology route, and a grapheme–word–phonology route (Figure 6.5). The grapheme–phoneme route is the laborious method by which we all learn to read, by sounding out each printed syllable, but more rapid reading requires the other two pathways. If grapheme–phoneme reading is the only method

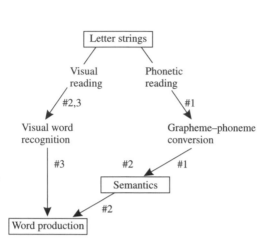

Figure 6.5 Three-part model of the reading system. In addition to the grapheme–phoneme reading and direct visual recognition–semantics reading pathways shown in Figure 6.4, this model suggests a third path to reading. Words are recognized and have direct access to output phonology, such that the subject can read aloud, but this third path does not have access to meaning. Patients can read aloud without necessarily understanding the words they read.

available, the patient has surface dyslexia. If it is lost, but both of the other two pathways are available, the patient has phonological dyslexia. If only the semantic route is available, the patient has deep dyslexia and can read only a few, common, imageable words.

AGRAPHIA: THE NEUROLOGY OF WRITING

Agraphia is defined as the disruption of previously intact writing skills by brain damage. Writing is generally very sensitive to impairment with acquired brain lesions, perhaps because it is the last learned and most complex language modality. In comparison to spoken language, writing requires the knowledge of how words are spelled. Most patients have less practice in writing as compared to speaking. In dementing illness and in acute confusional states, writing may be the most abnormal language function (Chedru and Geschwind 1972), and in mild aphasia the spelling errors in written productions may be the most sensitive key to the detection of these disorders.

Writing involves several elements: language processing, spelling, visual perception, visual–spatial orientation for graphic symbols, motor planning, and motor control of writing. A disturbance of any of these processes can impair writing, making the analysis of agraphia especially complex. Agraphia may occur by itself, or in association with aphasia, alexia, agnosia, and apraxia. Agraphia can also result from 'peripheral' involvement of the motor act of writing.

Dissociations in Speaking, Reading, Writing, and Spelling

Dissociations between reading and writing commonly occur. Not only can alexia exist without agraphia (see above), but agraphia can occur without alexia, a syndrome called pure agraphia. Disorders of reading and writing can also differ in the same syndrome, such as phonological dyslexia but surface agraphia (see below). The ability to spell can dissociate from the ability to write, or the ability to write in morse code, via typewriter, or in anagram letters may differ from standard writing. Patients have been described with preserved writing but impaired oral spelling (Kinsbourne and Warrington 1965), others with preserved spelling and impaired writing (Kinsbourne and Rosenfield 1974).

Classification of Agraphia

There are several ways to classify the agraphias (Lorch 1995). First, writing disorders can be classified by the underlying cognitive deficits: aphasic agraphia, apraxic agraphia, spatial agraphia. In addition, 'pure agraphia' indicates the absence of any other language or cognitive disorder. Another way of classifying agraphias is to divide writing into its component psycholinguistic steps and to analyze writing disorders according to the specific step that is disrupted. This classification is similar to the psycholinguistic categories of alexia discussed previously. In the psycholinguistic classification of agraphias, we first distinguish between 'central' agraphia, resulting from disorders of central language processing, and 'peripheral' agraphia, resulting from disorders of the motor aspect of writing. Central agraphias thus affect lexical (word choice), semantic (word meaning), and phonological processes, after which a 'graphemic' (written) version of the word is generated. The peripheral portion of writing involves selection of the proper letter string and the motor output to write it. The distinction between peripheral and central should not be taken as literal, neuroanatomical truth; peripheral agraphias frequently arise from central nervous system lesions (Ellis 1988). Rarely, patients may have both central and peripheral components of agraphia.

The agraphias are very complex, and it is not necessary for the average neurologist to commit all of the types of agraphia to memory. The principal classifications are included here for reference.

Central Agraphias
Aphasic Agraphia

For aphasic patients, writing is often the most severely impaired language modality. Writing tasks are typically more difficult for aphasics than either verbal or gestural tasks. Writing can be a very sensitive measure to detect mild aphasia (Critchley 1972). In aphasic patients, written language typically mirrors spoken language expression. In non-fluent aphasias (Broca's, global, and transcortical motor aphasia), speech is effortful and agrammatic, with short phrase length. Similarly, writing tends to be brief, effortful, clumsy, and lacking in syntax. Writing also permits the examination of the patient's spelling, which is often deficient as well (Wapner and Gardner 1979). Agrammatism is often more pronounced in patients' written than spoken language. An exception to this rule is aphemia, in which speech is non-fluent but writing is preserved. As discussed in Chapter 5, aphemia may not be a true aphasia, but rather a motor speech disorder akin to apraxia of speech.

The fluent aphasias, especially Wernicke's aphasia, also produce fluent errors in writing, and again the spelling errors are a sensitive measure of mild deficits. Some Wernicke's aphasics, unlike Broca's aphasics, write better than they speak. Occasional patients have dissociations between spoken and written language patterns, such as a patient with fluent, paraphasic speech but agrammatic written output with preserved nouns and verbs (Hier and Mohr 1977; Patterson and Shewell 1987).

As in the alexias, agraphias have been classified by the pattern of errors, which reflect the specific language-processing step that is deranged. The types of agraphia by this classification include phonological, deep, and surface agraphia. The parallel with the alexias should be obvious. Clinical neurologists who are not interested in linguistic approaches to the alexias and agraphias can skip the next sections.

Lexical (Surface, Orthographic) Agraphia   The syndrome of surface agraphia, also called lexical agraphia, is characterized by regularized spellings of words and phonologically plausible errors. Beauvois and Dérouesné (1981) described a patient with a left parieto-occipital arteriovenous malformation whose ability to write a word correctly depended on the frequency and regularity of the sound-to-spelling (phoneme-to-grapheme) correspondence. Errors typically consisted of phonologically plausible spellings (e.g. 'monsieur' was spelled as 'messieu'). The patient could spell pronounceable non-words. English speaking lexical (or surface) agraphic patients typically make errors in which words are misspelled but are phonologically plausible, such as 'spaid' for 'spade' or 'flud' for 'flood' (Hatfield and Patterson 1983) Lexical agraphia is associated with temporo-parieto-occipital lesions and posterior aphasia (Wernicke's, transcortical sensory, or anomic aphasia).

The cognitive deficit of lexical or surface agraphia is interpreted as an impairment in the ability to spell by access to word meanings; instead, words are accessed by knowledge of sound to spelling correspondence. Spelling is phonetic.

Phonological Agraphia   In phonological agraphia, irregular words or words with ambiguous spellings present no difficulty, but patients cannot spell non-words. These characteristics are in contrast to surface agraphia, in which non-words present no difficulty, but irregular words are spelled incorrectly. In addition, patients cannot spell words they did not know before their stroke or brain injury. Patients with phonological agraphia can spell and write words they know semantically, and they cannot use sound-to-spelling correspondences. Errors may visually resemble the target word (Hatfield 1985).

Phonological agraphia is typically seen in patients with lesions of the left supramarginal gyrus or underlying insula (Roeltgen *et al.* 1983). The type of aphasia varies with the exact size and location of lesion; phonological agraphia may be associated with Broca's, conduction, Wernicke's, or anomic aphasia (Alexander *et al.* 1992).

Deep Agraphia   Deep agraphia parallels deep dyslexia. As in phonological agraphia, patients have difficulty spelling non-words, but deep agraphics also show deficits in spelling certain classes of words. Words with concrete, imageable meanings are spelled more successfully than those with abstract meanings, and syntactic words (prepositions and conjunctions) present more difficulty than semantic words (nouns and verbs). The patient may occasionally be able to define a word he or she cannot spell. Errors may involve semantically related words, such as 'chair' for 'desk' or 'boat' for 'yacht' (Bub and Kertesz 1982). Lesions in deep agraphia generally involve the left parietal region, often including the supramarginal gyrus or insula but sparing the angular gyrus.

Semantic Agraphia   Patients with semantic agraphia have a selective inability to spell and write meaningful words, though they can spell irregular words and non-words. Often associated are aphasic deficits in comprehension. Semantic agraphics confuse homonyms in writing to dictation, even when given semantic information that should lead to the correct homonym. Examples of writing errors in semantic agraphia include 'not' instead of 'knot', 'lead' instead of 'led', or 'doe' instead of 'dough'. Similar errors occur in patients with surface agraphia or dementia, and in normals ('slips of the pen').

A variant of 'semantic agraphia' is the patient with 'asemantic writing' described by Patterson (1986). This patient, who had aphasia affecting auditory comprehension, could not write spontaneously but did write to dictation. He could not spell non-words. This pattern suggests that writing to dictation was being carried out through a direct auditory-to-graphemic whole word translation, without access to meaning. This writing performance is similar to the reading of patients with phonological dyslexia, who can sometimes read words without understanding them, or to the repetition ability of patients with mixed transcortical aphasia.

Unilateral (Callosal, Hemigraphia) Agraphia
In most cases of agraphia, the right and left hands are assumed to be equally impaired in writing, except for unilateral weakness or sensory loss resulting from the lesion causing the agraphia. In patients with surgical transection of the corpus callosum, writing is normal with the right hand but severely impaired with the left hand (Bogen 1969).

Unilateral agraphia may be aphasic agraphia or apraxic agraphia. Right-handers with left unilateral agraphia typically produce an illegible scrawl. The strong lateralization of written language in the left hemisphere for right-handers is underscored by the left hemispherectomy case of Burklund and Smith (1977). They observed that writing was initially the most impaired of language functions after left hemispherectomy, and that it recovered the most slowly postoperatively.

Writing and spelling are more variably affected in left-handed patients, as is the case with crossed aphasia (see Chapter 3).

Non-aphasic, peripheral agraphias occur in right-handers from right hemisphere lesions (see spatial agraphia, below.) A patient with Broca's aphasia may be unable to write with the left hand, in the presence of right hemiparesis. Although the patient's premorbid ability to write with the left hand might be questioned, most neurologically normal persons can write legibly, if awkwardly, with the left hand if forced to switch by a fracture, writer's cramp, or other abnormality of the right arm.

Writing prostheses resembling skates have been used to help right hemiparetic patients write with the weak arm, by means of partially spared proximal muscles. Interestingly, writing with the right, hemiplegic limb plus prosthesis is often better than that with the left, non-paralyzed limb. In one such patient (Whurr and Lorch 1991), treatment with the prosthesis reduced the spasticity in the hemiplegic right limb, after which the patient could write with the right hand unaided. The poorer performance with the left hand is not well understood, but may reflect non-linguistic factors such as apraxia.

Peripheral Agraphias

Peripheral agraphias are distinct from the central agraphias detailed above. The processes that go awry in the peripheral agraphias occur after the successful retrieval of a word and its spelling. Deficits may reflect difficulty with holding this graphemic information in a memory store (graphemic buffer) or in the subsequent stages of motor planning, programming and production of handwriting, oral spelling, or typing (Papagno 1992).

Graphemic Buffer Agraphia One type of peripheral agraphia is related to impairment in the graphemic buffer. The patient writes words no better than non-words, writes or types with equal success, and generally has a performance dependent on the length of the word. Errors occur more frequently in the middle of the word than at the beginning or end, reflecting difficulty with the memory store. Short words may be spelled correctly regardless of other variables. The lesion typically involves the angular gyrus.

The graphemic buffer is thought to represent letter identities and letter positions in the sequence. Information for each of these two variables may be lost selectively. The spellings may consist of the correct letters in transposed order. Alternatively, the patient may indicate the correct number of letters but not the specific letter names. Katz (1991), for example, reported a patient who could write only the first two or three letters correctly, regardless of the length of the target word. His accuracy was closely related to the temporal order in which the letters were written. This pattern of performance suggests that information on letter identity rapidly faded from the graphemic memory store. The lesion involved the left temporoparietal region, including the supramarginal gyrus, angular gyrus and posterior limb of the internal capsule. The patient had associated conduction aphasia, and his reading was classified as phonological dyslexia. In addition, the patient was unable to spell words aloud, involving a deficit in letter naming. In his written productions, the patient often mixed upper and lower case letters within a word (see ideational agraphia, below, for other letter case difficulties).

Allographic (Ideational, Physical-Letter-Code) Agraphia Patients with allographic agraphia have intact oral spelling and can type or use block letters successfully. Some patients have difficulty remembering which letter shapes correspond to which letter identities, but they can write individual letters well. The writing contains words with letter omissions, substitutions, insertions, and reversals, indicating that the sequence of letters is affected. Some letters, especially the most common ones, may be utilized better than other letters.

In cursive writing, letter shapes vary depending on the preceding and following letters, a pattern referred to as allographic variation. Patients with allographic agraphia have difficulties at the allographic level, when letter shape is determined in the context of the whole word. Similarly, patients may make errors in using capital versus small letters, or cursive versus printed letters, as well as in selection of the incorrect letter.

Baxter and Warrington (1986) reported a patient with a bilateral parieto-occipital tumor who could spell words orally but could not write even individual letters. She wrote upper case letters better than lower case ones in spontaneous productions, but she copied accurately. The patient showed no limb apraxia, and could draw objects from memory. She could often describe the letters she could not write. This agraphia is occasionally referred to as 'ideational agraphia' to draw an analogy to ideational apraxia (see Chapter 7).

Apraxic Agraphia (Transitional Agraphia)

Apraxic agraphia refers to writing difficulty caused by limb apraxia (see Chapter 7). In apraxic agraphia, writing to dictation is impaired but copying and oral spelling are preserved. Apraxic agraphia can be considered a peripheral agraphia, with difficulty in the motor production of the strokes necessary to produce letters. In contrast to the writing of patients with ideational agraphia, letters may be ill formed, but the differences between cases and print and script is maintained. Individual letter strokes can present difficulties, and letters may be written on top of one another. Letter substitutions are often determined by similarity in shape, such as 'H' for 'K' or 'u' for 'n'.

The term 'transitional agraphia' refers to the difficulty in transition from letter codes to graphomotor patterns. Letter imagery deficits may also occur. Lesions typically involve the left posterior parietal parasagittal region.

Spatial (Visuospatial, Afferent, Constructional) Agraphia

Spatial agraphia is typically associated with spatial difficulties in reading and calculations. The units of writing or calculation are spatially disorganized. The spatial array of letters on a page is disturbed. Individual letters may be erroneously separated or run together, and letters may have extra loops. Written lines may slant on the page. Writing may be crowded to the right, or an increasingly large left margin may be used in successive lines, a phenomenon related to neglect of the left half of space. The beginnings of words and lines may have more errors than the ends of words or lines. Even in typing, the patient may ignore the left side of the keyboard. Baxter and Warrington (1983) reported a patient with a right parietal lesion who could not write at all and made errors on word beginnings. The authors surmised that the problem was in deficient ability to visualize the word and then 'read' the letters orally, a spatial difficulty attributable to the right parietal lesion. This has been called 'neglect dysgraphia'. Spatial agraphia usually arises from a posterior right hemisphere lesion, and is often related to other 'constructional impairments' (Caramazza and Hillis 1990) (see Chapter 9).

Pure Agraphia

Pure agraphia results when the disturbance affects a component of writing not shared by other language functions. Pure agraphia is sometimes used to refer to writing disturbances arising from focal lesions, in contrast to 'isolated agraphia', which refers to writing disturbances arising from multifocal or diffuse disorders. Pure agraphia is often found as the only residual language disturbance after the recovery of a more general aphasia. A disproportionately large number of left-handers are found among patients with pure agraphia.

The incidence of pure agraphia is as rare as 2% of aphasic cases. At one time a writing area was thought to exist in the middle frontal gyrus, termed 'Exner's area' (Exner 1881). Figure 6.6 shows a CT scan from a patient with pure agraphia secondary to a left frontal lesion, though it would be difficult to specify a precise gyrus localization from this case. Lesions in the left middle frontal gyrus have only inconsistently been associated with pure agraphia. Parasagittal parietal lesions have also been associated with pure agraphia, and even subcortical lesions have been described. The wide range of lesion localizations that result in pure agraphias underscores the complexity of the processes involved in writing and spelling independent of those involved in spoken language and reading.

Pure agraphia following superior parietal damage may be associated with a defect of visually-guided hand movements. Auerbach and Alexander (1981) reported a patient with impaired production of writing spontaneously, to dictation, and copying, with good oral spelling. Spelling errors involved omission, substitution and repetition. Letters were poorly formed, with crossed lines and inappropriate loops. The lesion was in the left superior parietal lobe, an area thought to be responsible for the integration of cross-modal sensory information. The heteromodal parietal cortex overlies white matter pathways connecting visual association cortex (area 19) and motor association cortex (area 6).

The patient's native language also influences pure agraphia. Italian, for example, is entirely regular in spelling, and certain writing deficits might therefore be difficult to detect in Italian patients. English has many irregularly spelled words and is more sensitive to writing errors. Japanese writing has two separate systems of pictograms, kanji (pictorial ideograms), and kana, (phonograms more

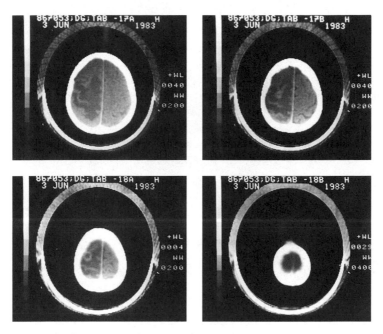

Figure 6.6 CT scan from a patient with pure agraphia. A small, ring-enhancing tumor in the left superior frontal region is surrounded by massive edema, or brain swelling. The patient had inability to write with virtually no other language deficits.

similar to English writing). A patient with pure kanji agraphia had a lesion in the foot of the middle frontal gyrus and adjacent portion of the precentral gyrus, while the patient with pure agraphia for kana had a lesion in the posterior two-thirds of the middle frontal gyrus only (Sakurai *et al.* 1997). The selectivity of these deficits parallels the separate processes of morphological (word recognition) and phonological (grapheme-phoneme) reading, as we saw in the syndromes of deep and surface alexia. These separate processes are more evident in Japanese than in English, because of the two systems of writing. Although the basic cognitive processes involved in producing meaningful graphic language are thought to be universal, different writing systems in specific languages reveal these underlying mechanisms of agraphia.

Isolated agraphia has been reported in diffuse encephalopathies and in confusional states associated with acute right middle cerebral artery infarctions (Chedru and Geschwind 1972).

CONCLUSION

Reading and writing disorders are highly complex in their clinical phenomenology and in the psycholinguistic classifications and models reviewed above. Psycholinguistic analysis of reading and writing performance is not needed in the typical behavioral neurology patient. For purposes of research, however, the behavioral complexity of the deficits has not yet been matched by precision in neuroanatomical analysis of lesions, and even single case research can make contributions. The most important aspect of reading and writing disorders is the necessity of testing these functions to detect deficits. Deficits in reading and writing are important in localization of brain lesions. In addition, they impair patients' ability to function in the world. A personal case of pure alexia discovered his own deficit only after going home from a hospitalization during which his stroke was not detected. Hence at least brief consideration to the patient's ability to read and write is important as part of the bedside mental status examination.

REFERENCES

Ajuriaguerra J, Hecaen H. La restauration functionelle après lobectomie occipitale. J Psychol (Paris) 1951;44:510–540.

Albert ML, Yamadori A, Gardner H, Howes D. Comprehension in alexia. Brain 1973;96: 317–328.

Alexander MP, Benson DF. The aphasias and related disturbances. 1999 In RJ Joynt (ed.), Clinical Neurology. Philadelphia: Lippincott, 1998:1–58.

Alexander MP, Friedman RB, Loverso F et al. Lesion localization in phonological agraphia. Brain Lang 1992;43:83–95.

Auerbach S, Alexander M. Pure agraphia and unilateral optic ataxia associated with a left superior parietal lobe lesion. J Neurol Neurosurg Psychiatry 1981;44:430–432.

Baxter D, Warrington E. Neglect dysgraphia. J Neurol Neurosurg Psychiatry 1983;46: 1073–1078.

Baxter D, Warrington E. Ideational agraphia; a single case study. J Neurol Neurosurg Psychiatry 1986;49:369–374.

Beauvois MF, Dérouesné J. Lexical or orthographic agraphia. Brain 1981;104;21–49.

Benson DF. The third alexia. Archives of Neurology 1977;34:327–331.

Benson DF, Ardila A. Aphasia: A clinical perspective. New York: Oxford University Press, 1996.

Benson DF, Denckla MB. Verbal paraphasia as a cause of calculation disturbances. Arch Neurol 1969;21:96–102.

Benson DF, Brown J, Tomlinson EB. Varieties of alexia: word and letter blindness. Neurology 1971;21:951–957.

Benson DF, Marsden CD, Meadows JC. The amnestic syndrome of posterior cerebral artery occlusion. Acta Neurol Scand 1974;50:133–145.

Benson DF, Cummings JC, Tsai SI. Angular gyrus syndrome simulating Alzheimer's disease. Arch Neurol 1982;39:616–620.

Benton AL. The fiction of the 'Gerstmann syndrome'. J Neurol Neurosurg Psychiatry 1961;24:176–181.

Benton AL. Gerstmann's syndrome. Arch Neurol 1992;49:445–447.

Bogen J. The other side of the brain: dysgraphia and dyscopia following cerebral commissurotomy. Bull LA Neurol Soc 1969;34:191–220.

Boller F, Grafman J. Acalculia: historical development and clinical significance. Brain Cogn 1983;2:205–223.

Bub D, Kertesz A. Deep agraphia. Brain Lang 1982;17:146–165.

Burklund C, Smith A. Language and the cerebral hemispheres: observations of verbal and non-verbal responses during 18 months following left ('dominant') hemispherectomy. Neurology 1977;27:627–633.

Caramazza A, Hillis A. Spatial representation of words in the brain implied by studies of a unilateral neglect patient. Nature 1990;346:267–269.

Chedru F, Geschwind N. Writing disturbances in acute confusional states. Neuropsychologia 1972;10:343–354.

Coltheart M, Patterson K, Marshall JC. Deep Dyslexia. London: Routledge & Kegan Paul, 1980.

Critchley M. The enigma of Gerstmann's syndrome. Brain 1966;89:183–198.

Critchley M. The detection of minimal dysphasia. In M Critchley, JL O'Leary, B Jennett (eds), Scientific Foundations of Neurology. London: Heinemann Medical Books, 1972. Reprinted in Critchley M. The Divine Banquet of the Brain. New York: Raven Press, 1979;63–71.

Croisile B, Laurent B, Michel D et al. Pure agraphia after deep left hemisphere hematoma. J Neurol Neurosurg Psychiatry 1990;53:263–265.

Damasio AR, Damasio H. The anatomic basis of pure alexia. Neurology 1983;33: 1573–1583.

Damasio A, Damasio H. Hemianopsia, hemiachromatopsia, and the mechanisms of alexia. Cortex 1986;22:161–170.

Damasio AR, McKee J, Damasio H. Determinants of performance in color anomia. Brain Lang 1979;7:74–85.

Dejerine J. Sur un cas de cecite verbale avec agraphie, suivi d'autopsie. Mem Soc Biol 1891;3:197–201.

Dejerine J. Contribution a l'étude anatomo-pathologique et clinique des differentes varietes de cecite verbale. Mem Soc Biol 1892;4:61 90.

Deloche G, Andreewsky E, Desi M. Surface dyslexia: a case report and some theoretical implications to reading models. Brain Lang 1982;15:12–31.

Devinsky O, Bear D, Volpe BT. Confusional states following posterior cerebral artery infarction. Arch Neurol 1988;45:160–163.

Ellis A. Normal writing processes and peripheral acquired dysgraphias. Lang Cogn Proc 1988;3:99–127.

Exner S. Untersuchungen über die lokalisation der funktionen. In Des Grosshirnrinde des Menschen. Vienna: Wilhelm Braumuller, 1881.

Friedman RB. Two types of phonological alexia. Cortex 1995;31:397–403.

Gardner H, Zurif E. Bee but not be: oral reading of single words in aphasia and alexia. Neuropsychologia 1975;13:181–190.

Gerstmann J. Zur symptomatologie der Hirnlasionen im Ubergangsgebiet der unteren Parietal- und mittleren Occipitalwindung (Das Syndrom: Fingeragnosie, Rechts-Links-Storung, Agraphie, Akalkulie). Nervenartzt 1930;691–695. Translated In Rottenberg DA, Hochberg FH (ed.), Neurological Classics in Modern Translation. New York: Hafner Press, 1977;150–154.

Geschwind N. Disconnection syndromes in animals and man. Brain 1965;88:237–294, 585–644.

Geschwind N, Fusillo M. Color-naming defects in association with alexia. Arch Neurol 1966;15:137–146.

Grafman J, Passafiume D, Faglioni P, Boller F. Calculation disturbances in adults with focal hemispheric damage. Cortex 1982;18:37–50.

Greenblatt S. Alexia without agraphia or hemianopsia. Brain 1973;96:307–316.

Greenblatt S. Subangular alexia without agraphia or hemianopsia. Brain Lang 1977;3:229–245.

Hatfield FM, Patterson K. Phonological spelling. Quart J Exp Psychology 1983;35: 451–458.

Hatfield F. Visual and phonological factors in acquired agraphia. Neuropsychologia 1985;23:13–29.

Hécaen H, Angelergues R. Etude anatomo-clinique de 280 cas de lesions retrorolandiques unilaterales des hemispheres cerebraux. Encephale 1961;6:533–562.

Heilman KM, Saffran E, Gewchwind N. Closed head trauma with aphasia. J Neurol Neurosurg Psychiatry 1971;34:265–269.

Hier DB, Mohr JP. Incongruous oral and written naming: Evidence for a subdivision of the syndromes of Wernicke's aphasia. Brain Lang 1977;4:115–126.

Hinshelwood J. Letter-, Word-, and Mind-Blindness. London, HK Lewis & Co Ltd, 1900.

Jackson M, Warrington EK. Arithmetic skills in patients with unilateral cerebral lesions. Cortex 1986;22:611–620.

Johansson T, Fahlgren H. Alexia without agraphia: lateral and medial infarction of left occipital lobe. Neurology 1979;29:390–393.

Kapur N, Perl NT. Recognition reading in paralexia. Cortex 1978;14:439–443.

Katz RB. Limited retention of information in the graphemic buffer. Cortex 1991;27:111–119.

Kinsbourne M, Rosenfield D. Agraphia selective for written spelling. Brain Lang 1974;1: 215–225.

Kinsbourne M, Warrington EK. A disorder of simultaneous form perception. Brain 1962; 86;461–486.

Kinsbourne M, Warrington E. A case showing selectively impaired oral spelling. J Neurol Neurosurg Psychiat 1965;28:563–566.

Kirshner HS, Webb WG. Word and letter reading and the mechanism of the third alexia. Arch Neurol 1982;39:84–87.

Kirshner HS, Staller J, Webb W, Sachs P. Transtentorial herniation with posterior cerebral artery territory infarction. A new mechanism of the syndrome of alexia without agraphia. Stroke 1982;13:243–246.

Levine DN, Calvanio R. A study of the visual defect in verbal alexia-simultanagnosia. Brain 1978;101:65–81.

Lhermitte J, deMassary J, Hugeuenin R. Syndrome occipital avec alexia pure d'origine traumatique. Rev Neurol (Paris) 1929;2:703–707.

Lorch MP. Disorders of writing and spelling. In HS Kirshner (ed.), Handbook of Neurological Speech and Language Disorders. New York: Marcel Dekker, Inc., 1995; 295–324.

Marshall JC, Newcombe F. Patterns of paralexia – a psycholinguistic approach. J Psycholing Res 1973;2:175–199.

Mazzoni M, Pardoni L, Giorgetti V, Arena R. Gerstmann's syndrome: a case report. Cortex 1990;26:459–467.

Milner B, Teuber HL. Alteration of perception and memory in man. In L Weiskrantz (ed.), Analysis of Behavioral Change. New York: Harper & Row, 1968.

Mohr JP. An unusual case of dyslexia with dysgraphia. Brain Lang 1976;3:324–334.

Morris HH, Luders H, Lesser RP et al. Transient neuropsychological abnormalities (including Gerstmann syndrome) during cortical stimulation. Neurology 1984;34:877–883.

Newcombe F, Marshall JC. On psycholinguistic classifications of the acquired dyslexias. Bull Orton Soc 1981;31:29–46.

Papagno C. A case of peripheral dysgraphia. Cogn Neuropsychol 1992;9:259–270.

Patterson KE. Neuropsychological approaches to the study of reading. Br J Psychiatry 1981;72:151–174.

Patterson KE. Lexical but nonsemantic spelling? Cogn Neuropsychol 1986;3:341–367.

Patterson K, Kay J. Letter-by-letter reading: psychological descriptions of a neurological syndrome. Q J Exp Psychol 1982;34A:411–441.

Patterson KE, Shewell C. Speak and spell: dissociations and word-class effects. In M Coltheart, G Sartori, R Job, eds. The cognitive neuropsychology of language. London: Erlbaum, 1987.

Price CJ, Howard D, Patterson K et al. A functional neuroimaging description of two deep dyslexic patients. J Cog Neurosci 1998;10:303–315.

Roeltgen D, Sevush S, Heilman K. Phonological agraphia: writing by the lexical-semantic route. Neurology 1983;33:755–765.

Roeltgen DP, Sevush S, Heilman KM. Pure Gerstmann's syndrome from a focal lesion. Arch Neurol 1983;40:46–47.

Rothi LJ, Heilman KM. Alexia and agraphia with spared spelling and letter recognition abilities. Brain Lang 1981;12:1–13.

Saffran EM, Marin OSM. Reading without phonology: evidence from aphasia. Q J Exp Psychol 1977;29:515–525.

Sakurai Y, Matsumura K, Iwatsubo T *et al*. Frontal pure agraphia for kanji or kana: dissociation between morphology and phonology. Neurology 1997;946–952.

Staller J, Buchanan D, Singer M, *et al*. Alexia without agraphia: an experimental case study. Brain Lang 1978;5:378–387.

Turgman J, Goldhammer Y, Graham J. Alexia without agraphia, due to brain tumor: a reversible syndrome. Ann Neurol 1979;6:265–268.

Varney NR. Gerstmann syndrome without aphasia: a longitudinal study. Brain Cogn 1984;3;1–9.

Vincent FM, Sadowsky CH, Saunders RL, Reeves AG. Alexia without agraphia, hemianopsia, or color-naming defect: a disconnection syndrome. Neurology 1977;27:689–691.

Wapner W, Gardner H. A study of spelling in aphasia. Brain Lang 1979;7:363–374.

Warrington EK, Rabin P. Visual span of apprehension in patients with unilateral cerebral lesions. Quart J Exp Psychology 1971;23:423–431.

Warrington EK, Shallice T. Word-form dyslexia. Brain 1980;103:99–112.

Whurr M, Lorch M. The use of a prosthesis to facilitate writing in aphasia. Aphasiology 1991;5:411–418.

7

Apraxia

So far as I know, it has not yet been observed – or at least not yet reported – that a human being might act with his right extremities as if he were a total imbecile, as if he understood neither questions nor commands, as if he could neither understand the value of objects nor the sense of printed or written words, yet prove by an intelligent use of his left extremities that all of those seemingly absent abilities were in reality present.

(Liepmann 1900)

Apraxia refers to a loss of the ability to carry out skilled or learned movements, as a result of brain disease. The German physician Hugo Liepmann (1900), who is generally credited with the original description of apraxia, considered the deficit a 'motor asymbolia', or loss of the symbolism for learned movements. Liepmann formulated neuroanatomic models to explain apraxia, much as Wernicke and Dejerine did for aphasia and alexia. Norman Geschwind (1975) revisited Liepmann's concepts and defined the apraxias as 'disorders of the execution of learned movement which cannot be accounted for either by weakness, incoordination, or sensory loss, or by incomprehension of or inattention to commands'. This definition says a great deal about what apraxia is not, but it does not provide much feeling for what it is. In practical terms, the apraxic patient cannot perform a motor act to command, yet he or she can understand the command and can perform the same act in another context, e.g., in response to imitation or with use of the actual object. The patient must also be demonstrated to understand the command, either by a verbal description of the act, or by choice of the correct act from a series of choices pantomimed by the examiner.

Liepmann described three principal varieties of apraxia: ideomotor apraxia, ideational apraxia, and limb-kinetic apraxia. Apraxia has been a confusing subject, for a large part because the term has been applied to a series of other motor phenomena. Table 7.1 lists the major disorders that have been called apraxias. The three Liepmann categories, ideomotor, ideational, and limb-kinetic apraxia,

Table 7.1 Types of apraxia

Traditional apraxias
Ideomotor apraxia
Ideational apraxia
Limb-kinetic apraxia

Other disorders called 'apraxia'
Apraxia of speech
Oral (buccolingual) apraxia
Constructional apraxia
Dressing apraxia
Oculomotor apraxia
Apraxia of eyelid opening
Gait apraxia

---

will be discussed in this chapter. The remaining apraxias do not all adhere to the Liepmann–Geschwind definition of apraxia, given above, and will be referred to only briefly.

'Apraxia of speech', or verbal apraxia, as discussed in Chapter 5, involves a motor programming disorder for sequential speech. Speech apraxia differs from dysarthria in that the phoneme errors are not consistent distortions, but rather a variable pattern of phoneme substitutions. Apraxia of speech is rarely seen in isolation, in which case comprehension and writing are normal, but usually it is mixed with aphasia. As to whether speech apraxia is a true apraxia, it is difficult to establish the criterion that the motor function of speech can be carried out normally in another context, other than speech itself. Controversy persists as to the apraxic nature of the disorder or whether it differs from aphemia (see Chapter 5), but the phenomena themselves remain important. Oral or bucco-facial apraxia, on the other hand, is a form of ideomotor apraxia involving the oral, facial, and tongue muscles. Oral apraxia is clearly analogous to ideomotor apraxia of the limbs, though the two can be dissociated in individual patients.

'Constructional apraxia' and 'dressing apraxia' are seen in patients with right hemisphere lesions, reflecting disordered visual–spatial perception and faulty body image rather than primary motor dysfunction. These topics are discussed in Chapter 9. Oculomotor apraxia refers to an inability to direct voluntary, conjugate gaze. This disorder may be congenital, as in the syndrome of ataxia-telangiectasia, or it may be related to acquired bilateral brain lesions (see the discussion of Balint's syndrome, under visual agnosias, in Chapter 8). Apraxia of eyelid opening is seen in some movement disorders (Goldstein and Cogan 1965) and rarely as an isolated disorder (Dewey and Maraganore 1994). Gait apraxia refers to an inability to walk, or an awkward gait, in the absence of muscular weakness or ataxia, as is seen in bilateral frontal lobe disease and hydrocephalus (Meyer and Barron 1960; Sudarsky 1990). Some patients have difficulty in initiating gait but perform better as they continue to walk. Normal gait involves a complex sequence of muscle contractions, easily deranged by the motor planning deficits seen in frontal lobe syndromes. Since it is difficult to prove that a motor sequence as complex as gait can be performed in a different context, it is more accurate to use the term 'frontal gait disorder' rather than 'gait apraxia'.

IDEOMOTOR APRAXIA

Ideomotor apraxia is the principal apraxia described by Liepmann, a separation of the idea of a movement from its execution. The diagnosis of ideomotor apraxia requires that the patient: (1) cannot carry out a motor command; (2) can be shown to understand the command; and (3) can perform the same motor act in a different context. For example, apraxic patients who are asked to demonstrate the use of a hammer may make no response or an incorrect response, such as pounding an imaginary nail with their fist ('use of the body part as object') or running their hand through their hair. Patients can show their understanding of the command, however, by describing verbally the act of hammering or by selecting the correct action from multiple choices demonstrated by the examiner. In addition, they perform the identical action either by manipulation of a real hammer or by imitation of the examiner's pantomime. In general, patients with ideomotor apraxia perform poorly to command, better but still clumsily to imitation, and best in using the actual object. Ideomotor apraxia is thus a separation of the idea of a movement from its execution, though both the idea itself and the movement itself are intact. This apraxia is evident more in the testing situation than in real life, but it may cause an examiner to misinterpret the failure to follow the command as a failure of comprehension (aphasia rather than apraxia). Asking the patient a series of yes/no questions will quickly establish that language comprehension is normal.

The phenomena of ideomotor apraxia are closely tied to the concept of cerebral dominance for skilled movement. According to this concept, the left premotor cortex of a right-handed person not only programs the more adept right limbs in learned motor patterns, but also the less adept left limbs. Dominance for skilled movement does not always correlate with language dominance, and not always even with handedness. These functions can be teased out in left-handed patients with 'crossed dominance'. Heilman and colleagues (1973), for example, reported a left-handed patient with left hemiparesis secondary to a right hemisphere stroke. The patient was not aphasic, but showed apraxia for commands involving the non-paralyzed right limbs. He thus appeared to have 'crossed' dominance in the left hemisphere for language, but in the right hemisphere for skilled motor actions. Studies on patients with surgical section of the corpus callosum also support left hemisphere dominance for skilled movement. For example, patients with corpus callosum section have more difficulty in programming movement of the right hand from visual displays of hand postures flashed to the right hemisphere (or left visual field) than in programming movement of the left hand from similar inputs to the left hemisphere (Gazzaniga *et al.* 1967).

Ideomotor apraxia is one of the classic disconnection syndromes, in which the behavioral disturbance can be explained not by direct damage to a cortical center, but by disconnection between two centers. Geschwind (1975) provided a simple neuroanatomic model for understanding apraxia, similar to the model for conduction aphasia presented in Chapter 5. The model consists of a series of steps, which are illustrated in Figure 7.1. When a patient carries out a spoken command, the command must first be heard, then decoded into language in Wernicke's area, then transmitted, via the arcuate fasciculus, to the left prefrontal cortex, which is dominant for skilled movement. If the command requires use of the right extremities, the left premotor area activates the appropriate motor neurons in the left motor cortex; if the act requires the left extremities, the information is transmitted across the corpus callosum to the right premotor area, which in turn activates the right motor cortex. Heilman *et al.* (1982) suggested an additional way-station in the left parietal lobe, a center for 'visuokinesthetic engrams' of skilled movements. The phenomena of ideomotor apraxia can be accounted for by lesions along the pathway from Wernicke's area to the motor cortex.

A lesion in the left temporal lobe, or Wernicke's area, renders the patient aphasic, unable to follow commands because of the failure to understand them. Such patients may have apraxia in addition to aphasia, however, in that they fail not only to follow commands, but also to imitate movements demonstrated by the examiner (DeRenzi *et al.* 1980; Kertesz and Hooper 1982). This failure of imitation can be considered as ideomotor apraxia, resulting from a disconnection of the perceived action from its execution in the left prefrontal area. The apraxia

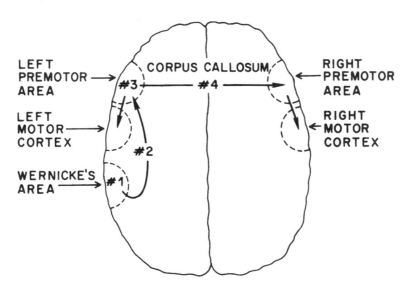

Figure 7.1 Lesion sites and pathways involved in ideomotor apraxia according to the Liepmann–Geschwind model. (1) Wernicke's area; (2) arcuate fasciculus; (3) left premotor cortex; (4) anterior part of the corpus callosum.

involves movement of both sides of the body, as neither motor cortex can be properly activated, and also movement of the face and lips, or 'oral apraxia'. Since most patients with Wernicke's aphasia have no hemiparesis, the apraxia is uncomplicated by weakness.

The second lesion involves the arcuate fasciculus, between the temporal lobe and the prefrontal cortex. This lesion classically causes conduction aphasia (see Chapter 5). Benson and colleagues (1973) pointed out that cases of conduction aphasia with parietal lesions also manifest ideomotor apraxia, while those with temporal lesions do not. While this apraxia should involve both the right and left extremities and the face, some patients have an associated right hemiparesis, and the apraxia is then evident only in the non-paralyzed, left extremities.

A lesion of the left premotor cortex itself usually results in Broca's aphasia and right hemiparesis. Many Broca's aphasics have intact comprehension, yet they perform commands clumsily with their non-paralyzed left limbs. This abnormal motor performance may be mistaken for poor comprehension or dismissed as normal for the non-dominant extremities. Normal people who are forced to use their left hand to write because of broken arms or similar injuries, however, rapidly become skillful in using the non-dominant hand. Geschwind (1975) considered this clumsy use of the left limbs in patients with left frontal lesions as the most common example of ideomotor apraxia, resulting from the lack of proper programming of learned movements by the damaged left prefrontal cortex.

The final lesion associated with ideomotor apraxia involves the anterior part of the corpus callosum, or the deep frontal white matter of either hemisphere, disconnecting the left from right premotor cortex. This 'callosal apraxia' is a selective apraxia of the left limbs; since the pathway for comprehension of commands, transmission to the left prefrontal cortex, and activation of the left motor cortex is intact, the patient can move the right limbs normally to command. Callosal apraxia is important to our understanding of the function of the corpus callosum in connecting the two cerebral hemispheres.

Examples of callosal apraxia date back to Liepmann and Maas (1907), who described a patient with a right hemiplegia and apraxia and agraphia of the non-paralyzed left limbs. At autopsy, the patient had an infarction in the left pons, accounting for the right hemiplegia, and a second lesion in the territory of the left anterior cerebral artery, including parts of the left frontal lobe and anterior corpus callosum, disconnecting the intact right premotor area from input from the left hemisphere. Geschwind and Kaplan (1962) rediscovered the callosal syndrome with a patient who had a left hemisphere glioblastoma and postoperative infarction of the anterior portion of the corpus callosum. This patient had profound apraxia of the left limbs. Other patients have been described involving either spontaneous lesions (Watson and Heilman 1983; Goldenberg *et al.* 1985; Graff-Radford *et al.* 1987) or surgical section of the corpus callosum, performed for treatment of intractable epilepsy. These surgical cases have shown a more variable degree of apraxia, often milder than the syndromes described by Liepmann and Maas (1907) and Geschwind and Kaplan (1962). For example, some patients could not indicate with the fingers of the left hand the corresponding areas touched on the right hand by the examiner. These patients also showed apraxia in imitating pictures of hand postures flashed tachistoscopically to the left visual field, suggesting that the right hemisphere had difficulty in programming fine movements of the ipsilateral, right hand. Patients with surgical section of the corpus callosum generally have a mild apraxia of the left hand, especially involving fine finger movements in response to verbal commands (Zaidel and Sperry 1977; Volpe *et al.* 1982). Corpus callosum lesions and behavioral deficits resulting from them are discussed further in Chapter 12.

As in aphasia, the detection of apraxia at the bedside can have practical importance in the localization of the responsible brain lesions. Recent studies on ideomotor apraxia have generally verified the lesion localizations predicted by the anatomic model of Liepmann and Geschwind, and also the close correlation between apraxia and aphasia. DeRenzi and colleagues (1980) studied 180 right-handed patients with unilateral brain lesions, examined for apraxia with a test involving only the imitation of the examiner's skilled movements. This methodology permits the diagnosis of apraxia even in patients with aphasia. Of patients with left brain lesions and aphasia, 80% also had apraxia, compared with only 5% of non-aphasic patients with left hemisphere lesions, and 20% of patients with right hemisphere lesions. The three most common aphasia types, global, Broca's, and Wernicke's aphasias, were all closely associated with apraxia; there were too few conduction aphasics for meaningful correlation. These correlations support the Liepmann–Geschwind anatomic model of apraxia, as depicted in Figure 7.1. The patients with right hemisphere lesions tended to have milder degrees of apraxia. DeRenzi *et al.* (1980), Kertesz *et al.* (1984), and Goodglass and Kaplan (1963) all found that the presence of aphasia and apraxia correlated closely, but the severity of the two deficits did not. Some patients had mild aphasia and severe apraxia, others had severe aphasia and mild apraxia. Recently, Meador and colleagues (1999) have correlated praxic errors and language errors during intracarotid amobarbital tests, used to determine language dominance preparatory to epilepsy surgery. In this study, language and praxic errors were correlated more closely with each other than with handedness, though patients with atypical dominance have more bilateral representation for both language and praxis. In summary, the correlation between aphasia and apraxia likely relates to the anatomic proximity of the structures involved in language and praxis, rather than to the shared symbolic nature of language and praxic behavior.

The relationship between ideomotor apraxia and aphasia is not only of theoretical and neuroanatomic interest, but also has important implications for the use of gestural communication in aphasia. Because aphasic patients are often apraxic as well, their capacity for gestural communication is often limited. In addition, gestural languages such as American Sign Language (ASL) involve linguistic symbolism as well as the use of learned motor acts (Bellugi and Klima 1979), and hence aphasic patients might be expected to be more deficient in this gestural system than in the simple gestures tested in bedside measures of praxis. In fact, however, gestural performance in aphasic patients has not correlated well with the symbolic content of the gestures (Pieczuro and Vignolo 1967; Kimura

1977). Even global aphasics may have the ability to learn simple gestural systems (Gardner *et al.* 1976; Helm-Estabrooks *et al.* 1982), as in Visual Action Therapy (Helm-Estabrooks *et al.* 1982), and more elaborate sign language can be useful in selected partial aphasic syndromes (Kirshner and Webb 1981; Peterson and Kirshner 1981). For example, patients with deficient auditory comprehension but preserved reading may be able to comprehend gestures, which share with reading the visual nature of the stimuli (Heilman *et al.* 1979; Varney 1978; Kirshner *et al.* 1981; Kirshner and Webb 1981). Gestural communication is being used increasingly in patients with acquired language disorders.

Oral or buccofacial apraxia refers to an inability to produce learned movement of the lips, mouth, and tongue in response to commands. As stated earlier, oral apraxia is considered a variety of ideomotor apraxia. In studies, however, oral apraxia does not always correlate with limb apraxia (Basso *et al.* 1987a; Raade *et al.* 1991). Left frontal lesions are most closely associated with oral apraxia, while both frontal and parietal lesions cause limb apraxia (Raade *et al.* 1991; Tognola and Vignolo 1980).

The disconnection model does not easily explain the occurrence of apraxia in patients with right hemisphere lesions. Right hemisphere lesions could cause apraxia by three possible mechanisms: (1) involvement of the deep frontal connections to the right premotor area; (2) right hemisphere dominance for skilled movement; or (3) faulty spatial perception and direction of movement. The right hemisphere might especially contribute to clumsy movements on tests of imitation, in which the subject must watch a movement and then reproduce the same movement pattern, as in the study of DeRenzi and colleagues (1980). Barbieri and DeRenzi (1988) attempted to tease out these factors by distinguishing the 'executive' aspect of motor performance, in an imitation test, from the 'ideational' aspect, as tested by asking the patient to gesture the use of an object. Of 56 patients with left hemisphere lesions, 57% scored in the apraxic range on the imitation test, 50% on the use of objects test. Of 38 patients with right hemisphere lesions, 34% scored in the apraxic range by the imitation test, but only 13% were apraxic by the use of objects test. Imitation testing is thus more sensitive to right hemisphere damage than apraxia testing to command.

Ideomotor apraxia has been reported not only with cortical lesions, but also with lesions of the basal ganglia (Agostoni *et al.* 1983; DeRenzi *et al.* 1986; Basso *et al.* 1987a). In a major review of apraxia in basal ganglia and subcortical lesions, Pramstaller and Marsden (1996) found only rare descriptions of apraxic behavior in lesions that purely affected the basal ganglia, but more frequent reports in combined lesions of the basal ganglia and deep white matter. These authors suggested that lesions in the vicinity of the putamen and anterior limb of the internal capsule impinge on the arcuate or superior longitudinal fasciculus, the white matter bundle connecting the temporoparietal and frontal lobes. Subcortical lesions may thus produce apraxia by a similar disconnection mechanism to that described above for cortical lesions (Geschwind 1975). Rarely, lesions of the thalamus have been associated with apraxia (Graff-Radford *et al.* 1984; Nadeau *et al.* 1994).

Ideomotor apraxia is also a feature of dementing illnesses (Foster *et al.* 1986; Rapcsak *et al.* 1989). Rapcsak and colleagues (1989) found apraxic deficits in patients with Alzheimer's disease, involving the pantomiming of transitive limb movements more than intransitive limb movements or movements of the trunk. As in patients with focal lesions of the left hemisphere, the presence of apraxia correlated with language deficits, especially auditory comprehension. Ideomotor apraxia has also been reported in the corticobasal degeneration syndrome (Graham *et al.* 1999). Cases of isolated, progressive apraxia have been reported in neurodegenerative illnesses, analogous to the syndrome of primary progressive aphasia (Leger *et al.* 1991; Azouvi *et al.* 1993; Rapcsak *et al.* 1995; Fukui *et al.* 1996).

The analysis of ideomotor apraxia is practically useful in the diagnosis and localization of left hemisphere lesions. Only deliberate testing reveals this information, as patients rarely complain of ideomotor apraxia. Recognition of the apraxic nature of deficits is important to the understanding of the functional difficulties these patients experience. In Broca's aphasia, for example, apraxic deficits may be mistaken for comprehension difficulty, and communication with the patient can be lost. Since ideomotor apraxia also occurs in patients with right hemisphere lesions and diffuse dementias, testing for apraxia is important in virtually all patients suspected of having cortical lesions.

IDEATIONAL APRAXIA

Ideational apraxia, the second of Liepmann's three varieties of apraxia, involves the loss of the 'idea' or concept of a movement. In practice, ideational apraxia has been defined in two major ways. Liepmann's (1900) original definition was the failure to carry out a sequential motor activity, when each component step could be performed separately. For example, the patient may be unable to use a coffee pot, coffee, and water to brew and pour a cup of coffee. The performance of a sequential act, of course, is more complex than a single action. Sequential acts require not only skilled movement, but also memory storage and sequential motor planning, which requires the normal functioning of the frontal lobes. For these reasons, apraxia for sequential actions is very sensitive to frontal lobe disease and is also commonly seen in dementing diseases (Rapcsak *et al.* 1989).

A second definition of ideational apraxia is a loss of ability to manipulate actual objects (DeRenzi *et al.* 1968; Ochipa *et al.* 1989, 1992; Heilman *et al.* 1997). Apraxia for real object use is a very different disorder from ideomotor apraxia, in that this apraxia interferes with everyday activities. Patients thus afflicted may be unable to care for themselves. Ochipa *et al.* (1992) have proposed the term 'conceptual apraxia' for this type of ideational apraxia.

DeRenzi and Luchelli (1988) investigated ideational apraxia in 20 right-handed patients with left hemisphere lesions. The testing involved sequential actions involving real objects. Most of the errors involved omission, misuse, or incorrect location of the part of the object to be acted upon, while only a small minority of errors involved faulty sequencing of steps. Thus ideational apraxia may be the same, whether defined as an inability to carry out a sequential action or a single action requiring use of a real object. In DeRenzi and Luchelli's patients (1988), ideational apraxia correlated poorly with ideomotor apraxia, suggesting a true separation between these two types of apraxia. Most of the patients with ideational apraxia had lesions of the posterior left temporoparietal junction.

Ochipa and colleagues (1989) studied the phenomena of ideational apraxia in a left-handed patient with a large left hemisphere stroke. This patient spontaneously misused objects, such as attempting to eat with a toothbrush or brush his teeth with a spoon. Although he had some aphasia, his language skills improved to the point that he could name objects, thus excluding an agnosic deficit or a failure to recognize the items, and he could point to objects on command, excluding a language comprehension deficit. In contrast, he was unable to identify objects by their function, to describe verbally the use of the objects, or to pantomime the use of the objects, and he could not demonstrate use of the actual objects. This patient thus appeared to have a loss of the 'how' knowledge of an object's use, despite preservation of the 'what' knowledge of the object's identity. This case is unusual because of the apparent crossed dominance for these two aspects of object knowledge. In the typical right-handed patient with a left hemisphere stroke, both aspects are impaired, and the patient's loss of object knowledge is masked by aphasia (inability to name objects or comprehend commands regarding their use). Patients with large left hemisphere strokes often misuse objects, but the nature of this misuse is unclear and is often referred to as 'confusion' rather than ideational apraxia. Heilman *et al.* (1997) also investigated 'conceptual apraxia' or tool-use apraxia in a series of right and left hemisphere stroke patients. In this study, conceptual apraxia correlated strongly with left hemisphere lesions, but no specific locus of injury could be determined. Ideational or conceptual apraxia also occurs in Alzheimer's disease (Ochipa *et al.* 1992).

LIMB-KINETIC APRAXIA

Limb-kinetic apraxia, the third of Liepmann's apraxia types, involves a motor disability of one limb, in the absence of gross weakness or ataxia. Often the patient has difficulty with fine finger movements and manipulation of small objects, though gross strength in the hand and arm is normal. Many stroke patients recover muscle strength but remain clumsy in fine movements and rapid manipulations with the affected limbs. Many neurologists regard this deficit as a mild pyramidal tract dysfunction, or elementary motor disorder, and not a true apraxia (Geschwind 1965). Heilman *et al.* (2000) investigated apraxic errors (referred to as a 'loss of deftness') during Wada testing in patients being evaluated for epilepsy surgery. Limb-kinetic apraxic errors, involving timing and sequence difficulties, could be differentiated from ideomotor errors. In patients with typical left hemisphere dominance, left hemisphere intracarotid barbiturate infusions produced limb-kinetic errors in both hands, whereas right hemisphere infusions affected only the left hand. The authors postulated that the dominant hemisphere programs the fine control of movements with either hand. In patients with atypical dominance (e.g. left-handedness), infusions in either hemisphere affected only the contralateral hand. This study can be taken as evidence for limb-kinetic apraxia as more than a subtle corticospinal tract deficit. Denes and colleagues (1998) also presented evidence from five cases that limb-kinetic apraxia has validity as a 'degradation of the innervatory patterns' of skilled motor actions. The deficit, unlike ideomotor apraxia, is consistent, occurring both with actions performed to command and those performed spontaneously. It usually involves the hand and arm, not the leg or oral apparatus. Most of the cases have involved neurodegenerative diseases, and in particular corticobasal degeneration, formerly called 'corticodentatorubral degeneration with neuronal achromasia' (Rebeiz et al. 1968; Leiguarda et al. 1994).

CONCLUSION

Apraxia is an intersection between cognitive and motor disorders, involving deficits in the concept and planning of skilled movements. It is an important window into the organization of the motor system in humans, and into the connections between the two hemispheres via the corpus callosum. Apraxia also affords understanding of the behavioral deficits of patients with strokes, other focal brain lesions, and neurodegenerative diseases. As in other areas of behavioral neurology, failure to test for apraxia can lead to an incomplete understanding of the patient's difficulty functioning in the world.

REFERENCES

Agostoni E, Coletti A, Orlando G, Tredici G. Apraxia in deep cerebral lesions. J Neurol Neurosurg Psychiat 1983;46:801–808.

Azouvi P, Bergego C, Robel L et al. Slowly progressive apraxia: two case studies. J Neurol 1993;240:347–350.

Barbieri C, DeRenzi E. The executive and ideational components of apraxia. Cortex 1988;24:535–543.

Basso A, Della Sala S, Farabola M. Aphasia arising from purely deep lesions. Cortex 1987a;23:29–44.

Basso A, Capitani E, Della Sala S et al. Recovery from ideomotor apraxia: a study on acute stroke patients. Brain 1987b;110:747–760.

Bellugi U, Klima ES. Language: perspectives from another modality. Ciba Found Symp 1979;69:99–117.

Benson DF, Sheremata WA, Bouchard R et al. Conduction aphasia. Arch Neurol 1973;18:339–346.

Denes G, Mantovan MC, Gallana A, Cappelletti JY. Limb-kinetic apraxia. Movement disorders 1998;13:468–476.

DeRenzi E, Luchelli F. Ideational apraxia. Brain 1988;111:1173–1185.

DeRenzi E, Pieczuro A, Vignolo LA. Ideational apraxia: a quantitative study. Neuropsychologia 1968;6:41–52.

DeRenzi E, Motti F, Nichelli P. Imitating gestures: a quantiative approach to ideomotor apraxia. Arch Neurol 1980;37:6–10.

DeRenzi E, Faglioni P, Scarpa M, Crisi G. Limb apraxia in patients with damage confined to the left basal ganglia and thalamus. J Neurol Neurosurg Psychiatry 1986;49: 1030–1038.

Dewey RB, Maraganore DM. Isolated eyelid-opening apraxia: report of a new levodopa-responsive syndrome. Neurology 1994;44:1752–1754.

Foster NL, Chase TN, Patronas NJ *et al.* Cerebral mapping of apraxia in Alzheimer's disease by positron emission tomography. Ann Neurol 1986;19:139–143.

Fukui T, Sugita K, Kawamura M *et al.* Primary progressive apraxia in Pick's disease. A clinicopathologic study. Neurology 1996:47:467–473.

Gardner H, Zurif EB, Berry T, Baker E. Visual communication in aphasia. Neuropsychologia 1976;14:275–292.

Gazzaniga MS, Bogen JE, Sperry RW. Dyspraxia following division of the cerebral commissures. Arch Neurol 1967;16:606–612.

Geschwind N. Disconnection syndromes in animals and man. Brain 1965;88:237–294, 585–644.

Geschwind N. The apraxias: neural mechanisms of disorders of learned movement. Am Sci 1975;63:188–195.

Geschwind N, Kaplan E. A human cerebral deconnection syndrome. Neurology 1962;12:675–685.

Goldenberg G, Wimmer A, Holzner F, Wessely P. Apraxia of the left limbs in a case of callosal disconnection: the contribution of medial frontal lobe damage. Cortex 1985; 21:135–148.

Goldstein JE, Cogan DG. Apraxia of eyelid opening. Arch Ophthalmol 1965;73:155–159.

Goodglass H, Kaplan E. Disturbance of gesture and pantomime in aphasia. Brain 1963; 86;703–720.

Graff-Radford NR, Eslinger PJ, Damasio AR, Yamada T. Nonhemorrhagic infarction of the thalamus: behavioral, anatomic, and physiologic correlates. Neurology 1984;34: 14–23.

Graff-Radford NR, Welsh K, Goderski J. Callosal apraxia. Neurology 1987;37:100–105.

Graham NL, Zeman A, Young AW *et al.* Dyspraxia in a patient with corticobasal degeneration: the role of visual and tactile inputs to action. J Neurol Neurosurg Psychiatry 1999;67:334–344.

Heilman KM, Coyle JM, Gonyea EF, Geschwind N. Apraxia and agraphia in a left-hander. Brain 1973;96:21–28.

Heilman KM, Rothi L, Campanella D, Wolfson S. Wernicke's and global aphasia without alexia. Arch Neurol 1979;36:129–133.

Heilman KM, Rothi LJ, Valenstein E. Two forms of ideomotor apraxia. Neurology 1982; 32:342–346.

Heilman KM, Maher LM, Greenwald ML, Rothi LJG. Conceptual apraxia from lateralized lesions. Neurology 1997;49:457–464.

Heilman KM, Meador KJ, Loring DW. Hemispheric asymmetries of limb-kinetic apraxia: a loss of deftness. Neurology 2000;55:523–526.

Helm-Estabrooks N, Fitzpatrick PM, Barresi B. Visual action therapy for global aphasia. J Speech Hear Disord 1982;47:385–389.

Kertesz A, Hooper E. Praxis and language: the extent and variety of apraxia in aphasia. Neuropsychologia 1982;20:276–286.

Kertesz A, Ferro JM, Shewan CM. Apraxia and aphasia: the functional–anatomical basis for their dissociation. Neurology 1984;34:40–47.

Kimura D. Acquisition of a motor skill after left-hemisphere damage. Brain 1977;100: 527–542.

Kirshner HS, Webb WG. Selective impairment of the auditory–verbal modality in an acquired communication disorder: benefit from sign language therapy. Brain Lang 1981;13:161–170.

Kirshner HS, Webb WG, Duncan GW. Word deafness in Wernicke's aphasia. J Neurol Neurosurg Psychiatry 1981;44:197–201.

Leger JM, Levasseur M, Benoit N *et al.* Apraxie d'aggravation lentement progressive: étude par IRM et tomographie a positons dans 4 cas. Rev Neurol (Paris) 1991;147:3: 183–191.

Leiguarda R, Lees AJ, Merello M *et al.* The nature of apraxia in corticobasal degeneration. J Neurol Neurosurg Psychiatry 1994;57:455–459.

Liepmann H. Das Krankheitsbild der apraxie ('motorischen asymbolie'). Monatschr Psychiatr Neurol 1900;8:15–44, 102–132, 182–197. Translated in part in Rottenberg DA and Hochberg FA. Neurological Classics in Modern Translation. New York: Hafner, 1977;155–181.

Liepmannn H, Maas O. Fall von linksseitiger Agraphie und Apraxie bei rechtsseitiger Lahmung. Z Psychologie Neurol 1907;10:214–227.

Meador KJ, Loring DW, Lee K *et al.* Cerebral lateralization. Relationship of language and ideomotor praxis. Neurology 1999;53:2028–2031.

Meyer JS, Barron DW. Apraxia of gait: a clinicophysiological study. Brain 1960;83: 261–284.

Nadeau SE, Roeltgen DP, Sevush S *et al.* Apraxia due to a pathologically documented thalamic infarction. Neurology 1994;44:2133–2137.

Ochipa C, Rothi LJG, Heilman KM. Ideational apraxia: a deficit in tool selection and use. Ann Neurol 1989;25:190–193.

Ochipa C, Gonzalez Rothi LJ, Heilman KM. Conceptual apraxia in Alzheimer's disease. Brain 1992;115:1061–1071.

Peterson LN, Kirshner HS. Gestural impairment and gestural ability in aphasia: a review. Brain Lang 1981;14:333–348.

Pieczuro A, Vignolo LA. Studio sperimentale sull' aprassia ideomotoria. Sist Nerv 1967; 19:131–143.

Pramstaller PP, Marsden CD. The basal ganglia and apraxia. Brain 1996;119:319–340.

Raade AS, Gonzalez-Rothi LJ, Heilman KM. The relationship between buccofacial and limb apraxia. Brain Cogn 1991;16:130–146.

Rapcsak SZ, Croswell SC, Rubens AB. Apraxia in Alzheimer's disease. Neurology 1989;39:664–668.

Rapcsak SZ, Ochipa C, Anderson KC, Poizner H. Progressive ideomotor apraxia: evidence for a selective impairment of the action production system. Brain Cogn 1995;27:213–236.

Rebeiz JJ, Kolodny EH, Richardson EP. Corticodentatonigral degeneration with neuronal achromasia. Arch Neurol 1968;18:20–33.

Sudarsky L. Geriatrics: gait disorders in the elderly. New Engl J Med 1990;322: 1441–1445.

Tognola G, Vignolo LA. Brain lesions associated with oral apraxia in stroke patients: a clinico-neuroradiological investigation with the CT scan. Neuropsychologia 1980; 18:257–272.

Varney N. Linguistic correlates of pantomime recognition in aphasic patients. J Neurol Neurosurg Psychiatry 1978;41:564–568.

Varney NR. Gerstmann syndrome without aphasia: a longitudinal study. Brain Cogn 1984;3:1–9.

Volpe BT, Sidtis JJ, Holtzman JD *et al.* Cortical mechanisms involved in praxis and observation following partial and complete section of the corpus callosum in man. Neurology 1982;32:645–650.

Watson RT, Heilman KM. Callosal apraxia. Brain 1983;106:391–403.

Zaidel E, Sperry RW. Some long-term effects of cerebral commisurotomy in man. Neuropsychologia 1977;15:193–203.

8

Agnosias

Sometimes a student would present himself, and Dr. P. would not recognize him; or, specifically, would not recognize his face. The moment the student spoke, he would be recognized by his voice. Such incidents multiplied, causing embarrassment, perplexity, fear – and, sometime, comedy. For not only did Dr. P. increasingly fail to see faces, but he saw faces when there were no faces to see: genially, Magoo-like, when in the street, he might pat the heads of water-hydrants and parking-meters, taking these to be the heads of children; he would amiably address carved knobs on the furniture, and be astounded when they did not reply.

(Sacks 1985)

Agnosias are disorders of recognition, as in Sacks' patient, who not only failed to recognize his wife's face but also mistook it for a hat (Sacks 1985). Sigmund Freud (1891) is generally credited with originating the term 'agnosia' in describing disturbances in the ability to recognize and name objects. Milner and Teuber (1968) defined agnosia as a 'normal percept...stripped of its meaning'. The agnosic patient perceives an object correctly, but fails to identify it or recognize what it is.

In order to meet diagnostic criteria for agnosia, the patient must: (1) fail to recognize or identify an object; (2) perceive the object normally, excluding an elementary sensory disorder; (3) name the object once it is recognized, excluding anomia as the cause of the failure to identify the object; and (4) not manifest a generalized dementia sufficient to explain the deficit. In practice, agnosias usually affect one sensory modality, and the patient is able to recognize the object when it is presented in a different sensory modality. For example, a patient with visual agnosia cannot identify a key ring by sight, but readily identifies it when touching the key ring or hearing the keys jingle.

Agnosias are defined in terms of the specific sensory modality affected: visual, auditory, and tactile. Agnosias may be selective for one class of items within a sensory modality, such as agnosia for colors, agnosia for visual objects, or agnosia for faces ('prosopagnosia'). In each case, it is necessary to establish that the agnosia is separable from primary sensory disorders and from other cognitive dysfunctions such as aphasia or dementia. The examiner must establish the preservation of normal sensory perception by performing tests of visual acuity, visual fields, auditory, and sensory functions as part of the standard neurological examination; the examiner likewise ensures the absence of aphasia and dementia by performing the bedside mental status examination. Naming deficits in aphasia or dementia should not be restricted to one sensory modality (see exceptions below), but rather should occur with all sensory stimuli.

Clinically, the agnosias are less common than the aphasias, alexias, or even apraxias. They are complex in behavioral description and in theoretical explanation. The lesions that produce agnosias are frequently diffuse or bilateral, as in hypoxic encephalopathy, multiple strokes, major head injuries, and neurodegenerative disorders and dementias. For this reason, agnosias are of less direct usefulness in lesion localization than the aphasias. The diagnosis of agnosia, however, does have considerable clinical importance. First, to delineate an agnosia is to create an important understanding of the patient's behavior. Second, the agnosias are fascinating windows into the workings of the brain and the processes of sensory perception and recognition. Third, these disorders may in some cases be the presenting symptoms of a bihemispheral degenerative disease.

The agnosias have aroused controversies since their first description. Agnosias are difficult to distinguish from primary sensory deficits on the one hand, and from cognitive dysfunctions such as aphasia or dementia on the other. In the visual modality, for example, cortical blindness is considered a primary visual disturbance, but patients with less complete loss of vision may show clear disorders of recognition and awareness. Visual perceptual deficits thus blend almost imperceptibly into the visual agnosias. In each modality, therefore, we shall begin with primary perceptual disorders and then proceed to the agnosias.

VISUAL AGNOSIAS
Cortical Visual Disturbances

Patients with bilateral occipital lobe damage may have complete blindness ('cortical blindness'), which is considered a primary sensory disorder rather than an agnosia (Aldrich *et al.* 1987). Some patients with cortical blindness are unaware that they cannot see and even confabulate the objects that they 'see', a phenomenon known as Anton's syndrome (Anton 1899). Such patients may attempt to walk and then bump into objects. Some confabulate visual experiences when asked what they see, whereas others admit to poor vision but blame it on incorrect glasses or poor lighting. Anton (1899) attributed the lack of awareness of blindness to interruption of white matter pathways from the occipital cortex to other sites. Although the absence of a subjective perception of 'blackness' or loss of vision seems surprising, loss of sensation secondary to cortical lesions frequently does not announce itself to the patient's subjective awareness. Even in normal individuals the limits of the visual fields are not consciously present; we are not consciously aware of a 'gap' in vision behind our heads, and we know instinctively to turn around when we hear a noise from behind. Patients with loss of vision from ocular disease are usually very aware of their visual loss, but patients with central visual loss are less so. Patients with hemianopias from occipital lesions frequently bump into objects in their blind fields, much more so than patients with ocular visual loss. Figure 8.1 shows a CT scan from a patient who suffered first a left and then a right occipital infarction. The patient had an initial deficit of pure alexia without agraphia (see Chapter 6) after the first stroke, then became totally blind, with neglect of blindness and severe short-term memory loss, after the second stroke.

Cortical blindness does not always involve a total absence of response to visual stimuli, despite the lack of subjective visual experience. In other words, some patients with bilateral occipital damage show evidence of residual vision of which they are not aware. This residual vision has been termed 'blindsight' or 'inverse Anton's syndrome' (Poppel *et al.* 1973; Perenin *et al.* 1980; Hartmann *et al.* 1991). Blindsight may be considered as an agnosic deficit, since the patient fails to recognize what little he or she sees. Such residual vision is generally absent in blindness secondary to diseases of the eyes, optic nerves, or optic tracts anterior to the lateral geniculate bodies. Primitive aspects of vision such as brightness, size, and movement of stimuli may be partially appreciated, whereas finer attributes such as shape, color, and depth fail to be perceived. (Brindley *et al.* 1969; Perenin

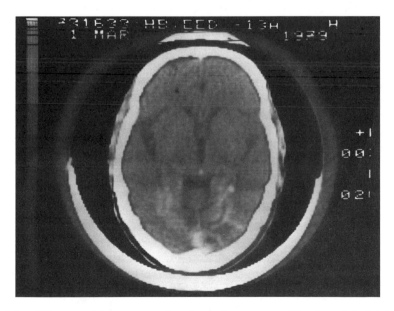

Figure 8.1 CT scan with contrast, showing enhancement of both occipital lobes. The patient had first left then right posterior cerebral artery territory infarctions, and had cortical blindness with neglect of deficit.

et al. 1980). Subjects may initiate eye movements towards objects they cannot see (Poppel *et al.* 1973). Milner and colleagues (1991) reported a woman with cortical blindness secondary to anoxia who could catch a ball she could not see, and she could insert a card into a slot, though she could not report the location or orientation of the slot. Blindsight may be mediated by subcortical connections, such as those from the optic tracts to the midbrain (Brindley *et al.* 1969).

Lesions causing cortical blindness may also be accompanied by visual hallucinations. Irritative lesions of the visual cortex (Brodmann area 17, striate or calcarine cortex) may produce unformed hallucinations of lines or spots, whereas more anterior stimulation in the occipital or temporal lobes may produce formed visual images (Forster 1936; Penfield and Perot 1963). Visual hallucinations in blindness are referred to as Bonnet's syndrome (McNamara *et al.* 1982). Although Bonnet originally described this phenomenon in a patient (his grandfather) with ocular blindness, it occurs more prominently in cortical forms of visual loss. Complex and varied visual hallucinations have been reported in patients with occipital lesions, presumably related to defective visual processing, or as a part of seizure activity (Manford and Andermann 1998). Visual hallucinations can occur during recovery from cortical blindness, and PET scanning has shown metabolic activation in the parieto-occipital cortex during such hallucinations, suggesting a hyperexcitability of the previously hypometabolic, recovering visual cortex (Wunderlich *et al.* 2000).

In practice, we diagnose cortical blindness by the absence of ocular pathology, preservation of the pupillary light reflexes, and the presence of associated neurological symptoms and signs. In addition to visual loss, patients with cortical blindness frequently manifest agitation, confusion, and short-term memory loss. Memory impairment is especially common in patients with bilateral strokes within the posterior cerebral artery territory, since this territory involves not only the occipital lobe, but also the medial temporal region, including the hippocampus. In the syndrome of 'top of the basilar embolus', cortical blindness may develop all at once, whereas other cases show first a hemianopia from a unilateral PCA stroke, then cortical blindness when the second side is affected (Ter Braak *et al.* 1971; Caplan 1980). Cortical blindness can also occur as a transient phenomenon after head trauma (Griffith and Dodge 1968; Greenblatt 1973), migraine (Hachinski *et al.* 1973), epileptic seizures (Barnet *et al.* 1970), and as a complication of arteriography (Stoddard *et al.* 1981) or myelography (Smirniotopoulos *et al.* 1984). Cortical blindness can develop in the setting of hypoxic–ischemic encephalopathy (Barnet *et al.* 1970; Milner *et al.* 1991; Wunderlich *et al.* 2000), meningitis (Barnet *et al.* 1970), systemic lupus erythematosis (Brandt *et al.* 1975), dementing conditions such as the Heidenhain variant of Creutzfeldt–Jakob disease (Heidenhain 1928) or the 'posterior dementia' variant of Alzheimer's disease (Cogan 1985; Benson *et al.* 1988; Victoroff *et al.* 1994), or in other disorders affecting both occipital lobes.

Cortical Visual Distortions

A myriad of positive visual phenomena have been described in syndromes of incomplete cortical visual loss. In both unilateral and bilateral visual field defects, distortions of vision occur, such as 'metamorphopsia' or distortion of shape (Bender and Kanzer 1941; Brau *et al*. 1986). Especially vivid examples of visual distortions occur in migraine, most commonly involving visual field defects (scotomas), often accompanied by positive, bright scintillating illusions or complex shapes such as 'fortification spectra' (teichopsia) (Richards 1971; Melen *et al*. 1978). Less common visual distortions in migraine include macropsia and micropsia or apparent enlargement or reduction of visual images (Hachinski *et al*. 1973; Cohen *et al*. 1994), and peculiar perversions of shape and size known as the 'Alice in Wonderland' syndrome (Golden 1979). Visual disturbances in migraine may relate to ischemia secondary to vasospasm or to spreading cortical depression, an electric depolarization that propagates slowly across the cerebral cortex at a rate that closely approximates the spread of the migraine aura. Other cortical visual disturbances described with disorders of the occipital cortex include achromatopsia or loss of color vision (Pearlman *et al*. 1979; Damasio *et al*. 1980; Zeki 1990); akinetopsia or loss of perception of motion (Zihl *et al*. 1983; Zeki 1991); palinopsia, or perseveration of visual images after the perceived objects have disappeared (Critchley 1951; Bender *et al*. 1968; Meadows *et al*. 1977; Michel and Troost 1980); and visual allesthesia, or spread of a visual image from a normal to a partially hemianopic visual field (Jacobs 1980). Occasionally, duplications of visual objects (polyopia or diplopia) also occur in occipital lobe disorders (Bender 1945). All of these deficits are considered to be disturbances of higher visual perception rather than agnosias.

Disorders of Color Vision

Two types of color vision deficit are associated with occipital lesions. Complete loss of color vision, or achromatopsia, may occur either bilaterally or in one hemifield with occipital lesions that spare the primary visual cortex (Brodmann area 17) but involve portions of the visual association cortex (Brodmann areas 18 and 19) (Pearlman *et al*. 1979; Damasio *et al*. 1980). Achromatopsia is a loss of color perception, not a color agnosia. As noted in Chapter 6, patients with pure alexia and lesions of the left occipital lobe may have a separate deficit of inability to name colors, though their color perception is normal (Geschwind and Fusillo 1966; Damasio *et al*. 1979). When asked to name a colored object, these patients may confabulate incorrect color names in a nearly random fashion. This deficit is sometimes called 'color anomia', but there is no anomia for the colors of familiar objects named from memory, such as the color of the sky or the inside of a watermelon. Rather, the color deficit of these patients meets the Milner and Teuber criterion of a 'percept without a meaning', for which the term 'color agnosia' is appropriate.

Balint's Syndrome and Simultanagnosia

In 1909, Balint described a syndrome in which patients appeared blind, yet were able to describe fine details of objects in central vision. The disorder is usually associated with bilateral occipital lobe lesions. Patients with Balint's syndrome often act totally blind, even bumping into walls as they walk, yet they can describe fine details of one small area of central vision.

The syndrome involves a triad of deficits: (1) psychic paralysis of gaze, or difficulty directing the eyes away from central fixation, also called 'ocular motor apraxia' (Cogan and Adams 1953); (2) 'optic ataxia', or incoordination of extremity movement under visual control, in the presence of accurate movement under proprioceptive control (for example, the patient may have difficulty reaching the cereal bowl with his spoon, but no difficulty bringing it back to his mouth); and (3) impaired visual attention. These deficits result in the perception of only small details of a visual scene, with loss of the ability to scan and perceive the 'big picture'. Patients with Balint's syndrome literally cannot see the forest for the trees. Some patients have visual field deficits, while others, with more anterior lesions, have full fields (Hecaen and Ajuriaguerra 1954).

Testing of patients with higher visual disturbances should include having the patient describe a complex drawing or photograph. Experimentally, Tyler showed that patients with Balint's syndrome make deficient eye movements when scanning a picture, explaining much of their visual disability (Tyler 1968). Patients with all three elements of Balint's syndrome generally have lesions of both parieto-occipital regions, sometimes with associated frontal lesions as well (Hecaen and Ajuriaguerra 1954; Hausser et al. 1980).

Partial deficits related to Balint's syndrome have also been described. For example, cases of isolated optic ataxia of one (Levine et al. 1978; Rizzo et al. 1992) or both (Boller et al. 1975; Damasio and Benton 1979) upper limbs have been seen with unilateral or bilateral parietal lesions. These disorders involve a difficulty with visually guided reaching towards a target. The mechanism of optic ataxia presumably involves disruption of visual information that must be transmitted to the premotor areas for visual direction of motor acts. Anatomically, optic ataxia may result from destruction of the visual areas or of the parietal centers for visuomotor integration, or 'disconnection' of visual and visuomotor centers from their frontal projections (Damasio and Benton 1979).

Another partial Balint's syndrome deficit is that of simultanagnosia, or loss of ability to perceive more than one item at a time (Wolpert 1924; Kinsbourne and Warrington 1962). This deficit amounts to a tendency to see details or parts of pictures or objects rather than the whole. Most such patients have left occipital lesions and associated pure alexia without agraphia (Levine and Calvanio 1978). The ability of pure alexics to read one letter at a time but not to recognize a word as a whole is a manifestation of the same type of perceptual deficit (Kinsbourne and Warrington 1962). Luria and colleagues also pointed out that faulty visual exploration by eye movements also contributes to simultanagnosia (Luria et al. 1963; Karpov et al. 1968). Robertson and colleagues (1997), in detailed studies of a patient with bilateral parieto-occipital strokes, also underlined the importance of spatial organization in the visual perceptual deficits of patients with Balint's syndrome.

Visual Object Agnosia

Visual object agnosia is the cornerstone of the concept of visual agnosia: the failure of recognition of objects by vision, with preserved ability to recognize them through touch or hearing, and in the absence of impaired primary visual perception or of a dementia sufficient to explain the deficit.

Lissauer (1890), who described the first well-documented case of visual agnosia, distinguished two subtypes: 'apperceptive' and 'associative' visual agnosia. According to Lissauer, there are two separable stages in object recognition: (1) an apperceptive stage, in which the perceived elements of the object are synthesized into a whole image; and (2) an associative stage, in which the meaning of the stimulus is appreciated by recall of previous visual experiences.

Apperceptive Visual Agnosia

The first type, apperceptive visual agnosia, is difficult to separate from impaired perception or partial cortical blindness. Patients with apperceptive visual agnosia can pick out features of an object correctly, such as lines, angles, colors, or movement, but they fail to appreciate the whole object (Luria 1966; Benson and Greenberg 1969; Grossman *et al.* 1997). Luria's patient, for example, misnamed eyeglasses as a bicycle, pointing to the two circles and a crossbar. Some patients show surprisingly good ability to navigate through doors and hallways (Benson and Greenberg 1969). Efron (1968) thought that apperceptive visual agnosia might be a selective perceptual deficit for visual shapes. Warrington and Rudge (1995) pointed to the right parietal cortex as the locus of lesions affecting the ability to identify visual objects; they categorize many of the bilateral occipital cases of apperceptive agnosia as 'pseudoagnosic syndromes' associated with early visual processing deficits.

Another way of analyzing apperceptive visual agnosia is by the analysis of global versus local perception, or the perception of the forest versus the trees. Posner (1987) suggested that an impaired 'spotlight' of visual attention may be the key to the deficit. Thaiss and DeBleser (1992) distinguished two separable functions of visual attention: a 'wide-angle attentional lens', which takes in the figure generally but perceives only gross features, and a narrow angle 'spotlight', which focuses on the fine visual details of one small area. Their patient appeared to have a faulty wide-angle attentional beam, such that she could identify small objects within drawings but often missed the overall context. Fink and colleagues (1996) studied visual perception in normal subjects with PET scan evaluation of areas of cortical activation. These authors found that right hemisphere sites, particularly the lingual gyrus, activated during global processing of figures, whereas left hemisphere sites, particularly the left inferior occipital cortex, activated during more local processing (the trees rather than the forest). The ability of patients with apperceptive visual agnosia to perceive fine details but not the whole picture is closely related to Balint's syndrome and simultanagnosia, discussed above.

As with all of the cortical visual syndromes, apperceptive visual agnosia is usually seen in patients with bilateral occipital lesions. It may be seen as a stage in recovery from complete cortical blindness. Warrington and James (1988) studied faulty visual object recognition in patients with unilateral posterior right hemisphere lesions. These deficits were especially apparent with recognition of degraded images, such as drawings or silhouettes rather than actual objects. Warrington and Rudge (1995), as mentioned above, reviewed the right parietal localization of apperceptive visual agnosia. Visual agnosia can also be part of dementing syndromes (Cogan *et al.* 1985; Benson *et al.* 1988; see also Chapter 13).

Associative Visual Agnosia

Associative visual agnosia, Lissauer's second type, is more closely related to the aphasias than to primary disorders of vision. Some of these patients can copy or match drawings of objects they cannot name, thus excluding a primary defect of visual perception, even for shapes. The failure to name the object is not considered as an aphasic deficit, since the patients can identify the same object presented in the tactile or auditory modality (Rubens and Benson 1971). Patients with associative visual agnosia often have other related recognition deficits, such as color agnosia, prosopagnosia (inability to recognize faces), and alexia, though visual agnosia can be present without alexia (Albert *et al.* 1975; Levine 1978). With all of these deficits, bilateral posterior hemisphere lesions are usually found (Benson *et al.* 1974; Albert *et al.* 1979), often involving the fusiform or occipito-temporal gyri, sometimes the lingual gyri, and adjacent white matter.

Jankowiak and colleagues (1992) described an extreme variant form of associative visual agnosia. The patient had bilateral parieto-occipital craniotomies for gunshot injuries. Visual acuity was nearly normal, except for bilateral upper ('altitudinal') visual field defects. He had mild anomia and reading difficulty, but no other evidence of aphasia. He had difficulty recognizing and naming colors, and even more difficulty with faces, objects, and pictures. He could copy drawings that he could not recognize, and could draw from memory copies of images flashed via tachistoscope for 100 milliseconds. This patient thus had not only normal perception, but also the ability to perceive, extract, and reproduce the key features of a visual pattern after a brief presentation. He could draw typical objects from memory, despite inability to identify these same objects, and he could correctly categorize drawings as real or unreal objects and as members of a specific class, such as animals. The crux of this patient's deficit was an inability to 'match the internal visual percept "in his mind's eye" with his representations of real visual stimuli'. The problem was not in the perception itself, but in assigning meaning to the item perceived.

Geschwind (1965) postulated that the bilateral lesions in visual agnosia prevent visual information from both occipital lobes from reaching the left hemisphere language areas, a 'disconnection syndrome' akin to the explanation of color agnosia given in Chapter 5. In fact, one case of associative visual agnosia was described with a unilateral left posterior cerebral artery territory infarction (McCarthy and Warrington 1986). This lesion did not involve the splenium of the corpus callosum or the right hemisphere by MRI scan, leading the authors to reject a disconnection explanation for the syndrome. Two well-studied autopsied cases of associative visual agnosia (Benson *et al.* 1974; Albert *et al.* 1979), however, had involvement of the fusiform or occipitotemporal gyri bilaterally, even though the visual field deficit was present only on the right, interrupting connections between the visual cortex and the language areas (for naming), and the medial temporal region (for memory). The disconnection hypothesis of visual agnosia remains viable, at least as a good way to remember the syndrome.

The subject of visual agnosia has long been controversial. Some skeptics have sought to dismiss the agnosias as combinations of elementary perceptual disturbances and dementia (Bay 1953; Bender and Feldman 1972). The cases just discussed make it clear that there are agnosic patients who are not aphasic, demented, or impaired in primary visual perception, yet cannot recognize objects. Precise classification of individual cases in terms of the type of agnosia and the complete preservation of visual perception, however, is often difficult. Riddoch and Humphreys (1987), for example, described a patient who appeared to have impaired visual perception, as shown by improved performance with greater stimulus duration, yet he could copy objects that he could not recognize, an ability usually diagnostic of associative visual agnosia. The deficit could not be completely categorized as apperceptive or associative; the authors proposed a specific deficiency in 'integration' of visual form information.

Optic Aphasia

The syndrome of optic aphasia or optic anomia is intermediate between the agnosias and the aphasias. The patient with optic aphasia fails to name objects presented in the visual modality, yet he or she can demonstrate recognition of the objects by pantomiming or describing their use (Lhermitte and Beauvois 1973; McCormick and Levine 1983; Coslett and Saffran 1989a). This preserved recognition of the objects is what distinguishes optic aphasia from associative visual agnosia. Like visual agnosics, patients with optic aphasia can name objects presented in the auditory or tactile modalities, distinguishing them from anomic aphasics. In optic aphasia, information about the object must reach the semantic system, such that the object is recognized, but the information is not sufficiently accessible to the language cortex to permit naming (Coslett and Saffran 1989a). Patients with optic aphasia may confabulate incorrect names when asked to name an object they clearly recognize. This confabulation of incorrect names is also seen in color agnosia; the language cortex seems to supply a name of one of the correct class of items when the specific information is not forthcoming. As in other types of confabulation, the brain appears unaware of a lack of information or of the substitution of an incorrect but related item. Patients with optic aphasia frequently manifest the associated deficits of alexia without agraphia and color agnosia, suggesting a left occipital lesion.

According to Geschwind's disconnection model (1965), optic aphasia, like pure alexia without agraphia (Chapter 5), represents a disconnection between the visual cortex in the occipital lobe and the left hemisphere language cortex. Presumably, the right hemisphere can recognize the object but cannot transmit the information to the left hemisphere for naming (Coslett and Saffran 1989a, 1989b). Plaut and Shallice (1993) also discussed the disconnection mechanism of optic aphasia as a breakdown between visual perception and semantics (naming).

Optic aphasia bears great similarity to pure alexia without agraphia (Chapter 6). Just as optic aphasics may recognize objects they cannot name, pure alexics may recognize words they cannot read (Riddoch and Humphreys 1987; Coslett and Saffran 1989b). In both cases, the right hemisphere is able to recognize objects and words, but the information cannot be accessed by the left hemisphere language centers. Most patients with pure alexia do not have difficulty recognizing and naming objects; their deficits are restricted to reading and naming colors. Subtle deficits in visual object naming have been described, however, such as greater difficulty with two-dimensional than three-dimensional drawings of objects (Damasio et al. 1979).

Prosopagnosia

Prosopagnosia refers to the inability to recognize faces. Patients fail to recognize close friends and relatives or pictures of famous people, unless they memorize details of size, hairstyle or color, and clothing. Prosopagnosia is restricted not only to the visual modality, but also to the class of faces; patients can recognize familiar people by voice, by mannerisms, and by posture or gait patterns (Bodamer 1947; Bornstein et al. 1959; Hécaen and Angelergues 1962). Oliver Sacks brought this syndrome to popular attention in *The Man Who Mistook his Wife for a Hat* (1985).

Facial recognition is often tested by matching of pictures of unfamiliar faces, taken from different angles. DeRenzi and colleagues (1991) pointed out, however, that matching of unfamiliar faces is a different function from recognition of familiar faces. These authors suggested that failure to match new faces reflects an apperceptive facial recognition deficit ('apperceptive prosopagnosia'), while failure to recognize familiar faces is an 'associative prosopagnosia'. The two functions are dissociated in some patients with prosopagnosia (Benton and Van Allen 1972; Malone et al. 1982; DeRenzi et al. 1991). Others have examined the recognition of emotional facial expressions, a function that appears localized to the right hemisphere (Rapcsak et al. 1989). It is important to specify exactly which type of facial recognition is meant when describing deficits in prosopagnosia.

In clinical studies, prosopagnosia may be either an isolated deficit or a part of a more general visual agnosia for objects and colors. Even pure prosopagnosia may not be truly restricted to faces; deficits have been discovered in the recognition of other complex but familiar visual stimuli such as architectural landmarks or pets (Beyn and Knyazeva 1962; Whiteley and Warrington 1977; Levine et al. 1978; Damasio et al. 1982). Humphreys (1996) reviewed evidence that living things may be recognized in a different part of the occipital cortex from nonliving things; the paper is entitled 'The man who mistook his dog for a cat.' Faces may thus not be a truly unique class of items that these patients cannot recognize, but they are surely the most individualized of visual displays.

The anatomic localization of prosopagnosia has been long debated. Early studies postulated a right hemisphere lesion based on the frequent association of left visual field defects, constructional and dressing apraxia, and left neglect (Hécaen and Angelergues 1962). More recent studies have demonstrated bilateral lesions in the temporo-occipital regions, often involving the fusiform or occipitotemporal gyri (Benson *et al.* 1974; Meadows 1974; Cohn *et al.* 1977; Damasio *et al.* 1982). Cases with unilateral posterior right hemisphere lesions have also been described (Michel *et al.*, 1986; Landis *et al.* 1988).

The mechanism of prosopagnosia could reflect a more generalized visual agnosia, or a specific loss of the function of facial recognition, which may reside in the fusiform gyri (Whiteley and Warrington 1977). The disconnection hypothesis has also been invoked, as in visual agnosia: an interruption of fibers passing from the occipital cortices to the centers where memories of faces are stored (Damasio *et al.* 1982). Prosopagnosia can also occur in dementing illnesses (Kurucz and Feldmar 1979). The importance of the diagnosis of prosopagnosia, besides the understanding of the patient's symptoms, is the likely presence of a unilateral or bilateral temporo-occipital lesion.

The Kluver–Bucy Syndrome

Another form of visual agnosia is the 'psychic blindness' seen in the Kluver–Bucy syndrome (Kluver and Bucy 1939). This syndrome was originally described in monkeys with bilateral temporal lobectomies, but similar symptoms have been described in humans with bilateral temporal lobe lesions. An animal with the Kluver–Bucy syndrome may inappropriately try to eat or mate with objects, or fail to show customary fear or hostility when faced with a natural enemy. Human patients manifest visual agnosia and often prosopagnosia, together with marked memory loss, variable aphasic deficits, and changes in behavior such as placidity, altered sexual orientation, and excessive eating (Lilly *et al.* 1983). Cases of the human Kluver–Bucy syndrome have been reported with bitemporal damage from surgical ablation (Terzian and Dalle Ore 1955), Herpes simplex encephalitis (Marlowe *et al.* 1975; Lilly *et al.* 1983), and dementing conditions such as Pick's disease (Cummings *et al.* 1981; Lilly *et al.* 1983). Patients with Kluver–Bucy syndrome appear to have no major deficits of primary visual perception, but connections appear to be disrupted between vision and memory and limbic structures, so that visual percepts do not arouse their ordinary associations. The prominent changes in speech, memory, affect, behavior, and personality overshadow the visual deficits in the human Kluver–Bucy syndrome.

Visual Agnosia in Dementia

Visual agnosia can be seen in dementing illnesses such as Alzheimer's disease. A variant syndrome of 'posterior dementia' has been described, in which higher visual disturbances are the presenting or most prominent symptoms of the disease (Cogan 1985; Victoroff *et al.* 1994). These disorders will be discussed further in Chapter 13 (dementia).

AUDITORY AGNOSIAS

Like cortical visual syndromes, cortical auditory disorders are complex conditions, ranging from complete cortical deafness to partial deficits of recognition of specific types of sound. As with the visual agnosias, most cortical auditory deficits require bilateral cerebral lesions, in this case of both temporal lobes, especially Heschl's gyri.

Cortical Deafness

Profound hearing deficits are seen in patients with acquired lesions of both primary cortical auditory areas (Heschl's gyrus, Brodmann areas 41 and 42 in each superior temporal gurus) or of the auditory radiations projecting to these areas. In general, unilateral lesions of the auditory cortex do not have clinically appreciable effects on hearing. Most patients with complete cortical deafness have had bilateral strokes; often the hearing disorder becomes evident only after the second of two strokes (Jerger *et al.* 1969; Kanshepolski *et al.* 1973; Barraquer-Bondas *et al.* 1980; Kirshner and Webb 1981; Musiek and Lee 1988; Bahls *et al.* 1988). Rare patients appear completely deaf on first examination, failing to respond even to loud noises (Jerger *et al.* 1969). Only a few patients with cortical deafness have no hearing at all; some have nearly normal pure tone hearing, but have deficits in temporal sequencing or sound localization (Jerger *et al.* 1969). As in visual agnosia, the distinction between cortical auditory deficits and auditory agnosia is difficult.

A patient with auditory agnosia can hear noises but not appreciate their meanings, as in identifying animal cries or sounds associated with specific objects, such as the ringing of a bell. Most such patients also cannot understand speech or appreciate music. Auditory agnosias can be divided into: (1) pure word deafness; (2) pure non-verbal auditory agnosia; (3) pure amusia; and (4) mixtures of the other three deficits.

Pure Word Deafness

The syndrome of pure word deafness, as discussed in Chapter 5, refers to a failure of comprehension of spoken words, with preserved ability to hear and recognize non-verbal sounds. Patients with bilateral temporal lobe lesions and pure word deafness often manifest more general auditory deficits early in their course (Mendez and Geehan 1988) and have abnormalities of other auditory parameters such as temporal sequencing (Tanake *et al.* 1987), loudness discrimination and auditory threshold duration (Kanshepolsky *et al.* 1973), or auditory reaction time (Buchtel and Stewart 1989). Such deficits link pure word deafness to primary auditory disorders and to an apperceptive rather than associative form of agnosia, by Lissauer's (1890) dichotomy for visual agnosia.

As stated in Chapter 5, pure word deafness has generally been explained as a disconnection of both primary auditory cortices from the left hemisphere Wernicke's area. Coslett and colleagues (1984), however, suggested that pure word deafness is associated with bilateral lesions of the auditory cortex, while non-verbal auditory sound recognition may be mediated by other parts of the auditory system, perhaps auditory association areas. Indeed, Engelien and colleagues (2000) showed activation on PET scanning during auditory stimulation in a patient with extensive bilateral temporal lesions, a phenomenon they referred to as 'deaf hearing' (analogous to 'blind sight'). Unilateral left hemisphere lesions have also been associated with pure word deafness; Geschwind (1970) postulated that such lesions are strategically placed so as to disconnect both primary auditory cortices from Wernicke's area. A recent case of pure word deafness with such a lesion has been reported (Takahashi *et al.* 1992). As discussed in Chapter 5, some patients with Wernicke's aphasia have more severe involvement of auditory comprehension than reading, also resembling pure word deafness (Kirshner *et al.* 1989). In a review of pure word deafness, Goldstein (1974) found that most cases have had paraphasic speech, further linking the syndrome to Wernicke's aphasia. Figure 8.2 shows a CT scan from a patient with extensive bilateral infarctions

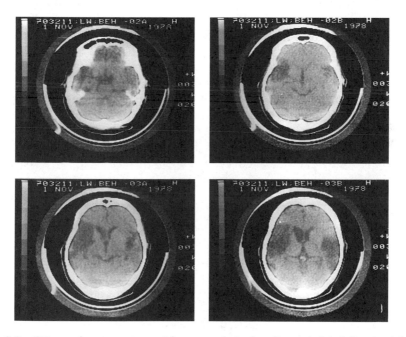

Figure 8.2 CT scan from a patient with severe cortical auditory deficit following bilateral middle cerebral artery strokes. Note the extensive damage to both temporal lobes. (Reprinted with permission from Kirshner and Webb 1981.)

involving the temporal lobes. The patient could hear pure tones and non-verbal sounds, but was completely unable to comprehend speech.

Auditory Non-Verbal Agnosia

Auditory non-verbal agnosia refers to patients who have lost the ability to identify meaningful non-verbal sounds but have preserved pure tone hearing and language comprehension. Such cases are rare but well documented (Spreen *et al.* 1965; Albert *et al.* 1972; Motomura *et al.* 1986), usually involving bihemispheral lesions. Vignolo (1982) distinguished a 'semantic-associative' type, with loss of ability to recognize familiar sounds, from a 'discriminative' type, involving failure to match two meaningless sounds. This distinction is closely related to the apperceptive–associative dichotomy of Lissauer (1890) for visual agnosia. Vignolo tested each function in patients with unilateral lesions, and found that the semantic–associative type correlated with aphasia and left hemisphere damage, while the discriminative type correlated with right hemisphere damage.

Amusias

The loss of musical abilities after focal brain lesions is complex, reflecting the complexity of musical appreciation and analysis. The evidence suggests that recognition of melodies and musical tones may be a right temporal function, whereas analysis of pitch, rhythm, and tempo involves the left temporal lobe (Bever and Chiarello 1974). Brain electrical activity mapping, an EEG technique, showed relative right hemisphere activation with melody, left temporal activation for scales (Breitling *et al.* 1987). The left hemisphere may be called on more when a trained musician listens to a musical piece, as compared with an untrained listener (Bever and Chiarello 1974), though a study using dichotic listening found only minimal differences between normal trained versus untrained subjects (Prior and Troup 1988). A recent study examined cortical activation by positron emission tomography scanning during musical performance in ten professional pianists (Sergent *et al.* 1992). Sight-reading of music activated both visual association cortices and the superior parietal lobes, areas distinct from those utilized in reading words. Listening to music activated both secondary auditory cortices, while playing of music activated frontal and cerebellar areas. The authors commented that, widespread as these areas were, the study did not examine the whole of musical experience, let alone the pleasure afforded by music.

The case studies of musical abilities in patients with focal brain lesions are surprisingly limited. Patients with bitemporal lesions and the syndromes of cortical deafness, auditory agnosia, and pure word deafness often have disturbance of musical abilities (Jerger *et al.* 1969). Selective loss of ability to appreciate and produce music, recognize familiar tunes, and even make simple judgments about musical pitch or rhythm have been associated with right hemisphere damage, especially right temporoparietal (McFarland and Fortin 1982) but also right frontal (Botez and Wertheim 1959) lesions. Right temporal lobectomy for epilepsy impairs perception of melody (Shankweiler 1966). Injection of barbiturates into the right carotid artery during the Wada test impairs singing (Gordon and Bogen 1974). Kinsella and colleagues (1988), however, found impaired singing with both left and right hemisphere lesions. Aphasic patients with left hemisphere damage may seem normally able to appreciate music and sing tones, but left hemisphere lesions may disturb the reading and writing of music (Brust 1980). The composer Maurice Ravel suffered an illness of progressive fluent aphasia, in association with which he lost the ability to read or write music, while he could still listen to and appreciate it (Alajouanine 1948; Sergent 1993). Polk and Kertesz (1993) have also reported progressive musical dysfunction in two professional musicians with dementing illness.

While musical functions do not appear localized to specific or even unilateral brain foci, the evidence from patients with focal lesions does suggest a relative right hemisphere dominance for perception of musical tones and of the left hemisphere for learned aspects of reading and writing music. Lesions of either hemisphere may affect singing. Considerable further research is needed on the complex relationships of music and the brain.

The preservation of unlearned musical abilities in patients with aphasia has been utilized in a form of speech therapy called 'Melodic Intonation Therapy' (Sparks *et al.* 1974). Many aphasic patients can hum melodies and sing familiar songs. They can be trained to intune words, even when they cannot say the words without music. With repetition, subjects gradually become able to say the words without singing. Presumably, right hemisphere musical abilities serve a facilitating role in the production of words.

TACTILE AGNOSIAS

As with the syndromes of cortical loss of auditory and visual perception, a range of sensory deficits is seen with cortical lesions. Patients with lesions of the parietal cortex may have preserved ability to feel pinprick, temperature, vibration, and proprioception, yet they fail to identify objects palpated by the contralateral hand or to recognize numbers or letters written on the opposite side of the body (Hécaen and David 1945; Semmes 1965). These deficits, called 'astereognosis' and 'agraphesthesia', respectively, are considered to represent cortical sensory loss rather than a true agnosia. Alternatively, they could be considered as apperceptive tactile agnosias. Rare cases have been described of patients who can describe the shape and features of a palpated object, yet cannot identify the object (Hécaen and David 1945). The patient can readily identify the object by sound or sight, thereby fulfilling the criteria for a true associative tactile agnosia.

Caselli (1991a) investigated 84 patients with unilateral hemisphere lesions for deficits in tactile perception. Seven patients were found with tactile agnosia for objects palpated by the contralateral hand. These deficits occurred in the absence of primary somatosensory loss. Some patients had severe hemiparesis or hemianopia yet performed well in tactile object recognition, but patients with neglect secondary to right hemisphere lesions tended to have more severe deficits. In a second study, Caselli (1991b) reported that only patients with neglect had bilateral tactile object recognition deficits, while patients with left parietal lesions had tactile agnosia only for items in the contralateral hand. Caselli did not study patients with bilateral lesions, however, and agnosia in the visual and auditory modalities is clearly more profound when bilateral lesions are present.

The mechanisms of tactile agnosia may vary. First, appreciation of shape and perception of a tactile figure or ideogram may be properties of the sensory cortex itself. Bottini and colleagues distinguished apperceptive versus associative aspects of somesthetic (tactile) processing, analogous to the same distinction discussed above for the visual and auditory systems (Bottini *et al.* 1995). Again, matching of meaningless shapes (the apperceptive task) was more sensitive to right hemisphere damage, whereas matching of meaningful shapes (the associative task) was more sensitive to left hemisphere lesions. Second, the right parietal cortex is also involved in spatial and topographical functions, and spatial disorders may account for some of the tactile recognition deficits of patients with right parietal lesions. Third, attentional deficits and neglect seen with right hemisphere lesions may increase the lack of tactile recognition (Caselli 1991b). Fourth, disconnection syndromes may be involved in tactile agnosia. The famous patient of Geschwind and Kaplan (1962) with a lesion of the corpus callosum could not identify objects with the left hand, but could point to the correct object in a group. Patients with surgical section of the corpus callosum have similar deficits (Sperry 1966–1967). Such patients clearly feel the characteristics of the object but cannot name it, presumably because the callosal lesion disconnects the right parietal cortex from left hemisphere language centers. Corpus callosum syndromes are discussed in more detail in Chapter 12.

Tactile Aphasia

Tactile aphasia is an inability to name a palpated object, despite intact recognition of the object and intact naming when the object is presented in another sensory modality (Beauvois *et al.* 1978). This syndrome is closely analogous to optic aphasia.

CONCLUSION

The agnosias are fascinating disorders of sensory perception. The precise mechanisms of the agnosias are difficult to analyze, because they span a spectrum between primary deficits of the sensory cortex and disorders of the association cortex, or disconnection syndromes between cortical areas. Recognition of objects requires not only primary sensation, but also association of the perceived item with previous memories in the same and other sensory modalities. The agnosias open a window into the brain's ability to perceive and recognize aspects of the world around us.

REFERENCES

Alajouanine T. Aphasia and artistic realization. Brain 1948;74:229–241.

Albert ML, Sparks R, von Stockert T, Sax D. A case study of auditory agnosia: linguistic and non-linguistic processing. Cortex 1972;8:427–443.

Albert M, Reches A, Silverberg R. Associative visual agnosia without alexia. Neurology 1975;25:322–326.

Albert ML, Soffer D, Silverberg R, Reches A. The anatomic basis of visual agnosia. Neurology 1979;29:876–879.

Aldrich MS, Alessi AG, Beck RW, Gilman S. Cortical blindness: etiology, diagnosis, and prognosis. Ann Neurol 1987;21:149–158.

Anton G. Ueber die Selbstwahrnehmungen der Herderkrankungen des Gehirnsdurch den Kranken bei Reihdenblindheit und Rindentaubheit. Arch Psychiatr 1899;32:86–127.

Bahls FH, Chatrian GE, Mesher RA *et al.* A case of persistent cortical deafness: clinical, neurophysiologic, and neuropathologic observations. Neurology 1988;38:1490–1493.

Balint R. Die seelenlahmung des 'Schauens': Optische ataxia, Raumliche Storung des Aufmerksamkeit. Monatschr Psychiatr Neurol 1909;1:51–81.

Barnet AB, Manson JI, Wilner E. Acute cerebral blindness in childhood: six cases studied clinically and electrophysiologically. Neurology 1970;20:1147–1156.

Barraquer-Bandas L, Pena-Casanova J, Pons-Irazabal L. Central deafness without aphasic disorders due to bilateral temporal lesion. Acta Neurol Latinoam 1980;26:165–174.

Bay E. Disturbances of visual perception and their examination. Brain 1953;76:515–551.

Beauvois MF, Saillant B, Meininger V, Lhermitte F. Bilateral tactile aphasia: a tacto-verbal dysfunction. Brain 1978;101:381–401.

Bender MB. Polyopia and monocular diplopia of cerebral origin. Arch Neurol 1945;54: 323–328.

Bender MB, Feldman M. The so-called 'visual agnosias'. Brain 1972;95:173–186.

Bender MB, Kanzer MG. Metamorphopsia and other psychovisual disturbances in a patient with a tumor of the brain. Arch Neurol Psychiatry 1941;45:481–485.

Bender MB, Feldman M, Sobin MJ. Palinopsia. Brain 1968;91:321–338.

Benson DF, Greenberg JP. Visual form agnosia: a specific defect in visual recognition. Arch Neurol 1969;20:82–89.

Benson DF, Segarra J, Albert M. Visual agnosia–prosopagnosia: a clinicopathologic correlation. Arch Neurol 1974;30:307–310.

Benson DF, Davis RJ, Snyder BD. Posterior cortical atrophy. Arch Neurol 1988;45:789–793.

Benton AL, Van Allen MW. Prosopagnosia and facial discrimination. J Neurol Sci 1972; 15:167–172.

Bever TG, Chiarello RJ. Cerebral dominance in musicians and non-musicians. Science 1974;185:537–539.

Beyn ES, Knyazeva GR. The problem of prosopagnosia. J Neurol Neurosurg Psychiatry 1962;25:154–158.

Bodamer J. Die Prosop-Agnosie (die Agnosie des Physiognomieerkennens). Archiv fur Psychiatrie und Nervenkrankheiten 1947;179:6–53.

Boller F, Cole M, Kim Y, Mack J, Patawaran C. Optic ataxia: clinico-radiological correlations with the EMI scan. J Neurol Neurosurg Psychiatry 1975;38:954–958.

Bornstein B, Kidron DP. Prosopagnosia. J Neurol Neurosurg Psychiatry 1959;22:124–131.

Botez MI, Wertheim N. Expressive aphasia and amusia following right frontal lesion in a right-handed man. Brain 1959;82:186–202.

Bottini G, Cappa SF, Sterzi R, Vignolo LA. Intramodal somaesthetic recognition disorders following right and left hemisphere damage. Brain 1995;118:395–399.

Brandt KD, Lessell S, Cohen AS. Cerebral disorders of vision in systemic lupus erythematosus. Ann Intern Med 1975;83:163–169.

Brau RH, Lameiro J, Llaguno AV, Rifkinson. Metamorphopsia and permanent cortical blindness after a posterior fossa tumor. Neurosurgery 1986;19:263–266.

Breitling D, Guenther W, Rondot P. Auditory perception of music measured by brain electrical activity mapping. Neuropsychologia 1987;25:765–774.

Brindley GS, Gautier-Smith PC, Lewin W. Cortical blindness and the function of the non-geniculate fibers of the optic tracts. J Neurol Neurosurg Psychiat 1969;32:259–264.

Brust JCM. Music and language: musical alexia and agraphia. Brain 1980;103:367–392.

Buchtel HA, Stewart JD. Auditory agnosia: apperceptive or associative disorder? Brain Lang 1989;37:12–25.

Caplan LR. 'Top of the basilar' syndrome. Neurology 1980;30:72–79.

Caselli RJ. Rediscovering tactile agnosia. Mayo Clin Proc 1991a;66:129–142.

Caselli RJ. Bilateral impairment of somesthetically mediated object recognition in humans. Mayo Clin Proc 1991b;66:357–364.

Cogan DG. Visual disturbances with focal progressive dementing disease. Am J Ophthal 1985;100:68–72.

Cogan DG, Adams RD. A type of paralysis of conjugate gaze (ocular motor apraxia). Arch Ophthalmol 1953;50:434–442.

Cohen L, Gray F, Meyrignac C et al. Selective deficit in visual size perception: two cases of hemimicropsia. J Neurol Neurosurg Psychiatry 1994;57:73–78.

Cohn R, Neumann MA, Wood DH. Prosopagnosia: a clinicopathological study. Ann Neurol 1977;1:172–182.

Coslett HB, Saffran EM. Preserved object recognition and reading comprehension in optic aphasia. Brain 1989a;112:1091–1110.

Coslett HB, Saffran EM. Preserved reading in pure alexia. Brain 1989b;112:327–359.

Coslett HB, Brashear HR, Heilman KM. Pure word deafness after bilateral primary auditory cortex infarcts. Neurology 1984;34:347–352.

Critchley M. Types of visual perseveration: 'palinopsia' and 'illusory visual spread'. Brain 1951;74:267–299.

Cummings JL, Duchen LW. Kluver–Bucy syndrome in Pick's disease: clinical and pathological correlations. Neurology 1981;31:1415–1422

Damasio AR, Benton AL. Impairment of hand movements under visual guidance. Neurology 1979;29:170–178.

Damasio AR, McKee J, Damasio H. Determinants of performance in color anomia. Brain Lang 1979;7:74–85.

Damasio A, Yamada T, Damasio H, Corbett J, McKee J. Central achromatopsia: behavioral, anatomic, and physiologic aspects. Neurology 1980;30:1064–1071.

Damasio AR, Damasio H, Van Hoesen GW. Prosopagnosia: anatomic basis and behavioral mechanisms. Neurology 1982;32:331–341.

DeRenzi E, Faglioni P, Grossi D, Nichelli P. Apperceptive and associative forms of prosopagnosia. Cortex 1991;27:213–221.

Efron R. What is perception? In R Cohen, M Wartofsky (eds), Boston Studies in the Philosophy of Science, Vol 4. New York: Humanities Press, and the Netherlands: O Reidel, 1968.

Engelien A, Huber W, Silbersweig D et al. The neural correlates of 'deaf-hearing' in man: conscious sensory awareness enabled by attentional modulation. Brain 2000;123:532–545.

Fink GR, Halligan PW, Marshall JC et al. Where in the brain does visual attention select the forest and the trees? Nature 1996;382:626–628.

Forster O. Sensible cortical felder. In Bumke O, Forster O (eds), Handbuch des Neurologie. Berlin: Julius Springer, 1936.

Freud S. On Aphasia (originally published in 1891; trans. E. Stengel). London: Imago, 1953.

Geschwind N. Disconnexion syndromes in animals and man. Brain 1965;88:237–294, 585–644.

Geschwind N. The organization of language and the brain. Science 1970;170:940–944.

Geschwind N, Fusillo M. Color-naming deficits in association with alexia. Arch Neurol 1966;15:137–146.

Geschwind N, Kaplan E. A human deconnection syndrome. Neurology 1962;12:675–685.
Golden GS. The Alice in Wonderland syndrome in juvenile migraine. Pediatrics 1979;63: 517–519.
Goldstein MN. Auditory agnosia for speech ('pure word-deafness'). A historical review with current implications. Brain Lang 1974;1:195–204.
Gordon HW, Bogen JE. Hemispheric lateralization of singing after intracarotid sodium amylobarbitone. J Neurol Neurosurg Psychiatry 1974;37:727–738.
Greenblatt SH. Post-traumatic transient cerebral blindness: association with migraine and seizure diathesis. JAMA 1973;225:1073–1076.
Griffith JF, Dodge PR. Transient blindness following head injury in children. N Engl J Med 1968;278:648–651.
Grossman M, Galetta S, D'Esposito M. Object recognition difficulty in visual apperceptive agnosia. Brain Cognition 1997;33:306–342.
Hachinski VC, Porchawka J, Steele JC. Visual symptoms in the migraine syndrome. Neurology 1973;23:570–579.
Hartmann JA, Wolz WA, Roeltgen DP, Loverso FL. Denial of visual perception. Brain Cogn 1991;16:29–40.
Hausser CO, Robert F, Giard N. Balint's syndrome. Can J Neurol Sci 1980;7:157–161.
Hécaen H, Ajuriaguerra J. Balint's syndrome (psychic paralysis of visual fixation) and its minor forms. Brain 1954;77:373–400.
Hecaen H, Angelergues R. Agnosia for faces (prosopagnosia). Arch Neurol 1962;7:92–100.
Hecaen H, David M. Syndrome parietale traumatique: asymbolie tactile et hemisomatognosie paroxystique et douloureuse. Rev Neurol (Paris) 1945;77:113–123.
Heidenhain A. Klinische und anatomische Untersuchungen uber eine eigenartige organische Erkrankung des Zentralnerven Systems im Praesenium. Z Neurol Psychiatr 1928;118:49–60.
Humphreys GW. Object recognition: The man who mistook his dog for a cat. Current Biology 1996;6:821–824.
Jacobs L. Visual allesthesia. Neurology 1980;30:1059–1063.
Jankowiak J, Kinsbourne M, Shalev RS, Bachman DL. Preserved visual imagery and categorization in a case of associative visual agnosia. J Cog Neurosci 1992;4: 119–131.
Jerger J, Weiker NJ, Sharbrough FW, Jerger S. Bilateral lesions of the temporal lobe: a case study. Acta Otolaryngol 1969;258(Suppl.):1–51.
Kanshepolsky J, Kelley JJ, Waggener JD. A cortical auditory disorder. Clinical, audiological and pathologic aspects. Neurology 1973;23:699–705.
Karpov BA, Luria AR, Yarbuss AL. Disturbances in the structure of active perception in lesions of the posterior and anterior regions of the brain. Neuropsychologia 1968;6: 157–166.
Kinsbourne M, Warrington EK. A disorder of simultaneous form perception. Brain 1962; 85:461–486.
Kinsella G, Prior M, Murray G. Singing ability after right and left sided brain damage. A research note. Cortex 1988;24:165–169.
Kirshner HS, Webb WG. Selective involvement of the auditory-verbal modality in an acquired communication disorder: Benefit from sign language therapy. Brain Lang 1981;13:161–170.
Kirshner HS, Casey PF, Henson J, Heinrich JJ. Behavioural features and lesion localization in Wernicke's aphasia. Aphasiology 1989;3:169–176.
Kluver H, Bucy PC. Preliminary analysis of functions of the temporal lobes in monkeys. Arch Neurol Psychiatry 1939;42: 979–1000.
Kurucz J, Feldmar G. Prosopo-affective agnosia as a symptom of cerebral organic disease. J Am Geriatr Soc 1979;27:225–230.
Landis T, Regard M, Bliestle A, Kleihues P. Prosopagnosia and agnosia for non-canonical views. Brain 1988;111:1287–1297.

Levine DN. Prosopagnosia and visual object agnosia: a behavioral study. Brain Lang 1978;5:341–365.

Levine DN, Calvanio R. A study of the visual defect in verbal alexia-simultanagnosia. Brain 1978;101:65–81.

Levine DN, Kaufman KJ, Mohr JP. Inaccurate reaching associated with a superior parietal lobe tumor. Neurology 1978;28:556–561.

Levine D, Calvanio R, Wolf E. Disorders of visual behavior following bilateral posterior cerebral lesions. Psychol Res 1980;41:217–234.

Lhermitte F, Beauvois MF. A visual-speech disconnexion syndrome. Brain 1973;96: 695–714.

Lilly R, Cummings JL, Benson DF, Frankel M. The human Kluver–Bucy syndrome. Neurology 1983;33:1141–1145.

Lissauer H. Ein Fall von Seelenblindheit nebst einem Beitrag zur Theorie derselben. Archiv fur Psychiatrie und Nervenkrankenheit 1890;21:222–270.

Luria AR. Higher Cortical Functions in Man. London: Tavistock Publishers, 1966.

Luria AR, Pravdina-Vinarskaya EN, Yarbuss AL. Disorders of the ocular movements in a case of simultanagnosia. Brain 1963;86:219–228.

Malone DR, Morris HH, Kay MC, Levin HS. Prosopagnosia: a double dissociation between the recognition of familiar and unfamiliar faces. J Neurol Neurosurg Psychiatry 1982;45:820–822.

Manford M, Andermann F. Complex visual hallucinations. Clinical and neurobiological insights. Brain 1998;121:1819–1840.

Marlowe WB, Mancall EL, Thomas TJ. Complete Kluver–Bucy syndrome in man. Cortex 1975;11:53–59.

McCarthy RA, Warrington EK. Visual associative agnosia: a clinico-anatomical study of a single case. J Neurol Neurosurg Psychiatry 1986;49:1233–1240.

McCormick GF, Levine DA. Visual anomia: a unilateral disconnection. Neurology 1983;33:664–666.

McFarland HR, Fortin D. Amusia due to a right temporoparietal infarct. Arch Neurol 1982;39:725–727.

McNamara ME, Heros R, Boller F. Visual hallucinations in blindness: the Charles Bonnet syndrome. Int J Neurosci 1982;17:13–15.

Meadows JC. The anatomical basis of prosopagnosia. J Neurol Neurosurg Psychiatry 1974;37:489–501.

Meadows JC, Munro SSF. Palinopsia. J Neurol Neurosurg Psychiatry 1977;40:5–8.

Melen O, Olson SF, Hodes BL. Visual disturbances in migraine. Postgrad Med 1978; 64:139–143.

Mendez M, Geehan GR. Cortical auditory disorder: clinical and psychoacoustic features. J Neurol Neurosurg Psychiatry 1988;51:1–9.

Michel EM, Troost BT. Palinopsia: cerebral localization with computed tomography. Neurology 1980;30:887–889.

Michel F, Perenin MT, Sieroff E. Prosopagnosie sans hemianopsie apres lesion unilaterale occipito-temporale droite. Rev Neurol 1986;142:545–549.

Milner AD, Perrett DI, Johnston RS et al. Perception and action in 'visual form agnosia'. Brain 1991;114:405–428.

Milner B, Teuber HL. Alteration of perception and memory in man. In L Weiskrantz (ed.), Analysis of Behavioral Change. New York: Harper and Row, 1968.

Motomura N, Yamadori A, Mori E, Tamaru F. Auditory agnosia. Analysis of a case with bilateral subcortical lesions. Brain 1986;109:379–391.

Pearlman AL, Burch J, Meadows JC. Cerebral color blindness: an acquired defect in hue discrimination. Ann Neurol 1979;5:253–261.

Penfield W, Perot P. The brain's record of auditory and visual experience. Brain 1963;86: 595–696.

Plaut DC, Shallice T. Perseverative and semantic influences on visual object naming errors in optic aphasia: a connectionist account. J Cog Neurosci 1993;5:89–117.

Perenin MT, Ruel J, Hecaen H. Residual visual capacities in a case of cortical blindness. Cortex 1980;605–612.

Polk M, Kertesz A. Music and language in degenerative disease of the brain. Brain Cogn 1993;22:98–117.

Poppel E, Held R, Frost D. Residual visual function after brain wounds involving the central visual pathways in man. Nature 1973;243:295–296.

Posner MI. Orientation of attention. Q J Exp Psychol 1987;32:3–25.

Prior M, Troup GA. Processing of timbre and rhythm in musicians and non-musicians. Cortex 1988;24:451–456.

Rapcsak SZ, Kaszniak AW, Rubens AB. Anomia for facial expressions: evidence for a category specific visual–verbal disconnection syndrome. Neuropsychologia 1989; 27:1031–1041.

Richards W. The fortification illusions of migraines. Sci Am 1971;224:88–96.

Riddoch MJ, Humphreys GW. A case of integrative visual agnosia. Brain 1987;110: 1431–1462.

Rizzo M, Rotella D, Darling W. Troubled reaching after right occipito-temporal damage. Neuropsychologia 1992;30:711–722.

Robertson L, Treisman A, Friedman-Hill *et al*. The interaction of spatial and object pathways: Evidence from Balint's syndrome. J Cogn Neurosci 1997;9:295–317.

Rubens AB, Benson DF. Associative visual agnosia. Arch Neurol 1971;24:305–316.

Sacks O. The Man who Mistook his Wife for a Hat and Other Clinical Tales. New York: Summit Books, 1985;7–21.

Semmes J. A non-tactual factor in astereognosis. Neuropsychologia 1965;3:295–315.

Sergent J. Music, the brain and Ravel. TINS 1993;16:168–172.

Sergent J, Zuck E, Terriah S, MacDonald B. Distributed neural network underlying musical sight-reading and keyboard performance. Science 1992;257:106–109.

Shankweiler D. Effects of temporal lobe damage on perception of dichotically presented melodies. J Comp Physiol Psychol 1966;62:115–119.

Smirniotopoulos JG, Murphy FM, Schellinger D *et al*. Cortical blindness after metrizamide myelography. Arch Neurol 1984;41:224–226.

Sparks R, Helm N, Albert M. Aphasia rehabilitation resulting from melodic intonation therapy. Cortex 1974;10:303–316.

Sperry RW. Mental unity following surgical disconnection of the cerebral hemispheres. Harvey Lect 1966–1967;62:293–323.

Spreen O, Benton AL, Rincham RW. Auditory agnosia without aphasia. Arch Neurol 1965;13:84–92.

Stoddard WE, David DD, Young SW. Cortical blindness after cerebral angiography: case report. J Neurosurg 1981;54:240–244.

Takahashi N, Kawamura M, Shinotou H *et al*. Pure word deafness due to left hemisphere damage. Cortex 1992;28:295–303.

Tanake Y, Yamadori A, Mori E. Pure word deafness following bilateral lesions. A psychophysical analysis. Brain 1987;110:381–403.

Ter Braak JWG, Schenk VWD, Van Vliet AGM. Visual reactions in a case of long-lasting cortical blindness. J Neurol Neurosurg Psychiatry 1971;34:140–147.

Terzian H, Dalle Ore G. Syndrome of Kluver and Bucy reproduced in man by bilateral removal of the temporal lobes. Neurology 1955;5:373–380.

Thaiss L, DeBleser R. Visual agnosia: a case of reduced attentional 'spotlight'? Cortex 1992;28:601–621.

Tyler HR. Abnormality of perception with defective eye movements (Balint's syndrome). Cortex 1968;4:154–171.

Victoroff J, Ross GW, Benson DF *et al*. Posterior cortical atrophy. Neuropathologic correlations. Arch Neurol 1994;51:269–274.

Vignolo LA. Auditory agnosia. Philos Trans R Soc Lond B Biol Sci 1982;25:49–57.

Warrington EK, James M. Visual apperceptive agnosia: a clinico-anatomical study of three cases. Cortex 1988;24:13–32.

Warrington EK, Rudge P. A comment on apperceptive agnosia. Brain Cognition 1995;28: 173–177.

Whiteley AM, Warrington EK. Prosopagnosia: a clinical, psychological, and anatomical study of three patients. J Neurol Neurosurg Psychiatry 1977;40:395–403.

Wolpert I. Die Simultanagnosie-Storung der Gesamtauffasung. Zeitsch Neurol Psychiat 1924;93:397–415.

Wunderlich G, Suchan B, Volkmann J et al. Visual hallucinations in recovery from cortical blindness. Imaging correlates. Arch Neurol 2000;57:561–565.

Zeki S. A century of cerebral achromatopsia. Brain 1990;113:1721–1777.

Zeki S. Cerebral akinetopsia (visual motion blindness). A review. Brain 1991;114: 811–824.

Zihl J, von Cramon D, Mai N. Selective disturbance of movement vision after bilateral brain damage. Brain 1983;106:313–340.

9

Disorders of the Right Hemisphere

I wish to draw attention to an observation I have had the opportunity to make of a mental disturbance associated with cerebral hemiplegia, in which the patients ignore, or seem to ignore, the existence of a paralysis that afflicts them...I will permit myself the use of a neologism in calling this state anosognosia. I have also observed several hemiplegics who, although not ignoring the existence of their paralysis, seemed to attach no importance to it as if it were an insignificant bother – a state that might be called anisodiaphoric (indifference, insouciance).

(Babinski 1914)

The right hemisphere is often called the minor or non-dominant hemisphere, because it is not the site of language in right-handed or in most left-handed people. The 'minor' hemisphere, however, has many important functions of its own. These functions, moreover, are just as crucial as language in making us who we are. Right hemisphere lesions produce clinically important and fascinating behavioral syndromes, readily assessed by bedside examination techniques. Attention to right hemisphere functions on the mental status examination is as important as the testing of language in localizing brain lesions.

Behavioral impairments caused by right hemisphere injury include constructional and dressing difficulties, spatial and topographical disorientation, inattention to the left side of the body and of space, neglect and denial of neurological deficits, emotional changes, and difficulties in the emotional and prosodic aspects of communication. Deficits in facial recognition and musical abilities associated with right hemisphere and bilateral lesions are discussed in Chapter 8. The major right hemisphere behavioral syndromes are listed in Table 9.1.

CONSTRUCTIONAL IMPAIRMENT

Patients with right parietal lesions frequently perform poorly on tests of drawing and copying figures such as a clock or a house. This deficit is often called

Table 9.1 Right hemisphere behavioral syndromes

Constructional impairment
Dressing impairment
Spatial and topographical disorientation
Hemineglect and anosognosia
Emotional indifference
Language alterations, aprosodias

'constructional apraxia'. In general, we think of visuoconstructional functions as involving appreciation and reproduction of spatial relationships rather than as skilled motor acts; for this reason, constructional apraxia is not clearly an 'apraxia' (see Chapter 7), and we prefer the term 'constructional impairment'. The bedside examination outlined in Chapter 4 includes several visuoconstructional tasks: clock drawing and placement of the hands, copying of geometric figures, location of cities on a map, and bisection of lines. Constructional impairments must be tested deliberately, as patients infrequently complain of them. These functions are closely related to those measured by psychologists on standard tests such as the block design subtest of the Wechsler Adult Intelligence Scale, the Bender Gestalt drawings, the Rey–Osterreith figure, and the Benton Visual Retention Test (Lezak 1983).

The drawings of patients with right hemisphere lesions frequently manifest both a failure to perceive spatial relationships and a relative inattention to the left side. Figure 9.1 shows drawings of a clock and a Greek cross by a patient with a right parietal stroke; the patient's CT scan is shown in Figure 9.2. All 12 clock numbers are crowded into the right side of the clock face, and the left side of the cross is missing. Drawings of patients with right hemisphere lesions also frequently contain misplaced lines or misaligned spatial relationships in two-dimensional geometric forms.

The deficits seen in these visuoconstructional tasks probably reflect a variety of behavioral impairments: altered visuospatial perception, poor conceptualization of spatial relationships, left-sided inattention, motor difficulties in the execution of drawings, and impersistence, or inability to sustain attention to a task. Because these impairments may differ in degree, more than one visuoconstructional task should be tested.

The anatomic localization of constructional impairment is most typically in the right parietal lobe. As noted in Chapter 6, however, posterior left hemisphere lesions, especially those in the vicinity of the angular gyrus, may also impair constructional ability (Benson et al. 1982). Several studies have documented that constructional impairment occurs with lesions of either hemisphere, more with posterior than anterior lesions (Benton 1967, 1973; Black and Strub 1976). Constructional impairment from left hemisphere lesions correlates closely with receptive language deficits, and is infrequent with purely

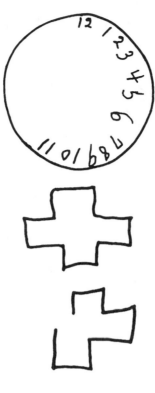

Figure 9.1 Spontaneous clock drawing (top) and copying of a Greek cross (bottom) by a patient with a right hemisphere stroke. Note the neglect of the left side of space in both drawings.

expressive or no language dysfunction (Benton 1973). More complex visuoconstructional tasks, such as the copying of drawings or three-dimensional block designs, are impaired more frequently by right than left hemisphere lesions, though deficits in simple block design may occur with equal incidence in the presence of lesions of the two hemispheres (Benton 1967). In a CT scan study of neuropsychological deficits in 41 right hemisphere stroke patients, Hier and colleagues (1983) found a close correlation among impaired block design, poor performance on the Rey figure, and unilateral neglect in drawing; all three deficits were associated with right parietal lesions posterior to the rolandic fissure.

Constructional impairment is a common accompaniment of right hemisphere lesions, occurring in 36–93% of patients (Benton 1967; Hier *et al.* 1983). Constructional impairment can be taken to indicate a disorder of the right parietal lobe, until proved otherwise. The examiner must keep in mind that impairments on constructional tasks also occur with left parietal and with bilateral or diffuse cerebral diseases. The most useful aspect of constructional impairments, however, is that they clearly indicate a cerebral lesion and exclude a spinal cord or peripheral nerve lesion. A patient who presents with left arm weakness but cannot draw a clock can be presumed to have

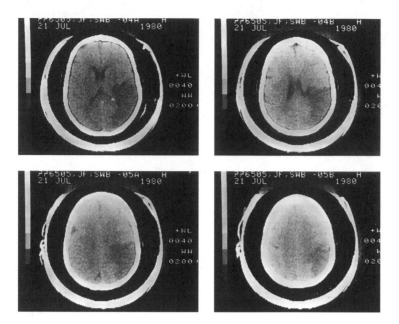

Figure 9.2 CT scan of the patient whose drawings are shown in Figure 9.1. A large area of infarction is seen in the right temporoparietal region, within the territory of the middle cerebral artery. Despite the severe cortical deficits and left hemianopia, the patient had only mild left-sided weakness and sensory loss.

a right hemisphere disorder, and not a lesion of the cervical cord or cervical nerve roots.

DRESSING IMPAIRMENT

Patients with right hemisphere lesions frequently have difficulty dressing themselves, a deficit often referred to as 'dressing apraxia'. Dressing impairment comprises both an inability to conceptualize the spatial relationships of articles of clothing to parts of the body and a tendency to neglect the left side (Brain 1941). Whereas constructional impairment must be brought out by testing, dressing impairment is evident to the patient and especially to the family. The presence of dressing impairment can usually be ascertained during the medical history. In the observational portion of the bedside examination (see Chapter 4), decreased neatness and grooming may be noted on the left side of the body, or the left side of the face may be unshaved.

The localization of dressing impairment, even more than constructional impairment, is usually in the right parietal lobe. In the study of Hier *et al.* (1983), dressing impairment correlated with both left-sided neglect and visuospatial and visuoconstructional deficits, and the localization by computerized tomography (CT) scan was nearly always right parietal.

SPATIAL AND TOPOGRAPHICAL DISORIENTATION

Patients with right hemisphere lesions frequently manifest spatial disorientation for both the body image and external space. They may become lost when traveling familiar routes or when navigating the halls of a hospital. As discussed in Chapter 4, simple questions about the location of the nurses' station or shower room or the route to the patient's home may reveal spatial disorientation. Patients also manifest topographical impairment when drawing maps and locating cities on a map drawn by the examiner. Benton and co-workers recommended the use of a test of judgment of line orientation as a means of assessing spatial disorientation (Benton *et al.* 1975). Although cumbersome for use in the routine bedside examination, this test is of value in experimental studies and in neuropsychological test batteries. Spatial and topographical deficits have a strong association with disease of the right parietal lobe, though they occur occasionally in left-hemisphere-damaged patients (Benton *et al.* 1974).

The mechanisms underlying spatial and topographical disorientation are incompletely understood. Inattention to or neglect of the left side of the body and space is doubtless a contributing factor; this hemi-inattention leads to incorrect choices of direction in route-finding and impairs map drawing and topographical localization. In addition, the right parietal lobe appears to have direct involvement in the sense of the body image, its relationship to external space, and topographical relationships outside the body (Ettlinger *et al.* 1957). Takahashi *et al.* (1997) described three patients with focal intracerebral hemorrhages in the retrosplenial area of the right hemisphere, extending into the medial parietal lobe. All lost the ability to recall spatial relationships of streets and buildings, despite intact memory for and recognition of the buildings, the furniture and objects contained in them, and the streets themselves. One previous patient with a glioma of the splenium of the corpus callosum had similar topographical disorientation (Bottini *et al.* 1990). Takahashi and colleagues (1997) postulated that the retrosplenial region of the right parietal lobe is closely involved with the function of topographical localization in space.

A deficit closely related to topographical disorientation is the phenomenon of 'reduplicative paramnesia', in which patients mistakenly and repeatedly give the location of the hospital as in or near their home town or former place of residence. Such patients may be oriented in other respects and not globally confused. This deficit occurs most frequently after head trauma in which bilateral damage is likely, but the frequent association with left hemiparesis suggests predominant right hemisphere involvement (Benson *et al.* 1976). One of the author's patients manifested prolonged and consistent reduplicative paramnesia, thinking he was both in the hospital in Nashville but also in his hometown of Knoxville, Tennessee. He repeatedly said that Vanderbilt Hospital was in Knox County. This patient had suffered a stroke that, clinically and by CT scan, was restricted to the right hemisphere. Another recent patient watched a political speech on TV, recalling substantive details of the speech but insisting that she had been present in the Congress for the presentation. She then relocated both her farm and our medical center to Washington, DC. The phenomenon of reduplicative paramnesia may also be related to more global confusional states seen after right hemisphere injuries (Levine and Grek 1984).

Bisiach and Luzzatti (1978) studied the neglect of visual space in imaginary, as opposed to actual, visual situations. These investigators asked patients to describe, from memory, the Piazza del Duomo in Milan, Italy. Patients described more details on the imagined right side of the Piazza than on the left. When they were asked what they imagined from a vantage point at the other end of the Piazza, however, they then described the buildings on the other side of the square, which they had previously neglected. Marshall and Halligan (1993) have shown that neglect of actual and imaginary spaces do not necessarily parallel each other; neglect can be selective for either actual or imagined space. Beschin and colleagues (1997) have also reported a patient with 'representative' or imaginary neglect, without neglect for actually perceived scenes.

HEMINEGLECT AND ANOSOGNOSIA

Unilateral neglect and inattention are the most striking abnormalities manifested by patients with right hemisphere lesions. Patients with an acute right hemisphere stroke are frequently seen lying on their right side, with head and eyes turned to the right. They attend to stimuli coming from the right but not the left. A patient may ignore an examiner approaching from the left until he or she crosses into the right visual field. Left hemianopsia may or may not be present; some patients can see stimuli in the left visual field but pay no attention to them ('visual neglect'). As noted earlier, a patient with a right hemisphere lesion may neglect the left side of the body when dressing or shaving. The patient may eat the food on the right side of a dinner plate or hospital tray but leave the left side untouched, stumble into walls or objects on the left side, leave out words at the beginning of a line in reading, and fail to notice cars approaching from the left. Hemineglect is thus a deficit of great functional importance in the activities of daily living.

Neglect can involve the left side of the body or the left side of space (Calvanio et al. 1987). Neglect is usually discussed in terms of visual stimuli, but to a large extent it is a 'supramodal' phenomenon that affects all sensory modalities. Neglect can be visual, tactile, auditory, and even olfactory (Bellas et al. 1988) for stimuli on the contralateral side of the body or space. Related to this phenomenon is 'extinction' of left-sided stimuli when bilateral stimuli are presented (Critchley 1966). As mentioned in Chapter 3, functional MRI studies have shown activation of the right occipital cortex in response to left-sided visual stimuli that are extinguished and not consciously seen by the subject; these stimuli are thus perceived cortically but not brought to conscious awareness (Rees et al. 2000).

Perhaps even more striking than this left inattention is the neglect of the deficit itself, termed 'anosognosia' by the French neurologist Babinski (1914). Patients with acute right hemisphere strokes frequently have left hemiparesis but appear unaware of their weakness. When asked to raise both hands only the right comes up, yet the patient may deny that he has any weakness. When asked to show the examiner the left hand, the patient may point vaguely toward the left side or grope with the right hand toward the left shoulder. The patient is also unconcerned about the paralysis, a phenomenon termed 'anisodiaphoria' by Babinski (1914), and later by Critchley (1966). In the most severe stages of the neglect syndrome, patients may even deny that their left limbs belong to them. If the examiner lifts the patient's left arm, the patient may maintain that it is the examiner's arm, although still recognizing his or her own wristwatch. In lesser degrees of neglect or after recovery has begun, patients do not deny their limbs and may even be able to state verbally that their limbs are weak. Patients at this stage often speak of the paralysis in emotionless, impersonal terms, such as 'They say my left side is paralyzed', suggesting that complete subjective awareness of the deficit is still lacking. They may also repeatedly attempt to get up and fall to the left, as if 'forgetting' the deficit. Finally, in the mildest stage of neglect, patients are aware of the deficit but appear unconcerned, with a bland affect. Thus a stroke patient who faces the loss of livelihood and ability to walk makes jokes with the examiner and speaks unrealistically about the future.

These gradations of anosognosia and anisodiaphoria are extremely common in acute or rapidly developing right hemisphere lesions. In practical terms, they interfere greatly with rehabilitative therapies, which often fail until the neglect begins to resolve (Denes *et al.* 1982).

In addition to neglect of motor deficits, patients with right hemisphere lesions frequently manifest abnormalities of sensory function. They may neglect sensory stimuli emanating from the left side, or they may extinguish or ignore the left-sided stimulus when both sides of the body are touched simultaneously (Critchley 1966). Some patients may appreciate a single stimulus applied to the left side of the body but report it as coming from the right, a phenomenon known as 'allesthesia' (Bender and Teuber 1949). Some patients may grimace when pinched on the left limbs but are unable to localize the source of pain. Occasional patients with right hemisphere lesions experience peculiar sensations of the left limbs, e.g. amputation or phantom limb feeling or the presence of 'extra' limbs in their beds. The family of one such patient actually complained to the hospital administration that their relative had been forced to share a bed with another patient (F. R. Freemon, personal communication 1983).

Neglect and Delirium

Acute right hemisphere lesions occasionally cause a global confusional state, with agitation, disorientation, and hallucinations. This can occur either immediately following a right middle cerebral artery territory stroke (Mesulam *et al.* 1976) or after a delay (Levine and Finklestein 1982), possibly related to seizure activity. Although these observations are of interest, it should be stressed that global confusion usually implies dysfunction of both cerebral hemispheres (see Chapter 14). Levine and Grek (1984) presented evidence that pre-existing cerebral atrophy, as judged by CT scan, might have a role in the development of confusion after a right hemisphere stroke. Rabins and colleagues (1991) found that delusions and hallucinations were more likely to occur in stroke patients with the following risk factors: older age; family history of psychiatric disorder; right hemisphere lesions, particularly involving the temporo-parieto-occipital junction; cortical atrophy; and seizures. Caplan and colleagues (1986) described agitated delirium in association with acute infarction of the inferior division of the right middle cerebral artery, a stroke syndrome often not associated with hemiparesis. The authors called this the 'mirror image of Wernicke's aphasia' in the left hemisphere.

Anatomy of Hemineglect

The anatomical lesions reported to cause neglect, anosognosia, and aniso-diaphoria have been quite varied and controversial. The first issue is the apparent association of neglect with right as opposed to left hemisphere disease. Denny-Brown and colleagues related neglect to poor integration of sensory information from the contralateral side of the body, a function deranged by a lesion of either parietal lobe (Denny-Brown et al. 1952). Others have suggested that the apparent association of neglect with right hemisphere lesions is artifactual, in that aphasic deficits caused by left hemisphere lesions prevent detection of the neglect syndrome. Numerous studies, however, have found hemineglect to be more frequent and more severe in right than in left hemisphere lesions (Brain 1941; Battersby et al. 1956; Denny-Brown and Chambers 1958; Critchley 1966; Hecaen 1969; Gainotti et al. 1972; Schwartz et al. 1979; Cutting 1978; Denes et al. 1982). The dysproportionate occurrence of neglect with right hemisphere lesions also seems evident from personal experience with stroke patients; neglect is very common in acute right middle cerebral artery territory strokes but is seen infrequently with similar strokes in the left hemisphere. Aphasic patients are frequently both aware of and depressed about their deficits, a phenomenon originally described by Kurt Goldstein (1948) under the term 'catastrophic reaction'. Such patients, even though unable to speak, clearly have awareness of their hemiparesis; for example, they repeatedly exercise the paralyzed right arm passively with the left.

Within the right hemisphere, a number of separate lesion sites can produce neglect behavior. The right parietal lobe (Hier et al. 1972, 1983; Brain 1941; Denny-Brown et al. 1952; Ettlinger et al. 1957), and particularly the inferior parietal lobule (Denny-Brown and Chambers 1958; Critchley 1966), have been implicated. In the study of Hier et al. (1983), those patients with strokes associated with neglect and denial of deficit had large infarcts, usually involving much of the parietal lobe. A recent study by Samuelsson and colleagues (1997) found a close correlation between visuospatial neglect and lesions of the middle temporal gyrus and temporoparietal paraventricular white matter; 12 of 18 right hemisphere stroke patients with neglect had lesions involving one or both of these areas, whereas 1 of 35 patients without neglect had a lesion of these areas. Another CT scan study (Egelko *et al.* 1988), however, found that visual neglect correlated only with lesions of the right parietal, temporal, or occipital lobes; the parietal lobe had no more association with visual neglect than did the temporal and occipital lobes. A recent study by Karnath and colleagues (2001) found that isolated left hemispatial neglect correlated best with lesions of the right superior temporal gyrus. The authors cited similar evidence from primate studies, though in primates the temporal lesions associated with neglect could be in either hemisphere. Isolated right frontal lesions have also been associated with neglect (Heilman and Valenstein 1972; Damasio *et al.* 1980). The lesions in these cases involved either the medial or dorsolateral surfaces of the frontal lobe or the cingulate gyrus, the gray matter gyrus located just above the corpus callosum in each hemisphere. Deep subcortical lesions in the right hemisphere, specifically in the striatum and deep white matter (Hier *et al.* 1977; Damasio *et al.* 1980; Healton *et al.* 1982; Bogousslavsky *et al.* 1988), posterior limb of the internal capsule (Ferro and Kertesz 1984), and thalamus (Watson and Heilman 1979; Watson *et al.* 1981) have been associated with left-sided neglect. As in the aphasic syndromes associated with left hemisphere subcortical lesions (see Chapter 5), these lesions may disrupt the functions of the overlying cerebral cortex either by pressure effects, as in intracerebral hemorrhages or tumors, or by interruption of ascending and descending neural pathways. SPECT studies in patients with subcortical neglect (Bogousslavsky *et al.* 1988) have shown hypoperfusion of the right parietal lobe as well as of the subcortical structures directly involved in CT scans.

Mechanism of Hemineglect

The cerebral mechanisms underlying neglect and hemi-inattention have been the subject of intense speculation. Early theories revolved largely around afferent sensory defects, including altered sensation (Battersby *et al.* 1956), impaired sensory integration Horenstein ('amorphosynthesis', Denny-Brown *et al.* 1952), or disordered body schema. Pure sensory theories of neglect, however, have difficulty accounting for impaired motor acts, e.g. omission of the left side of a drawing, and denial of hemiparesis.

A second possible mechanism of neglect is a disorder of attention. Both Brain (1941) and Critchley (1966) early cited the importance of right hemisphere function in maintaining attention. Heilman and colleagues, in a series of animal and human studies, extended this theory into an 'attention-arousal' hypothesis. Anatomically, the frontal and inferior parietal cortical areas associated with neglect have abundant connections both to each other and to the reticular activating system, the ascending system of neurons in the brainstem and thalamus that alerts the brain (Heilman and Watson 1977). Lesions anywhere in this circuit may impair the alerting or orienting responses to contralateral stimuli. Damage to this ascending system may explain the neglect seen with thalamic and other subcortical lesions (Watson and Heilman 1979; Watson *et al.* 1981). Because right hemisphere lesions cause neglect more often than left hemisphere lesions, the attention-arousal theory requires right hemisphere 'dominance' for attention. Otherwise stated, the right hemisphere may have a capacity for alerting both hemispheres, such that damage to the left hemisphere alone does not result in neglect. In the presence of right hemisphere damage, however, the left hemisphere cannot alert the right, and neglect appears. Heilman and colleagues presented experimental evidence for this decreased arousal in right hemisphere lesions by recording the galvanic skin response (GSR) in the hand ipsilateral to the lesion after stimulation of this same hand. GSRs were less in patients with right hemisphere lesions and neglect than in either normal controls or patients with left hemisphere lesions and aphasia (Heilman *et al.* 1978). Similarly, electroencephalographic (EEG) desynchronization in the parietal lobe of normal subjects, another measure of arousal, occurred in the right parietal lobe after stimulation of either side of the body, whereas the left parietal lobe desynchronized only after right-sided stimulation (Heilman and Van Den Abell 1980). A dominant role of the right hemisphere in attention is also suggested by the finding that reaction times are more slowed by right than left hemisphere lesions (DeRenzi and Faglioni 1965; Howes and Boller 1975). Clinically, patients with acute right hemisphere strokes often seem more apathetic, or hypovigilant, than do patients with left hemisphere strokes.

A third cerebral mechanism related to neglect is unilateral hypokinesia, or decreased spontaneous motor use of either the left limbs or of all limbs in the left side of space. This mechanism can be thought of as the motor aspect of neglect, or 'intentional' neglect as opposed to 'attentional' neglect, discussed above (Adair *et al.* 1998). Occasional patients with neglect have clinically evident hypokinesia of the left limbs, even in the absence of weakness or sensory extinction (Valenstein and Heilman 1981). Hemiakinesia may also explain the omission of left-sided details in the spontaneous drawings of patients with right hemisphere lesions. In clinical usage, line bisection tasks are thought to show attentional neglect, whereas 'cancellation tasks' (cross out every letter 'S' in a display of letters) reveal intentional deficits (Na *et al.* 1998). Coslett and Heilman (1989) suggested that the right hemisphere is dominant for motor intention of both sides, whereas the left hemisphere is dominant only for motor intention of the right side of the body. These authors matched nine patients with similar infarcts in the middle cerebral artery territory of the right and left hemispheres; the right hemisphere group had much less elevation of the contralateral shoulder when subjects were asked to lift both shoulders than did the left.

Experimental evidence also favors motor akinesia as a factor in neglect behavior. Heilman and colleagues demonstrated unilateral or hemispatial hypokinesia in three separate experimental paradigms. First, patients were tested on a line bisection task after being asked to read a letter on the right or left end of the line. Looking to the left or right before bisecting the line had very little effect on performance, whereas moving the entire line into the subject's left hemispace produced much more neglect than placement of the line in the midline or to the right. The authors interpreted these findings as more consistent with hemispatial hypokinesia than with a sensory or attentional mechanism (Heilman and Valenstein 1979). Second, patients were asked to point directly in front of their chests, with their eyes closed, to what they thought was the midline. In this task, patients with right hemisphere lesions erred more to the right of midline than those with left hemisphere lesions erred to the left. The authors again interpreted this result as a motor phenomenon, as the task, in their opinion, did not require any visual or somatosensory input from the left side (Heilman *et al.* 1983). The third experimental model involved monkeys with lesions in either the right frontal (Watson, Miller, and Heilman, 1978) or right temporoparietal (Valenstein *et al.* 1982) cortex, both of which produced neglect but no paralysis. The animals were required to move the right upper limb, ipsilateral to the lesion, when stimulated on the left, and the contralateral (left) upper limb when stimulated on the right. Only stimulation on the side ipsilateral to the lesion produced abnormal motor responses. Because the ipsilateral side would be expected to have normal sensation, this deficit too appeared more consistent with hypokinesia than with sensory loss as the mechanism of neglect. Husain and colleagues (2000) have also confirmed the role of the parietal lobe in planning motor reaching to the contralateral space, from human stroke cases as well as animal models.

Mesulam (1981) attempted to synthesize the behavioral and neuroanatomical data on neglect in a 'network' approach. In this model, the right inferior parietal region contains the sensory schema for the contralateral body, and hence right parietal lesions produce sensory inattention, extinction, and abnormalities of spatial and topographical function. The frontal lobe subserves movement and exploration in contralateral space, and hence right frontal lesions produce inattention and hypokinesia. The cingulate gyrus, a limbic structure also implicated in neglect (Heilman and Valenstein 1972), relates to the motivation to explore or attend to contralateral space. The cingulate gyrus has extensive connections to other limbic structures thought related to motivation and rewards. Finally, the reticular activating system in the brain stem and thalamus is necessary for arousal, vigilance, and attention, especially as directed to the contralateral body and space. Support for a right hemisphere network subserving attention has also come from PET studies (Fiorelli *et al.* 1991), which showed hypometabolism throughout the frontal, temporal, and parietal cortex and subcortical structures in right hemisphere stroke patients with neglect, even if the anatomic lesion was much smaller. This 'network' theory brings together the three mechanisms of sensory alteration, inattention, and hypokinesia, and takes into account much of the clinical and experimental evidence relating to neglect.

Recovery and Therapy of Hemineglect

Neglect is a disabling deficit in patients with strokes and other right hemisphere injuries. Frequently, progress in rehabilitation is minimal until the patient can recognize the deficits in the neglected side of the body and work actively to correct them. Neglect is often variable, coming and going in the same patient on the same tests (Small and Ellis 1994), perhaps related to alertness, fatigue, motivation, and presence of other stimuli on the left side (Seki *et al.* 1996). Neglect is temporarily reduced by vestibular stimulation via cold liquids infused into the ear canal (Cappa *et al.* 1987; Rode *et al.* 1998). A study of recovery of visual neglect after stroke (Stone *et al.* 1992) found that most patients had recovered from neglect at 3 months post-onset. The most rapid recovery occurred in the first 10 days. Amphetamine stimulation may facilitate motor recovery, possibly via alleviation of neglect (Crisostomo *et al*, 1988; Walker-Batson *et al.* 1995; Grade *et al.* 1998). A prospective trial of amphetamines in stroke patients undergoing rehabilitation has recently been initiated. These and other methods are used in rehabilitation programs to try to help patients recognize their deficits, so that they can work to adapt to or overcome them.

Motor Impersistence

A right hemisphere syndrome related to neglect is 'motor impersistence', or the tendency for patients to cease a motor task even when asked to continue it. Such impersistence is seen even in simple tasks such as closing the eyes, opening the mouth, protruding the tongue, or gazing to the left (Kertesz *et al.* 1985). Hier and colleagues (1983) tested motor impersistence as one of the symptoms in their study of right hemisphere stroke patients; like neglect, motor impersistence correlated with right parietal lesions. Motor impersistence is a functionally important deficit when it interferes with rehabilitation or the carrying out of life or work activities.

EMOTIONAL INDIFFERENCE

In addition to the phenomena of visuospatial-constructional impairment, hemi-inattention, and denial of deficit, patients with right hemisphere lesions frequently manifest changes in emotional state. These changes are evident in the patient's affect and mood, as assessed during the medical history (see Chapter 4). When sustained over weeks and months, they constitute an alteration in the patient's entire personality. Patients with acute right hemisphere strokes often seem indifferent, unconcerned, and apathetic, despite major neurological impairments that threaten their jobs and family security. This emotional flatness may persist despite the return of at least partial intellectual understanding of the situation. Some right hemisphere stroke patients seem generally unmotivated and unselfconscious, lying passively in bed, neglecting their personal hygiene, and failing to cover themselves when visitors enter. One normally fastidious patient continued to eat his dinner, allowing food to dribble down the left side of his chin, and repeatedly scratched his genitals while the physician attempted to discuss the prognosis with the patient and his wife. These emotional aspects of right hemisphere dysfunction, together with hemi-inattention and neglect, are frequently more difficult for families to adjust to than the aphasic deficits associated with left hemisphere disease.

Human emotion is a complex phenomenon, not clearly localized to specific regions of the brain. Focal brain lesions, however, do affect emotional states in specific and predictable ways, and emotion therefore is an important part of the behavioral neurology assessment. Chapter 17 will explore this subject in further detail. Left hemisphere lesions are frequently associated with heightened emotional responses. As mentioned in Chapter 5, patients with left frontal lesions and Broca's or global aphasia frequently appear severely withdrawn and depressed, a symptom complex termed the 'catastrophic reaction' by Goldstein (1948). Patients with left temporoparietal lesions and Wernicke' s aphasia often seem angry and frustrated that they are not being understood, and over time they may become aggressive or paranoid (Benson 1973). These left hemisphere emotional states contrast strikingly with the decreased emotional responsiveness seen with right hemisphere disease. As will be discussed in Chapter 10, patients with bilateral frontal lobe dysfunction show an even more marked emotional flatness than patients with right hemisphere lesions, a state termed 'akinetic mutism' or 'abulia'. These differences in emotional state with lesions in different brain regions have been validated in several large studies (Gainotti 1972; Gasparrini *et al.* 1978; Robinson and Price 1982; Robinson *et al.* 1984). Robinson and colleagues (1984) found that depression correlated not only with left hemisphere localization as compared to right, but also to anterior hemisphere as compared to posterior lesions. Many subsequent studies, however, have failed to confirm either a left hemisphere or an anterior lesion preponderance in post-stroke depression (Dam *et al.* 1989; House *et al.* 1990; Pohjasvaara *et al.* 1998; Gainotti *et al.* 1999). Some of the discrepancy may have to do with the timing of assessment, as right hemisphere stroke patients may be indifferent and flat in affect in the early post-stroke period but then become depressed over time. Hospitalized patients are also more likely to be depressed than community patients (Robinson, 2000). In one study, the Minnesota Multiphasic Personality Inventory showed more marked depression in left- as opposed to right-hemisphere-damaged patients despite approximately equal degrees of cognitive loss as measured by a neuropsychological test battery (Gasparrini *et al.* 1978). In a series of stroke patients, ischemic lesions in the right frontal region were most likely to be associated with emotional indifference, whereas patients with more posterior right hemisphere damage manifested depression nearly as often as patients with left hemisphere damage (Robinson *et al.* 1984). One biochemical marker of depression, the failure of adrenal cortisol secretion to be suppressed after a test dose of dexamethasone, has shown more frequent abnormalities after left than after right hemisphere strokes. Four patients with right hemisphere lesions and the 'indifference reaction' had normal dexamethasone suppression tests (Finklestein *et al.* 1982).

The cerebral mechanisms underlying the decreased emotional responsiveness of right hemisphere dysfunction are incompletely understood. Heilman and his colleagues have related the 'indifference reaction' to the decreased arousal seen with right hemisphere lesions (Heilman *et al.* 1978; Heilman and Bowers 1982), as discussed in the previous section with reference to neglect. Considerable clinical and experimental evidence has pointed to a dominant role of the right hemisphere in emotional processes. Patients with right hemisphere lesions have difficulty perceiving the emotional expression of faces (DeKosky *et al.* 1980; Kolb and Taylor 1981). Right-hemisphere-damaged patients also have difficulty expressing and comprehending the emotional tone of speech, a subject discussed in the next section. Studies in normal subjects have demonstrated superiority of the right hemisphere for perception of emotional faces, as tested by flashing pictures very rapidly by means of a tachistoscope into only the left or right visual field. The left visual field, and hence the right hemisphere, was consistently more accurate in identifying facial emotions (Suberi and McKeever 1977; Ley and Bryden 1979). Normal subjects have also shown greater emotional responses to scenes of surgical operations presented in the left visual field (Dimond *et al.* 1976). Emotional expression in normal people may also be more intense on the left side of the face (Sackheim *et al.* 1978).

Another source of evidence concerning hemispheric specialization for emotion has come from studies of patients with partial complex or temporal lobe epilepsy, a subject discussed in Chapter 19. Patients with epileptic foci in the right temporal lobe more frequently manifest mood changes or aggressive behavior, whereas those with left temporal foci show altered thought patterns and intellectual–philosophical concerns (McIntyre *et al.* 1976; Bear and Fedio 1977; Flor-Henry 1979). Bear (1983) suggested that the specialization of the left inferior parietal region for the intermodality associations needed for language has caused the analogous region of the right hemisphere to become dominant for the surveillance of the environment for drive-related stimuli. This specialization may account for the superior spatial abilities and enhanced affective responses of the right hemisphere (Bear 1983).

RIGHT HEMISPHERE FUNCTIONS IN LANGUAGE AND COMMUNICATION

Although the left hemisphere is usually dominant for language, considerable evidence has accumulated that the right hemisphere also has important functions in communication. First, left-handed patients often have partial or complete right hemisphere dominance for language (Subirana 1969). Rarely, right-handed persons have 'crossed' dominance for language and develop clinically obvious aphasia after right hemisphere lesions (see Chapter 5). More importantly, the right hemisphere may have some language capability even in the great majority of persons who are right-handed and left hemisphere-dominant for language. Evidence for some language capability in the right hemisphere has come from patients with surgical removal of the left hemisphere for tumor (Smith 1966), from 'split-brain' (commissurotomy) studies (Gazzaniga and Sperry 1967; Sidtis *et al.* 1981), and from language recovery in patients with extensive left hemisphere damage (Cummings *et al.* 1979; Landis *et al.* 1982). Mild deficits in semantic comprehension and naming have been reported in patients with right hemisphere lesions (Rivers and Love 1980; Gainotti *et al.* 1981). Although some of these deficits can be attributed to neglect or visuospatial impairments (Rivers and Love 1980; Cavalli *et al.* 1981), others appear to reflect a true language disturbance (Gainotti *et al.* 1981). Stimulation of the exposed right hemisphere in patients undergoing neurosurgical procedures has also produced errors in naming and completion of sentences (Bhatnagar and Andy 1984). Overall, however, patients with right hemisphere injury and an intact left hemisphere retain largely normal linguistic abilities.

In contrast to the limited role of the right hemisphere in linguistic processes, the non-verbal or emotional aspects of communication are severely affected by right hemisphere injury. Patients may understand 'what is said but not how it is said' (Tucker *et al.* 1977). Heilman and colleagues demonstrated that patients with right temporoparietal lesions and neglect had markedly reduced ability to perceive the emotional tone of dictated sentences compared to patients with left hemisphere lesions and aphasia (Heilman *et al.* 1975). These authors referred to the deficit as an 'affective agnosia'. Later studies have shown that the expression as well as the comprehension of emotional tone is impaired by right hemisphere lesions (Tucker *et al.* 1977; Ross and Mesulam 1979). Ross has proposed bedside tests of expression, comprehension, and repetition of emotional tone. In a manner analogous to the classification of the aphasias, he grouped these emotional deficits into 'motor', 'sensory', and 'transcortical' forms (Ross 1981). Ross has termed these disorders 'aprosodias', in that the prosody or musical quality of speech is lost. Aprosodia has also been described after a right hemisphere subcortical infarct (Ross *et al.* 1981). A recent comparison of 20 right hemisphere and 18 left hemisphere normal subjects did confirm the presence of affective prosody disturbance in all 20 patients, but comparisons between expressive and receptive aprosodia and lesion localization were not meaningful (Wertz *et al.* 1998). Although the division into these separate categories of aprosodia may exceed the practical usefulness of the concept, the recognition of a loss of emotional aspects of communication in right hemisphere disease is very important to the understanding of the behavior of these patients. The emotional flatness of speech doubtless plays a role in the 'indifference reaction' described in these patients. Prosody of speech, as affected by right hemisphere lesions, involves more than simply emotional tone. Mesulam and colleagues demonstrated that non-emotional aspects of prosody, such as the placement of stress or emphasis within a sentence or the ability to distinguish the intonations of a question and a statement, may be impaired in right-hemisphere-damaged patients (Weintraub *et al.* 1981). Other complex effects of right hemisphere disease in communication, such as an inability to detect humor or a failure of judgment of plausibility or logical relationships in sentences, have also been described (Wapner *et al.* 1981). Because comprehension of language depends heavily on intonations, emphasis, context, humor, and emotional tone, it is easy to see that patients with right hemisphere lesions are at a distinct disadvantage in interpersonal communication despite their preserved linguistic skills. Thus, although language seems intact in right hemisphere stroke patients, the pragmatics of communication, the organization of discourse, and the interplay of conversation can be seriously impaired. Rehabilitative efforts should include attention to these communication difficulties (Kirshner *et al.* 1999).

CONCLUSION

The impairments brought about by right hemisphere damage comprise a variety of behaviorally important dysfunctions. Some, such as dressing impairment, spatial disorientation, and neglect of deficit, make themselves obvious to both families and physicians. Others, such as constructional impairment, alterations in emotional state, and blunting of the prosodic and emotional aspects of language, are more subtle and may require deliberate testing for documentation. An awareness of the rich variety of dysfunctions seen with right hemisphere damage not only permits the physician to diagnose brain lesions but also helps in understanding the behavior of these patients.

REFERENCES

Adair JC, Williamson DJG, Schwartz RL et al. Dissociation of sensory-attentional from motor-intentional neglect. J Neurol Neurosurg Psychiatry 1998;64:331–338.

Babinski J. Contribution a l'étude des troubles mentaux dans l'hemiplegie organique cerebrale (Anosognosie). Revue neurologique 1914;22:845–848. Translated in DA Rottenberg, FH Hochberg. Neurological Classics in Modern Translation. New York: Hafner Press, 1977;131–135.

Battersby WS, Bender MB, Pollack M, Kahn RL. Unilateral spatial agnosia ('inattention') in patients with cerebral lesions. Brain 1956;79:68–92.

Bear DM. Hemispheric specialization and the neurology of emotion. Arch Neurol 1983; 40:195–202.

Bear DM, Fedio P. Quantitative analysis of interictal behavior in temporal lobe epilepsy. Arch Neurol 1977;34:454–467.

Bellas DN, Novelly RA, Eskenazi B, Wasserstein J. Unilateral displacement in the olfactory sense: a manifestation of the unilateral neglect syndrome. Cortex 1988;24: 267–275.

Bender MB, Teuber, HL. Allesthesia and disturbance of the body schema. Arch Neurol Psychiatry 1949;62:222–231.

Benson DF. Psychiatric aspects of aphasia. Br J Psychiatry 1973;123:555–566.

Benson DF, Gardner H, Meadows JC. Reduplicative paramnesia. Neurology (NY) 1976; 26:147–151.

Benson DF, Cummings JC, Tsai SI. Angular gyrus syndrome simulating Alzheimer's disease. Arch Neurol 1982; 39:616–620.

Benton AL. Constructional apraxia and the minor hemisphere. Confin Neurol 1967;29: 1–16.

Benton AL. Visuoconstructive disability in patients with cerebral disease: its relationship to side of lesion and aphasic disorder. Doc Ophthalmol 1973; 34:67–76.

Benton AL, Levin HS, Van Allen MW. Geographic orientation in patients with unilateral cerebral disease. Neuropsychologia 1974;12:183–191.

Benton AL, Hannay J, Varney NR. Visual perception of line direction in patients with unilateral brain disease. Neurology (NY) 1975;25:907–910.

Beschin N, Cocchini G, Della Sala S, Logie RH. What the eyes perceive, the brain ignores: a case of pure unilateral representational neglect. Cortex 1997;33:3–26.

Bhatnagar S, Andy OJ. Language in the nondominant right hemisphere. Arch Neurol 1984;40:728–731.

Bisiach E, Luzzatti C. Unilateral neglect of representational space. Cortex 1978;14:129–133.

Black FW, Strub RL. Constructional apraxia in patients with discrete missile wounds of the brain. Cortex 1976;12:212–220.

Bogousslavsky J, Miklossy J, Regli F *et al.* Subcortical neglect: neuropsychological, SPECT, and neuropathological correlations with anterior choroidal artery territory infarction. Ann Neurol 1988;23:448–452.

Bottini G, Cappa S, Geminiani G, Sterzi R. Topographic disorientation: a case report. Neuropsychologia 1990;28:309–312.

Brain WR. Visual disorientation with special reference to lesions of the right cerebral hemisphere. Brain 1941; 64:244–272.

Calvanio R, Petrone PN, Levine DN. Left visual spatial neglect is both environment-centered and body-centered. Neurology 1987;37:1179–1183.

Caplan LR, Kelly M, Kase CS *et al.* Infarcts of the inferior division of the right middle cerebral artery: mirror image of Wernicke's aphasia. Neurology 1986;36:1015–1020.

Cappa S, Sterzi R, Vallar G, Bisiach E. Remission of hemineglect and anosognosia during vestibular stimulation. Neuropsychologia; 1987;25:775–782.

Cavalli M, DeRenzi E, Faglioni P, Vitale A. Impairment of right brain-damaged patients on a linguistic cognitive task. Cortex 1981;17:545–556.

Coslett HB, Heilman KM. Hemihypokinesia after right hemisphere stroke. Brain Cogn 1989;9:267–278.

Crisostomo E, Duncan P, Propst M *et al.* Evidence that amphetamine with physical therapy promotes recovery of motor function in stroke patients. Ann Neurol 1988;23:94–97.

Critchley M. The Parietal Lobes. New York: Hafner, 1966.

Cummings JL, Benson DF, Walsh MJ, Levine HL. Left-to-right transfer of language dominance: a case study. Neurology (NY) 1979;29:1547–1550.

Cutting J. A study of anosognosia. Neurol Neurosurg Psychiatry 1978;41:548–555.

Dam H, Pedersen HE, Ahlgren P. Depression among patients with stroke. Acta Psychiaatr Scand 1989;80:118–124.

Damasio AR, Damasio H, Chui HC. Neglect following damage to frontal lobe or basal ganglia. Neuropsychologia 1980;18:123–132.

DeKosky S, Heilman K, Bowers D, Valenstein E. Recognition and discrimination of emotional faces and pictures. Brain Lang 1980;9:206–214.

Denes G, Semenza C, Stoppa E, Lis A. Unilateral spatial neglect and recovery from hemiplegia. Brain 1982;105:543–552.

Denny-Brown D, Chambers RA. The parietal lobe and behavior. Proc Assoc Res Nerv Ment Dis 1958;36:35–117.

Denny-Brown D, Meyers JS, Horenstein S. The significance of perceptual rivalry resulting from parietal lobe lesion. Brain 1952;75:433–471.

DeRenzi E, Faglioni P. The comparative efficiency of intelligence and vigilance detecting hemisphere damage. Cortex 1965;1:410–433.

Dimond SJ, Farrington L, Johnson P. Differing emotional response from right and left hemispheres. Nature 1976;261:690–692.

Egelko S, Gordon WA, Hibbard MR *et al.* Relationship among CT scans, neurological exam, and neuropsychological test performance in right brain-damaged stroke patients. J Clin Exp 1988;10:539–564.

Ettlinger G, Warrington E, Zangwill OL. A further study of visual–spatial agnosia. Brain 1957; 80:335–361.

Ferro JM, Kertesz A. Posterior internal capsule infarction associated with neglect. Arch Neurol 1984;41:422–424.

Finklestein S, Benowitz LI, Baldessarini RJ *et al.* Mood, vegetative disturbance, and dexamethasone suppression test after stroke. Ann Neurol 1982;12:463–468.

Fiorelli M, Blin J, Bakchine S *et al.* PET studies of diaschisis in patients with motor hemi-neglect. J Neurol Sci 1991;104:135–142.

Flor-Henry P. Schizophrenic-like reactions and affective psychoses associated with temporal lobe epilepsy. Am J Psychiatry 1979;126:400–403.

Gainotti G. Emotional behavior and hemispheric side of lesion. Cortex 1972;8:41–55.

Gainotti G, Messerli P, Tissot R. Qualitative analysis of unilateral spatial neglect in relation to laterality of cerebral lesions. J Neurol Neurosurg Psychiatry 1972;35: 545–550.

Gainotti G, Caltagirone C, Miceli G, Masullo C. Selective semantic-lexical impairment of language comprehension in right brain-damaged patients. Brain Lang 1981;13:201–211.

Gainotti G, Azzoni A, Marra C. Frequency, phenomenology and anatomical–clinical correlates of major post-stroke depression. Br J Psychiatry 1999;175;163–167.

Gasparrini W, Satz P, Heilman K, Coolidge F. Hemispheric asymmetries of affective processing as determined by the MMPI. J Neurol Neurosurg Psychiatry 1978;4:470–473.

Gazzaniga MS, Sperry RW. Language after section of the cerebral commissures. Brain 1967;90:131–148.

Goldstein K. Language and Language Disturbances. New York: Grune & Stratton, 1948.

Grade C, Redford B, Chrostowski J et al. Methylphenidate in early post-stroke recovery: a double-blind, placebo-controlled study. Arch Phys Med Rehabil 1998;79:1047–1050.

Healton EB, Navarro C, Bressman S, Brust JCM. Subcortical neglect. Neurology (NY) 1982; 32:776–778.

Hecaen H. Aphasic, apraxic, and agnostic syndromes in right and left hemisphere lesions. In PJ Vinken, GW Bruyn (eds), Handbook of Clinical Neurology, Vol. 4. Amsterdam: North Holland, 1969;291–311.

Heilman KM, Bowers D. Affective disorders induced by hemispheric dysfunction. In HS Kirshner, FR Freemon (eds), The Neurology of Aphasia. Amsterdam: Swets, 1982; 173–185.

Heilman KM, Valenstein E. Frontal lobe neglect in man. Neurology (NY) 1972;22: 660–664.

Heilman KM, Valenstein E. Mechanisms underlying hemispatial neglect. Ann Neurol 1979;5:166–170.

Heilman KM, Van Den Abell T. Right hemisphere dominance for attention: the mechanism underlying hemispheric asymmetries of inattention (neglect). Neurology (NY) 1980;30:327–330.

Heilman KM, Watson RT. Mechanisms underlying the unilateral neglect syndrome. Adv Neurol 1977;18:93–105.

Heilman KM, Scholes R, Watson RT. Auditory affective agnosia: disturbed comprehension of affective speech. J Neurol Neurosurg Psychiatry 1975;38:69–72.

Heilman KM, Schwartz HD, Watson RT. Hypoarousal in patients with neglect syndrome and emotional indifference. Neurology (NY) 1978;28:229–232.

Heilman KM, Bowers D, Watson RJ. Performance on hemispatial pointing task by patients with neglect syndrome. Neurology (NY) 1983;33:661–664.

Hier DB, Davis KR, Richardson EP, Mohr JP. Hypertensive putamenal hemorrhage. Ann Neurol 1977;1:152–159.

Hier DB, Mondlock J, Caplan LR. Behavioral abnormalities after right hemisphere stroke. Neurology (NY) 1983; 33:337–344.

House A, Dennis M, Warlow C et al. Mood disorders after stroke and their relation to lesion location: a CT scan study. Brain 1990;113:1113–1130.

Howes D, Boller F. Simple reaction times: evidence for focal impairment from lesions of the right hemisphere. Brain 1975;98:312–332.

Husain M, Mattingley JB, Rorden C et al. Distinguishing sensory and motor biases in parietal and frontal neglect. Brain 2000;123:1643–1659.

Karnath H-O, Ferber S, Himmelbach M. Spatial awareness is a function of the temporal not the posterior parietal lobe. Nature 2001;411:950–953.

Kertesz A, Nicholson I, Cancelliere A et al. Motor impersistence: a right-hemisphere syndrome. Neurology 1985;35:662–666.

Kirshner HS, Alexander M, Lorch MP, Wertz RT. Disorders of speech and language. Continuum 1999;5:1–237.

Kolb B, Taylor L. Affective behavior in patients with localized cortical excisions: role of lesion site and side. Science 1981;214:89–91.

Landis T, Graves R, Goodglass H. Aphasic reading and writing: possible evidence for right hemisphere participation. Cortex 1982;18:105–112.

Levine DN, Finklestein S. Delayed psychosis after right temporoparietal stroke or trauma: relationship to epilepsy. Neurology (NY) 1982;32:267–273.

Levine DN, Grek A. The anatomic basis of delusions after right cerebral infarction. Neurology (NY) 1984;34:577–582.

Ley R, Bryden M. Hemispheric differences in recognizing faces and emotions. Brain Lang 1979;1:127–138.

Lezak, M: Neuropsychological Assessment. 2nd Ed. New York: Oxford University 27. Press 1983.

Marshall JC, Halligan PW. Imagine only the half of it. Nature 1993;364:193–194.

McIntyre M, Prichard PB, Lombroso CT. Left and right temporal lobe epileptics: a controlled investigation of some psychological differences. Epilepsia 1976;17:377–386.

Mesulam M-M. A cortical network for directed attention and unilateral neglect. Ann Neurol 1981; 10:309–325.

Mesulam M-M, Waxman SG, Geschwind N, Sabin TD. Acute confusional states with right middle cerebral artery infarctions. J Neurol Neurosurg Psychiatry 1976;39:84–89.

Na DL, Adair JC, Williamson DJG et al. Dissociation of sensory-attentional from motor-intentional neglect. J Neurol Neurosurg Psychiatry 1998;64:331–338.

Pohjasvaara T, Leppavuori A, Siira I et al. Frequency and clinical determinants of post-stroke depression. Stroke 1998;29:2311–2317.

Rabins PV, Starkstein SE, Robinson RG. Risk factors for developing atypical (schizophreniform) psychosis following stroke. J Neuropsychiatry Clin Neurosci 1991; 36–39.

Rees G, Wojciulik E, Clarke K et al. Unconscious activation of visual cortex in the damaged right hemisphere of a parietal patient with extinction. Brain 2000;123: 1624–1633.

Rivers DL, Love RJ. Language performance on visual processing tasks in right hemisphere lesion cases. Brain Lang 1980;10:348–366.

Robinson RG. An 82 year-old woman with mood changes following a stroke. JAMA 2000;283:1607–1614.

Robinson RG, Price TR. Post-stroke depressive disorders: a follow-up study of 103 patients. Stroke 1982;13:635–641.

Robinson RG, Kubos KL, Starr LB et al. Mood disorders in stroke patients: importance of location of lesion. Brain 1984;107:81–93.

Rode G, Perenin MT, Honore J, Boisson D. Improvement of the motor deficit of neglect patients through vestibular stimulation: evidence for a motor neglect component. Cortex 1998;34:253–261.

Ross ED. The aprosodias: functional–anatomic organization of the affective components of language in the right hemisphere. Arch Neurol 1981;38:561–569.

Ross ED, Mesulam M-M. Dominant language functions of the right hemisphere? Prosody and emotional gesturing. Arch Neurol 1979;36:144–148.

Ross ED, Harney JH, deLacoste-Utamsing C, Purdy P. How the brain integrates affective and propositional language into a unified behavioral function: hypothesis based on clinico-anatomic evidence. Arch Neurol 1981;38:745–748.

Sackheim H, Gur R, Saucy M. Emotions are expressed more intensely on the left side of the face. Science 1978;202:434–436.

Samuelsson H, Jenson C, Ekholm S et al. Anatomical and neurological correlates of acute and chronic visuospatial neglect following right hemisphere stroke. Cortex 1997;33: 271–285.

Schwartz AS, Marchok PL, Kreinick CJ, Flynn RE. The asymmetric lateralization of tactile extinction in patients with unilateral cerebral dysfunction. Brain 1979;102:669–684.

Seki K, Ishiai S, Koyama Y, Fujimoto Y. Appearance and disappearance of unilateral spatial neglect for an object: influence of attention-attracting peripheral stimuli. Neuropsychologia 1996;34:819–826.

Sidtis JJ, Volpe BT, Wilson DH *et al.* Variability in right hemisphere language function after callosal section: evidence for a continuum of generative capacity. J Neurosci 1981;1:323–331.

Small M, Ellis S. Brief remission periods in visuospatial neglect: evidence from long-term follow-up. Eur Neurol 1994;34:147–154.

Smith A. Speech and other functions after left (dominant) hemispherectomy. J Neurol Neurosurg Psychiatry 1966;29:467–471.

Stone SP, Patel P, Greenwood RJ, Halligan PW. Measuring visual neglect in acute stroke and predicting its recovery: the visual neglect recovery index. J Neurol Neurosurg Psychiat 1992;55:431–436.

Suberi M, McKeever W. Differential right hemisphere memory storage of emotional and non-emotional faces. Neuropsychologia 1977;15:757–768.

Subirana A. Handedness and cerebral dominance. In PJ Vinken, GW Bruyn (eds), Handbook of Clinical Neurology, Vol. 4. Amsterdam: North-Holland, 1969;248–272.

Takahashi N, Kawamura M, Shiota J *et al.* Pure topographic disorientation due to right retrosplenial lesion. Neurology 1997;49:464–469.

Tucker DM, Watson RT, Heilman KM. Discrimination and evocation of affectively intoned speech in patients with right parietal disease. Neurology (NY) 1977;27:947–950.

Valenstein E, Heilman KM. Unilateral hypokinesia and motor extinction. Neurology (NY) 1981; 31:445–448.

Valenstein E, Van Den Abell T, Watson RT, Heilman KM. Non-sensory neglect from parietotemporal lesions in monkeys. Neurology (NY) 1982;32:1198–1201.

Walker-Batson D, Smith P *et al.* Amphetamine paired with physical therapy accelerates motor recovery after stroke. Further evidence. Stroke 1995;26:2254–2259.

Wapner W, Hamby S, Gardner H. The role of the right hemisphere in the apprehension of complex language materials. Brain Lang 1981;14:15–33.

Watson RT, Heilman KM. Thalamic neglect. Neurology (NY) 1979;29:690–694.

Watson RT, Miller BD, Heilman KM. Non-sensory neglect. Ann Neurol 1978;3:505–508.

Watson RT, Valenstein E, Heilman KM. Thalamic neglect: possible role of the medial thalamus and nucleus reticularis in behavior. Arch Neurol 1981;38:501–506.

Weintraub S, Mesulam M-M, Kramer L. Disturbances in prosody: a right hemisphere contribution to language. Arch Neurol 1981;38:742–744.

Wertz RT, Henschel CR, Auther L *et al.* Affective prosodic disturbance subsequent to right hemisphere stroke. J Neuroling 1998;11:89–102.

10

Frontal Lobe Syndromes

The equilibrium or balance... between his intellectual faculties and animal propensities seems to have been destroyed. He is fitful, irreverent, indulging at times in the grossest profanity..., manifesting but little deference for his fellows, impatient of restraint or advice when it conflicts with his desires, at times pertinaciously obstinate, yet capricious and vacillating, devising many plans of operation, which are no sooner arranged than they are abandoned in turn for others appearing more feasible. A child in his intellectual capacity and manifestations, he has the animal passions of a strong man... His mind was radically changed, so decidedly that his friends and acquaintances said he was 'no longer Gage'.

(Harlow 1868, describing Phineas Gage)

The frontal lobes make up a major portion of the human brain, greatly expanded in comparison to mammalian or even primate brains, yet their precise functions have been difficult to elucidate. The frontal regions are sometimes called 'silent', because large amounts of frontal brain tissue can be damaged or surgically resected without gross consequences in terms of motor, sensory, or even language and cognitive functions. A neurologist may examine a patient with frontal damage and find nothing wrong, yet the family sees drastic changes in the patient's behavior and personality; they may go so far as to declare, like Phineas Gage's friends, 'he is not the same person'. Changes in behavior after frontal lobe lesions may be extremely subtle, involving emotions and modes of behavior more than measurable higher cortical functions. On the other hand, mood and behavior changes involve our very personality, that which makes us who we are. Frontal lobe disorders are a true borderland between neurology and psychiatry, and a subject of great interest and controversy in behavioral neurology and neuropsychology.

Some investigators (Rylander 1939; Halstead 1947) have emphasized a critical relationship of the frontal lobes to higher mental functioning, but others (Hebb 1939; Teuber 1964; Smith 1966) have stressed the intactness of cognitive abilities after severe frontal lobe insults. Much of this discrepancy can be explained by three factors. First, many of the behavioral changes that accompany frontal lobe disease are extremely difficult to evaluate and quantify with formal tests. Second, the specific behavioral tasks are important; patients with frontal lobe lesions sometimes show markedly different performances when the tasks are varied by minor changes in procedures (Milner 1964). Third, the specific lesion and location in the frontal lobe can make an enormous difference in the behavioral consequences. Behavioral sequelae of a frontal lobe lesion vary as a function of the side (Benton 1968) and size (Luria 1969) of the lesion, the specific frontal regions affected (Milner 1964), the type of pathology (Luria 1969), the presence of distant effects from a mass lesion, increased pressure or diaschisis (Luria 1969), the extent of subcortical damage (Geschwind 1975), and the time course of the disease (Damasio *et al.* 1980).

Although the term 'frontal lobe syndrome' is in common usage, there is no single specific behavioral syndrome that regularly or consistently accompanies frontal lobe lesions. In fact, a wide variety of behavioral changes accompany frontal lobe lesions. These include some of the syndromes discussed in other chapters: altered consciousness (Chapter 3), aphasia (Chapter 5), apraxia (Chapter 7), dementia (Chapter 13), delirium (Chapter 14), and emotional changes (Chapter 17). As in these other behavioral syndromes, the information derived from the history and bedside examination is crucial for the evaluation of these sometimes subtle neurobehavioral syndromes.

This chapter reviews briefly the anatomy of the frontal lobes, and then considers the behavioral disturbances of frontal lobe disease. Frontal lobe disorders, outlined in Table 10.1, are divided into the categories of abstraction and judgment, attention and memory, language, spatial functions, motor functions, and personality or emotional changes. Finally, we shall discuss the specific diseases commonly associated with frontal lobe pathology.

FRONTAL LOBE ANATOMY

For practical purposes, the frontal lobes should not be regarded as a single functional unit. The frontal lobes are the largest of all of the lobes of the brain, constituting roughly one-third of the surface of each hemisphere (Carpenter 1972). Each frontal lobe is comprised of three major cortical areas: (1) the lateral convexity; (2) the medial surface; and (3) the inferior, orbital aspect. The primary motor cortex (Brodmann area 4) is the posterior-most part of the frontal lobe, lying immediately anterior to the central or Rolandic sulcus on the lateral convexity. Just in front of the primary motor area is the premotor area (Brodmann areas 6, parts of 8, 44, 45). Both the motor cortex and premotor area overlap the superior convexity and continue on the medial surface of the hemisphere, down to the cingulate sulcus. The premotor region is involved in motor planning. It includes the cortical eye fields and the supplementary motor area. On the inferior medial surface of the frontal lobe, between the cingulate sulcus and the corpus callosum, is the cingulate gyrus. The cingulate gyrus (Brodmann area 24) is

Table 10.1   Frontal lobe behavioral disturbances

Abstraction and judgment
   Normal IQ, memory
   Concrete proverb interpretation
   Decreased insight and judgment
   Perseveration
   Defective planning

Attention and memory
   Inattentiveness
   Normal memory, except 'recency' deficit

Language
   Non-fluency, transcortical motor aphasia
   Abulia, akinetic mutism

Visuospatial impairment
   Motor (intentional neglect) or 'planning' rather than perceptual deficit

Motor changes
   Abulia, akinetic mutism
   Motor perseveration
   'Utilization' and 'imitation' behavior
   Apraxia

Emotional and personality changes
   Apathy, inattentiveness
   Abulia, akinetic mutism
   Euphoria, facetiousness
   'Pseudodepressed' personality
   'Pseudopsychopathic' personality
   Pseudobulbar emotional lability

increasingly important to behavioral neurology; it comprises part of the Papez circuit of the limbic system and is involved in initiation of many types of behavior. The rest of the frontal cortex anterior to the premotor region is the 'prefrontal cortex'. The prefrontal cortex is the area to which most authors refer when they speak of the 'frontal lobes' in relation to behavioral changes. The prefrontal cortex includes Brodmann areas 9–13, 46, 47, and parts of 8 and 24 (Carpenter 1972).

   The best way to think of the functional anatomy of the frontal lobes is in a series of 'frontal-subcortical circuits', as summarized by Cummings (1993). All of these circuits have in common a loop beginning in the frontal cortex, projecting to the striatum (caudate and putamen), in turn to the globus pallidus and substantia nigra, then to the thalamus (especially the dorsomedial and centromedial nuclei), and finally back to the frontal cortex. There are five frontal-subcortical circuits, as shown in Table 10.2. The first is the motor circuit, familiar to most neurologists through its involvement in movement disorders such as Parkinson's disease. The second circuit is an oculomotor circuit, beginning in the frontal eye

Table 10.2 Frontal-subcortical circuits (Reprinted with permission from JL Cummings. Frontal-subcortical circuits and human behavior. ArchNeurol 1993;50:873–880)

No. 1 Motor	No. 2 Oculomotor	No. 3 Dorsolateral prefrontal	No. 4 Lateral orbitofrontal	No. 5 Anterior cingulate
Motor, SMA, premotor	Frontal eye fields (B8)	Lat prefrontal (B9,10)	Inferolateral prefrontal (B10)	Anterior cingulate gyrus (B24)
Putamen	Central caudate	Dorsolateral caudate	Ventromedial caudate	Ventral striatum (n accumbens)
VL globus pallidus	Dorsomedial GP, SN	Dorsomedial GP, SN	Dorsomedial GP, SN	Rostrolateral GP, SN
VL, VA, CM Thalamus	VA, MD thalamus	VA, MD thalamus	VA, MD thalamus	MD thalamus ventral tegmental, habenula,
hypothalamus				amygdala
Motor, SMA, premotor	Frontal eye fields	Lateral prefrontal	Orbital frontal	Anterior cingulate
Movement	Eye movements	Executive functions	Personality changes	Akinetic mutism

GP = globus pallidus; SN = substantia nigra; VL = ventrolateral nucleus of thalamus; VA = ventral anterior nucleus of thalamus; CM = centromedian nucleus of thalamus; MD = medial dorsal nucleus of thalamus; DM = dorsomedial nucleus of thalamus.

fields on the superior frontal convexity (Brodmann area 8). The last three circuits all originate in portions of the prefrontal cortex and are more heavily involved in behavior. The dorsolateral frontal circuit, beginning in Brodmann areas 9 and 10 of the lateral frontal convexity, is thought to be involved in executive functions, such as motor planning, deciding which stimuli to attend to, and shifting cognitive sets. This part of the frontal lobe is also important for attention span and working memory (see Chapter 11). The orbitofrontal circuit is heavily involved in emotional life and personality structure. Patients with lesions of this circuit may be irritable, tactless, inappropriately unconcerned, or fatuous in their sense of humor. They may exhibit an uninhibited tendency to pick up and use objects in their environment ('utilization behavior', Lhermitte *et al.* 1986), or to imitate in a slavish fashion the words and gestures of the examiner ('imitation behavior'). The anterior cingulate circuit, when lesioned, causes akinetic mutism or abulia. Disorders of these circuits encompass most of the psychopathology of frontal lobe diseases, as will be discussed in the rest of this chapter.

The afferent and efferent connections of the prefrontal cortex are important in explaining the functional importance of the frontal lobes in behavior.

Afferent connections to the frontal cortex arise from the sensory association cortex, either by direct projections or via the dorsomedial thalamic nuclei, and from subcortical structures including the dorsomedial and intralaminar nuclei of the thalamus, hypothalamus, hippocampus, amygdala, septum, and midbrain tegmentum (Nauta 1971). Through these systems the frontal lobes presumably receive neural information regarding both the external environment and the internal milieu of the individual. As discussed in Chapter 2, such interoceptive–interoceptive integration seems essential for consciousness; the 'supramodal association cortex' of the orbitofrontal region seems especially involved in this integration. Lesions of the orbitofrontal cortex are associated with profound alterations of consciousness. In addition, the extensive bi-directional connections of the frontal region to both the limbic system and the reticular activating system (in the thalamus and midbrain tegmentum) ensure a major role for the frontal lobes in the modulation of arousal, motivation, and affect. Specific cortical regions within the prefrontal area have distinctly different afferent and efferent connections. Hence lesions in different areas of the frontal lobe result in disparate behavioral manifestations.

OVERVIEW OF FRONTAL LOBE FUNCTIONS

Benson (1994) divided the behavioral effects of frontal lobe injury into five categories:

1. Sequencing
2. Drive
3. Executive control
4. 'Future memory' or planning for the future
5. Self-awareness.

These five areas of frontal functioning are fundamentally involved in frontal deficits in all of the more traditional categories of mental functioning listed in Table 10.1. They overlap considerably with each other, but an appreciation of these five functions helps to understand the richness of frontal lobe disorders.

Sequencing involves maintaining serial information in sets, integrating the information with previously learned facts, and attending to tasks in an order appropriate to solving the problem at hand. Sequencing is a form of attention or 'working memory', and is closely related to the concept of executive function (Goldman-Rakic 1996). The sequencing of behavior seems to depend critically on the lateral prefrontal convexity (Fuster 1985; Goldman-Rakic 1996). Patients who cannot carry out this sequencing activity become 'stuck' in one behavioral response mode, perseverating endlessly on tasks that are already irrelevant to the problem at hand. Stuss and Benson (1984) described a case of a middle-aged man with a bifrontal closed head injury who scored a Wechsler Full Scale IQ of 138, yet could not keep a job sorting mail. He even scored at the ninety-ninth percentile on the Raven's Progressive Matrices, but the Wisconsin Card Sort Test revealed perseverative tendencies and an inability to shift cognitive sets. "Drive, or the urge to seek gratification of basic human needs, derives from a system with cortical connections in the frontal lobes. Normal human beings learn to inhibit their drive-related activities within limitations prescribed by society. Some individuals with frontal lobe damage may either manifest a reduction of total behavioral activity (akinetic mutism, abulia, psychomotor retardation; Benson 1990). Others seem paradoxically hyperactive; more precisely, they lack normal inhibitions of behavior. The lack of activity with frontal lesions correlates best with lesions of the lateral frontal convexity. The converse, hyperactivity, appears related to midline and orbital frontal lesions, in the right but especially in both hemispheres. Cases of secondary hypomania have been described in patients with frontal lobe lesions (Cummings and Mendez 1984). Poor impulse control and irritability characterize the behavior of such patients" (Benson 1994).

Executive control involves planning behavior toward perceived goals, selecting the next response, anticipating future responses, and monitoring those behaviors already carried out. Working memory, attention, sequencing, and anticipation of the future are all aspects of this category of function. What we choose to attend to, out of the vast complexity of incoming stimuli from the external world and from our own bodies, and in what order, and with what response, summarizes the executive functions of the frontal lobes. To a large extent, executive control is the central function associated with the frontal lobes, and it integrates all of the other functions. Executive functions are almost always disturbed in the presence of frontal lobe lesions, even when more basic cognitive functions are intact (Benson 1994).

Also included in frontal executive control is the 'superego' function of inhibiting drive-related behavior. Daniel Weinberger, in an editorial in the *New York Times* (2001), presents this frontal function as follows: "The human brain has required many millennia and many evolutionary stages to reach its current complex status... As part of its capacity for achievement, it must also be able to exercise control that stops maladaptive behavior. Everyone gets angry; everybody has felt a desire for vengeance. The capacity to control impulses that arise from these feelings is a function of the prefrontal cortex. This is the part that distinguishes our brain most decisively from those of all other animals, even our closest relatives. It allows us to act on the basis of reason. It can preclude an overwhelming tendency for action (e.g., to run from a fire in a crowded theater), because an abstract memory (e.g., 'don't panic') makes more sense. It knows that all that glitters is not gold. Without a prefrontal cortex, it would be impossible to have societies based on moral and legal codes."

Future memory (Ingvar 1985) involves planning for future acts such that memory of already formulated plans is called into action. For example, when a person saves up money for an anticipated purchase, this requires advance planning and also some deferment of gratification. Patients with frontal lobe damage often appear surprised by entirely predictable occurrences, or they may simply fail to plan for the future. This function is closely related to executive control.

Self-awareness, by Benson's definition (1994), is 'the ability of the human mental system to monitor itself'. Synonyms include self-consciousness or self-analysis. When the individual plans or selects an act, this planning must involve both awareness of past actions, future potentials and goals, and a sense of the self. Imagination and fantasy of future consequences are also features of this self-awareness. Patients with frontal lesions may seem inadequately concerned about consequences of their actions on relationships with others. Other aspects of self-awareness include the inhibition of socially unacceptable drive-directed behaviors and 'reality-testing' of practical consequences of actions (Benson 1994). When we discussed consciousness in Chapter 3, the frontal cortex assumed prominence as a monitoring center for both internal drives and sensory stimuli and also as a center for the regulation of attention and action to the external world. These combined functions are necessary for the phenomenon of consciousness. Also in Chapter 3, we discussed recent research indicating that the right frontal lobe might be important for self-recognition. Subjects undergoing Wada tests looked at a 'morphed' photograph of self and a famous person. During right-sided anesthesia they chose the famous person, but during left-sided anesthesia they chose the self-photograph (Keenan *et al.* 2001).

In the rest of this chapter, these five themes of frontal lobe dysfunction shall be blended into the more traditional discussion of categories of behavior, as outlined in Table 10.1: abstraction and judgment, attention and memory, language, visuospatial functions, motor functions, and emotional and personality changes.

COGNITION, ABSTRACTION, AND JUDGMENT

The study of cognition in frontal lobe disorders is beset by the conundrum that most measurable cognitive functions are undisturbed by frontal lobe lesions, yet profound behavioral changes occur. Many neurologists and neuropsychologists in the early part of the twentieth century thought that the frontal lobes served a critical role in cognitive and intellectual abilities and abstract reasoning (Brickner 1934; Goldstein 1936; Rylander 1939; Halstead 1947). When neuropsychological testing became more routine in the era of World War II, some psychologists began to espouse a radically different viewpoint, denying the importance of the prefrontal structures in mediating cognitive activity. Hebb (1939), for instance, reported four cases from the Montreal Neurological Institute with extensive frontal lobe resections; postoperatively all patients had normal or near-normal Stanford–Binet IQ scores. Preservation of intellectual performance was particularly striking in Hebb's case 4, a 25-year-old man who had undergone a frontal lobectomy. Four years postoperatively his IQ was 152, in the very superior range. Subsequent studies have also documented that persons with large frontal lobe lesions often have normal performance on standard tests of intelligence and memory (Milner 1964; Smith 1966). A study (Black 1976) of Vietnam veterans with missile wounds to the brain indicated that the performance of patients with focal frontal lobe lesions was uniformly superior to that of patients with posterior lesions who were matched for age, education, and time since injury. The mean Wechsler Adult Intelligence Scale IQ scores and Wechsler Memory Scale Memory Quotient scores of the frontal lobe group were within the normal range. These studies do not mean that patients with frontal lesions never show changes in intelligence or memory. They do demonstrate, however, that young, previously healthy adults without other neurological disease can sustain a large injury to the frontal lobes and still seem intact not only in terms of 'hard' neurological signs but also in terms of cognitive functions.

As mentioned earlier, these normal test scores frequently contrast vividly to the family's reports of drastic changes in personality and behavior. Alterations in personality, motivation, insight, and social judgment overshadow cognitive changes in patients with frontal lobe damage. The examiner must carefully attend to these aspects of behavior during the bedside mental status examination whenever there is a possibility of frontal lobe dysfunction. In addition, the examiner must be sensitive to differences between artificial test results and actual behavior. In the area of judgment, for example, a patient may give an appropriate verbal response to a judgment question ('what would you do if you saw a fire in a movie theatre?'), yet in actual behavior may seem unable to govern actions by the same principle. The dissociation between verbal understanding and behavior is a hallmark of frontal lobe disturbance (Luria 1966).

Despite the limited usefulness of bedside cognitive testing in detecting frontal lobe dysfunction, some features of performance on tasks of cognition and abstraction are helpful. The ability to abstract is assessed during the bedside mental status examination by interpretation of familiar proverbs. Patients with frontal lobe disturbance, especially with bilateral lesions, typically show very concrete and simplistic proverb interpretation. Benton (1968) reported defective interpretation in 25% of patients with right frontal disease, 20% of patients with left frontal disease, and 71% of patients with bilateral disease. As discussed in Chapter 3, insight and judgment are practically assessed by the patients' reactions to and understanding of their own disease. Patients with frontal lobe disease are often inappropriately unconcerned about the major impact of the illness on their lives.

One of the problems with the diagnosis of frontal lobe disorders is the degree to which bedside neurological examinations can be normal. For this reason, neuropsychological testing has been especially valuable in the diagnosis of frontal disorders. Both experimentally and in neuropsychological assessment, the tests most likely to detect impairment in cognition and judgment are those reflecting ability to shift cognitive sets (Grant and Berg 1948; Cierone and Lazar 1983). Milner (1963) tested patients undergoing frontal lobectomy for intractable seizures with the Wisconsin Card Sorting Test. In this test, four stimulus cards show figures varying in color, form (shape), and number. The patient sorts the response cards, placing each card below a stimulus card on the basis of color, number, or form. The patient is told after each sort if the choice is correct. The first sorting criterion is color; sorting by any other rule is incorrect. After ten consecutive color-matched sorts have been made, the sorting criterion changes, without warning, to form rather than color. After ten according to form, the criterion changes to number, and then the entire cycle is repeated. Patients with dorsolateral frontal lesions performed more poorly than patients with other focal lesions. Frontal lobe patients were also found to have an excess of perseverative errors, or responses that would have been correct on the immediately preceding stage of the test. Both left and right frontal lobe resection patients demonstrated this tendency, a finding confirmed in other studies (Drewe 1974; Robinson *et al.* 1980). Impaired abstract reasoning and conceptual perseveration appeared to contribute to the poor performance of the frontal lobe group. Some patients were observed to verbalize correct sorting strategies even though they did not execute them in practice.

The Wisconsin Card Sort Test (WCST) has become a part of the standard armamentarium of neuropsychologists for assessment of frontal lobe disorders (Barcelo *et al.* 1997). The test probes the ability to form an abstract concept of the test goal, then to shift that concept as the criteria change. Multiple studies have confirmed that the test is sensitive to frontal lobe disorders (Nelson 1976; Spreen and Strauss 1998), but the precise anatomic locus of the critical lesion, whether dorsolateral or medial frontal, is unclear (Drewe 1974; Damasio 1983). Similar tests of ability to shift cognitive sets are the Categories Test of the Halstead–Reitan Battery (Lezak 1983), the Stroop test (five color names are presented, either with the letters themselves in five colors, or the words representing the color names, and the subject is instructed to cross out color names based on one or the other criterion), go–no go tests (See Chapter 4 for a simple example), and Trails B of the Trailmaking test of the Wechsler Adult Intelligence Scale (Mesulam 1986; Spreen and Strauss 1998).

The perseverative tendency observed in the Wisconsin Card Sorting Test is often striking in patients with significant frontal pathology. Perseveration should be carefully attended to during history taking, as well as during tests of memory, praxis, and visuoconstructive functions. Perseveration, or getting 'stuck' on one response, is evidence that the sequencing, executive control, and future memory categories of frontal function (Benson 1994) are impaired.

Another difficulty often described in patients with frontal lobe dysfunction is impaired ability to plan and organize everyday activities. Poor planning is better assessed by history than by performance on a standard mental status examination. The ability to plan and structure a sequential organization of activities can be assessed practically by asking the patient to discuss how he or she would carry out a task involving a series of steps. The examiner might ask a housewife how she would bake a cake, or a mechanic how to repair a flat tire. Deficits in planning and organization are also evidence of impaired sequencing, executive control, and future memory functions.

The ability to develop a strategy for organizing information into a meaningful sequence has consistently shown impairment in studies of patients with frontal lobe lesions (Rylander 1939; McFie and Thompson 1972; Petrides and Milner 1982). Petrides and Milner (1982), for example, asked normal controls and patients with focal cortical excisions to place in logical order a list of items presented repeatedly in varying sequences. The patient was asked to touch each item once in arriving at the logical order. Four lists were presented: abstract designs, representational designs, high-imagery words, and low-imagery words. Patients with left frontal excisions were impaired on all four lists, whereas patients with right frontal excisions showed impairment only on the non-verbal tasks. When questioned about how they approached the task, patients with frontal lobe lesions infrequently reported the use of any systematic strategy. The left frontal region appears to play an important role in the programming and organization of behavioral responses. This capacity for sequential ordering also underlies ideational apraxia or apraxia for series actions (Kimura and Archibald 1974; DeRenzi et al. 1980; see Chapter 7).

Difficulties in selecting and carrying out plans of action have been suggested by other studies. Patients with frontal lesions often have greatly impaired performance on maze learning tests (Milner 1964, 1965; Canavan 1983). The major factors resulting in poor maze learning appear to be impulsivity and a failure to respond appropriately to feedback. The failure of frontal lobe patients to utilize feedback from errors has been noted in other studies (Luria 1966; Konow and Pribram 1970). Patients with frontal lobe disease may be able to recognize their errors, but they fail to act to correct their mistakes.

Another area of deficit in frontal lobe syndromes is a lack of judgment. One example is a seemingly thoughtless or unreasonable response to questions requiring cognitive analysis or mental estimation. Shallice and Evans (1978) asked 31 patients a series of questions that required an estimated answer (e.g. 'How tall is the average English woman?' or 'How fast do race horses gallop?'). Patients with frontal lobe lesions tended to provide more bizarre answers than patients with posterior lesions. Such patients indicated that the length of the average spine was between 4 and 5 feet, or that a horse had five legs. This type of gross misestimate is reminiscent of the Ganser syndrome (Carney et al. 1987) discussed in Chapter 14. There was no laterality effect, and the defect could not be explained on the basis of a loss of 'general intelligence'. The bedside mental status described in Chapter 4 does not include specific material of this type, but the examiner should be attentive to bizarre or inappropriate answers during history taking, especially when patients estimate durations, amounts, and distances.

Dementia and Frontal Lobe Disease

No discussion of cognition in frontal lobe disease should omit some mention of dementia. Although patients with discrete frontal lesions without mass effect may have little if any generalized intellectual disturbance, large frontal or subfrontal tumors may result in frank and progressive dementia (Hecaen 1964; Maxwell and Chow 1977). Hecaen (1964) found that confusion and dementia were associated more often with frontal brain tumors than with tumors elsewhere in the brain. The subfrontal or olfactory groove meningioma is a classical though rare cause of dementia, without obvious focal neurological symptoms and signs. Hécaen's frontal lobe tumor patients had a higher incidence of raised intracranial pressure, however, suggesting diffuse as well as focal brain dysfunction. A focal frontal lobe lesion such as a tumor should be considered in all patients presenting with generalized dementia. Dementia in relation to mass lesions is further discussed in Chapter 13.

ATTENTION AND MEMORY

Impaired focusing and maintenance of attention is a central feature of frontal lobe dysfunction. Attention is critical to the sequencing and executive control categories of frontal lobe behavior. Attention is first evaluated in the bedside mental status examination by observing the patient's capacity to listen to and answer the examiner's questions. Mild inattention is evident when a patient sporadically fails to comprehend a question fully despite intact language capacity or asks that the question be repeated. More severe inattention is present when the patient completely loses the train of thought and has to be redirected. These lapses usually occur because attention is directed to another thought. External events may also trigger a lapse of attention; the patient may be unduly distracted by the hospital paging system or by a nurse attending to a patient in a nearby bed. Formal assessment of attention is obtained on the bedside examination by the serial sevens test and the digit span.

Salmaso and Denes (1982) demonstrated the critical role of the frontal lobes in the maintenance of attention by a simple signal detection task, in which patients were required to detect the appearance of a unique stimulus interspersed among other stimuli. Patients with frontal lobe lesions in either hemisphere performed more poorly on this task than patients with posterior lesions or normal controls. Luria and Homskaya (1964) cited the 'orienting reflex' as the neurophysiological basis for the impairment of attention in frontal lobe injuries. Under normal circumstances the presentation of a novel stimulus results in a variety of physiological changes, including depression of the electroencephalogram (EEG) alpha rhythm, increased galvanic skin response, constriction of peripheral blood vessels, and dilatation of cerebral blood vessels. After repeated stimulus presentation habituation occurs, and the orienting reflex diminishes and eventually disappears. Habituation is slowed, however, when a special meaning is given to the stimuli through verbal instruction. Luria and Homskaya (1964) reported that the orienting reflex was seriously disturbed in all patients with large cerebral tumors, regardless of mass effect. Patients with posterior brain lesions, however, were able to maintain the orienting reflex in response to verbal commands, e.g. 'count the signals', whereas patients with frontal tumors could not. Luria thought that the loss of the ability to focus attention selectively resulted from a reduced capacity for cortical activation of the reticular activating formation (Luria and Homskaya 1964). Immediate or 'working' memory, a large part of the ability to sustain attention, is clearly a frontal lobe function and is disturbed in patients and experimental animals with frontal lobe damage (Fuster 2000).

In general, frontal lobe lesions do not cause marked disturbance in either recent or remote memory (Teuber 1964; Black 1976; Ladavas *et al.* 1979; Delaney *et al.* 1980). In fact, the quantity of material that frontal lobe patients can remember on standardized memory tests can be quite normal. Talland *et al.* (1967) opined that patients with frontal lobe lesions and amnestic deficits probably have additional pathology in other brain areas involved in memory. On the other hand, practical experience with patients teaches that frontal lobe damage does affect memory. Despite the normal performance of most patients with frontal lesions on both standard and bedside memory tests, clinicians and family members often describe the behavior of patients as 'absent-minded'. Some patients show inconsistent performance on short-term memory tests, but some of the faulty performance may be related to reduced attention rather than to a true memory deficit. As mentioned previously, immediate memory or attention, as assessed by the digit span test, is frequently impaired in discrete left and right frontal lobe injuries (Black and Strub 1978). Failure to attend to stimuli, of course, disrupts later memory for these stimuli. On the bedside mental status examination, patients with frontal lesions often display a pattern of performance directly opposite to that of patients with the amnestic syndrome; immediate memory is impaired, but short-term and long-term memories are largely intact.

The frontal lobes have a more important effect on memory performance, which does not show up in some of the standard tests for short-term memory. The frontal lobes are involved in the selection of which items to remember, which to recall, and how to organize these memories. Moskovitch (1992) referred to these aspects of memory as 'working-with memory'. In general, patients with frontal lobe damage perform most normally on tests of recognition memory, less well on cued recall, and least well when they are required to recall a series of items ('free recall'); this pattern was clearly supported in a meta-analysis of studies of memory functions in frontal lobe-damaged patients by Wheeler *et al.* (1995).

Some authors have cited a deficit in semantic processing and semantic memory to explain the apparent memory loss of patients with frontal lobe damage, as an alternative to the 'working memory' theory. Gershberg (1997), however, showed experimentally that frontal lobe patients can perform normally in memory for word lists in some 'implicit' memory tasks, but abnormally in explicit tasks calling for cued recall of a list of similar items. The memory difficulties of patients with frontal lobe lesions are thus not well explained by semantic deficits.

A subtle sort of short-term memory impairment has been documented in patients with frontal lobe lesions when specific procedures known as recency tests are used. In these tests a series of stimuli are shown sequentially to a patient, and periodically a judgment must be made as to which of two stimuli has been most recently presented. The ability to judge the recency of information is impaired after focal frontal lesions but not after discrete temporal lesions. Performance on these tasks also shows that the defect observed is specific to the side of the lesion; left frontal lesions lead to impairment of verbal recency judgments, whereas right hemisphere lesions lead to impairment of non-verbal (abstract art reproduction) recency judgments. The impairment of recency judgment is likely related to the general sequencing deficit discussed earlier. In clinical practice, any patient showing significant difficulty in organizing a series of events during the history should be suspected of having frontal lobe dysfunction.

One striking exception to the pattern of relatively normal short-term memory in patients with frontal lobe damage is the syndrome of memory loss following rupture of aneurysms of the anterior communicating artery (Volpe and Hurst 1983; Alexander and Freedman 1984; Rousseaux *et al.* 1997). These patients suffer damage not only to the medial frontal lobe, but also to deep, midline structures such as the septal area, which are part of Papez's circuit (see Chapter 11). Some of the most profound syndromes of amnesia with confabulation are seen in patients with such lesions (Johnson *et al.* 1997).

The role of frontal structures in such memory-related disorders as confabulation (Mercer *et al.* 1977; Kapur and Coughlan 1980; Shapiro *et al.* 1981) and reduplicative paramnesia (Benson *et al.* 1976; Ruff and Volpe 1981) is discussed in Chapters 8 and 10.

LANGUAGE

Left frontal lesions in Broca's area or the supplementary motor area produce frank aphasia (see Chapter 5). Patients with left prefrontal lesions not involving these regions often perform normally during bedside evaluations of aphasia, except for a striking decrease in spontaneous speech (Bonner *et al.* 1951; Luria 1966; Zangwill 1966). In extreme forms, this reduced fluency, with normal repetition, comprises the syndrome of transcortical motor aphasia (see Chapter 5). Many patients with left frontal lesions show mild degrees of dysfluency. This tendency has been noted in speech analysis of left frontal lobectomy patients before and after surgery. Reduced fluency of speech represents a modality-specific form of the lack of spontaneity manifested generally by frontal lobe patients. When interviewed, patients with frontal lesions offer little information spontaneously and tend to initiate conversation only rarely. Responses to questions, though syntactically and semantically correct, tend to be brief and to the point. In extreme cases patients may be virtually mute; such syndromes are usually associated with a more generalized, severe lack of spontaneity (abulia or akinetic mutism) resulting from bilateral rather than unilateral frontal disease. These syndromes are discussed later in this chapter. In milder cases, patients may produce fluent sentences but fail to produce well-organized, paragraph-length discourse.

The impairment of fluency in frontal lobe patients has been objectively studied with standardized verbal fluency tests (Milner 1964; Benton 1968; Ramier and Hécaen 1970; Perret 1974; Pendleton *et al.* 1982; Dubois *et al.* 2000). For example, patients are asked to generate words beginning with a certain letter ('s') or belonging to a specific category (e.g. 'animals') as rapidly as possible. This task is closely analogous to the tests of free recall mentioned in the previous section on memory deficits in patients with frontal pathology. Patients with focal left frontal lesions are consistently more impaired on these tasks than patients with focal lesions elsewhere in the brain. Within the right hemisphere, frontal lesions affect performance more than posterior lesions. Fluency tasks detect a general difficulty in the spontaneous generation of information, a function of both hemispheres, and a more specific difficulty with the generation of verbal information, a preferential left hemisphere function.

A related language deficit seen in patients with frontal lobe damage is difficulty with the production and organization of discourse (Alexander *et al.* 1989). Discourse production is a language function hierarchically above the simple tasks of naming, word production, and comprehension seen in the aphasias. It requires the subject to organize several utterances to lead to a conclusion. This higher-level language function is affected in aging and dementia (Bayles 1995; see Chapter 13) and in patients with head injury (Ehrlich 1988; Chapman *et al.* 1992; see Chapter 20).

Luria (1966) postulated yet another deficit related to frontal lobe lesions with regard to language: a loss of the ability to govern simple motor responses on the basis of verbal rules. As mentioned earlier, patients with frontal lobe lesions are often able to verbalize the correct solution to a problem yet cannot perform in accordance with this verbalization (Milner 1964; Luria 1966; Konow and Pribram 1970). Luria also suggested that lesions of the left frontal convexity are especially associated with this uncoupling of verbal and motor behaviors (Luria 1969). Experimental studies have confirmed the dissociation between intact production of verbal rules and defective motor responding, but only on specific tasks (Canavan 1983; Drewe 1975). Luria's patients had large frontal tumors, many of which were associated with mass effect. The inability of patients with frontal lobe lesions to use overt verbalization to guide motor behavior is probably not as generalized or as localized as Luria hypothesized.

SPATIAL FUNCTIONS

Gross deficiencies in spatial abilities are not typically encountered after focal frontal lesions (McFie 1960; Black 1976). Patients with frontal lesions can often copy geometric figures at the bedside with reasonable accuracy. Nonetheless, characteristic changes on non-verbal spatial tasks have been reported after frontal lobe disturbance. Jones-Gotman and Milner (1978) required patients to generate novel, abstract, meaningless designs within a time limit. This task is a non-verbal analogue to the verbal fluency measures described above. Patients with right frontal lesions were most impaired, whereas milder impairment was found after left frontal and right temporal resections.

Benton (1968) reported that patients with right and bilateral frontal lobe disease show difficulty with three-dimensional block construction and design copying tasks. However, in later work (Benton *et al.* 1978) with the Judgment of Line Orientation Test, a spatial perception task without a motor component, virtually no patients with frontal involvement were impaired, whereas most patients with right posterior lesions performed defectively. It is difficult to compare these two studies, as the former included many patients with tumors and degenerative diseases whereas the latter included mainly patients with strokes, and the tasks employed in the two studies may have been of unequal difficulty. It does seem likely, however, that spatial tests with both sensory and motor components are susceptible to frontal dysfunction, whereas purely perceptual tasks are impaired only with posterior lesions.

In addition, the apparent deficits in spatial tasks seen in patients with right frontal lesions may involve defective planning rather than impaired spatial capabilities. Many patients with frontal lesions, when asked to copy a set of geometric shapes, copy each individual shape well but tend to align them poorly on the page, running one into the next. Such behavior supports a deficit in planning. The motor hypokinesia associated with right frontal lesions was discussed in Chapter 9.

Neglect phenomena, as discussed in Chapter 9, sometimes occur after right frontal lobe lesions (Heilman and Valenstein 1972; Damasio *et al.* 1980), though they are more frequently associated with right parietal lobe lesions. 'Frontal neglect' has been described in cases with both left and right frontal lesions, involving both the dorsolateral and medial aspects of the frontal lobes. Unilateral neglect after frontal disturbances, however, is generally less severe than neglect after parietal lobe lesions, and it recovers more rapidly and more completely.

MOTOR CHANGES

Frontal lesions produce motor changes that can be evaluated at the bedside. First, reduced spontaneous motor activity is often observed, representing another manifestation of the lack of spontaneity of patients with frontal lobe lesions. This lack of initiative, or abulia, is often extreme; the patient may sit listlessly in a chair and make little effort to do anything, despite adequate alertness, motor strength, and coordination. Families may report that the patient no longer carries out usual activities of daily living such as personal hygiene and eating. When coaxed, however, the patient is fully capable of these activities (Hécaen and Albert 1975). One recent patient with a bilateral frontal syndrome secondary to a ruptured anterior communicating artery aneurysm sat all day watching television, and lost all of his previous interest in hunting and gardening. This patient, who had been a very aggressive and enterprising businessman, had suffered a complete change in personality, as reported by his wife. Signs of poor grooming and hygiene are often observed in these patients. Motor changes are among the most sensitive indicators of frontal lobe disturbances (Reitan 1964), and most patients show at least some deficit in motor initiation or speed. Clinicians have long observed that patients with frontal lobe lesions show a striking lack of motor spontaneity in their facial expressions (Goldstein 1944). Experimental observation of patients with surgical resections confirms that patients with unilateral frontal lesions on either side are more likely to show a reduction in the number of spontaneous facial expressions than those with unilateral parietal or temporal lobe excisions (Kolb and Milner 1981).

Another common feature of motor behavior in frontal disease patients is motor perseveration. Many of the behavioral changes seen after frontal lobe lesions can be characterized as perseverative. Motor perseveration can be readily evaluated at the bedside by having the patient draw a repeating sequence consisting of alternating square and triangular elements (see Chapter 4), a test first described by Luria (1969). Patients with frontal lesions, particularly those involving the premotor areas, have difficulty switching smoothly from one component of the sequence to the next and often perseverate on one of them. Motor perseveration may also be elicited during constructional and writing tasks (see Chapter 9). Such motor perseveration is closely related to the cognitive perseveration discussed earlier in this chapter, with regard to Milner's studies with the Wisconsin Card Sorting Test.

The akinesia and abulia of frontal lobe disease can be extreme. Fisher (1968) described a number of patients with unilateral and bilateral strokes in the territory of the anterior cerebral artery. These patients intermittently fail to respond to questions or commands for periods of several seconds or minutes; when active, however, they can answer complex questions, follow commands, speak, and solve problems. The extreme of this abulia is called 'akinetic mutism' (Segarra and Angels 1970). Akinetic, mute patients are nearly totally unresponsive to the environment, lying motionless in bed, often with open eyes. They fail to perform even the simplest motor activities. Only vigorous stimulation elicits motor responses or speech. The patient may cease to eat or to ask for assistance with elementary biological needs. Manifestations of the disorder vary in severity. Akinetic mutism is usually associated with medial frontal lesions, particularly with bilateral involvement. Anterior cerebral artery territory infarction, especially when bilateral (Segarra and Angels 1970), bilateral frontal trauma (Hécaen and Albert 1975), and hydrocephalus are common causes of this syndrome. Destruction of Brodmann area 24 has been implicated as necessary for the development of akinetic mutism (Segarra and Angels 1970). These frontal syndromes are distinguished from a brainstem form of akinetic mutism, in which midbrain signs are present and consciousness is more impaired (Segarra and Angels 1970).

Teuber (1964) made major contributions to the experimental study and the theoretical understanding of the role of the frontal lobes in motor activity (Teuber 1964). He observed patients with penetrating gunshot wounds to the frontal lobes. These patients manifested no major defects in intelligence or memory, but showed selective deficits on specific experimental tasks. In the visuopostural task, for instance, patients were requested to set a rod to the vertical position under different conditions of body tilt. Patients with frontal lobe lesions performed defectively compared to those with posterior lesions and controls; when there was no body tilt, however, frontal lesion patients performed normally. In a second task involving visual search, a test field containing numerous geometrical shapes was presented to the patient; the patient was required to pick out as quickly as possible a pattern in the periphery of the field corresponding to a pattern flashed in the center of the field. Patients with frontal lesions showed prolonged searching times, particularly in the hemifield contralateral to their lesion. Drawing on data from these and other studies, Teuber hypothesized that a critical function of the frontal lobes was to maintain 'corollary discharge', a discharge from the motor to the sensory areas of the brain to prime sensory structures for an anticipated change, thereby allowing for adjustment of perception at or near the time of the motor act.

Imitation and Utilization Behavior

Lhermitte and colleagues (1986) pointed to two distinctive symptoms of frontal lobe dysfunction called 'imitation' and 'utilization' behavior. Patients with frontal lobe lesions often imitate gestures made by the examiner, even after being instructed specifically not to do so. Likewise, these patients often cannot seem to stop picking up and manipulating objects from the examiner's desk, despite occasional requests to leave them alone. These deficits were very common in patients with frontal lobe lesions in this series, though inferior frontal lobe lesions were more consistently associated with both imitation and utilization behavior than superior frontal lesions. The authors suggested an interruption of normally inhibitory connections from the frontal to the parietal lobes, thus 'disinhibiting' these parietal centers. The patient thus becomes a slave to external stimuli, whereas the frontal lobe mental activity normally inhibits response to these stimuli. Lhermitte (1986) also described an 'environmental dependency syndrome', in which patients seem constrained to act in ways prescribed by the environment in which they find themselves. A woman shown a table with trays of food immediately began acting as a hostess, passing out food and drinks to the physician and others in the room. Another patient shown a syringe and needle actually prepared to give the physician (Dr Lhermitte) the injection, when he pulled down his trousers. The frontal assessment battery referred to in Chapter 4 (Dubois *et al.* 2000) includes observation of the patient's response when the examiner puts his or her hands near those of the patient and says, 'do not take my hands'. Lhermitte considered imitation and utilization behavior a more complex behavioral expression of the same frontal disinhibition of parietal structures, rendering the patient completely dependent on the environment. Lhermitte (1986) went so far as to state that human autonomy and 'free will' require intact frontal lobes.

Apraxia

Apraxia is usually encountered in the context of left hemisphere lesions, but the frontal lobes appear to be important in the execution of nonrepresentational movement sequences (Kolb and Milner 1981b). Patients with both left and right frontal lesions (surgical excisions for epilepsy) had difficulty executing or imitating arm movements, though the deficits were not as severe as those suffered by patients with left parietal lesions. Initiation of facial movements was markedly impaired after unilateral lesions of either frontal lobe, whereas lesions elsewhere in the brain caused no difficulty. Although the cause of these motor problems is not entirely established, deficient motor programming has been postulated. Apraxia is discussed further in Chapter 7. Frontal gait disorders are also mentioned in Chapter 13 (normal-pressure hydrocephalus).

EMOTIONAL AND PERSONALITY CHANGES

Emotional and personality changes are the most striking and devastating effects of frontal lobe disorders. In addition, frontal lobe disorders may affect only these 'psychic' or mental spheres, without associated deficits in motor function, coordination, sensation, or even obvious cognitive dysfunction. Personality changes are readily apparent to friends and family members, but they may be less obvious to an examiner who does not know the patient. Attention to these symptoms during the history is essential to proper diagnosis of frontal lobe disorders.

One of the earliest descriptions of the alterations in personality subsequent to frontal lobe lesions was the case of Phineas Gage, described by Harlow (1868). The patient was a 25-year-old railroad worker who sustained a severe left frontal injury when a tamping iron was blown through his skull. He made an excellent physical recovery, but his personality was so radically changed that his friends described him as 'no longer Gage' (see the quotation at the beginning of this chapter). He became irritable, stubborn, and lacking in consideration for others. His speech became profane. He made many plans, but failed to execute them.

Feuchtwanger (1923) compared 200 patients with frontal gunshot wounds and 200 with non-frontal gunshot wounds. In the frontal lesion patients, defects in intellect appeared to be minor, but more prominent symptoms included apathy, irritability, euphoria, facetiousness (*Witzelsucht* or 'sick humor'), and impaired attention. Tactlessness, loss of moral valuation, and difficulty in planning were also described.

Holmes (1931) differentiated three frontal syndromes: (1) apathy, decreased initiative, passivity, inattention, and faulty memory (probably related to poor attention); (2) depression, dementia, drowsiness, and periods of stupor, akinesia, and incontinence; (3) restlessness, exuberance, euphoric lack of concern, immaturity, and labile affect.

Kleist (1934) attempted to relate the specific locations of frontal lesions to behavorial changes, and stressed the importance of orbital lesions in the genesis of immoral, deceitful, facetious, and defiant behavior. He also observed that the euphoria of patients with orbital frontal lesions was prominent early after injury, then dissipated with time, sometimes to be replaced by a more dysphoric disposition. He related the apathy and reduced motor activity to lesions of the frontal convexity. Kleist made these observations on the basis of *post-mortem* studies, long before the advent of modern neuroradiological techniques for lesion localization.

In a descriptive characterization of the personality changes associated with frontal lobe disturbance, Blumer and Benson (1975) described two distinct patterns: (1) a 'pseudodepressed' type characterized by apathy and indifference; and (2) a 'pseudopsychopathic' type characterized by euphoria and puerility. 'Pseudodepressed' patients show little interest or initiative; in more extreme instances they manifest frank abulia. They are usually slow to respond and rarely embark spontaneously on any activity, though they can respond to questions in a meaningful fashion and engage in intelligent conversation. 'Pseudopsychopathic' personality changes are marked by poor social tact and judgment. Affect is usually poorly modulated, and behavior is marked by irritability and impulsivity. Sporadic antisocial behavior, promiscuity, and uninhibited profanity in conversation are common. Blumer and Benson suggested that the 'pseudodepressed' changes tend to occur after convexity lesions, whereas the 'pseudopsychopathic' changes tend to occur after orbital destruction. Bilateral disease is usually required for the development of enduring personality changes (Blumer and Benson 1975).

In everyday practice, these variants of the frontal lobe personality change usually occur in mixed forms (Damasio 1983); for example, a patient who appears to be generally apathetic and indifferent may show irritability, impulsivity, or frank outbursts at times. Frontal lesions are rarely restricted to just the orbital surface or just the lateral convexity, rendering precise localization of these affective and personality changes difficult. Bilateral lesions produce personality changes more often than unilateral lesions (Damasio and Van Hoesen 1983). Most patients with significant personality changes following frontal lobe insults have an underlying shallow or labile mood (Massey and Coffey 1983); patients tend not to be consistently euphoric or depressed, but rather fluctuate unpredictably in mood.

Studies have differed with regard to the propensity of patients with frontal lobe damage to commit violent acts. Long-term follow-up studies of soldiers who sustained focal gunshot injuries in World War II found that brain-injured soldiers were no more likely than non-brain-injured soldiers to engage in criminal acts (Virkkunen *et al.* 1977). In the brain-injured group who had engaged in a criminal act, there was no specific association with lesions to the frontal areas (Virkkunen *et al.* 1976). In this study, frontal damage did not appear to result in true psychopathic personality changes despite clinical impressions to the contrary. Other studies, however, have found evidence for an association of frontal damage with violent behavior. Lishman (1968), for example, evaluated the presence of the 'frontal lobe syndrome' in soldiers with penetrating head injuries. He defined the 'frontal lobe syndrome' as having one of the following symptoms in severe degree: euphoria; lack of judgment; lack of concern, reliability, or foresight; facile or childish behavior; and disinhibition. Among the 32 patients who manifested one of these changes, nine had no lesions of the frontal lobes, and the remaining 23 had substantial frontal involvement.

Clinicians should be aware that a small minority of patients with frontal lobe disturbance present with symptoms suggestive of psychiatric disorders (Hecaen 1964). Psychiatric syndromes in frontal lobe patients have mimicked schizophrenia (Hunter *et al.* 1968; Thompson 1970; Carlson 1977; Andy *et al.* 1981; Ramani 1981); catatonia (Thompson 1970; Ruff and Russakoff 1980); hypomania (Hunter *et al.* 1968); and depression (Hunter *et al.* 1968; Carlson 1977). Mental status testing on these patients usually suggests frontal lobe pathology, though as discussed previously the cognitive abnormalities may be minimal. The sudden emergence of psychiatric signs and symptoms in previously normal adults should always raise the question of a frontal lobe syndrome.

Another specific type of affective change commonly encountered in patients with frontal lobe damage is pseudobulbar palsy. This term describes the clinical effects of bilateral involvement of the corticobulbar tracts that innervate the face, mouth, tongue, pharynx, and larynx. Facial weakness, dysarthria, dysphagia (difficulty swallowing), and exaggerated gag and jaw reflexes are the motor signs of this syndrome; the behavioral change is an extreme form of emotional lability characterized by uncontrollable laughter and crying. These outbursts often have only a slight connection with the patient's underlying feelings and do not reflect the intensity of the patient's mood at the time. The affective displays are intense and prolonged, yet may be triggered by a minimal stimulus. Some patients describe an inability to inhibit emotional expression such that the least, most fleeting emotional feeling is immediately expressed. The precise neuroanatomical pathology underlying this syndrome has not been clearly established. Poeck (1969) reviewed 30 patients with pathological laughter and crying; in all cases the lesions were primarily anterior, subcortical and located in the region of the internal capsule or basal ganglia. In no case was there an isolated cortical lesion, though in several cases the insular cortex was involved. No cases were found with isolated thalamic or upper brainstem lesions. Although the motor disturbances of pseudobulbar palsy are virtually always encountered in the context of bilateral lesions (Rondat 1969), Poeck found that both left and right unilateral lesions could result in pathological laughter and crying. A closely related syndrome is the opercular syndrome or Foix–Chavany–Marie syndrome, seen in patients with bilateral lesions. Patients with the opercular syndrome are usually mute, with apparent paralysis of the face, lips, tongue, and speech apparatus, but they can move their craniofacial muscles in reflex activities such as yawning and spontaneous laughter and crying. In contrast, they can follow commands to use their limbs. The lesions are classically bilateral cortical, but subcortical lesions have also been described (Bakar *et al.* 1998). Clinical observation suggests that mild forms of emotional lability are found in cerebral lesions generally, regardless of cause or location. Frontal lesions may be more likely than posterior lesions to result in these disturbances, but firm anatomical evidence is lacking. Emotional changes with brain disease are discussed in Chapter 17.

In addition to these emotional effects of frontal lobe injury, reference has previously been made to the depression commonly seen with left middle cerebral artery strokes and Broca's aphasia (see Chapter 5). The correlation of emotional indifference with right hemisphere lesions was discussed in Chapter 9.

DISEASES COMMONLY ASSOCIATED WITH FRONTAL LOBE SYNDROMES

Changes in behavior suggesting frontal lobe involvement can arise from a number of disease states. However, because many of these disorders do not respect classical anatomical boundaries the clinical presentation may vary widely from patient to patient.

Traumatic brain injury is probably the most frequent cause of frontal lobe damage. The two most frequent types of traumatic brain injury are missile injuries (e.g. gunshot wounds) and closed head injuries (Levin *et al.* 1982). Advances in emergency evacuation procedures and neurosurgical techniques have reduced the mortality of head trauma in recent years, and the number of patients surviving major head injuries is increasing. Head trauma is especially common in young adult males (Annegers *et al.* 1980). Multiple factors are involved in the type and location of pathology after a head injury. In serious closed head injury there is widespread stretching and shearing of nerve fibers throughout the brain.

Experimental studies (Holbourn 1943) and animal models (Ommaya and Gennarelli 1974) have suggested that the frontal and anterior temporal lobes are particularly vulnerable to the shearing and stretching damage of closed head injury. Contusions (Gurdjian and Gurdjian 1976) and intracerebral hematomas (Strich 1970) are distinctly common in the orbital frontal and frontal polar areas after closed head injury.

Even minor closed head injuries result in the 'postconcussive syndrome'. A recent study of 13 individuals with 'severe' traumatic brain injury but without abnormal CT or MRI scans (Fontaine *et al*. 1999) used PET scanning to evaluate the sites of dysfunction. In general, there was a strong correlation between frontal cognitive and behavioral disorders and damage to the prefrontal regions. Abnormalities of executive function and memory correlated best with lesions of the cingulate gyrus and both medial and lateral prefrontal areas. Alterations of behavior correlated best with cingulate and medial prefrontal hypometabolism. Behavioral effects of head trauma are discussed in Chapter 19.

Vascular disease is a common cause of frontal lobe disturbances, particularly in the elderly. Infarction in the territory of the anterior cerebral artery causes damage primarily to the medial frontal area, whereas distal middle cerebral artery infarctions involve the dorsolateral frontal lobe. Striking changes typically result from hemorrhage secondary to a rupture of the anterior communicating artery, as involvement in such cases is likely to be bilateral. Storey (1970) described long-term neurobehavioral sequelae of subarachnoid hemorrhage after ruptured aneurysms. Patients with anterior communicating aneurysms had relatively preserved intellectual functions but striking changes in emotion and personality, including disinhibition and apathy. Rousseaux *et al*. (1997), as well as earlier authors (see Chapter 11), have reported an amnestic-confabulatory state in patients with medial frontal damage secondary to ruptured anterior communicating artery aneurysms.

Tumors are another common cause of frontal lobe dysfunction. Many of the patients described by Luria (1966), who contributed much to our understanding of the frontal lobes and behavior, had intracranial tumors. Specific psychological changes are related to the type, size, and location of the tumor, as well as the degree of mass effect and raised intracranial pressure (Hécaen 1964). Gliomas and meningiomas are the most commonly encountered frontal tumors. As mentioned earlier, subfrontal or olfactory groove meningiomas can present with profound changes in personality or dementia.

Multiple sclerosis (MS) is another frequent cause of frontal lobe disturbances. In an autopsy study where material was obtained from 22 unselected cases of MS the frontal lobes had the second largest number of cerebral plaques (22% of the total), ranking behind only the periventricular area (where 40% were found). Plaques are located primarily in white matter. Euphoric mood in MS appears to be strongly related to cognitive impairment secondary to brain dysfunction (Surridge 1969). Clinically depressed mood (Schiffer and Babigian 1984) and memory loss (Grant *et al*. 1984; Rao *et al*. 1984) are also common in patients with this disease. Cognitive and behavioral effects of multiple sclerosis are discussed in Chapter 18.

Several degenerative diseases, including Pick's disease and Huntington's disease, show maximal involvement of the frontal lobes (Lishman 1968). Huntington's disease (HD) has a predilection for the frontal lobes and the basal ganglia, beginning in the medial caudate nucleus and then spreading laterally to the putamen (Vonsattel *et al.* 1985). The head of the caudate has extensive connections to the frontal cortex. In one series of HD patients, 37% had mood disturbances, 30% had irritability or temper outbursts, and 6% had antisocial personality disorder (Folstein 1989). Apathy and even obsessive-compulsive behavior are occasionally seen in HD (Cummings and Cunningham 1992). 'Frontal' cognitive dysfunction is common in patients with HD; examples include poor cognitive set shifting on the Wisconsin Card Sort Test (Weinberger *et al.* 1988), decreased verbal fluency, and memory/attentional deficits (Butters *et al.* 1978). Huntington's disease is discussed in Chapter 15.

Prior to the advances in adequate treatment for infectious diseases, neurosyphilis, which has a predilection for the anterior regions of the brain (Breutsch 1959), was a common cause of frontal lobe disease. Many of the clinical features of frontal disturbances were described in cases of neurosyphilis. Although the disease is less commonly encountered in modern-day practice, cases continue to be seen. Herpes simplex encephalitis selectively affects the cortical structures of the limbic system, including the orbital frontal, anterior cingulate, and medial temporal areas (Damasio and Van Hoesen 1984). Such patients often show a severe amnestic syndrome as the most prominent residual deficit, but frontal lobe symptoms also occur. Numerous other diseases affect the frontal lobes, many of which are discussed in Chapter 13 with the dementias.

CONCLUSION

The frontal lobes are a source of fascinating neurobehavioral syndromes, many of which pose a significant challenge to the clinician. Only frontal lobe lesions, among the neurobehavioral disorders discussed thus far in this volume, affect personality and mood more than cognitive functions. Attention to the euphoric or labile mood and perseverative tendencies of frontal lobe patients may lead an examiner to suspect frontal lobe disease, whereas purely psychiatric disease was suggested by the patient's symptoms. Nowhere in behavioral neurology is the 'borderland' of psychiatry and neurology more evident than in the disorders of the frontal lobes.

REFERENCES

Alexander MP, Freedman M. Amnesia after anterior communicating artery aneurysm rupture. Neurology 1984;34:752–757.

Alexander MP, Benson DF, Stuss DT. Frontal lobes and language. Brain Lang 1989;37:656–691.

Andy OJ, Webster, JS, Carranza J. Frontal lobe lesions and behavior. South Med J 1981;74:968–972.

Annegers JF, Graham JD, Kurland LT, Laws ER. The incidence, causes, and secular trends of head trauma in Olmsted County, Minnesota. Neurology 1980;30:912–919.

Bakar M, Kirshner HS, Niaz F. The opercular–subopercular syndrome: four cases with review of the literature. Behav Neurol 1998;11:97–103.

Barcelo F, Sanz M, Molina V, Rubia F. The Wisconsin Card Sorting Test and the assessment of frontal function: a validation study with event-related potentials. Neuropsychologia 1997;35:399–408.

Bayles KA. Language in aging and dementia. In HS Kirshner (ed.), Handbook of Neurological Speech and Language Disorders. New York: Marcel Dekker Inc., 1995;351–372.

Benson DF. Psychomotor retardation. Neuropsychiatry, Neuropsychology, and Behavioral Neurology 1990;3:36–47.

Benson DF. The neurology of higher mental control disorders. In DF Benson (ed.), The Neurology of Thinking. New York: Oxford University Press, 1994;208–226.

Benson DF, Gardner H, Meadows JC. Reduplicative paramnesia. Neurology 1976;26:47–151.

Benton, AL. Differential behavioral effects of frontal lobe disease. Neuropsychologia 1968;6:53–60.

Benton A, Varney NR, Hamsher KD. Visuospatial judgment. Arch Neurol 1978;35:364–367. 1978.

Black, FW. Cognitive deficits in patients with unilateral war-related frontal lobe lesions. J Clin Psychol 1976;32:366–372.

Black FW, Strub RL. Digit repetition performance in patients with focal brain damage. Cortex 1978;14:12–21.

Blumer D, Benson DF. Personality changes with frontal and temporal lobe lesions. In D Blumer, DF Benson (eds), Psychiatric Aspects of Neurologic Disease, Vol. 1. New York: Grune & Stratton, 1975;137–170.

Bonner F, Cobb S, Sweet WH, White JC. Frontal lobe surgery. Res Publ Assoc 1951; 31:392–421.

Breutsch WC. Neuropsychiatric conditions. In S Arieti, (ed.), American Handbook of Psychiatry, Volume 2. New York: Basic Books, 1959, 1003–1020.

Brickner, RM. An interpretation of frontal lobectomy. Res Publ Assoc Res Nerv Ment Dis 1934;13:259–351.

Butters N, Sax D, Montgomery K *et al.* Comparison of the neuropsychological deficits associated with early and advanced Huntington's disease. Arch Neurol 1978;35: 585–589.

Canavan, AGM. Stylus-maze performance in patients with frontal lobe lesions: effects of signal valency and relationship to verbal and spatial abilities. Neuropsychologia 1983; 21:375–382.

Carlson RJ. Frontal lobe lesions masquerading as psychiatric disturbances. Can Psychiatr Assoc J 1977;22:315–318.

Carney MWP, Chary TKN, Robotis P, Childs A. Ganser syndrome and its management. Br J Psychiatry 1987;151:697–700.

Carpenter, MD. Core Text of Neuroanatomy. Baltimore: Williams & Wilkins, 1972.

Chapman SB, Culhane KA, Levin HS *et al.* Narrative discourse after closed head injury in children and adolescents. Brain Lang 1992;43:42–65.

Cierone, KD, Lazar, RM. Effects of frontal lobe lesions on hypothesis sampling during concept formation. Neuropsychologia 1983;21:513–524.

Cummings JL Frontal-subcortical circuits and human behavior. Arch Neurol 1993;50: 873–880.

Cummings JL, Cunningham K. Obsessive-compulsive disorder in Huntington's disease. Biol Psychiatry 1992;31:263–270.

Cummings JL, Mendez MF. Secondary mania with focal cerebrovascular lesions. Am J Psychiatry 1984;141:1084–1087.

Damasio A. The frontal lobes. In KM Heilman, E Valenstein (eds), Clinical Neuropsychology (2nd edn). New York: Oxford University Press, 1983;360–412.

Damasio A, Van Hoesen GW. Emotional disturbances associated with focal lesions of the limbic frontal lobe. In K Heilman, P Satz (eds), Neuropsychology of Human Emotion. New York: Guilford Press, 1983;85–110.

Damasio AR, Damasio H, Chui HC. Neglect following damage to the frontal lobe or basal ganglia. Neuropsychologia 1980;18:123–132.

Delaney RC, Rosen AJ, Mattson RH. Memory function in focal epilepsy: a comparison of non-surgical unilateral temporal lobe and frontal lobe samples. Cortex 1980;16:103–117.

DeRenzi E, Matte R, Nichelli P. Imitating gestures: a quantitative approach to ideomotor apraxia. Arch Neurol 1980;37:6–10.

Drewe EA. The effect of type and area of brain lesion on Wisconsin Card Sorting Test performance. Cortex 1974;10:159–170.

Drewe EA. An experimental investigation of Luria's theory on the effects of frontal lobe lesions in man. Neuropsychologia 1975;13:421–429.

Dubois B, Slachevsky, Litvan I, Pillon B. The FAB: a frontal assessment battery at bedside. Neurology 2000;55:1621–1626.

Ehrlich JS. Selective characteristics of narrative discourse in head-injured and normal adults. J Commun Disord 1988;211–219.

Feuchtwanger E. Die Funkionen des Stirnhirns: Ihre Pathologie und Psychologie. Springer: Berlin, 1923.

Fisher CM. Intermittent interruption of behavior. Trans Am Neurol Assoc 1968;93:209–210.

Folstein SE. Huntington's Disease: A Disorder of Families. Baltimore MD: Johns Hopkins University Press, 1989.

Fontaine A, Azouvi P, Remy P et al. Functional anatomy of neuropsychological deficits after severe traumatic brain injury. Neurology 1999;53:1963–1968.

Fuster JM. Temporal organization of behavior. Human Neurobiology 1985;4:57–60.

Fuster JM. Prefrontal neurons in networks of executive memory. Brain Res Bull 2000;52:331–336.

Gershberg FB. Implicit and explicit conceptual memory following frontal lobe damage. J Cog Neurosci 1997;9:105–116.

Geschwind N. The apraxias: neural mechanisms of disorders of learned movement. Am Sci 1975;63:188–195.

Goldman-Rakic PS. The prefrontal landscape: implications of functional architecture for understanding human mentation and the central executive. Phil Trans R Soc London B 1996;351:1445–1453.

Goldstein, K. The significance of frontal lobes for mental performances. J Neurol Psychopathol 1936;17:27–40.

Goldstein, K. The mental changes due to frontal lobe damage. J Psychol 1944;17:187–208.

Grant DA, Berg EA. A behavioral. analysis of degree of reinforcement and ease of shifting to new responses in a Weigl-type card-sorting problem. J Exp Psychol 1948;38:404–411.

Grant I, McDonald WI, Trimble MR. Deficient learning and memory in early and middle phases of multiple sclerosis. J Neurol Neurosurg Psychiatry 1984;47:250–255.

Gurdjian ES, Gurdjian ES. Cerebral contusions: re-evaluation of the mechanisms of their development. J Trauma 1976;16:35–51.

Halstead WC. Brain and Intelligence: A Quantitative Study of Frontal Lobes. Chicago: University of Chicago Press, 1947.

Harlow, JM. Recovery from the passage of an iron bar to the head. Mass Med Soc 1868;2:328–347.

Hebb, DO. Intelligence in man after large removals of cerebral tissue: report of four left frontal lobe cases. J Gen Psychol 1939;21:73–87.

Hécaen H. Mental symptoms associated with tumors of the frontal lobe. In JM Warren, K Akert (eds), The Frontal Granular Cortex and Behavior. New York: McGraw-Hill, 1964, 335–352.

Hécaen H, Albert M. Disorders of mental functioning related to frontal lobe pathology. In Blumer D, Benson DF, eds. Psychiatric aspects of neurological disease. Vol. 1. New York: Grune & Stratton, 1975, 137–150.

Holbourn, AHS. Mechanics of head injuries. Lancet 1943;2:438–441.

Holmes G. Discussion on the mental symptoms associated with cerebral tumors. Proc R Soc Med 1931;24:997–1008.

Heilman KM, Valenstein E. Frontal lobe neglect in man. Neurology 1972;22:660–679.

Hunter R, Blackwood W, Bull J. Three cases of frontal lobe meningiomas presented psychiatrically. Br Med 1968;3:9–16.

Ingvar DH. Memory of the future: an essay on the temporal organization of conscious awareness. Human Neurobiol 1985;4:127–136.

Johnson MK, O'Connor M, Cantor J. Confabulation, memory deficits, and frontal dysfunction. Brain Cogn 1997;34:189–206.

Jones-Gotman M, Milner B. Design fluency: the invention on nonsense drawings after focal cortical lesions. Neuropsychologia 1978;15:653–674.

Kapur N, Coughlan AK. Confabulation and frontal lobe dysfunction. J Neurol Neurosurg Psychiatry 1980;43:461–463.

Keenan JP, Nelson A, O'Connor M, PascualLeone A. Self-recognition and the right hemisphere. Nature 2001;409:305–306.

Kimura D, Archibald Y. Motor functions of the left hemisphere. Brain 1974;97:337–350.

Kleist K. Gehirnpathologie. Leipzig: Barth, 1934.

Kolb B, Milner B. Observations on spontaneous facial expression after focal cerebral excisions and after intracarotid injection of sodium amytal. Neuropsychologia 1981a; 19:505–514.

Kolb B, Milner B. Performance of complex arm and facial movements after focal brain lesions. Neuropsychologia 1981b;9:491–503.

Konow A, Pribram K. Error recognition and utilization produced by injury to the frontal cortex in man. Neuropsychologia 1970;8:489–491.

Ladavas E, Umilta C, Provinciali L. Hemisphere-dependent performances in epileptic patients. Epilepsia 1979;20:493–502.

Levin H, Benton, AL Grossman RG. Neurobehavioral Consequences of Closed Head Injury. New York: Oxford University Press, 1982.

Lezak MD. Neuropsychological assessment. Second edition. New York: Oxford University Press, 1983, 480–482.

Lhermitte F. Human autonomy and the frontal lobes. Part II. Patient behavior in complex and social situations: the 'environmental dependency syndrome'. Ann Neurol 1986;19: 335–343.

Lhermitte F, Pillon B, Serdaru M. Human autonomy and the frontal lobes. Part I. Imitation and utilization behavior: a neuropsychological study of 75 patients. Ann Neurol 1986;19:326–334.

Lishman WA. Brain damage in relation to psychiatric disability after head injury. Br J Psychiatry 1968;114:373–410.

Luria, AR: Higher Cortical Functions in Man. London: Tavistock, 1966.

Luria, AR. Frontal lobe syndromes. In PJ Vinken, GW Bruyn (eds), Handbook of Clinical Neurology, Vol. 2. New York: American Elsevier, 1969;725–757.

Luria AR, Homskaya ED. Disturbance in the regulative role of speech with frontal lobe lesions. In JM Warren, K Akert (eds), The Frontal Granular Cortex and Behavior. New York: McGraw-Hill, 1964;353–371.

Massey EW, Coffey CE. Frontal lobe personality syndromes. Postgrad Med Res Publ Assoc 1983;73:99–106.

Maxwell RE, Chow SN. Aneurysmal tumors of the basifrontal region. J Neurosurg 1977; 46:438–445.

McFie J. Psychological testing in clinical neurology. J Nerv Ment Dis 1960;131:383–393.

McFie J, Thompson JA. Picture arrangement: a measure of frontal lobe function? Br J Psychiatry 1972;121:547–552.

Mercer B, Wapner W, Gardner H, Benson, DF. A study of confabulation. Arch Neurol 1977; 34:429–433.

Mesulam M-M. Frontal cortex and behavior. Ann Neurol 1986;19:320–325.

Milner, B. Effects of different brain lesions on card sorting. Arch Neurol 1963;9:90–100.

Milner, B. Some effects of frontal lobectomy in man. In JM Warren, K Akert (eds), The Frontal Granular Cortex and Behavior. New York: McGraw-Hill, 1964;313–334.

Milner B. Visually guided image learning in man: effects of bilateral hippocampal, bilateral frontal, and unilateral cerebral lesions. Neuropsychologia 1965;3:317–338.

Moskovitch M. Memory and working-with memory: a component process model based on modules and central systems. J Cog Neurosci 1992;4:257–267.

Nauta, WJH. The problem of the frontal lobe: a reinterpretation. J Psychiatr Res 1971;8: 167–187.

Nelson, HE. A modified card sorting test sensitive to frontal lobe defects. Cortex 1976;12: 313–324.

Ommaya AK, Gennarelli TA. Cerebral concussion and traumatic unconsciousness: correlation of experimental and clinical observations on blunt head injuries. Brain 1974;97:663–654.

Pendleton MG, Heaton RK, Lehman RAW, Hulihan D. Diagnostic utility of the Thurston Word Fluency Test in neuropsychological evaluation. J Clin Neuropsychol 1982;4: 307–317.

Perret E. The left frontal lobe of man and the suppression of habitual responses in verbal categorical behavior. Neuropsychologia 1974;12:323–330.

Petrides M, Milner B. Deficits of subject-ordered tasks after frontal and temporal lobe lesions in man. Neuropsychologia 1982;20:249–262.

Poeck K. Pathophysiology of emotional disorders associated with brain damage. In PJ Vinken, GW Bruyn (eds), Handbook of Clinical Neurology, Vol. 3. Amsterdam: North Holland, 1969;356–367.

Ramani SV. Psychosis associated with frontal lobe lesions and behavior. Southern Med J 1981;74:968–972.

Ramier AM, Hecaen H. Role respectiv des atteintes frontales et de la lateralisation lesionelle dans les deficits de la 'fluence verbale'. Rev Neurol (Paris) 1970;122:17–22.

Rao SM, Hammeke TA, McQuillen MP et al. Memory disturbance in chronic progressive multiple sclerosis. Arch Neurol 1984;41:625–631.

Reitan RM. Psychological deficits resulting from cerebral lesions in man. In JM Warren, K Akert K (eds), The Frontal Granular Cortex and Behavior. New York; McGraw-Hill, 1964;295–312.

Robinson AL, Heaton RK, Lehman RAW, Stilson DW. The ability of the Wisconsin Card Sorting Test in detecting and localizing frontal lobe lesions. J Consult Clin Psychol 1980;48:605–614.

Rondat P. Syndromes of central motor disorder. In PJ Vinken, GW Bruyn (eds), Handbook of Clinical Neurology, Vol. 1. Amsterdam: North Holland, 1969;169–217.

Rousseaux M, Godefroy O, Cabaret M et al. La memoire retrograde après rupture des aneurysms de l'artere communicante anterieure. Rev Neurol (Paris) 1997;153:659–668.

Ruff RL, Russakoff LM. Catatonia with frontal lobe atrophy. J Neurol Neurosurg Psychiatry 1980; 43:185–187.

Ruff R, Volpe BT. Environmental reduplication associated with right frontal lobe injury. J Neurol Neurosurg Psychiatry 1981;44:382–386.

Rylander, A. Personality Changes after Operations on the Frontal Lobes. London: Oxford University Press, 1939.

Salmaso D, Denes G. The frontal lobes on an attention task: a signal detection analysis. Percept Motor Skills 1982;54:1147–1152.

Schiffer RB, Babigian HM. Behavorial disorders in multiple sclerosis, temporal lobe epilepsy, and amyotrophic lateral sclerosis. Arch Neurol 1984;41:1067–1069.

Segarra JM, Angels JN. Presentation 1. In AL Benton (ed.), Behavior Change in Cerebrovascular Disease. New York: Harper & Row, 1970;3–14.

Shallice T, Evans ME. The involvement of the frontal lobes in cognitive estimation. Cortex 1978;14:294–303.

Shapiro BE, Alexander MP, Gardner H, Mercer B. Mechanisms of confabulation. Neurology 1981;31:1070–1076.

Smith A. Intellectual function in patients with lateralized frontal tumor. J Neurol Neurosurg Psychiatry 1966;29:52–59.

Spreen O, Strauss E. A Compendium of Neuropsychological Tests. Administration, Norms, and Commentary. New York: Oxford University Press, 1998.

Storey PB. Brain damage and personality change after subarachnoid hemorrhage. Br J Psychiatry 1970;117:129–142.

Strich JJ. Lesions in the cerebral hemispheres after blunt head injury. In S Sevitt, HB Stoner (eds), The Pathology of Trauma. London: BMA House, 1970;166–171.

Stuss DT, Benson DF. Neuropsychological studies of the frontal lobes. Psychological Bull 1984;95:3–28.

Surridge D. An investigation into some psychiatric aspects of multiple sclerosis. Br J Psychiatry 1969;115:749–764.

Talland GA, Sweet WH, Ballantine HT. Amnesia syndrome with anterior communicating artery aneurysm. J Nerv Ment Dis 1967;145:179–192.

Teuber HL. The riddle of frontal lobe function in man. In JM Warren, K Akert (eds), The Frontal Granular Cortex and Behavior. New York: McGraw-Hill, 1964;410–444.

Thompson G. Cerebral lesions simulating schizophrenia: three case reports. Biol Psychiatry 1970;2:59–64.

Virkkunen M, Nuutila A, Huusho S. Effect of brain injury on social adaptability. Acta Psychiatr Scand 1976;53:168–172.

Virkkunen M, Nuutila A, Huusho S. Brain injury and criminality. Dis Nerv Syst 1977;38: 907–908.

Volpe BT, Hirst W. Amnesia following the rupture and repair of an anterior communicating artery aneurysm. J Neurol Neurosurg Psychiat 1983;46:704–709.

Vonsattel J-P, Myers RH, Stevens TJ et al. Neuropathological classification of Huntington's disease. J Neuropathol Exp Neurol 1985;44:559–577.

Weinberger DR. A brain too young for good judgment. New York Times, March 10, 2001.

Weinberger DR, Berman KF, Ladorola M et al. Prefrontal cortical blood flow and cognitive function in Huntington's disease. J Neurol Neurosurg Psychiatry 1988;51: 94–104.

Wheeler MA, Stuss DT, Tulving E. Frontal lobe damage produces episodic memory impairment. J Int Neuropsychol Soc 1995;1:525–536.

Zangwill OL. Psychological deficits associated with frontal lobe lesions. Int J Neurol 1966;5:395–402.

11

Amnesias: Focal Syndromes of Memory Loss

And suddenly the memory revealed itself. The taste was that of the little piece of Madeleine which on Sunday mornings at Combray..., my aunt Leonie used to give me, dipping it first in her own cup of tea or tisane. The sight of the little Madeleine had recalled nothing to my mind before I tasted it... But when from a long-distant past nothing subsists, after the people are dead, after the things are broken and scattered, taste and smell alone, more fragile but more enduring, more immaterial, more persistent, more faithful, remain poised a long time, like souls, remembering, waiting, hoping, amid the ruins of all the rest; and bear unflinchingly, in the tiny and almost impalpable drop of their essence, the vast structure of recollection.

(Proust 1913)

The amnesias are clinical syndromes in which memory loss occurs out of proportion to any other cognitive impairment. Memory refers to the ability of the brain to store and retrieve information, a function required for learning and therefore important to all human intellectual activities. Some memories are vivid, a virtual reliving of a prior experience, as in Marcel Proust's sudden, complete recollections of childhood events on experiencing the taste and smell of a madeleine. Other memories are less direct, more a recollection of a series of facts rather than a sensory perception. Memory has been divided into types, stages, and modalities, which has led to considerable confusion. We shall discuss these subdivisions of the memory system later in this chapter. Amnesias involve both a loss of memory for prior events and an inability to learn, or to store and retrieve, new information. The amnesic patient is confined to the present, unable to recall the recent past and forced to repeat daily experiences without learning from them.

The amnesias can be divided into four categories:

1. The 'amnestic syndrome', a specific dysfunction of memory storage and retrieval
2. Partial amnesias, in which only specific classes or modalities of memory are lost
3. Amnesia as part of a more generalized cognitive dysfunction or dementia;
4. Functional or psychogenic amnesias.

Within these categories, amnesias can occur in temporary or permanent forms. As in other disorders in behavioral neurology, memory dysfunction is first categorized behaviorally by the bedside examination, then matched with the patient's history, and finally a diagnosis is established.

MEMORY STAGES

Clinical neurologists divide memory into three stages: immediate, recent, and remote. The first stage, immediate memory, corresponds to attention span, or to Baddeley's (1992) concept of 'working memory'. Immediate memory denotes the amount of information a subject can keep in conscious awareness, without active memorization. A normal person can retain seven digits in the active memory span (Miller 1956), perhaps by coincidence the number of digits in a local telephone number. Most normal people can hear a telephone number, walk across the room, and dial the number without having to 'memorize' (rehearse) it. Numbers of more than seven digits, called 'supraspan numbers', require active memory processing, as does remembering digits in reverse order ('reverse digit span').

Disorders of attention affect digit span, as in dementia and delirium. In addition, focal lesions of the superior frontal cortex, affecting Brodmann areas 8 and 9, have profound effects on immediate memory (Goldman-Rakic 1996). Many patients with Broca's aphasia secondary to left frontal lesions have impaired immediate memory, with digit spans often reduced to three or four items (Gordon 1983). The items in immediate memory are normally forgotten as soon as the subject's attention switches to another topic; telephone numbers, once looked up and dialed, are completely forgotten, unless the subject actively memorizes them.

The second stage of memory, referred to by clinicians as short-term memory, involves the ability to register and recall specific items such as words or events after a delay of a few minutes to hours. One confusing aspect of the literature on memory is that some cognitive neuroscientists refer to immediate memory span as short-term, and recent memory as long-term. We will use the clinical stages of immediate, short-term, and long-term memory in this chapter. The second or short-term stage of memory has also been called 'declarative' or 'episodic' memory (Squire and Zola 1996). Clinicians also refer to short-term memory as 'recent' memory, meaning the ability to recall events from the past few hours or days.

Short-term memory involves a series of processes occurring over time: (1) the recording or 'registration' of memory items; (2) a period of 'consolidation' of the memory traces, without which they may fade; and (3) the later retrieval of the items, called 'recall' if the subject has to state it directly, or 'recognition' if the subject merely has to pick the item from a group of choices. The first two processes, registration and consolidation, can be thought of as 'storage'. If a head injury suddenly disrupts consolidation, those memories undergoing consolidation are lost, a phenomenon called 'retrograde amnesia'. In addition, new memories cannot be recorded for a time after the trauma; this inability to learn new memories is called 'anterograde amnesia'. For example, a football player who is 'dinged' on the field will lose a few seconds of memory before the injury, almost always including the injury itself, and will also fail to form any new recollections for a few minutes to hours afterwards. The duration of retrograde amnesia is roughly related to the severity of the injury. In one study of football concussions, players recalled their injuries when questioned immediately afterwards but not 20 minutes later, suggesting that non-consolidated memories fade within seconds to minutes (Lynch and Yarnell 1973). In more severe traumatic brain injuries, there is often an initial period of confusion, during which a much longer period of retrograde amnesia is evident. As the patient recovers, anterograde memory returns, and the period of retrograde amnesia 'shrinks' (Benson and Geschwind 1963), such that partial cues can help the patient recall some forgotten events. The phenomenon of 'shrinking retrograde amnesia' and the effectiveness of memory cues suggest that this longer period of retrograde amnesia reflects a failure of retrieval of items that were previously registered and consolidated (Benson and Geschwind 1963). The retrograde and anterograde memory losses reflect the disruption of the short-term memory system.

There is considerable animal and human evidence that short-term memory requires the function of the hippocampus and parahippocampal areas of the medial temporal lobe for both storage and retrieval. The amygdala, an adjacent structure of the medial temporal cortex, is not essential for episodic memory but seems crucial for recall of emotional contexts of specific events and the reactions of fear or pleasure that are associated with these events. We shall return to the neuroanatomy of short-term memory in more detail later.

For the purposes of bedside testing, short-term memory is tested by anterograde tasks such as the recall of three unrelated memory words at 5 minutes. The examiner can also test non-verbal short-term memory by asking the subject to remember the locations of three hidden coins. Retrograde short-term memory is tested by the recall of recent events, such as medical tests, visits to doctors, and symptoms leading up to the patient's hospitalization.

The third stage of memory, which we shall call 'long-term' or 'remote' memory, refers to long known information such as where one grew up, who was one's first grade teacher, or the names of grandparents. Recall of famous figures such as presidents is also used as a test of remote memory, but these questions actually probe the subject's fund of information, which can be continuously replenished by reading and conversation. The separation in time between recent and remote memory is arbitrary, but remote memory generally refers to events dating back months to years. Remote memory, as we shall see later, is resistant to the effects of medial temporal damage; once memory is well stored, probably in the neocortex, it can be retrieved without use of the hippocampal system. Electrical stimulation of specific areas of the cortex in Wilder Penfield's laboratory produced vivid, sensory-specific memories reminiscent of Proust's biting into the madeleine. For example, stimulation of the occipital lobe in one patient produced such a vivid visual image of a fluttering butterfly that the subject reached out his hand to catch it. Stimulation of the temporal lobe produced smells and complex sounds such as orchestra performances. 'A patient might report a feeling tone, or a sense of familiarity, or a full retrieval of an experience of many years previous playing back in his mind, simultaneously but in no conflict with his awareness of being in an operating room conversing with a physician' (Sagan 1977).

OTHER TYPES OF MEMORY (NON-DECLARATIVE OR IMPLICIT MEMORY)

The three-stage model of immediate, short-term, and long-term memory discussed above has proved inadequate to describe the complexity of human memory. Unfortunately, a bewildering array of classifications and terminologies of memory has arisen, as listed in partial form in Table 11.1. Some aspects of memory do not involve the conscious recall involved in the three memory stages recounted above. A simple example is motor memory, such as the ability to ride a bicycle, which is remarkably resistant to hippocampal damage. Such motor memories probably reside in the basal ganglia and cerebellum. In Squire and Zola's (1996) classification, motor memories of this type are called 'procedural' or 'non-declarative' memories.

Another term for the whole class of memories for which subjects have no conscious awareness is 'implicit' memory, contrasted to the 'explicit' memory of episodic events. Implicit memories have in common the fact that their storage and retrieval do not involve the hippocampal system, and perhaps for this reason the subject has no conscious knowledge of them. Several types of implicit memory

Table 11.1   Types of memory and their localizations

Types of recent memory	Localization
Declarative (explicit)	
Facts, events	Medial temporal lobe
Non-declarative (implicit)	
Procedural skills	Basal ganglia, frontal lobes
Classical conditioning	Cerebellum (+ amygdala)
Probabilistic classification learning	Basal ganglia
Priming	Neocortex

have been described. The first type of implicit memory is procedural memory. Squire and colleagues (Cohen and Squire 1980; Squire *et al*. 1984) demonstrated that memories based on rules and procedures ('knowing how' rather than 'knowing that') are spared in the amnestic syndrome. Patients not only retain previously learned motor skills, such as riding a bicycle, but can also learn new skills such as solving a maze or learning a mirror drawing technique (Corkin 1968; Starr and Phillips 1970; Cohen and Squire 1980). A patient reported by Starr and Phillips (1970) learned to play new melodies on the piano, though he recalled no memory of the pieces until prompted with the first few bars. The much-studied patient H.M., amnestic following bilateral temporal lobe excisions for epilepsy, even learned perceptual tasks such as mirror drawing and discrimination of circles from ellipses, though he could not give any verbal description of the task he was about to perform (Sidman *et al*. 1968).

A second type of implicit memory is classical conditioning, in which an unconditioned stimulus becomes associated with a reward or punishment given when the conditioned stimulus is presented (Thompson and Kim 1996). The conditioning itself clearly involves the cerebellum, though the emotional aspect of the reward or punishment stimulus may reside in the amygdala. Classical conditioning can continue to function after bilateral hippocampal damage (Weiskrantz and Warrington 1979). Brust (2000), as mentioned in Chapter 3, cited a 1911 patient with severe amnesia who, after being jabbed by the examiner, withdrew her hand whenever he approached, though she could not say why she did so.

Squire and Zola (1996) outlined other types of non-declarative memory that take place independent of the hippocampal system. 'Probabilistic classification learning', such as predicting the weather from a combination of cues that are regularly associated with sunny or rainy weather, is unaffected by hippocampal damage but impaired in diseases of the basal ganglia such as Huntington's and Parkinson's diseases. Another implicit memory function is artificial grammar learning, which can also take place in otherwise amnestic patients. In all of these types of implicit memory, subjects have no awareness of knowing how they can answer the questions. One last form of implicit or non-declarative memory is called 'priming'. Priming involves the presentation of a stimulus associated with the word or idea to be remembered, such that the priming stimulus aids in the retrieval of the item. For example, if the word 'doctor' has appeared as a word to remember, presentation of the word 'nurse' will trigger the memory more than a neutral word. Priming appears to involve the neocortex (Thompson and Kim 1996). Schacter has shown that deliberate use of priming can help amnestic patients compensate for their memory loss in everyday life (Schacter 1996a; Schacter and Buckner 1998).

The Amnestic Syndrome

The amnestic syndrome refers to a profound and selective loss of the second stage of recent or short-term memory, in the absence of generalized cognitive dysfunction or dementia. The principal features of the amnestic syndrome are

Table 11.2 Features of the amnestic syndrome

Impaired recent memory
  Anterograde
  Retrograde
  Global amnesia
  Spared procedural memory
Preserved immediate memory
Preserved remote memory
Intact general cognitive function
Disorientation to time, place
Confabulation

listed in Table 11.2. The memory deficit involves the short-term memory system (explicit, episodic memory) in both its retrograde and anterograde aspects. Two other variable features of the amnestic syndrome are: (1) disorientation to time and sometimes place but virtually never to person; and (2) confabulation, a tendency to 'make up' information to fill in gaps in memory. Memory loss is global, or not restricted to any class or modality of declarative memory items. Patients with the amnestic syndrome, most of whom have bilateral hippocampal damage, have normal immediate memory span and largely normal ability to recall remote memories such as their childhood upbringing and education. In experimental studies in which amnestic subjects with the alcoholic Korsakoff syndrome are shown famous people from past decades, a 'temporal gradient' has been found in which subjects have excellent memory for remote personages but recall progressively less from periods dating up to the recent past (Seltzer and Benson 1974; Marslen-Wilson and Teuber 1975; Albert *et al.* 1979). Similar findings have been reported in patients rendered amnestic by electroconvulsive therapy (Squire *et al.* 1979). Warrington and colleagues have criticized this point, on the grounds that tests of remote memory are not usually as detailed as those of recent memory. In both normal subjects (Warrington and Sanders 1971) and amnestic patients (Sanders and Warrington 1971), major deficits in remote memory have nearly matched more recent memory deficits. The relative preservation of remote memories in amnestic patients, however, is clinically striking, and it should be a part of the clinical definition of the syndrome.

  The preservation of other cortical functions distinguishes amnestic patients from those with delirium or dementia. An amnestic patient can take an IQ test, score in the normal range, and shortly afterwards fail to remember the psychologist or the experience of taking the test. Patients with the amnestic syndrome live in an eternal present, in which they can interact, speak intelligently, and reason appropriately, yet they do not remember anything about the interaction a few minutes after it ends. These patients are condemned to repeat the same experiences without learning from them.

The recent memory deficit of the amnestic syndrome is considered global, not restricted to any one class of memories or to any one sensory modality. Syndromes of partial amnesia, e.g. disorders of verbal versus non-verbal memory or amnesias restricted to a single sensory modality, are considered later in this chapter. The global nature of the memory deficit, however, does not include those implicit memories that are virtually always spared in the amnestic syndrome, including procedural memories, probabilistic classification learning, artificial grammar learning, and priming.

Confabulation

The last feature of the amnestic syndrome, confabulation, is probably the least understood. In Berlyne's (1972) classification, confabulations are divided into two forms: (1) momentary confabulations, in which an incorrect answer is supplied to a specific question; and (2) fantastic confabulations, in which the stories are offered spontaneously, exceed any specific request for information, and typically have an adventurous, grandiose, or fantastic quality. Both types of confabulation occur in patients with the amnestic syndrome and in demented patients with severe memory loss. In the amnestic syndrome, confabulation is most evident just after onset and often disappears with time, even if some memory deficit persists. Momentary confabulations are more common and often consist of true events, displaced from earlier periods of time, used to fill in gaps in recent memory. Wartime experiences and other remote memories with strong affective content are frequently represented, and the confabulation appears more often in response to questions concerning recent than remote events (Mercer *et al.* 1977).

Experimental studies have suggested that confabulation tends to occur when a patient feels called on to give a response, when a correct memory is lacking, when an affectively important memory comes readily to mind, and when the patient has defective ability to monitor the logical content of the responses (Mercer *et al.* 1977; Shapiro *et al.* 1981). This last characteristic, poor monitoring of responses for accuracy or plausibility, seems especially important, as responses to successive questions may be mutually contradictory. For example, a patient may give the correct current year but state that he has just returned from the Vietnam War, or he may know that he is in the hospital yet report being in another city the same morning.

The 'fantastic confabulator' may embellish questions about presidents or famous personages by stating that he knows them personally or has spent time with them recently. Perhaps related to these confabulations are the 'reduplications' of place and persons discussed previously in Chapter 9. Patients with reduplicative paramnesia state repeatedly that they are in a different place, often in or nearer to their homes, or that familiar people are 'different' or even imposters. The refusal to recognize familiar people, sometimes called the Capgras syndrome, has often been considered a functional psychosis, but it is seen also in patients with diffuse and especially right hemisphere brain damage (Alexander *et al.*

1979). Staton and colleagues (1982) suggested that reduplication is a result of recent memory loss, such that the patient expects people and surroundings to appear as they did in the past.

In general, confabulation should serve as a useful clue to the presence of memory deficits. Confabulation is not clearly useful, however, in distinguishing specific etiologies of amnesia or in separating the amnestic syndrome from more diffuse, dementing illnesses.

Neuropsychological Mechanism of the Amnestic Syndrome

The neuropsychological mechanism of the amnestic syndrome primarily involves deficient transfer of items in immediate memory to the short-term store (storage, or consolidation) (McGaugh 2000). Immediate span itself is normal, but delays of even a few seconds prevent later recall (Cermak *et al.* 1971). The patient is confined to the present, forgetting events as soon as they pass out of immediate memory. Deliberate memorization can keep the items in immediate memory longer, but the introduction of a distractor disrupts the memories, a phenomenon called 'proactive interference' (Cermak and Butters 1972). Similarly, the patient may remember only the first item of a list ('primacy effect') or just the last item ('recency effect').

Cognitive scientists have disagreed on whether the memory deficit in the amnestic syndrome is exclusively a disorder of storage or of retrieval. The phenomenon of proactive interference suggests a storage defect. Further evidence for a storage defect comes from studies of patients with Korsakoff's syndrome. When such patients are tested by recognition of previously presented pictures, they require many more trials than normals to register the items, but once learned the items are forgotten at a rate no faster than that of normals (Huppert and Piercy 1978). Butters and colleagues (1973) suggested that verbal encoding of memories might be the deficient step in Korsakoff's syndrome, as these patients recall fewer verbal than non-verbal items at brief intervals after presentation, whether the items are visual, auditory, or tactile. Another study (Kovner *et al.* 1981) demonstrated deficits in word definitions and semantic memory in patients with both Korsakoff's syndrome and post-traumatic amnesia. On the other hand, evidence for a retrieval defect also exists in the amnestic syndrome. Warrington and Weiskrantz (1970), for example, pointed out the usefulness of memory cues, such as the first letter of a word the subject cannot remember, in eliciting lost memories. It may be that both storage and retrieval deficits exist in the amnestic syndrome, as well as both verbal and non-verbal memory encoding problems, and that these factors may differ in different etiologies and lesion localizations in patients with the amnestic syndrome (Squire 1981; Winocur *et al.* 1984).

For the clinical neurologist, it is sufficient to be aware of the general features of the amnestic syndrome (see Table 11.2) and to recall that immediate memory is preserved, that transfer into short-term memory is deficient, that proactive interference disrupts and memory cues improve recall, and that some non-verbal or motor types of learning can still occur in amnestic patients.

Neuroanatomy and Neurochemistry of Short-Term Memory

The neuroanatomy of the amnestic syndrome is one of the best-studied areas of cognitive neuropsychology. In animal models, bilateral lesions of the hippocampus, parahippocampal gyrus, and entorhinal cortex produce profound amnesia (Squire and Zola 1996). Studies on human patients have provided confirmation of the importance of the hippocampus and related structures to memory. Human patients undergoing temporal lobectomy for epilepsy have shown very similar syndromes to animals in whom the medial temporal structures were ablated (see below).

Evidence from both animal experiments and human patients with amnesia indicates that the hippocampus alone, even when damaged bilaterally, is not sufficient to produce a full-blown amnestic syndrome. Vargha-Khadem and associates (1997) reported that children with bilateral hypoxic damage restricted to the hippocampi have difficulty with explicit memory of episodic events and experiences, yet they are able to learn in a general way about the world, and they are able to make progress in schooling. Semantic memory is generally spared in amnestic patients, but these patients seem able to learn new semantic memories without use of the hippocampal system. Verfaellie and colleagues (2000) contrasted two patients, one with bilateral hippocampal and parahippocampal damage from herpes simplex encephalitis, the other with isolated bilateral hippocampal damage from hypoxia. The first patient had a complete amnestic syndrome, including the inability to learn new semantic information, whereas the second patient showed above-chance performance on new semantic memory testing. The authors postulate that the subhippocampal cortex is important in semantic learning. The authors state that this non-effortful type of learning, or recognition of familiarity, may be related to priming.

The precise role of the hippocampus has been controversial. Horel (1978) reviewed both animal and human evidence and concluded that the medial temporal stem, a structure containing connections between the temporal lobe and thalamus, was the source of memory loss associated with medial temporal lobe surgery. Mishkin (1978, 1982), in animal experiments, however, showed that combined resection of the hippocampus and amygdala does produce permanent short-term memory loss. Isolated resections of the temporal stem did not produce memory loss (Zola-Morgan *et al.* 1979).

The anatomy of memory storage and retrieval in the human brain is shown in Figure 11.1. The hippocampus on each side projects via the fornix to the deep medial frontal region, especially the septal areas. Cutting of the fornix in neurosurgery has been reported to cause amnesia (Sweet *et al.* 1959), though other authors have not confirmed an essential role of the fornix in memory (Woolsey and Nelson 1975). Damage to the septal areas, as in ruptured anterior communicating

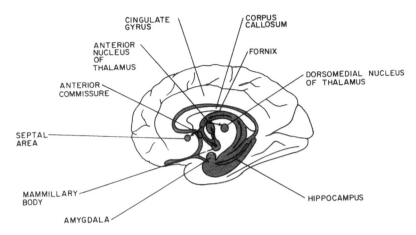

Figure 11.1 Diagram of the memory circuit of the right hemisphere (Papez's circuit). The principal projections are from hippocampus to mammillary body, via the fornix, with a way station in the septal area, from the mammillary body to the anterior thalamic nucleus, from the anterior thalamus to the cingulate gyrus (not shown), and from the cingulate gyrus back to the hippocampus.

artery aneurysms, does cause memory loss (see below). The septal areas are waystations on the pathway from the hippocampus to the mammillary bodies. These in turn project to the anterior nucleus of the thalamus via the mammillothalamic tract of Vic D'Azyr. From the thalamus, fibers project to the cingulate gyrus of the frontal lobe, and then back to the hippocampus. This circuit (Papez's circuit) is critical for short-term memory registration and retrieval (Papez 1937).

Recently, functional brain imaging in patients undergoing memory testing has contributed to our knowledge of the anatomy of memory. According to one PET study, six brain regions show consistent activation in normal subjects during memory tasks:

1. The prefrontal cortex, especially on the right
2. The hippocampal and adjacent medial temporal regions
3. The anterior cingulate cortex
4. The posterior midline regions of the cingulate, precuneate, and cuneate gyri;
5. The inferior parietal cortex, especially on the right
6. The cerebellum, particularly on the left (Cabeza and colleagues 1997).

Preliminary analyses of the functions of these areas in memory are as follows: the prefrontal cortex appears to relate to retrieval activation and probably to attention, the hippocampi to conscious recollection, the cingulate cortex to the activation of memory and selection of a specific response, the posterior midline regions to visual imagery, the parietal cortex to spatial awareness, and the cerebellum to voluntary, self-initiated retrieval. The right prefrontal cortex is particularly involved in 'intentional or effortful search' for memories, whereas the hippocampus is essential for conscious recollection (Schacter and Buckner 1998). This anatomic schema may be an oversimplification, but it indicates the widespread networks involved in memory. In subjects asked to recognize previously presented pairs of associated words, the right prefrontal cortex, anterior cingulate cortex, and inferior parietal region activated the most. When the subject had to recall the words, the basal ganglia and left cerebellum also became active. Peterson and colleagues (1997), in studies of the recognition of visual designs, found that the medial temporal cortex activates more during new learning tasks than during previously trained and practiced memory tasks. The hippocampal, medial temporal structures thus appear more critical for the storage of new memories than for the activation of older memories. Other areas activated during the new learning task included the prefrontal and anterior cingulate areas, more on the right side, and the parieto-occipital lobes bilaterally, as well as the right infero-occipito-temporal region. These findings correlate with human studies indicating that overlearned memories gradually become less dependent on the hippocampus. Rugg and colleagues (1997) reported greater activation of the left medial temporal cortex in tasks in which the subject remembered words by 'deep encoding' of their meaning, as compared to more simple, 'shallow' encoding of the words, without meaning. Other investigations have also indicated that the deeper the encoding of a word's meaning, the better the subject remembers it (see Schacter 1996a). This research can be interpreted as partial confirmation of the earlier evidence from Butters and colleagues (1973) that verbal encoding is important in the memory deficit of the amnestic syndrome.

Basic research on animals has begun to unravel the fundamental biochemical processes involved in memory. Animal models have contributed greatly to our understanding of the memory functions of the hippocampus and related structures. The consolidation process in which immediate memory is converted to short-term storage appears to be virtually synonymous with long-term potentiation in the hippocampus. The formation of memories can be blocked by injection of inhibitors of protein synthesis into the hippocampus or by surgical ablation of the hippocampus (McGaugh, 2000). Calcium-calmodulin-dependent protein kinase II, or CaMKII is an enzyme related to this process, and inhibitors of CaMKII interfere with memory formation. Another enzyme, protein kinase C or PKC, is involved with late protein synthesis in the hippocampus, and blockade of this enzyme also disrupts the consolidation of memories. PKC, in turn, appears to be involved in the activation of the CREB gene, discovered by Kandel and colleagues (1996) in studies of memory formation in the giant snail, *aplysia*. Development of long-term potentiation, a correlate of memory in this species, requires activation of a gene called CREB (cyclic AMP response element binding protein) in sensory neurons. In this system and also in similar studies on the fruitfly *drosophila*, and more recently in mammals such as the mouse, gene activation and protein synthesis are necessary for memory formation (Silva *et al.* 1998). While similar studies have not been performed in humans, it is likely that similar gene activation and protein synthesis, perhaps beginning in the hippocampi but proceding through its neocortical connections, is necessary for the transition from immediate 'working memory' to longer-term storage of memory (Bear 1997). The actual memory traces, or the specific content of memories, likely reside in specific areas of the neocortex, especially the association cortex for specific sensory modalities, as discussed earlier. The hippocampal system is necessary to store the memories initially or to retrieve them into active thought processes, at least for a time. The scientific investigation of memory storage and retrieval holds promise for the development of drugs to enhance memory storage.

Finally, the amygdala is involved in modulating memory function, especially in enhancing the storage of emotionally important memories. The amygdala, and in particular the basolateral nucleus of the amygdala, is the intermediary structure by which epinephrine and glucocorticoids also enhance memory formation; ablation of the amygdala or infusion of beta-adrenergic receptor antagonists blocks the enhancement of emotionally charged memories (McGaugh 2000).

Diseases Associated with the Amnestic Syndrome

The amnestic syndrome can result from a number of disease states, all involving the limbic structures of the medial temporal lobe or their connections via Papez's circuit. All produce global impairment of short-term memory, with sparing of both immediate and remote memory, as well as of general intellectual functioning. Confabulation may be present to variable degrees.

Wernicke–Korsakoff Syndrome

Wernicke–Korsakoff syndrome is a striking amnestic-confabulatory disorder seen in thiamine-deficient, chronic alcoholics. It is probably the most studied syndrome of memory loss, and one that results entirely from damage to extrahippocampal parts of the memory circuit. S. S. Korsakoff, a Russian psychiatrist of the late nineteenth century, described an amnestic syndrome in alcoholics with peripheral neuropathy (Victor and Yakovlev 1955; Levin *et al*. 1983). At about the same time, in Germany, Karl Wernicke (1881) described an acute syndrome of delirium, ataxia, nystagmus, and extraocular muscle palsies, associated with hemorrhagic, necrotic lesions in deep gray matter structures around the third ventricle, brainstem and cerebellum (Brierly 1977). Later neurologists, especially Maurice Victor, Raymond Adams and colleagues (Victor *et al*. 1971), linked the two conditions together. In their studies of the Wernicke–Korsakoff syndrome, the nystagmus, ataxia, and extraocular muscle palsies correlated with lesions of the brainstem and anterior cerebellum, whereas the amnestic deficits were associated with bilateral lesions of the diencephalon, especially the mammillary bodies, fornices, and thalamic nuclei, including most prominently the dorsomedial, anteroventral, and pulvinar groups. Although previous authors had emphasized the mammillary body pathology, Victor and colleagues found that the dorsomedial nucleus of the thalamus was the most consistently damaged structure in amnestic patients. The etiology of the Wernicke–Korsakoff syndrome is now known to be a deficiency of vitamin B1, or thiamine. Although the syndrome occurs most often in alcoholics, it can also result from states of malnutrition such as the excessive vomiting of pregnancy hyperemesis gravidarum, (Lavin *et al.* 1983) and gastric plication surgery (Haid *et al.* 1982). The double vision and ataxia associated with acute Wernicke's encephalopathy may reverse after thiamine treatment, but the memory loss of Korsakoff's syndrome may remain permanently, after the initial delirium has cleared.

Amnesia Secondary to Medial Temporal Ablations

In the early years of surgical resection of the medial temporal lobes for treatment of epilepsy a few patients were deliberately subjected to bilateral medial temporal ablations, with disastrous results for memory, as seen in the famous patient H.M. (Scoville and Milner 1957; Penfield and Milner 1958). In two of the 90 unilateral surgery cases of Penfield and Milner, severe postoperative amnesia developed. The authors postulated that these patients had damage to the medial temporal cortices from birth, called 'medial temporal sclerosis' and a frequent cause of temporal lobe epilepsy. In one such case, an autopsy many years after the second of two unilateral, left temporal lobe surgeries showed pre-existing damage to the contralateral, right hippocampus (Penfield and Mathieson 1974). In general, bilateral damage to the hippocampus and surrounding structures is necessary to produce permanent, severe amnesia. Planning for resection of the medial temporal cortex for treatment of epilepsy now involves extensive evaluation, such as the Wada test of intracarotid barbiturate infusion, to ensure that ablation of one hippocampus will not result in the amnestic syndrome. Even in these carefully selected patients, however, partial memory deficits still occur.

The precise anatomic substrate of the amnestic syndrome in patients with surgical ablation of the medial temporal structures has not been completely elucidated. The resections generally include not only the hippocampus, but also the amygdala, parahippocampal regions, and uncus. Removal of the uncus and amygdala, even bilaterally, does not appear to cause amnesia (Penfield and Milner 1958; Andy *et al.* 1975). Isolated cases of purely hippocampal resections have not been reported in humans. More extensive, bilateral temporal lobe excisions cause the Kluver–Bucy syndrome of placidity, oral and sexual aberrations, and visual agnosia (Terzian and Ore 1955; see Chapter 7).

Penfield and Milner (1958) also studied the results of electrical stimulation of temporal structures. Electrical stimulation of the medial structures, such as the hippocampus, caused a temporary disruption of memory, whereas stimulation of the lateral temporal cortex activated previously stored memories of sensory experiences. As mentioned earlier, these observations were important in the development of our concepts of the hippocampus as the activator of previously stored memories, whereas the neocortex is the site of stored memories.

Other Diseases Associated with Amnesia

Other diseases of the medial temporal cortex also cause amnesia. Herpes simplex encephalitis has a predilection for the orbital frontal and temporal lobes.

Bilateral temporal lobe damage secondary to Herpes simplex encephalitis may leave patients permanently amnestic (Drachman and Adams 1962; Hierons et al. 1978). Other behavioral deficits after herpes simplex encephalitis include aphasia, agnosia, and the Kluver–Bucy syndrome. Pathological studies have shown damage to the hippocampus, amygdala, uncus, cingulate gyrus, and orbital frontal gyri, all structures closely associated with the limbic system and with memory.

Cerebral tumors in the region of the third ventricle and diencephalon have produced relatively selective amnestic syndromes (Squire 1981; Sprofkin and Sciarra 1952; Williams and Pennypacker 1954). The responsible lesions are usually large, midline tumors, such as thalamic gliomas, craniopharyngiomas, colloid cysts of the third ventricle, and large pituitary adenomas.

Hypoxic brain damage in systemic hypotension, cardiac arrest, or hypoxemia is a frequent cause of the amnestic syndrome in severely ill, hospitalized patients. The hippocampus is known to be selectively vulnerable to hypoxic damage, but typically there is associated cortical damage, and a more generalized cognitive dysfunction accompanies the memory loss.

Head injury, or traumatic brain injury (see Chapter 20) is a frequent cause of memory loss. Initial delirium often gives way to more isolated short-term memory loss, and the period of retrograde amnesia then shrinks with time (Benson and Geschwind 1963). In general, the severity of the head injury correlates with the length of the retrograde amnesia.

Strokes are frequent causes of memory loss. The classical case is a bilateral infarction in the posterior cerebral artery (PCA) territory, affecting the medial temporal lobes (Victor et al. 1961; Benson et al. 1974, Trillet et al. 1980). In older patients, even a unilateral posterior cerebral artery stroke regularly causes memory loss, often following a more generalized confusional state (Devinsky et al. 1988; Von Cramon et al. 1988; Ott and Saver 1993).

One patient with an autopsy-documented, unilateral left PCA territory stroke had stable amnesia until his death 82 days later (Mohr et al. 1971). Older individuals may have enough neuronal loss in both medial temporal regions to prevent the spared hippocampus from compensating for the loss of the other. Left PCA strokes are usually easy to diagnose, based on the association of a right visual field defect, reading and color naming difficulties (see Chapter 6), and memory loss. Right PCA strokes may produce only visual field defects and confusion or memory loss. Bilateral infarctions of the thalamus also cause memory loss (Winocur et al. 1984).

Another cerebrovascular cause of memory loss is a ruptured aneurysm of the anterior communicating artery, with damage to the deep, medial frontal areas such as the septal nuclei (D'Esposito et al. 1996; Diamond et al. 1997). Like Korsakoff's syndrome, the memory loss after ruptured anterior communicating artery aneurysms is commonly associated with confabulation.

Memory loss is seen in a host of other neurological diseases, including white matter diseases such as multiple sclerosis (see Chapter 18), neurodegenerative disorders such as Parkinson's disease and related disorders (see Chapter 16), and the diffuse encephalopathies and dementias (see below). In general, the isolated nature of the memory loss in the amnesias distinguishes them from these other diseases.

Memory Loss in Delirium and Dementia

Amnesia classically results from focal lesions of the medial temporal-diencephalic memory circuit, but memory is also prominently affected in diffuse brain disorders such as delirium and dementia. These disorders are discussed in Chapters 13 and 14, but a few comparative statements regarding their memory deficits are in order here. Delirious patients often cannot form memories, but the diagnosis is usually obvious because of the presence of other behavioral deficits and signs of physiological hyperactivity, e.g. agitation, restlessness, tachycardia, hypertension, sweating, tremor, and fever. In the case of dementia, these physiological changes are usually absent. The bedside examination, however, reveals deficits of other higher cortical functions, such as aphasia, acalculia, visuospatial impairments, and loss of insight and judgment, not present in the pure amnestic syndrome. Deficits of recent memory in Alzheimer's disease may be nearly as severe as those of the amnestic syndrome, probably because of the predilection of Alzheimer's disease to affect the hippocampus, as well as the deep frontal nuclei and the neocortex.

Another way of looking at the difference between amnesia and dementia is the distinction drawn by Tulving and Donaldson (1972) between 'semantic' and 'episodic' memory. Semantic memory refers to the set of rules by which we organize new information, and episodic memory refers to the recall of specific events. The amnestic syndrome, as we have seen, impairs recent episodic memory but spares both remote episodic memory and semantic memory. Patients with dementia, on the other hand, suffer the loss of both semantic and episodic memory (Weingartner *et al.* 1983). Demented patients, like amnestic ones, seem to recall remote better than recent episodic memories. One study, however, found that demented patients showed rather large deficits in remote memories as well as recent ones and lacked the clear 'temporal gradients' found in Korsakoff syndrome patients (Wilson *et al.* 1981). Memory loss was most severe for the most recent one or two decades, however, possibly because anterograde memory loss had already begun during this period.

In general, careful bedside testing readily distinguishes the amnestic syndrome from both delirium and dementia. Only occasional patients pose clinical difficulty, such as those with very early dementia or mild cognitive impairment, in whom recent memory is more affected than other cognitive functions (see Chapter 13).

SYNDROMES OF PARTIAL MEMORY LOSS

In contrast to the global amnesia seen in the amnestic syndrome, patients have been described who have memory loss for specific classes of memories or for a single sensory modality. For example, patients with left temporal lobectomy for intractable epilepsy usually have detectable impairment of short-term verbal memory, whereas those undergoing right temporal resection have impairment only of non-verbal memory (Milner 1958; Novelly et al. 1984; Ojemann and Dodrill 1985; Davies et al. 1998). Cortical lesions not involving the deep memory structures also produce selective memory deficits. In many cases these partial amnesias seem more closely related to dysfunctions of specific cortical functions such as aphasia or agnosia than to the global amnestic syndrome. In general, if a matching task can be performed with simultaneous comparison of the sample to the choices, but not when a delay is interposed, the deficit can be considered a disorder of memory.

Amnesia for words, or deficient verbal memory, is a characteristic feature of the aphasias. Immediate memory for digits or words is typically reduced in aphasia (Gordon 1983), and this deficit may be one reason for the difficulty with repetition seen in many aphasic patients. Conduction aphasia (see Chapter 5), for example, can be considered a selective deficit of auditory–verbal immediate memory, restricted not only to the class of words but also to the auditory modality (Shallice and Warrington 1977). Most aphasics show not only deficits of immediate verbal span, but also reduced verbal short-term memory, or reduced ability to learn and retain words (Coughlan 1979; Riege et al. 1980; Risse et al. 1984) or to recall verbal sequences (Albert 1976). Reduced verbal memory likely plays a role in the language dysfunction of these patients, particularly in comprehension of complex sentences and in following commands of multiple steps; these tasks may exceed the patient's verbal memory capacity. An aphasic patient does not show a global amnestic syndrome, performing well on non-verbal memory tasks such as memory for visual designs (Riege et al. 1980), spatial locations of items in a visual display (Grober 1984), auditory patterns such as bird calls (Riege et al. 1980), and the frequency with which specific words have appeared on a test (Grober 1984). Aphasic patients do, however, show deficits on some higher level tasks that do not obviously involve verbal encoding, such as Raven's progressive matrices (Boller and DeRenzi 1967; Goodglass et al. 1974; Kelter et al. 1977). These conceptually difficult tasks may require 'covert verbal mediation', or silent verbal encoding, and they may therefore be susceptible to left hemisphere damage involving the language cortex. Patients with right hemisphere strokes typically show deficits in non-verbal memory out of proportion to any deficits of verbal memory (Coughlan 1979; Riege et al. 1980).

Memory deficits may also be restricted to a single sensory modality. Ross (1980a, 1980b) described partial memory deficits in the visual and tactile modalities. Two patients with bilateral occipital lesions had difficulty finding their way around the hospital ward and in learning new spatial relationships, yet they could draw the floor plan of their own homes or the map of the state. Bedside memory tests showed an inability to learn and recall visual stimuli, although verbal memory was intact. Both patients had bilateral occipitotemporal lesions; Ross postulated bilateral disconnection of the visual cortices from the medial temporal memory circuit. Ross (1980a) proposed the following criteria for diagnosis of a selective visual recent memory disorder: (1) documentation of normal visual perception; (2) absence of aphasia sufficient to impair testing; (3) intact immediate visual memory; (4) intact remote visual memory; and (5) normal recent memory in other modalities.

Ross (1980b) also described a unilateral tactile memory disorder in three patients with unilateral medial temporal lesions. These patients were able to perform stereognosis tasks immediately but could not match a non-verbalizable shape, palpated by the contralateral hand, to a series of choices after a 3-minute delay. Intact immediate but impaired delayed performance indicated a memory deficit, in this instance restricted to the tactile modality. Ross postulated a disconnection explanation for this syndrome as well, this time a unilateral disconnection between the somatosensory cortex in the parietal lobe and the medial temporal memory system. This tactile memory syndrome is usually transitory, perhaps because connections to the medial temporal memory structures of the other hemisphere can develop over time (Ross 1980b).

Comment

The cases discussed above make clear that memory is not a single function, but rather involves the storage and retrieval of a variety of specific memories, in different classes and sensory modalities. The description of the sensory-specific memory syndromes is ingenious, but the syndromes are rare and little attention has been devoted to these disorders. On the other hand, memory dysfunction for specific classes of items is clinically significant in patients with cortical lesions. Even the separation of the left from the right hippocampus, in terms of verbal versus non-verbal memory, is clinically significant in temporal lobe lesions such as temporal lobectomy for epilepsy.

TRANSIENT AMNESIA

Transient amnesia is a temporary version of the amnestic syndrome. The familiar features of retrograde and anterograde amnesia, preservation of remote memories and of intellect, and disorientation, sometimes accompanied by confabulation, are present during the episode. Additional characteristics of transient amnesia include the 'shrinking' of the retrograde amnesia after the transitory event, and the recovery of anterograde memory function. After recovery, a permanent gap in memory remains, equal to the sum of the retrograde amnesia plus the period of anterograde amnesia after onset.

The causes of transient amnesia are numerous (see Table 11.2). All have in common temporary disruption of the memory storage system secondary to either generalized brain dysfunction or focal disruption of the medial temporal-diencephalic memory circuit. Head trauma has already been discussed as a cause of transient amnesia. Epileptic seizures, especially of the complex partial type involving the medial temporal structures, frequently disrupt memory (Gilbert

1978; Dugan *et al.* 1981). If the seizure itself is not witnessed, the patient may present with the clinical problem of an unexplained episode of amnesia. Usually recurrent seizure episodes make the diagnosis clear. Electroconvulsive therapy produces temporary amnesia by a similar mechanism. Transient ischemia of the posterior cerebral artery territory can produce a temporary amnesia (Poser and Ziegler 1960). Cases of transient amnesia during coronary arteriography probably result from either unilateral or bilateral ischemia of the hippocampal complex (Shuttleworth and Wise 1973). Transient amnestic states in patients with migraine, usually followed by severe headache, also likely reflect an ischemic mechanism (Gilbert and Benson 1972; Olivarius and Jensen 1979; Caplan *et al.* 1981). Drug intoxications, especially those with benzodiazepines (Gilbert and Benson 1972; Schmidtke and Ehmsen 1998) are among the more common causes of transient amnesia, presumably by temporarily depressing the activity of the memory system. Of course, physicians use this property of benzodiazepines deliberately in pre-anesthesia with midazolam (Versed) before esophagogastroscopies and similar procedures. Three physicians reported on their own transient amnesia following airplane travel in which they took triazolam (Halcion) for sleep and also consumed alcoholic beverages. 'Alcoholic blackouts' have a similar mechanism (Goodwin *et al.* 1969). Shelly Berman's recording of *The Morning after the Night Before* contains humorous evidence of the fact that persons under the influence of alcohol may be awake and engaging in all sorts of behavior for which they have no memory the following day. Occasionally, transient amnesia occurs in patients with brain tumors, perhaps on the basis of seizures (Hartley *et al.* 1974; Lisak and Zimmerman 1977). Finally, transient amnesia can be of psychogenic cause, as in hysterical fugue states. Psychogenic amnesia is discussed later in this chapter.

Transient Global Amnesia

The most striking example of transient amnesia is the syndrome of transient global amnesia (TGA), initially described by Bender (1956) and later Fisher and Adams (1964). TGA is diagnosed after all of the known causes of transient amnesia have been excluded. TGA typically occurs in an elderly or middle-aged patient, lasts from 1 to 24 hours, and then resolves spontaneously and completely. Precipitating events such as cold temperature, sexual intercourse, and compromising situations (e.g. an elderly man in the midst of an extramarital affair) have been reported in some cases. When examined during the episode, an otherwise cognitively intact individual suddenly loses memory for recent events, asks repeated questions about his or her whereabouts and how he or she got there, forgets the answers, and immediately asks the same questions again. Remote memories and knowledge of personal identity remain intact, though there may initially be a period of retrograde amnesia dating back years. Acutely, the patient has both anterograde and retrograde amnesia, as in the permanent amnestic syndrome, but as recovery occurs the retrograde portion 'shrinks' to a brief period. The patient is left with a permanent gap in memory, consisting of the brief retrograde amnesia before the episode and the period of no learning during the episode. Recurrent episodes occur in only a minority of cases (Nausieda and Sherman 1979; Shuping *et al.* 1980), though one study found a 23.8% recurrence rate (Miller *et al.* 1987). Focal neurological symptoms and signs are usually absent during the episode.

Transient global amnesia is quite common in clinical practice. Miller and colleagues (1987) reported an overall incidence in Rochester, Minnesota of about 5 cases per 100,000 of population, though in patients above the age of 50 years the incidence was more than 20 per 100,000.

The etiology of transient global amnesia is unknown. Fisher and Adams (1964) initially favored an epileptic cause, but seizure activity is not witnessed during or after the episode. The low recurrence rate of TGA also argues against an epileptic etiology. EEG recordings have been normal even during the episode (Jaffe and Bender 1966). A second theory of TGA is vascular (Mathew and Meyer 1974). As mentioned above, transient amnesia can occur in migraine (Gilbert and Benson 1972; Olivarius and Jensen 1979; Caplan *et al.* 1981; Schmidtke and Ehmsen 1998) and with presumed transient ischemic attacks (Poser and Ziegler 1960; Shuttleworth and Wise 1973). TGA does tend to occur in middle-aged and elderly patients, who frequently have risk factors for cerebrovascular disease, but follow-up studies have not indicated a high incidence of TIAs or stroke (Nausieda and Sherman 1979; Shuping *et al.* 1980; Miller *et al.* 1987). Also contrary to the vascular hypothesis is the absence of focal neurological signs, such as visual field defects, during the TGA episode.

Recently, ultrasensitive brain imaging modalities such as diffusion weighted MRI and PET have been performed in patients with TGA. Strupp and colleagues (1998) reported that seven of ten patients imaged during TGA episodes showed abnormal diffusion MRI signal in the left hippocampus; of these seven cases, three had bilateral hippocampal abnormalities. The authors postulated that reduced extracellular space caused by edema or spreading depression might be the cause; permanent infarctions were not found. Other investigators have found frontal lobe abnormalities by diffusion-weighted MRI (Ay *et al.* 1998) or PET imaging (Eustache *et al.* 1997). These studies, however, do not prove an ischemic etiology for TGA; rather, they indicate transient dysfunction in either the hippocampal system or its connections (Papez's circuit), as would be expected. The last four patients observed at our hospital with TGA have had negative diffusion-weighted MR studies, even though all were elderly patients with vascular risk factors. In summary, transient global amnesia is a syndrome of unknown cause, or perhaps multiple causes, though it is closely mimicked by transient amnesia caused by migraine, ischemia, seizures, or trauma.

The evaluation of a patient with transient amnesia should include observation of the patient until the symptoms have passed. Brain imaging with CT or MRI is usually performed to exclude other causes of memory loss, but these are probably not necessary in patients with typical TGA. EEG and drug screening should also be performed if there is clinical suspicion of seizures or drug abuse.

PSYCHOGENIC AMNESIA

Patients are occasionally encountered in whom amnesia appears to be the result of psychogenic (functional) rather than physical (organic) causes. Such syndromes are usually transitory, though cases of permanent psychogenic amnesia have been reported (Pratt 1977).

One interesting subset of psychogenic memory disorders is the group of patients with amnesia for personal identity. Such patients are frequently featured in the news media; the patient is found wandering, with no recollection of how he got there, of prior events, or of his own name or identity. Pictures are shown in the hope that family members or friends will be able to identify the errant patient. Many such patients show normal anterograde memory function and are even able to learn new jobs and form identities while not recalling any details of their childhood, school or military experiences, prior occupations, or spouses and children. In effect, the retrograde amnesia extends back to the earliest childhood memories, although anterograde memory is normal. Some such patients show a loss of personal memories, with preservation of non-personal ones. One patient recalled important public events such as the assassination of President Kennedy, but he could not recall what he was doing during these events. These features of total retrograde amnesia, normal anterograde memory, and the selective impairment of personal memories are not seen in organic amnesias. In general, patients with amnesia for personal identity are virtually never proved to have an organic cause of their amnesia. Careful exploration often reveals a stressful event or circumstance just before the onset of amnesia, and discovery of this event often results in the disappearance of the amnesia. Such patients may develop amnesia either consciously, through malingering and deliberate avoidance of a compromising situation, or through an unconscious mechanism, or hysterical conversion reaction. This distinction, though important to psychiatric diagnosis, seems impossible to make with certainty unless the patient admits to malingering.

The most common psychogenic amnesias are transient losses of memory. Patients may 'forget' or repress uncomfortable memories, and attempts to recall these memories are painful and are inevitably met with resistance. The role of the unconscious and the influence of repressed memories on behavior, of course, form much of the basis of Freudian psychology. In forensic medicine, persons accused of committing violent or criminal acts often claim amnesia for the event. Occasionally such patients have temporal lobe epilepsy (see Chapter 19) or alcoholic blackouts (Goodwin et al. 1969), but psychogenic amnesia of either the conscious or unconscious type should always be considered.

Another variant of transient psychogenic amnesia is the 'fugue state'. These patients suddenly 'awaken' from a state of amnesia and find themselves in strange circumstances, without memory of how they got there. Often they have walked or driven during the spell, with apparently intact motor performance. The fugue state resembles the first type of psychogenic amnesia, the loss of personal identity, except that the patient who awakens from a fugue state has normal retrograde memory, with a gap only for the period of the fugue itself. Few reports are available of patients examined during fugue states, but in general such patients go about their business and do not seek help or complain of amnesia (Pratt 1977). Occasionally fugue states follow traumatic events such as accidents or wartime experiences. Some fugues may be organic, especially those related to head injury, confusional migraine (Gascon and Barlow 1970; Ehyai and Fenichel 1978), or temporal lobe seizures (Mayeux *et al*. 1979). Episodes of wandering in temporal lobe epilepsy, with amnesia for the episode, are called 'poriomania' (Mayeux *et al*. 1979). The majority of fugue states, however, are psychogenic, again related either to malingering or to hysterical dissociative states (Kirshner 1973). The distinction between organic and psychogenic fugue states, although difficult, rests on the association of other organic symptoms such as migraines or seizures in organic fugues, and on other evidence of psychodynamic factors in the psychogenic cases.

Closely related to the fugue states are the rare syndromes of dual or multiple personalities. Such a patient can recall the history of only the personality currently assumed, with total unawareness of the alternate personality. Most of these cases are psychogenic, though rare syndromes approaching this picture may occur in partial complex epilepsy.

A last topic related to psychogenic memory loss is the opposite symptom, the recall of 'false memories' or the false recognition of people or events that the subject believes have been seen or experienced before. A familiar example is the long-repressed memory of child sexual abuse claimed by a man against Father Bernardin, a Catholic priest and bishop in Chicago. The man later confessed that his childhood memories were not real. Schacter (1996a) has emphasized the fragility of memory and the ease with which normal people can make a false recognition of an emotionally charged memory. Schacter (1996b) reviewed the evidence that right frontal activation is involved in the conscious, voluntary search for memory; he cited a case of a 65-year-old man with a right frontal stroke who showed no major memory disturbance except for a tendency to false recognition. Older adults may also show false recognitions more frequently than younger adults (Schacter 1996b). This tendency is obviously problematic in legal cases, where 'eye-witness' accounts are usually believed.

CONCLUSION

The subject of memory brings behavioral neurologists to the crossroads of the behavioral description of human cognitive deficits and the research into basic brain mechanisms by cognitive neuroscientists, in studies of animal models and human functional brain imaging. The student is left with a respect for the complexity of the human memory system, its fragility in disease states and normal aging, and its potential for 'false recognition' even in normal persons. The research cited in this chapter is a good model for the interrelatedness of descriptions of behavior in human diseases such as Wernicke–Korsakoff syndrome and transient global amnesia, research with animal ablation models, and human memory experiments with functional brain imaging. Molecular neuroscience, coupled with behavioral neurology, promises to delineate the exact mechanisms of memory, in terms of brain structure and molecular processes, in the near future.

REFERENCES

Albert ML. Short–term memory and aphasia. Brain Lang 1976;3:26–33.

Albert MS, Butters N, Levin J. Temporal gradients in the retrograde amnesia of patients with alcoholic Korsakoff's disease. Arch Neurol 1979;36:211–216.

Alexander MP, Stuss DT, Benson DF. Capgras syndrome: a reduplicative phenomenon. Neurology 1979;29:334–339.

Andy OJ, Jurko MF, Hughes JR. Amygdalotomy for bilateral temporal seizures. South Med J 1975;68:743–748.

Ay H, Furie KL, Yamada K. Diffusion-weighted MRI characterizes the ischemic lesion in transient global amnesia. Neurology 1998;51:901–903.

Baddeley A. Working memory. Science 1992;255:556–559.

Bailey CH, Bartsch D, Kandel ER. Toward a molecular definition of long-term memory storage. Proc Natl Acad Sci 1996;93:13445–13452.

Bear MF. How do memories leave their mark? Nature 1997;385:481–482.

Bender MB. Syndrome of isolated episode of confusion with amnesia. J Hillside Hosp 1956;5:212–215.

Benson DF. Approaches to Intellectual Memory Impairments. In WG Bradley, RB Daroff, GM Fenichel, CD Marsden (eds), Neurology in Clinical Practice (2nd edn). Boston: Butterworth-Heinemann, 1996;71–81.

Benson DF, Geschwind N. Shrinking retrograde amnesia. J Neurol Neurosurg Psychiatry 1963;30:539–544.

Benson DF, Marsden CD, Meadows JC. The amnestic syndrome of posterior cerebral artery occlusion. Acta Neurol Scand 1974;50:133–145.

Berlyne N. Confabulation. Br J Psychiatry 1972;120:31–39.

Boller F, DeRenzi E. Relationships between visual memory defects and hemispheric locus of lesion. Neurology 1967;17:1052–1058.

Brierly JB. Neuropathology of amnestic states. In CWM Whitty, OL Zangwill (eds), Amnesia (2nd edn). London: Butterworth, 1977;199–223.

Brust JCM. The non-Freudian unconscious. Neurologist 2000;6:224–231.

Butters N, Lewis R, Cermak LS, Goodglass H. Material-specific memory deficits in alcoholic Korsakoff patients. Neuropsychologia 1973;11:291–299.

Cabeza R, Kapur S, Craik FIM et al. Functional neuroanatomy of recall and recognition: a PET study of episodic memory. J Cog Neurosci 1997;9:254–265.

Caplan L, Chedru F, Lhermitte F, Mayman C. Transient global amnesia and migraine. Neurology 1981;31:1167–1170.

Cermak LS, Butters N. The role of interference and encoding in the short-term memory deficits of Korsakoff patients. Neuropsychologia 1972;10:89–95.

Cermak LS, Butters N, Goodglass H. The extent of memory loss in Korsakoff patients. Neuropsychologia; 1971;9:307–315.

Chan J-L, Ross ED. Alien hand syndrome: influence of neglect on the clinical presentation of frontal and callosal variants. Cortex 1997;33:287–299.

Cohen NJ, Squire LR. Preserved learning and retention of pattern-analyzing skill in amnesia; dissociation of knowing how and knowing that. Science 1980;210:207–210.

Corkin S. Acquisition of motor skill after bilateral medial temporal lobe excision. Neuropsychologia 1968;6:255–265.

Coughlan AK. Effects of localized cerebral lesions and dysphasia on verbal memory. J Neurol Neurosurg Psychiatry 1979;42:914–923.

Davies KG, Bell BD, Bush AJ, Wyler AR. Prediction of verbal memory loss in individuals after anterior temporal lobectomy. Epilepsia 1998;39:820–828.

D'Esposito M, Alexsander MP, Fischer R *et al*. Recovery of memory and executive function following anterior communicating artery rupture. J Int Neuropsychol Soc 1996;2: 565–570.

Devinsky O, Bear D, Volpe BT. Confusional states following posterior cerebral artery infarction. Arch Neurol 1988;45:160–163.

Diamond BJ, DeLuca J, Kelley SM. Memory and executive functions in amnesic and non-amnesic patients with aneurysms of the anterior communicating artery. Brain 1997;120:1015–1025.

Drachman DA, Adams RD. Herpes simplex and acute inclusion-body encephalitis. Arch Neurol 1962;7:45–63.

Dugan TM, Nordgren RD, O'Leary P. Transient global amnesia associated with bradycardia and temporal lobe spikes. Cortex 1981;17:633–638.

Ehyai A, Fenichel GM. The natural history of acute confusional migraine. Arch Neurol 1978;35:368–369.

Eustache F, Desgranges B, Petit-Taboue MC. Transient global amnesia: implicit/explicit memory dissociation and PET assessment of brain perfusion and oxygen metabolism in the acute stage. J Neurol Neurosurg Psychiatry 1997;63:357–367.

Fisher CM, Adams RD. Transient global amnesia. Acta Neurol Scand 1964;40(Suppl. 9):1–83.

Gascon G, Barlow C. Juvenile migraine, presenting as an acute confusional state. Pediatrics 1970;45:628–635.

Gilbert GJ. Transient global amnesia: manifestation of medial temporal lobe epilepsy. Clin Electroencephalogr 1978;9:147–152.

Gilbert GJ, Benson DF. Transient global amnesia: report of two cases with definite etiologies. J Nerv Ment Dis 1972;154:461–464.

Goldman-Rakic PS. The prefrontal landscape: implications of functional architecture for understanding human mentation and the central executive. Phil Trans R Soc Lond B (1996);351:1445–1453.

Goodglass H, Denes G, Calderone M. The absence of covert verbal mediation in aphasia. Cortex 1974;10:264–269.

Goodwin DW, Crane JB, Guze SB. Alcoholic blackouts: a review and clinical study of 100 alcoholics. Am J Psychiatry 1969;126:191–198.

Gordon WP. Memory disorders in aphasia. I. Auditory immediate recall. Neuropsychologia 1983;21:325–339.

Grober E. Nonlinguistic memory in aphasia. Cortex 1984;20:67–73.

Haid RW, Gutmann L, Crosby TW. Wernicke–Korsakoff encephalopathy after gastric plication. JAMA 1982;247:2566–2567.

Hartley TC, Heilman KM, Garcia-Bengochia F. A case of a transient global amnesia due to a pituitary tumor. Neurology 1974;24:998–1000.

Hierons R, Janota I, Corsellis JAN. The late effects of necrotizing encephalitis of the temporal lobes and limbic areas: a clinico-pathological study of 10 cases. Psychol Med 1978;8:21–42.

Horel JA. The neuroanatomy of amnesia: a critique of the hippocampal memory hypothesis. Brain 1978;101:403–445.

Huppert FA, Piercy M. Dissociation between learning and remembering in organic amnesia. Nature 1978;275:317–318.

Jaffe R, Bender MD. EEG studies in the syndrome of isolated episodes of confusion with amnesia "transient global amnesia." J Neurol Neurosurg Psychiatry 1966;29:472–474.

Kelter S, Cohen R, Engel D *et al*. Verbal coding and visual memory in aphasics. Neuropsychologia 1977;15:51–60.

Kirshner LA. Dissociative reactions: an historical review and clinical study. Psychiatr Scand 1973;49:698–711.

Kovner R, Mattis S, Gartner J, Goldmeier E. A verbal semantic deficit in the alcoholic Korsakoff syndrome. Cortex 1981;17:419–426.

Lavin PJM, Smith D, Kori SH, Ellenberger C. Wernicke's encephalopathy: a predictable complication of hyperemesis gravidarum. Obstet Gynecol 1983;62:13S–15S.

Levin HS, Peters BH, Hulkonen DA. Early concepts of anterograde and retrograde amnesia. Cortex 1983;19:427–440.

Lisak RP, Zimmerman RA. Transient global amnesia due to a dominant hemisphere tumor. Arch Neurol 1977;34:317–318.

Lynch S, Yarnell PR. Retrograde amnesia: delayed forgetting after concussion. Am Psychol 1973;86:643–650.

Marslen-Wilson WD, Teuber HL. Memory for remote events in anterograde amnesia: recognition of public figures from news photographs. Neuropsychologia 1975;13: 347–352.

Mathew NT, Meyer JS. Pathogenesis and natural history of transient global amnesia. Stroke 1974;5:303–311.

Mayeux R, Alexander MP, Benson DF et al. Poriomania. Neurology 1979;29:1616–1619.

McGaugh JL. Memory – a century of consolidation. Science 2000;287:248–251.

Mercer B, Wapner W, Gardner H, Benson DF. A study of confabulation. Arch Neurol 1977;34:429–433.

Miller GA. The 'magical' number 7, plus or minus two: some limits on our capacity for processing information. Psychol Rev 1956:63:81–97.

Miller JW, Peterson RC, Metter EJ. Transient global amnesia: clinical characteristics and prognosis. Neurology 1987;37:733–737.

Milner B. Psychological defects produced by temporal lobe excision. Res Publ Assoc Res Ner Ment Dis 1958;36:244–257.

Mishkin M. Memory in monkeys severely impaired by combined but not by separate removal of amygdala and hippocampus. Nature 1978;297–298.

Mishkin M. A memory system in the monkey. Philos Trans R Soc Lond B 1982;298:85–95.

Mohr JP, Leicester J, Stoddard LT, Sidman M. Right hemianopsia with memory and color deficits in circumscribed left posterior cerebral artery territory infarction. Neurology 1971;21:1104–1113.

Nausieda PA, Sherman IC. Long-term prognosis in transient global amnesia. JAMA 1979;241:392–393.

Novelly RA, Augustine EA, Mattson RH et al. Selective memory improvement and impairment in temporal lobectomy for epilepsy. Ann Neurol 1984;15:64–67.

Ojemann GA, Dodrill CB. Verbal memory deficits after left temporal lobectomy for epilepsy. Mechanism and intraoperative prediction. J Neurosurg 1985;62:101–107.

Olivarius B, Jensen TS. Transient global amnesia in migraine. Headache 1979;19:335–338.

Ott BR, Saver JL. Unilateral amnesic stroke. Six new cases and a review of the literature. Stroke 1993;24:1033–1042.

Papez JW. A proposed mechanism of emotion. Arch Neurol Psychiatry 1937;38:725–743.

Penfield W, Milner B. Memory deficit produced by bilateral lesions in the hippocampal zone. Arch Neurol Psychiatry 1958;79:475–497.

Penfield W, Mathieson G. Memory. Autopsy findings and comments on the role of hippocampus in experiential recall. Arch Neurol 1974;31:145–154.

Peterson KM, Elfgren C, Ingvar M. A dynamic role of the medial temporal lobe during retrieval of declarative memory in man. Neuroimage 1997;6:1–11.

Poser CM, Ziegler DK. Temporary amnesia as a manifestation of cerebrovascular insufficiency. Trans Am Neurol Assoc 1960;85:221–223.

Pratt RTC. Psychogenic loss of memory. In CWM Whitty, OL Zangwill (eds), Amnesia (2nd edn). London: Butterworth, 1977;224–232.

Proust M. Remembrance of Things Past. Vol. 1. Swann's Way (originally published 1913; trans. CKS Moncrieff, T Kilmartin). New York: Modern Library, 1992;63–64.

Riege WH, Metter EJ, Hanson WR. Verbal and non-verbal recognition memory in aphasic and non-aphasic stroke patients. Brain Lang 1980;10:60–70.

Risse GL, Rubens AB, Jordan LS. Disturbances of long-term memory in aphasic patients. Brain 1984;107:605–617.

Ross ED. Sensory-specific and fractional disorders of recent memory in man. I. Isolated loss of visual recent memory. Arch Neurol 1980a;37:193–200.

Ross ED. Sensory-specific and fractional disorders of recent memory in man. II. Unilateral loss of tactile recent memory. Arch Neurol 1980b;37:267–272.

Rugg MD, Fletcher PC, Frith CD et al. Brain regions supporting intentional and incidental memory: a PET study. NeuroReport 1997;8:1283–1287.

Sagan C. The Dragons of Eden. Speculations on the Evolution of Human Intelligence. New York: Random House, 1977;31.

Sanders HI, Warrington EK. Memory for remote events in amnesic patients. Brain 1971; 94:661–668.

Schacter DL. Searching for Memory. The Brain, the Mind, and the Past. New York: Basic Books, 1996a.

Schacter DL. Illusory memories: a cognitive neuroscience analysis. Proc Natl Acad Sci 1996b;93:13527–13533.

Schacter DL, Buckner RL. On the relations among priming, conscious recollection, and intentional retrieval: evidence from neuroimaging research. Neurobiol Learning Memory 1998;70:284–303.

Schmidtke K, Ehmsen L. Transient global amnesia and migraine. A case control study. Eur Neurol 1998;40:9–14.

Scoville WB, Milner B. Loss of recent memory after bilateral hippocampal lesions. J Neurol Neurosurg Psychiatry 1957;20:11–21.

Seltzer B, Benson DF. The temporal pattern of retrograde amnesia in Korsakoff's disease. Neurology 1974;24:527–530.

Shallice T, Warrington EK. Auditory–visual short-term memory impairment and conduction aphasia. Brain Lang 1977;4:479–491.

Shapiro BE, Alexander MP, Gardner H, Mercer B. Mechanisms of confabulation. Neurology 1981;31:1070–1076.

Shuping JR, Rollinson RD, Toole JF. Transient global amnesia. Ann Neurol 1980;7: 281–285.

Shuttleworth EC, Wise GR. Transient global amnesia due to arterial embolism. Arch Neurol 1973;29:340–342.

Sidman M, Stoddard LT, Mohr JP. Some additional quantitative observations of immediate memory in a patient with bilateral hippocampal lesions. Neuropsychologia 1968;6:245–254.

Silva AJ, Kogan JH, Frankland PW, Kida S. CREB and memory. Annu Rev Neurosci 1998; 21:127–148.

Sprofkin BE, Sciarra D. Korsakoff psychosis associated with cerebral tumors. Neurology 1952;2:427–434.

Squire LR. Two forms of human amnesia: an analysis of forgetting. J Neurosci 1981;1: 635–640.

Squire LR, Zola SM. Structure and function of declarative and nondeclarative memory systems. Proc Natl Acad Sci 1996;93:13515–13522. (See also Squire LR, Zola-Morgan S. The medial temporal lobe memory system. Science 1991;253:1380–1386.)

Squire L, Slater PC, Chace PM. Retrograde amnesia: temporal gradient in very long-term memory following electroconvulsive therapy. Science 1979;187:77–79.

Squire LR, Cohen NJ, Zouzounis JA. Preserved memory in retrograde amnesia: sparing of a recently acquired skill. Neuropsychologia 1984;22:145–152.

Starr A, Phillips L. Verbal and motor memory in the amnestic syndrome. Neuropsychologia 1970;8:75–88.

Staton RD, Brumback RA, Wilson H. Reduplicative paramnesia: a disconnection syndrome of memory. Cortex 1982;18:23–36.

Strupp M, Bruning R, Wu RH *et al.* Diffusion-weighted MRI in transient global amnesia: elevated signal intensity in the left mesial temporal lobe in 7 of 10 patients. Ann Neurol 1998;43:164–170.

Sweet WH, Talland GA, Ervin FR. Loss of recent memory following section of the fornix. TAm Neurol Assoc 1959;84:76–82.

Teng EL, Chui, HC. The modified mini-mental state (3MS) examination. J Clin Psychiatry 1987;48:314–318.

Terzian H, Ore GD. Syndrome of Kluver and Bucy reproduced in man by bilateral removal of the temporal lobes. Neurology 1955;5:373–380.

Thompson RF, Kim JJ. Memory systems in the brain and localization of a memory. Proc Natl Acad Sci 1996;93:13438–13444.

Trillet M, Fischer C, Serclerat *et al.* Le syndrome amnesique dans ischemies cerebrales posterieures. Cortex 1980;16:421–434.

Tulving E, Donaldson W. Organization of Memory. New York: Academic Press, 1972.

Vargha-Khadem F, Gadian DG, Watkins KE *et al.* Differential effects of early hippocampal pathology on episodic and semantic memory. Science 1997;277:376–380.

Verfaellie M, Koseff P, Alexander MP. Acquisition of novel semantic information in amnesia: effects of lesion location. Neuropsychologia 2000;38:484–492.

Victor M, Yakovlev PI. Translation of SS Korsakoff's psychic disorder in conjunction with peripheral neuritis. Neurology 1955;5:394–406 (originally 1889).

Victor M, Angevine JB, Mancall EL, Fisher CM. Memory loss with lesions of the hippocampal formation. Arch Neurol 1961;5:244–263.

Victor M, Adams RD, Collins GH. The Wernicke–Korsakoff syndrome. Philadelphia: Davis, 1971.

Von Cramon DY, Hebel N, Schuri U. Verbal memory and learning in unilateral posterior cerebral artery infarction. A report on 30 cases. Brain 1988;111:1061–1077.

Warrington EK, Sanders HI. The fate of old memories. Q J Exp Psychol 1971;23:432–442.

Warrington EK, Weiskrantz L. Amnestic syndrome: consolidation or retrieval? Nature 1970;228:628–670.

Weingartner H, Grafman J, Boutelle W *et al.* Forms of memory failure. Science 1983;221: 380–382.

Weiskrantz L, Warrington EK. Conditioning in amnestic patients. Neuropsychologia 1979;17:187–194.

Wernicke C. Acute hemorrhagic poliioencephalitis superior. In DA Rottenberg, FH Hochberg (eds), Neurological Classics in Modern Translation (originally published 1881). New York: Hafner, 1977.

Williams M, Pennypacker J. Memory disturbance in third ventricular tumors. J Neurol Neurosurg Psychiatry 1954;17:115–128.

Wilson RS, Kaszniak AW, Fox JH. Remote memory in senile dementia. Cortex 1981; 17:41–48.

Winocur G, Oxbury S, Roberts R *et al.* Amnesia in a patient with bilateral lesions of the thalamus. Neuropsychologia 1984;22:123–143.

Woolsey R, Nelson JS. Asymptomatic destruction of the fornix in man. Arch Neurol 1975;32:566–568.

Zola-Morgan S, Squire LR, Mishkin M. The neuroanatomy of amnesia – hippocampus versus temporal stem. Science 1979;218:1337–1339.

12

Syndromes of the Corpus Callosum

The two hemispheres of the brain are really and in fact two distinct and complete organs, and each respectively as complete (indeed more complete) and as fully perfect in all its parts, for the purposes it is intended to perform, as are the two eyes. The corpus callosum, and the other commissures between them, can with no more justice be said to constitute the two hemispheres into one organ, than the optic commissure can be called an union of the two eyes into one organ.

(Wigan 1844, p. 19)

If...one brain be a perfect instrument of thought – if it be capable of all the emotions, sentiments, and faculties, which we call in the aggregate, mind – then it necessarily follows that man must have two minds with two brains; and however intimate and perfect their unison in their natural state, they must occasionally be discrepant, when influenced by disease, either direct, sympathetic, or reflex.

(Wigan 1844, pp. 201–202)

The concept of two separate cerebral hemispheres, linked by the corpus callosum, subserving one consciousness has been the center of most thought about brain, behavior, and consciousness over the past 150 years. This concept, given early criticism by Wigan in 1844, has undergone major revision in the era of corpus callosum section surgery for epilepsy.

The history of our conception of the corpus callosum is an interesting one. Nineteenth-century physicians thought in terms of connections via the corpus callosum in analyzing neurobehavioral deficits. As discussed in Chapter 7, Liepmann (Liepmann 1900; Liepmann and Maas 1907) analyzed ideomotor apraxia in terms of disconnection via the corpus callosum of the concepts of movement in the left hemisphere and the execution of the movement by the right hemisphere motor cortex. The patient of Liepmann and Maas had a right hemiparesis from a pontine lesion; apraxia resulted from a lesion of the anterior corpus callosum, disconnecting the right hemisphere motor centers from the left hemisphere language cortex. Similarly, Dejerine (1892) described a disconnection at the level of the splenium of the corpus callosum as the basis of the syndrome of pure alexia without agraphia (see Chapter 6); in this syndrome, visual information from the intact right occipital lobe is disconnected from the left hemisphere centers involved in reading. Figure 12.1 shows the anatomy of the corpus callosum.

After the promising beginnings in the nineteenth century of interest in the corpus callosum as the source of behavioral deficits, interest in the subject of interhemispheric transfer waned in the early twentieth century. Exceptions were Trescher and Ford (1937) and Maspes (1948), who reported deficits in patients who underwent partial section of the corpus callosum for removal of tumors in the vicinity of the third ventricle. These patients had difficulty in naming letters placed in the left hand or shown in the left visual field. Neurosurgeons such as Akalaitis (1944) developed the technique of surgical section of the corpus cal-

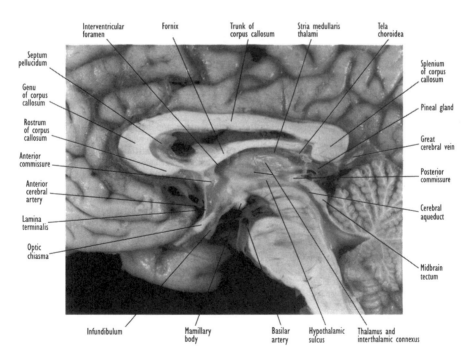

Figure 12.1 Midline sagittal section of the brain, showing the corpus callosum, a dense band of fibers connecting the two cerebral hemispheres. (Reprinted with permission of JL Wilkinson. Neuroanatomy for Medical Students. Boston: Butterworth-Heinemann, 1986;130.)

losum to prevent the spread of epilepsy. Akalaitis (1943, 1944) reported no significant neurobehavioral consequences from corpus callosotomy.

In 1962, Geschwind and Kaplan rekindled interest in the corpus callosum with a detailed case study of a 41-year-old man who underwent surgery for a left frontal glioblastoma multiforme; postoperatively it was noted that he could write with his right hand, but not with the left. In testing, he could name objects or cardboard letters placed in his right but not his left hand. He could demonstrate how to manipulate an object placed in his left hand: for example, he turned a key to show its use to start a car, but he could neither say the name 'key' nor say what it was used for, stating 'erasing a blackboard with a chalk eraser'. Likewise, he held a pair of scissors and showed a cutting movement but said 'I'd use that to light a cigarette'. If he opened his eyes, however, he could name the object in his left hand. He followed commands to move his right hand correctly, but he made many errors in commands involving his left hand. Clearly all of these deficits reflect failure of transmission of information from the right hemisphere to the left hemisphere language areas. At autopsy, the patient had residual tumor of the left frontal lobe but also an infarction of the anterior corpus callosum, which apparently resulted from sacrifice of the anterior cerebral artery during surgery. Geschwind and Kaplan cited the animal experiments of Roger Sperry (1961), who had demonstrated similar failures in animals subjected to section of the optic chiasm and cerebral commissures. This human patient was the first modern case of a corpus callosum syndrome. Along with the animal experiments of Sperry, it opened the contemporary era of research into corpus callosum function.

THE CORPUS CALLOSOTOMY SYNDROME

The next chapter in the story of corpus callosum syndromes came from human research on patients undergoing corpus callosum surgery by Sperry and his associates, including Michael Gazzaniga, Philip Vogel, and Joseph Bogen (Sperry 1966–1967). The publication of these studies caught the attention of the scientific community and even the general public, and Sperry was later awarded the Nobel Prize for the research. Many 'pop psychology' notions of right brain and left brain processing have come from the 'split-brain' research.

Like the patient described by Geschwind and Kaplan (1962), the first few commissurotomy patients showed an inability to follow simple commands to use the left hand or identify objects in the left hand. As the surgical technique improved, however, patients presented much less obvious deficits. Some patients are temporarily mute after the surgery but recover quickly (Sussman *et al.* 1983). One 12-year-old male patient joked on the day after surgery that he had a 'splitting headache'. These patients were tested in an apparatus in which visual stimuli could be projected via a tachistoscope into just the left or right visual field, and the subject could palpate objects out of sight with either hand. During such testing, the patients misreported visual stimuli projected into the left visual field, while correctly naming stimuli projected to the right visual field. It was as if the 'verbal hemisphere' was aware only of the right visual field, and the 'non-verbal hemisphere' could not communicate information available to it. If a series of objects was presented tactily to the left hand, however, the subject could readily match the stimulus projected to the left visual field with the object palpated by the left hand, indicating that the subject saw the object with the right hemisphere but could not transfer the information to the left hemisphere language areas to talk about it. In another experiment, the subject was shown a square in the left visual field and a triangle in the right visual field. The subject was asked to draw what he saw with the left and then the right hand. As one might guess, the left hand drew a square (while the patient said he was drawing a triangle), and the right hand drew a triangle. In Sperry's words, 'these people have, in effect, not one inner visual world any longer like the rest of us, but rather two separate and independent inner visual worlds – one for the right and one for the left half field of vision, each in their separate hemispheres'. Wigan's (1844) prophetic statements cited at the beginning of the chapter have thus found confirmation in studies of patients with surgical section of the corpus callosum.

Language in Corpus Callosotomy Patients

Testing of split-brain patients has also revealed interesting language disorders. Corpus callosum surgery patients failed to name objects palpated by the left hand, though they could match them with other palpated items, and they had no difficulty naming objects palpated by the right hand. Interestingly, one subject said that his ability to match objects with the left hand that he could not identify verbally must have been done 'unconsciously' (Sperry 1966–1967). This statement brings up the concept of separate consciousnesses in the two cerebral hemispheres. To the patient, the right hemisphere's ability to perform tasks not available to the left hemisphere consciousness means that the non-verbal hemisphere is 'unconscious'. Yet the right hemisphere can perform sophisticated tasks such as matching items between the tactile and visual modalities, or even choosing an item from a similar semantic class; for example, if the subject saw a picture of a cigarette in his left visual field, he would choose an ashtray or box of matches from a group of tactile items, if no cigarette was present. Similarly, a subject shown a dollar sign in the left visual field would pick a coin from a group of objects to touch with the left hand. The right hemisphere of these subjects thus appeared to have considerable language ability. One mystery yet to be solved is why patients with left hemisphere damage and aphasia cannot seem to utilize this right hemisphere capability; does the intact corpus callosum somehow inhibit the right hemisphere from carrying out its inherent language functions?

Another area of evidence from the initial studies of patients with surgical section of the corpus callosum (Sperry 1966–1967) was the capability of the right hemisphere for comprehension of language. As in the other tests, the subject had to be tested by methods that permitted the right hemisphere to express itself in ways other than by speaking or writing its responses. The right hemisphere appeared able to process printed phrases such as 'kitchen utensil', 'container for liquids', or 'used for slicing', projected into the left visual field, in matching them to a spatula, jug, or knife palpated with the left hand, or in indicating which one was correct when the examiner said the correct word aloud. Likewise, if a picture of a face was projected to the left visual field with an arrow pointing to any specific facial feature, the subject could point with the left hand to the correct feature on his own face, but he could not do so with the right hand. In addition, he could not name the feature aloud until after he had completed the pointing movement with the left hand. The ability of the right hemisphere to read words and phrases is in stark contrast to descriptions of patients with alexia without agraphia (see Chapter 6), who cannot read words at all in their left visual field. It may be that some such reading goes on but remains 'unconscious', just as it does in the corpus callosum surgery patients. Sperry (1966–1967) commented that the upper limit of the right hemisphere for language comprehension has not been discovered. Again, these findings suggest that the right hemisphere either had more language capacity than normal in these patients with lifelong epilepsy, or that the right hemisphere is somehow inhibited from making language processing available to the left hemisphere in patients with intact corpus callosa and left hemisphere lesions.

Zaidel (see Zaidel 1990) has studied the language capacity of the separated right hemisphere more extensively in the years since Sperry's landmark research. The right hemisphere cannot speak, but it appears to have an extensive auditory vocabulary, and a somewhat more limited visual vocabulary. It can understand not only nouns, but also verbs, adjectives, and even some simple grammatical constructions. It has major deficits on tests of grammatical comprehension such as the Token Test (see Chapter 5), but Zaidel (1990) argues that much of this deficit relates to a shortened immediate memory span, approximating three items in the isolated right hemisphere, as compared to seven in the isolated left hemisphere. Similar information on the language capacity of the isolated right hemisphere has been presented from patients in Gazzaniga's series from Dartmouth (Myers 1984; Sidtis *et al.* 1981).

Other more subtle deficits have been shown to occur in patients with corpus callosum section. These largely reflect the lack of participation of the right hemisphere in language tasks. For example, patients have difficulty describing their emotional experiences (Ten Houten *et al.* 1986) or reading paragraph-length text (Zaidel 1990), and they may seem inappropriate in their conversational style, just as right-hemisphere-damaged patients sometimes do (see Chapter 9, also Zaidel 1990). Wechsler verbal IQ tends to be undiminished after surgery (Campbell *et al.* 1981), though verbal memory deficits may occur (Zaidel and Sperry 1974). Specifically, deficits in right hemisphere tasks such as appreciation of prosody, understanding pictorial metaphor, pragmatics of communication, ability to recognize emotional intonation, and discourse have all been reported in commissurotomy patients (Zaidel 1990).

Praxis in Commissurotomy Patients

Another set of tasks in the corpus callosum surgery patients probed praxis, or the ability of either hemisphere to program movements such as hand postures. The subject was asked to imitate finger postures projected into either visual field. Again, the subjects did better in moving the right fingers to right visual field stimuli or the left fingers to left visual field stimuli, indicating superior performance of either hemisphere for contralateral as opposed to ipsilateral movements. Subjects had much more difficulty with ipsilateral motor control, but control of the left hand from the left hemisphere seemed better than that of the right hand from the right hemisphere, indicating that the left hemisphere was at least partially dominant for learned motor acts (see Chapter 7 for a similar discussion of motor dominance from study of apraxic patients).

Memory in Commissurotomy Patients

Zaidel and Sperry (1994) published the first study on memory functions in patients after corpus callosum section. They found that memory performance was consistently below IQ. There were specific deficiencies in the non-verbal, visual task of the Wechsler Memory Scale (WMS), the word association task, and the short story passages of the WMS. Huppert (1981) and Bentin and colleagues (1984) confirmed similar memory impairments in their split-brain patients. The basis for memory impairments in patients with corpus callosum section could be damage to extracallosal structures such as the fornix. It appears likely, however, that the corpus callosum or interhemispheric associations may be essential to memory function, particularly in word associations and recollection of details of stories.

Spatial Functions in Callosotomy Patients

In general, studies of patients with surgical section of the cerebral commissures have confirmed the evidence (see Chapter 9) that the right hemisphere is superior to the left in visuospatial tasks. Bogen and Gazzaniga (1965) first reported that the left hand was superior to the right in split-brain patients in copying cubes or constructing Koh's block designs. Ledoux and colleagues (1978) also found that subjects performed block design copying better when the designs were flashed in the left as opposed to right visual field. Levy-Agresti and Sperry (1968) suggested that spatial tasks that require *gestalt* recognition favored the right hemisphere, whereas those that require analytical steps in processing favored the left. Recognition of a partial arc as part of a specific circle (Nebes 1971) or a pattern of dots as representing a line or shape (Nebes 1973) was also performed more efficiently by the left visual field–right hemisphere than by the right visual field–left hemisphere. Mental rotation of images was also performed better in the left than right visual field (Corballis and Sergent 1988). Memory for spatial designs presented in the tactile modality favored the left over the right hand (Milner and Taylor 1972; Kumar 1977). These differences in right versus left hemisphere processing styles have also entered the lexicon of pop psychology.

One surprising finding from the corpus callosum section research is that neglect of the left side of the body or the left side of space has not been reported (Bogen and Gazzaniga 1965; Plourde and Sperry 1982). Zaidel and colleagues (1981) pointed out that section of the corpus callosum, leaving the left hemisphere without important input from the right hemisphere, is not equivalent to damage to the right hemisphere in the presence of an intact callosum.

Consciousness in Callosotomy Patients

Perhaps the most important implications of the corpus callosum research relate to the cognitive capacity of the 'unconscious' right hemisphere. Sperry (1966–1967) pointed out that the right hemisphere can associate tactile with visual stimuli in a characteristically human manner, concentrate on tasks at hand and carry them out to the correct conclusion, even when the left hemisphere is supplying 'distracting comments and giving erroneous advice'. Reaction time tests can be performed by split-brain patients simultaneously in both hemispheres as fast as in either hemisphere alone, which is not true of normal subjects. The right hemisphere can respond to emotional or startling stimuli. For example, subjects were shown pictures of nudes in the left visual field; they did not verbally acknowledge seeing anything unusual, but they might giggle, blush, or say something like 'that's some machine you have there!'. Similarly, when the verbal hemisphere misidentifies an object, the subject might frown or shake his head. At times, the right hemisphere seems able to program spoken responses from the left hemisphere, even when the left hemisphere is unaware of having the knowledge to respond (Gazzaniga *et al.* 1987). All of these behaviors suggest that the right hemisphere indeed has its own consciousness, at least in these split-brain patients.

EFFECTS OF PARTIAL SECTION OF THE CORPUS CALLOSUM

The practical implications of the corpus callosum disconnection studies must be tempered by the importance of complete section for lasting deficits. In general, patients who undergo corpus callosum surgery do not show major disconnection syndromes unless nearly all of the corpus callosum and also the anterior commissures are sectioned. Goldstein and Joynt (1969) reported a woman who had corpus callosum surgery, but sparing part of the splenium of the corpus callosum. This patient could perform bimanual coordination tasks, name or select objects palpated with either hand. She did fail to select objects with the right hand when the images of the objects were flashed visually to her left visual field, indicating a partial callosal syndrome. Gordon and colleagues (1971) studied two patients with section of the anterior commissure and the anterior two-thirds of the corpus callosum; as in the cases of Akelaitis, no major disconnection deficits could be found. On the other hand, a Japanese patient (Abe *et al.* 1986) with a self-inflicted ice-pick stab wound of the splenium and genu of the corpus callosum showed hemialexia for information in the left visual field; this case is the behavioral converse of the Goldstein and Joynt (1969) case in which section of all of the corpus callosum except for the splenium permitted intact transmission of visual information (Gordon 1990). Volpe and colleagues (1982) also described preservation of interhemispheric transfer in patients with section of the anterior corpus callosum, sparing the splenium. Lesser sections of the callosum near the splenium have no gross sensory hemiagnosia or apraxia, as described in the complete commissurotomy patients, though there may be subtle differences in the latency of identification of letters flashed by tachistiscope into the left or right visual field (Levine and Calvanio 1980). Even these subtle changes were not detected in a similar case reported by Greenblatt *et al.* (1980). In addition, children with agenesis of the corpus callosum or even those with corpus callosotomy in early childhood did not show the disconnection phenomena described by Sperry and colleagues (Lassonde *et al.* 1991). The requirement of complete section of the posterior portions of the corpus callosum may account for the lack of major behavioral deficits in the patients studied by Akalaitis (1941).

ALIEN HAND SYNDROME

A striking syndrome described in association with damage to the corpus callosum is the alien hand syndrome. Brion and Jedynak (1972) first used this term to refer to the neglect of the left arm in patients with corpus callosum tumors. Bogen (1979) used the term somewhat differently, to indicate involuntary behavior of the left hand of patients with corpus callosum section. In some cases, the left hand might behave completely independently of the right. Subjects have been described after corpus callosum surgery with behavior as goal-directed and conflicting as a woman selecting a casual outfit from a rack with the left hand, while the right hand tried to select a conservative dress. The left hand might withdraw cash from the cash register, as the right hand attempted to deposit it. Usually, the behavior of the 'alien hand' is not this purposeful or goal-directed. The conflicting behavior between the left and right hand has also been referred to as intermanual conflict, diagonistic dyspraxia, or wayward hand (Tanaka *et al.* 1996; Chan and Ross 1997). The patient may verbally describe the movements of the left hand as 'alien'. Cases of alien hand and related phenomena have been described in patients with strokes in the anterior cerebral artery territory, involving the corpus callosum as well as some frontal lobe damage (Feinberg *et al.* 1992; Tanaka *et al.* 1996; Chan and Ross 1997). Cases of alien hand phenomena have also been described in neurodegenerative diseases such as corticobasal degeneration (see Chapter 16; Doody and Jankovic 1992). Feinberg and colleagues (1992) distinguished two types of alien hand syndrome. The first, associated with damage to the anterior corpus callosum, was the same as described by Bogen (1979) and always involved the left hand. The second, associated with damage both to medial frontal structures and to the anterior corpus callosum, usually involved the right hand, with involuntary grasping and manipulation of objects.

CONCLUSION

Damage to connections within the corpus callosum helps to explain several complex neurobehavioral syndromes, for example ideomotor apraxia and alexia without agraphia. The study of patients with surgical section of the corpus callosum has provided important information on the function of the separate cerebral hemispheres in man. These studies have generally confirmed the dominance of the left hemisphere for language and praxis, and the right hemisphere for emotional and visuospatial processes. The right hemisphere, however, appears to have greater language capacity than expected from the literature on patients with aphasia secondary to destructive left hemisphere lesions. Perhaps most importantly, 'split-brain' research has opened a window into the separate consciousnesses of the cerebral hemispheres, a topic that has changed our very understanding of consciousness itself.

REFERENCES

Abe T, Nakamura H, Sugishita M *et al*. Partial disconnection syndrome following penetrating stab wound of the brain. Eur Neurol 1986;25:233–239.

Akelaitis AJ. Studies on the corpus callosum. VII. Study of language function (tactile and visual lexia and graphia) unilaterally following action of the corpus callosum. J Neuropathol Exp Neurol 1943;2:226–262.

Akelaitis AJ. A study of gnosis, praxis and language following section of the corpus callosum and anterior commisure. J Neurosurg 1944;1:94–101.

Bentin S, Sahar A, Moscovitch M. Interhemispheric information transfer in patients with lesions in the trunk of the corpus callosum. Neuropsychologia 1984;22:601–611.

Bogen JE. The callosal syndrome. In KM Heilman, E Valenstein (eds), Clinical Neuropsychology (1st edn). New York: Oxford University Press, 1979;333–334.

Bogen JE, Gazzaniga MS. Cerebral commissurotomy in man: minor hemisphere dominance for certain visuospatial functions. J Neurosurg 1965;23:394–399.

Brion S, Jedynak CP. Troubles du transfert interhemispherique. Revue Neurol (Paris) 1972;126:257–266.

Campbell AL, Bogen JE, Smith A. Disorganization and reorganization of cognitive sensorimotor functions in cerebral commissurotomy: compensatory roles of the forebrain commissures. Brain 1981;104:493–511.

Chan J-L, Ross ED. Alien hand syndrome: influence of neglect on the clinical presentation of frontal and callosal variants. Cortex 1997;33:287–299.

Corballis MC, Sergent J. Imagery in a commissurotomized patient. Neuropsychologia 1988;26:13–26.

Dejerine J. Contribution a l'etude anatomo-pathologique et clinique des differentes varietes de cecite verbale. Mem Soc Biol 1892;4:61–90.

Doody RS, Jankovic J. The alien hand and related signs. J Neurol Neurosurg Psychiatry 1992;55:806–810.

Feinberg TE, Schindler RJ, Flanagan NG, Haber LD. Two alien hand syndromes. Neurology 1992;42:19–24.

Gazzaniga MS, Holzman JD, Smylie CS. Speech without conscious awareness. Neurology 1987;37:682–685.

Gazzaniga MS, Risse GL, Springer SP et al. Psychologic and neurologic consequences of partial and complete cerebral commissurotomy. Neurology 1975;25:10–15.

Geschwind N, Kaplan E. A human cerebral deconnection syndrome: a preliminary report. Neurology 1962;12:675–685.

Goldstein MN, Joynt RJ. Long-term follow-up of a callosal-sectioned patient. Arch Neurol 1969;20:96–102.

Gordon HW. Neuropsychological sequelae of partial commissurotomy. In RD Nebes (ed.), Handbook of Neuropsychology, Vol. 4. Amsterdam: Elsevier, 1990;85–97.

Gordon HW, Bogen JE, Sperry RW. Absence of deconnexion syndrome in two patients with partial section of the neocommissures. Brain 1971;94:327–336.

Greenblatt SH, Saunders RL, Culver CM, Bogdanowicz W. Normal interhemispheric transfer with incomplete section of the splenium. Arch Neurol 1980;37:567–573.

Huppert FA. Memory in split-brain patients: a comparison with organic amnesic syndromes. Cortex 1981;17:303–312.

Kumar S. Short-term memory for a non-verbal tactual task after cerebral commissurotomy. Cortex 1977;13:55–61.

Lassonde M, Sauerwein H, Chicoine A-J, Geoffroy G. Absence of disconnexion syndrome in callosal agenesis and early callosotomy: brain reorganization or lack of structural specificity during ontogeny? Neuropsychologia 1991;29:481–495.

Ledoux JE, Wilson DH, Gazzaniga MS. Block design performance following callosal sectioning: observations on functional recovery. Arch Neurol 1978;35:506–508.

Levine DN, Calvanio R. Visual discrimination after lesion of the posterior corpus callosum. Neurology 1980;30:21–30.

Levy-Agresti J, Sperry RW. Differential perceptual capacities in the major and minor hemispheres. Proc Natl Acad Sci 1968;61:1161–1174.

Liepmann H. Das Krankheitsbild der Apraxie ('Motorischen Asymbolie'). Monatschr Psychiatr Neurol 1900;8:15–44,102–132, 182–197. (Translated in part in Rottenberg DA, Hochberg FA. Neurological Classics in Modern Translation. New York: Hafner, 1977;155–181.)

Liepmann H, Maas O. Fall von linksseitiger Agraphie und Apraxie bei rechtsseitiger Lahmung. Z Psychologie Neurol 1907;10:214–227.

Maspes PE. Le syndrome experimental chez l'homme de la section du splenium du corps calleux alexia visualle pure hemianopsique. Rev Neurol 1948;80:100–113.

Milner B, Taylor L. Right hemisphere superiority in tactile pattern recognition after commissurotomy: evidence for nonverbal memory. Neuropsychologia 1972;10:1–15.

Myers JJ. Right hemisphere language: science or fiction? Am Psychol 1984;39:315–320.

Nebes RD. Superiority of the minor hemisphere in commissurotomized man for the perception of part–whole relations. Cortex 1971;11:333–349.

Nebes RD. Perception of dot patterns by the disconnected right and left hemisphere in man. Neuropsychologia 1973;11:285–290.

Plourde G, Sperry RW. Left hemisphere involvement in left spatial neglect from right-sided lesions: a commissurotomy study. Brain 1982;107:95–106.

Sidtis JJ, Volpe BT, Wilson DH et al. Variability in right hemisphere language functions: evidence for a continuum of generative capacity. J Neurosci 1981;1:323–331.

Sperry RW. Cerebral organization and behavior. Science 1961;133:1749–1757.

Sperry RW. Mental unity following surgical disconnection of the cerebral hemispheres. Harvey Lectures 1966–1967;62:293–323.

Sussman NM, Gur RC, Gur RE, O'Connor MJ. Mutism as a consequence of callosotomy. J Neurosurg 1983;59:514–519.

Tanaka Y, Yoshida A, Kawahata N et al. Diagonistic dyspraxia: clinical characteristics, responsible lesion and possible underlying mechanism. Brain 1996;119:859–873.

Ten Houten WD, Hoppe KD, Bogen JE, Walter DO. Alexithymia: an experimental study of cerebral commissurotomy patients and normal control subjects. Am J Psychiatry 1986;143:312–316.

Trescher JH, Ford FR. Colloid cyst of the third ventricle. Report of a case; operative removal with section of posterior half of corpus callosum. Arch Neurol Psychiatry 1937;37:959–973.

Volpe BT, Sidtis JJ, Holtzman JD *et al.* Cortical mechanisms involved in praxis: observations following partial and complete section of the corpus callosum in man. Neurology 1982;32:645–650.

Wigan AL. A New View of Insanity: The Duality of the Mind, proved by the Structure, Functions, and Diseases of the Brain and by the Phenomena of Mental Derangement, and shown to be Essential to Moral Responsibility. London: Longman, Brown, Green and Longmans, 1844 (reprinted by Joseph Simon Publisher, 1985).

Zaidel E. Language functions in the two hemispheres following complete cerebral commissurotomy and hemispherectomy. In RD Nebes (ed.), The Commissurotomized Brain. Handbook of Neuropsychology, Vol. 4. Amsterdam: Elsevier, 1990;115–150.

Zaidel D, Sperry RW. Memory impairment after commissurotomy in man. Brain 1974;97:263–272.

Zaidel E, Zaidel DW, Sperry RW. Left and right intelligence: case studies of Raven's Progressive Matrices following brain bisection and hemidecortication. Cortex 1981; 17:167–186.

PART III

Generalized, Diffuse, Multifocal and 'Psychiatric' Disorders

13

Dementia and Aging

There is not much left of the acumen of the mind which helped them in their youth, nor of the faculties which served the intellect, and which some call judgment, imagination, power of reasoning and memory. They see them gradually blunted by deterioration and see that they can hardly fulfill their function.

(Aristotle, quoted by Berchtold and Cotman 1998)

"It is our duty to resist old age; to compensate for its defects by a watchful care; to fight against it as we would fight against disease....Much greater care is due to the mind and soul; for they, too, like lamps, grow dim with time, unless we keep them supplied with oil....Intellectual activity gives buoyancy to the mind...Old men retain their mental faculties, provided their interest and application continue."

(Cicero, quoted by Berchtold and Cotman 1998)

Of all the neurobehavioral syndromes discussed in this book, dementia and related aging changes are the most common and the most detrimental to the overall health of the population. As many as 10–15% of persons over the age of 65 years have detectable intellectual deterioration, and 5% have dementia severe enough to interfere with self-care (Wang 1977). Dementia accounts for approximately half of the million patients confined to nursing homes in the USA, and the economic loss brought about by early retirement and medical and custodial care runs into billions of dollars (Terry 1978; Ernst and Hay 1994). In the case of Alzheimer's disease (AD), the most common dementing illness, the incidence is less than 1% at age 65, the prevalence 3%; above age 85, the incidence is over 8% per year, and prevalence may reach nearly 50% (Slooter and van Duijn 1997). Over 4 million persons in the USA are thought to suffer from AD. As the population ages, the number of persons suffering from dementia continues to increase; it is estimated that as many as 14 million Americans will have dementia by 2050. Dementia also decreases life expectancy. Although dementia is infrequently cited on death certificates, it may represent the fourth or fifth leading cause of death in the USA (Go *et al.* 1978). Dementia is a source of tragic losses for patients, families, and society as a whole. Many people in our society have friends or family members with dementia. If reductions in mental capacity with normal aging are included, this illness touches nearly everyone.

The two quotations above express the two poles of common attitudes towards aging and cognitive deterioration. Aristotle seems to regard cognitive loss as an inevitable accompaniment of aging, whereas Cicero sounds an optimistic, 'use it or lose it' note, a hope that mental exercise can preserve active minds into advanced age. These two attitudes towards aging persist today.

AGING AND COGNITION

Cognitive function declines with normal aging, though to an extent not considered clinically important. Performance on an IQ test at age 70 requires only half the correct answers as the same score at age 20. Some cognitive functions are very resistant to aging (Burke and MacKay 1997; Cullum and Rosenberg 1998); these include practiced skills and motor abilities, professional facts, autobiographical information, semantic knowledge (vocabulary, oral reading, and language comprehension), ability to recall the 'gist' of information, and ability to recall items with priming (such as recalling the word 'doctor' when 'nurse' is given as a cue; Schacter and Buckner 1998). Vocabulary and oral reading are so resistant to aging that they are used to estimate premorbid intelligence in demented patients. The group of preserved intellectual functions is sometimes referred to as 'crystallized intelligence'.

Other functions deteriorate more quickly with age. These include new learning of unfamiliar material, language expression (naming and especially series naming), abstract content, and 'remembering to remember' – such as remembering to bring back a roast from the freezer when on a trip to the basement for a hammer. These more age-sensitive functions are sometimes referred to as 'fluid intelligence'. Cockburn and Smith (1991) studied the influence of aging with the Rivermead Behavioural Memory Test, a 13-item test consisting of simple memory tasks but also three 'prospective memory tests': remembering to ask for the return of a hidden belonging on completion of the test; remembering to ask for an appointment on hearing a kitchen timer; and following a route, with a reminder to deliver a message. The three prospective memory tests were heavily affected by age but not by 'crystallized IQ' estimated by years of education or oral reading performance. An index of the degree of participation in community activities did seem to protect against the decline in prospective memory with age; this finding supports the 'use it or lose it' attitude espoused by Cicero. Similar encouragement can be taken from a study by Shimamura and associates (1995) of aging university professors; these individuals appeared to retain the ability to analyze and recall new factual information related to their professional fields better than younger subjects without their formal training, though the professors fared worse than young controls on unrelated items. Oliver Sacks (1997) reminds us of the accomplishments of aged professionals such as Erik Erikson, Grandma Moses, and the neurologist MacDonald Critchley, who died aged 97 while still actively writing.

Katzman and Terry (1983) reviewed several longitudinal studies that showed little decline over long periods of time in tests of vocabulary, verbal abilities, language comprehension, and judgment. Performance on measures dependent on speed of response, on the other hand, show a more rapid decline with age. Memory tests show less decline with age if meaningful concepts are presented for memory, as opposed to rote items.

The loss of short-term memory with normal aging, considered a normal phenomenon, borders on the abnormal syndrome of 'mild cognitive impairment' (see below). The baby boomer syndromes of 'post-it note dependency' and 'lost-car-in-the-parking-lot' probably belong within the category of normal aging.

Mild Cognitive Impairment

Intermediate between normal aging and dementia is a group of patients with minor memory loss; this group has been referred to under various terms including 'benign senescent forgetfulness' (Kral 1962), 'mild cognitive impairment' (Petersen *et al.* 1999), or 'age associated memory impairment' (Hanninen and Soininen 1997). Many patients with mild cognitive impairment (MCI) remain relatively stable over periods of several years. A small percentage develop dementia each year, more than the incidence of a normal elderly group (Cullum and Rosenberg 1998; Petersen *et al.* 1999; Ritchie *et al.* 2001). The category of mild cognitive impairment thus appears to include both patients with static mild memory loss associated with aging and patients with the earliest stage of dementia or Alzheimer's disease; controversy continues as to whether most or all patients with MCI will eventually develop Alzheimer's disease. At present, it is not possible to distinguish MCI from early AD with certainty by clinical or behavioral methods (Petersen *et al.* 2001). One recent study (Chen *et al.* 2000) found that delayed word recall and performance of the Trails B test of the Halstead – Reitan battery distinguished normal controls from elderly subjects who developed Alzheimer's disease during a follow-up period. This study did not include specific reference to patients who showed memory deficits but did not develop dementia. A recent autopsy study found no evidence by neuropsychological testing of detectable cognitive dysfunction in a group of patients with pathological changes of preclinical Alzheimer's disease (Goldman *et al.* 2001).

The relationship of MCI to the normal memory loss of aging is problematic. Patients should not receive the diagnosis of MCI unless they fall below age-related norms for memory. Many later develop dementia, perhaps related to the rates of deterioration of individual patients. Morris and colleagues (2001) have stated their belief that most cases of MCI actually have early-stage Alzheimer's disease.

DEMENTIA

Dementia is defined as a deterioration of previously intact intellectual function caused by diffuse disease of the cerebral hemispheres (Wells 1977). This definition implies three important prerequisites: (1) the prior attainment of normal cognitive functions (excluding mental retardation or developmental cognitive disorders); (2) dysfunction of multiple higher cortical functions localized to different areas of the brain; and (3) evidence of organic brain disease rather than a primary psychogenic or affective disorder. Some definitions of dementia also require a progressive course, as is usually seen in neurodegenerative diseases such as Alzheimer's disease and even in many vascular causes of dementia. Severe traumatic brain injury, hypoxemic encephalopathy after cardiac arrest, or deficits resulting from major strokes may rob a patient of mental faculties, yet the course may be relatively static. The distinction of these cases from dementia is artificial and of questionable usefulness. The first goal of diagnosis of dementing illnesses, of course, is the identification of treatable causes of dementia.

Unlike the focal neurobehavioral syndromes discussed in earlier chapters of this book, dementia is a multifocal or diffuse process. Instead of localizing a lesion, the bedside examination serves to document the multiplicity of the deficits, not localized to any single brain region. Although dementing diseases differ from one another, some general patterns of behavioral deficits hold true regardless of etiology. Forgetfulness is often the earliest symptom, made manifest in the clinical examination when the patient turns to a spouse or relative for answers to questions. The patient refers to notes, asks frequently for reminders, and tells the same stories over and over. Language and communication are more or less intact at this early stage, except for memory for names (Appell. 1982; Kirshner et al. 1984a). Mood may be normal or depressed, and the patient often has enough insight to be troubled and to attempt to hide the deficit. The patient may perform other cognitive functions at a relatively normal level, except that most tasks are performed slowly. As mentioned earlier, it is difficult to distinguish the patient with early dementia secondary to Alzheimer's disease from the normal aging patient with mild memory loss or MCI. One of the traditional hallmarks of dementia is the loss of self-awareness of deficit. One recent study (Lopez et al. 1994) found considerable variability of awareness of deficit in 181 patients with presumed Alzheimer's disease. In general, unawareness of deficit correlated with the severity of the cognitive deficits themselves; i.e., the more the patient becomes demented, the less aware he or she is of the cognitive loss. On the other hand, awareness of deficit had a poor correlation with depression.

Later in the progression of dementia, the presence of diffuse disease becomes evident. Memory loss becomes more severe, to the point of disorientation to time and place. Forgetfulness takes more malignant forms, such as misplacing important items, leaving stove burners on, and forgetting frequently traveled routes. Other cortical functions are more definitely affected, and syndromes of aphasia, agnosia, and visuospatial impairment develop. Occasionally, apparently isolated syndromes of aphasia (Mesulam et al. 1982; Kirshner et al. 1984b, 1987) or constructional apraxia (Crystal et al. 1982) may be the presenting symptoms of what later proves to be a progressive illness, but usually the impairments are multiple from the beginning.

Language and communication are abnormal in a majority of patients with dementia (Sim and Sussman 1962; Ferm 1974; Sjogren *et al.* 1974). Speech and voice characteristics change with aging; Shakespeare depicted alterations in voice and in articulation in the 'seven ages of man' oration from *As You Like It*: 'and his manly voice turning again toward childish treble pipes, and whistles in his sound.' Early on, naming is the most sensitive language function, and the patient fails to recall proper names and names of uncommon objects. Generic names or generic words like 'thing' replace specific names. The novelist Mordechai Richler created dialogue by a character with early dementia, epitomizing the anomia: 'that city in Germany where Hitler led the march on Parliament. You know, the British prime minister with the umbrella was there. Peace in our time is what he promised. Damn damn damn. It's the city where they have the famous beer festival. Pilsner? Molson's? No. It sounds like the name of the little people in *The Wizard of Oz*. Or like that painting *The Shout* [*The Scream*] by . . . by Munch Munich' (Richler 1998). As dementia progresses, utterances become devoid of abstract content and impoverished of vocabulary (Critchley 1964; Appell *et al.* 1982). The mechanics of speech, such as utterances of phonemes, repetition, and reading aloud tend to be preserved. In general, reading comprehension and written expression deteriorate more rapidly than auditory comprehension and speech (Albert 1980; Appell *et al.* 1982; Kirshner 1982). Although the grammatical construction of language remains intact, meaningful communication is greatly reduced; in the words of Schwartz *et al.* (1977), 'the instrumentalities of language can remain intact, though no longer in the service of cognition'.

Calculations, praxis, and visuospatial – constructional tasks also deteriorate in most patients with dementia. The patient may easily become lost in familiar surroundings. Insight and judgment are usually impaired at this stage, and mood shows labile fluctuations from elation to tearfulness to anger, without the normal inhibitions of a healthy cerebrum (Kirshner 1982). Some patients can still mask their deficits to some extent with social graces and 'cocktail party' conversation, but any discussion of factual information quickly reveals the extent of the intellectual deterioration.

Behavior also changes in the course of dementing illnesses. Some patients have episodic confusion, with hallucinations, delusional or paranoid thinking, and agitation (Cohen *et al.* 1993). A recent survey found hallucinations and delusions in 20% of diagnosed AD patients at 1 year, increasing to over 50% at 4 years (Paulsen *et al.* 2000). These symptoms correlated both with cognitive loss and with Parkinsonian motor signs. Behavioral symptoms are among the most troublesome aspects of dementing illness for caregivers and family members. Along with physical symptoms such as urinary and fecal incontinence, these are the leading reasons for admission to a chronic care facility (Steele *et al.* 1990).

In the last stages of dementia, patients become less spontaneous, speaking only in answer to questions or to express immediate biological needs. They become incapable of dressing themselves, feeding themselves, or taking care of personal hygiene and toileting. Mood changes become blunted, with an overall apathetic affect. Such patients require custodial care and are susceptible to such secondary medical complications as pneumonia, urinary tract infections, and decubitus ulcers. These are the immediate causes of death in demented patients, but the stage is already set by the dementia itself.

These 'stages' of dementia, while discussed by many authors, are in truth oversimplifications of a group of disorders with complex and variable symptoms. Indeed, the richness of the behavioral and cognitive manifestations of dementia parallel the richness and complexity of the human nervous system itself. Although memory loss is usually the first stage in a dementing illness, occasional patients present with psychiatric symptoms such as hallucinations, agitation, or paranoia; others present with focal language disorder; still others with topographical disorientation, becoming lost easily in familiar routes. Part of the variability is masked by the specialties of the physicians who see the patient; those patients with behavior problems go first to psychiatrists, while those with memory or language disorders are likely to see neurologists.

DISTINGUISHING DEMENTIA FROM OTHER DISORDERS

In addition to the documentation of a multifocal cerebral abnormality on the bedside examination, the behavioral neurologist must distinguish dementia from other conditions that present features suggestive of diffuse dysfunctions. These are: (1) affective disorder or 'pseudodementia'; (2) acute encephalopathy or delirium; and (3) cortical dysfunction related to a focal lesion.

Depression and 'pseudodementia'

Since Kiloh's initial report on 'pseudodementia'(Kiloh 1961), clinicians have been concerned by the apparent memory and cognitive deficits of elderly patients with depression. The pendulum has shifted somewhat, however, from a consideration of depression mimicking dementia to one of depression as a contributing factor to the cognitive impairment of dementia.

Wells (1979) presented the clinical features of depressive cognitive impairment in ten carefully studied clinical cases. The general findings were: (1) complaints of both recent memory loss and more global cognitive difficulty occur in depression and other psychiatric disorders; (2) the resemblance of these syndromes to dementia may be close; and (3) improvement is possible with treatment of the psychiatric disorder. Wells provided a number of helpful bedside techniques for distinguishing depressed from demented patients. Features suggestive of pseudodementia include recent or abrupt onset, history of previous psychiatric disease, and complaints by patients themselves, rather than by the family, of memory loss. On bedside testing, patients highlight their disabilities and frequently give 'I don't know' responses to questions. Overall, the behavioral performance is variable, with areas of very high level functioning, generally not in keeping with the level of subjective complaints. Most importantly, the patients' affect is depressed, with considerable and consistent expression of distress. Weight loss, anorexia, and insomnia frequently accompany depression. In contrast, demented patients usually have a gradual onset of disability, complained of more by the family than by the patient. The patient cooperates with testing, with consistently deficient performance. 'Near-miss' answers are more typical than 'I don't know' responses. The affect is more often labile than consistently depressed. Nocturnal worsening of the cognitive dysfunction ('sundowning') is also typical (Wells 1979).

The concept of pseudodementia has been largely abandoned, for several reasons. First, the term 'pseudo' implies that there is no genuine cognitive dysfunction, whereas depression clearly interferes with intellectual performance. New learning and memory, particularly immediate memory, are especially sensitive to depression (Sternberg and Jarvik 1976). 'Depression-induced organic mental disorder' may be a better term for this syndrome (McAllister 1983). Second, depressed patients with pseudodementia are usually elderly, and hence some degree of organic dementia may coexist with a reversible decline brought on by depression. On the other hand, patients with primary dementia may be appropriately depressed. Patients with such combined disorders have been reported in whom treatment of depression improved cognitive function, though not to normal levels (Shraberg 1978; Snow and Wells 1981). The important issue in such patients is thus not whether the diagnosis is depression or dementia, but whether or not depression is producing a further treatable deterioration of an already abnormal mental status (Jones and Reifler 1994). Such judgments can be made only by careful clinical observation, and sometimes by trials with antidepressant therapy. Neurodiagnostic tests do not provide simple answers. Computed tomography (CT) scans, for example, may show brain atrophy even in elderly patients who are not demented (Wells and Duncan 1977). If the clinician is in doubt, empiric treatment for depressed mood is warranted in elderly patients with cognitive impairment.

Delirium

Delirium, or acute encephalopathy, is difficult to distinguish from dementia. Chapter 14 explores delirium further. Usually the time course of delirium is much shorter and the onset more abrupt than dementia. Clouding of consciousness, varying from lethargy to stupor, is much more common than in dementia, in which the patient usually appears alert. Excitement, restlessness, and hypomanic behavior are also more common in delirium. Finally, most causes of delirium also produce autonomic nervous system hyperactivity; such signs as sweating, tremor, tachycardia, flushing, and fever are more common in delirium than dementia. In the terminology of the nineteenth-century neurologist Hughlings Jackson, 'positive' neurological phenomena are the hallmark of delirium, whereas the 'negative' phenomena of loss of intellect and judgment are more typical of dementia but apply to both conditions. Considerable overlap occurs between dementia and delirium; in doubtful cases, etiologies of both disorders should be considered.

Focal Brain Lesion

The third pitfall in the diagnosis of dementia is the misinterpretation of a focal neurological deficit as a more diffuse disorder. Focal mass lesions such as brain tumors or subdural hematomas may produce apparently diffuse syndromes because of raised intracranial pressure and compression of normal brain structures. Lesions associated with edema or hydrocephalus can be especially troublesome to localize. Benign mass lesions such as meningiomas, subdural hematomas, and colloid cysts of the third ventricle are important 'treatable causes' of dementia. Meningiomas of the falx, sphenoid bone, or olfactory groove may present with frontal lobe syndromes and dementia; absence of the sense of smell in one nostril may be a telltale sign. Subdural hematoma should be considered whenever an elderly patient has an abrupt deterioration of mental status, often engrafted on a pre-existing but well-compensated dementia. The history of a head injury or fall may not be forthcoming from the patient at diagnosis. Tumors such as colloid cysts, which present largely via hydrocephalus, may be difficult to distinguish from idiopathic or 'normal pressure hydrocephalus,' to be discussed later.

Aphasia secondary to focal lesions of the left hemisphere may pose a special problem in the differential diagnosis of dementia. Aphasia renders the testing of other cortical functions difficult, and a diagnosis of diffuse dementia may erroneously be made. Lesions of the left angular gyrus, as discussed in Chapter 6, can produce a syndrome of multiple deficits, including fluent aphasia, alexia, agraphia, calculation disturbance, and constructional apraxia; the resemblance to dementia may be very close (Benson *et al.* 1982). As mentioned earlier, some dementing illnesses also begin as apparently focal syndromes of aphasia, agnosia, or constructional apraxia. Whenever a patient's examination findings suggest a single focal abnormality as the predominant deficit, brain imaging is essential to exclude a potentially treatable focal lesion.

DIFFERENTIAL DIAGNOSIS OF DEMENTIA

Once the diagnosis of dementia is established, the specific disease process must be sought. As in other neurobehavioral syndromes, associated neurological signs are frequently helpful in pointing to a specific diagnosis, as are symptoms and signs of disease in other organs of the body. We divide dementing diseases into three categories: (1) dementias secondary to medical illness; (2) primary neurological diseases involving both the cerebral cortex and other neurological systems; and (3) primary dementias with signs largely restricted to the higher functions. A distinction between 'treatable' and 'non-treatable' causes of dementia should also be kept in mind. Most but not all of the treatable dementias are in the first category. Laboratory tests are frequently necessary to arrive at a specific diagnosis. After discussion of the specific dementing diseases, we shall present a battery of tests useful in the diagnosis of dementia.

DEMENTIAS SECONDARY TO MEDICAL DISEASES

Many systemic diseases affect the brain in diffuse or multifocal patterns, and classification of these diseases comprises most of the categories of systemic disease. Many of these disorders present as acute confusional states rather than as dementias, depending on the timing of neurological involvement. In slowly developing syndromes, a picture of typical dementia, described earlier in this chapter, may be closely followed.

Specific systemic diseases producing dementia are too numerous to discuss with more than brief comments. Table 13.1 lists some of the more common medical causes of dementia.

Table 13.1   Medical diseases associated with dementia

1. Metabolic, nutritional, endocrine, toxic disorders
   a. Metabolic disorders
      1. Hyponatremia, hypocalcemia
      2. Renal, hepatic, pulmonary failure, dialysis dementia
   b. Nutritional disorders (pernicious anemia, pellagra, thiamine deficiency)
   c. Endocrinopathies (hypothyroidism, hyperthyroidism, Hashimoto's encephalopathy, Cushing's, hyperparathyroidism)
   d. Toxic disorders
      - Heavy metals, chemicals
      - Drug encephalopathies
      - Polypharmacy
      - Alcoholism
      - Marchiafava – Bignami syndrome

2. Infections
   a. Neurosyphilis
   b. Chronic meningitis (Listeria, fungi, brucellosis, tuberculosis, sarcoid)
   c. Cysticercosis, other parasitic diseases
   d. Viral encephalitis
   e. Subacute sclerosing panencephalitis (SSPE)
   f. Progressive multifocal leukoencephalopathy (PML)
   g. Creutzfeldt–Jakob disease
   h. Adult immunodeficiency syndrome (AIDS)

3. Vascular diseases
   a. Multiinfarct dementia (large infarcts, lacunar state)
   b. Binswanger's disease
   c. Cholesterol emboli
   d. Collagen vascular diseases
   e. Arteriovenous malformation
   f. Subacute diencephalic angioencephalopathy

4. Neoplasms
   a. Mass lesions, increased intracranial pressure, hydrocephalus
   b. Multiple metastases
   c. Meningeal carcinomatosis
   d. Chemotherapy, radiation effects
   e. Limbic encephalitis

Metabolic, Nutritional, Endocrine, and Toxic Disorders

Metabolic disturbances associated with mental deterioration include electrolyte disturbances (particularly hyponatremia), hypo- and hypercalcemia, and organ failure syndromes (hepatic, renal, and pulmonary). In most instances these produce acute encephalopathy or delirium (see Chapter 14).

One interesting metabolic dementia that has already come and gone is dialysis dementia, or Alfrey's syndrome. This unique disorder of modern medical treatment was first described during the 1970s in chronic hemodialysis patients (Alfrey *et al.* 1976). The disease begins with stuttering, dysarthria, muteness, and myoclonic jerking. These symptoms occur transiently at first, after each dialysis, but then become chronic and progressive. The speech abnormality includes not only a motor speech disorder but also syllable substitutions and aphasic deficits (Madison *et al.* 1977). Confusion, dementia, and seizures ensue, usually progressing to death within weeks to months (Lederman *et al.* 1978; Dewberry *et al.* 1980). Intermittent, rhythmic frontal slow wave activity and spike or sharp wave discharges are characteristically seen on electroencephalography (EEG), but other neurodiagnostic tests are unrevealing. Although most cases occur in association with dialysis, the syndrome has occasionally developed in chronic renal failure without dialysis and even after renal transplantation (Madison *et al.* 1977). Increased aluminum levels have been reported in brain tissue (Alfrey *et al.* 1976); in most centers the use of deionized water has resulted in disappearance of the syndrome (Rozas *et al.* 1978). Occasional syndromes of confusion and memory loss, without the full-blown picture of dialysis dementia, have continued to appear despite removal of aluminum from the water and aluminum-containing antacids from the diet (Dewberry *et al.* 1980; Harrington *et al.* 1994). Once developed, dialysis dementia is a progressive and largely untreatable illness.

Of the nutritional disorders, vitamin deficiencies still rank as important treatable causes of dementia. Vitamin B12 deficiency, or pernicious anemia, frequently produces mental changes that can include predominant mood changes ('megaloblastic madness'; Smith 1960), confusion, or dementia. The neurological signs of subacute combined systems degeneration, including posterior column, lateral corticospinal tract, and peripheral nerve degeneration, may develop before or after the mental changes. Anemia may be absent in early stages; the diagnosis can then be made by macrocytic changes in the peripheral blood smear, high mean corpuscular volumes, low vitamin B12 serum levels, and reduced B12 absorption on the Schilling test. Vitamin B12 injections can be curative. Pellagra, a vitamin deficiency associated with rash and diarrhea, was a common cause of dementia in the past, though it is rarely diagnosed today. Vitamin B1 (thiamine) deficiency produces the Wernicke – Korsakoff syndrome. As discussed in Chapter 11, this syndrome is more properly classified as a focal amnestic syndrome than as a dementia.

Endocrine causes of dementia include thyroid, adrenal, and parathyroid disorders. Hypothyroidism is the most common such disorder, characteristically producing slowing of mentation, which may progress to frank dementia. Neurological signs of hypothyroidism are extremely variable, and may include weakness, myopathy, delayed rebound of reflexes, peripheral neuropathy, and ataxia (Swanson *et al*. 1981). Because thyroxine levels are often in the lower range of normal in elderly patients, the presence of an elevated thyroid-stimulating hormone (TSH) level may be needed to confirm the diagnosis. Hyperthyroidism may also produce mental changes in the elderly, often without the tachycardia, tremor, and excitation seen in younger patients ('apathetic hyperthyroidism').

The syndrome of Hashimoto's encephalopathy involves confusion, memory loss, seizures, and mood changes, occurring in patients with a history of hypothyroidism but not correlating well with the degree of endocrine dysfunction (Shaw *et al*. 1991; Seipelt *et al*. 1999). The syndrome appears to be mediated by anti-thyroid antibodies, and the dementia or confusional state may improve with corticosteroid therapy. This syndrome is probably underdiagnosed and definitely treatable, though in the author's experience very high doses of steroids may be required.

Cushing's disease, or excessive production of adrenal corticosteroids, may be associated with mental changes (Starkman and Schteingart 1981). Hyperparathyroidism may produce a variety of neurological and mental disturbances, including fatigue and cognitive deficits (Cogan *et al*. 1978).

Toxic causes of dementia are of obvious importance to the prevention and treatment of dementia. Heavy metal poisoning, especially with lead and other environmental toxins, is often sought but rarely discovered as a cause of dementia in adults, except when exposures are known to have occurred. Much more common are toxic effects of medications. A few specific drugs cause encephalopathies that, with chronic use, can resemble dementia. Alpha-methyldopa (Aldomet, an antihypertensive), cimetidine (Tagamet, a histamine blocker), and anticholinergic drugs can all cause reversible mental changes. Anticholinergic drugs are omnipresent in modern medical care; they include over-the-counter sleep medications, antispasmodics for abdominal pain or neurogenic bladder, antivertigo drugs such as scopolamine, tricyclic antidepressants, and antipsychotics such as phenothiazines or haloperidol. Psychiatric patients who are confused, moreover, may be treated with increased antipsychotics, only to become more confused. One patient referred for hallucinations complicating Parkinson's disease was taking trihexyphenidyl (Artane) for tremor, haloperidol (Haldol) for confusion, oxybutynin (Ditropan) for incontinence, and nortriptyline (Pamelor) for depression, all of which share anticholinergic properties. Discontinuation of all medications resulted in complete resolution of the confusion. Another common cause of a dementia-like picture is 'polypharmacy'. An elderly patient may seek a sleeping pill from one physician, an analgesic from another, a tranquilizer from a third, and then treatment for hypertension from yet another. The individual physicians prescribe rationally and in good faith but are ignorant of each other's ministrations. The combined effects of all of these drugs may produce profound mental slowing. In one series of dementia cases, polypharmacy ranked as one of the most frequent treatable causes of dementia (Freemon 1976). Elderly patients are more sensitive to medications than younger ones, and patients with mild cognitive loss may deteriorate dramatically under the effect of even a single drug. This same 'sensitivity' of the nervous system in mildly demented patients underlies the familiar decompensations that occur in response to fever, infection, or even the change to an unfamiliar environment.

Alcoholic dementia is a controversial subcategory of toxic dementia. The Wernicke–Korsakoff amnestic syndrome, as discussed in Chapter 11, is not a true dementia, but rather a focal, amnestic syndrome. Wernicke–Korsakoff syndrome is caused by thiamine deficiency rather than by toxic effects of alcohol. Chronic alcoholics, however, frequently have generalized neuropsychological deficits not limited to memory (Ron 1977), and CT scans of alcoholic patients frequently demonstrate cortical atrophy (Carlen et al. 1981). The existence of alcoholic dementia is clear not only from research studies but also from everyday clinical experience. The causative factors, however, may be multiple, including nutritional deficiencies, incidental head trauma, chronic psychiatric illness, and other substance abuse in addition to the toxic effects of alcohol itself.

One additional disease, the Marchiafava–Bignami syndrome, is considered a toxic or nutritional deficiency disease, though the pathogenesis is unknown. This rare disorder, reported most commonly in Italian red wine drinkers, involves necrosis of white matter pathways, particularly the rostral corpus callosum (Ironside et al. 1961). Mental deterioration is prominent, with associated frontal lobe signs and gait disorder. According to one report, a callosal disconnection syndrome may be found, with apraxia and agraphia of the left arm and anomia for items presented in the left visual field or by touch to the left limbs (Barbizet et al. 1978). The disease is not well characterized clinically, and is usually diagnosed only at autopsy.

Infectious Dementias

Infectious diseases associated with dementia include neurosyphilis, chronic meningitis, parasitic infestations, and encephalitis. During the nineteenth century, neurosyphilis was one of the most common causes of both psychosis and dementia. General paresis, a form of tertiary syphilis associated with diffuse pathology of the cerebral cortex, produced generalized cognitive loss and affective changes, often including an inappropriate euphoria suggestive of frontal lobe disease. The disease also mimics functional psychoses. The advent of penicillin resulted in treatment of most cases of syphilis prior to neurological involvement, but the disease is making a comeback in the age of AIDS and venereal diseases. Whereas one survey suggested that the currently appearing forms of neurosyphilis were all reported during the pre-antibiotic era (Luxon et al. 1979), another reported non-classical, less obvious presentations of the disease, perhaps because of the omnipresent use of antibiotics that may modify the infection but not cure it (Hooshmand et al. 1972). The disease is still encountered, in both HIV-positive and HIV-negative patients (Russouw et al. 1997). In HIV-positive patients, syphilis can also take atypical forms or have a more accelerated course from primary to tertiary stages (Johns *et al.* 1987). Another spirochetal disease, Lyme borreliosis, has also been reported to result in late dementia, though milder degrees of memory loss are more common (Gaudino *et al.* 1997).

In the current era, infection with the human immunodeficiency virus (HIV) has become the leading infectious cause of dementia. This dementia, called the 'AIDS dementia complex', is often listed with 'subcortical dementias' because of the prominent mental slowing, rather than complete loss of cognitive function. Short-term memory difficulty, difficulty with attention and concentration, and inability to read often make up the early symptoms; later in the course, impaired balance and other focal signs can develop. Behavioral changes such as apathy and social withdrawal tend to be prominent in AIDS dementia complex, though they are often misdiagnosed as depression; occasionally, frank mood changes such as depression or mania can be present (Simpson and Berger 1996; Bouwman *et al.* 1998). Late in the course, profoundly reduced behavior with psychomotor retardation and obvious neurological problems such as paraparesis, seizures, and tremor make the diagnosis more obvious (Simpson and Berger 1996). Most patients have already experienced AIDS-defining infectious illnesses by the time they develop dementia, though occasional patients present with neurological symptoms and signs. Even asymptomatic HIV-positive patients may have subtle neuropsychological deficits (Maj *et al.* 1994). White matter changes predominate on MRI scans, though deep atrophy and ventricular enlargement develop over time. The exact pathophysiology is unclear; HIV-infected mononuclear cells can be found in the brain, but the virus does not appear to infect neurons directly (Simpson and Berger 1996). The CSF may contain oligoclonal bands. Antiretroviral drugs may slow the progression of the dementia or even bring about improvement. Recognition of the AIDS dementia complex is therefore of clinical importance.

Among meningeal infections, the chronic fungal, tuberculous, or parasitic forms are the most likely to result in dementia. Bacterial meningitis is usually an acute, fulminating infection characterized by high fever, stiff neck, severe headache, delirium, and then stupor or coma. Patients with partial or delayed treatment may suffer enough cerebral damage to result in dementia. Occasional cases of meningitis secondary to the bacterium *Listeria monocytogenes* are associated with an insidious, subacute mental decline. Hydrocephalus after meningitis of any cause may also cause delayed mental deterioration.

A rare, bacterial cause of dementia is Whipple's disease, a disorder of mental changes and ataxia or ocular palsies, often in association with a malabsorption syndrome. Bacillus-like organisms are found in jejunal biopsies. Antibiotic treatment may be effective in reversing the neurological symptoms (Singer 1998).

Fungal meningitis secondary to Cryptococcus, Coccidioides, Candida, histoplasmosis, or blastomycosis may be indolent over months or even years, with chronic headaches and mental changes as the predominant symptoms (Lewis and Rabinovich 1972; Ellner and Bennett 1976; Bonza *et al.* 1981). Brucellosis (Larbrisseau *et al.* 1978), tuberculosis (Kennedy and Fallon 1979), and sarcoidosis (Delaney 1977) may also be associated with chronic meningitis. The parasitic disease cysticercosis, related to the pork tapeworm, is an increasingly common cause of multifocal cystic cerebral lesions, particularly in developing countries (McCormick *et al.* 1982). In all of these diseases except cysticercosis, a lumbar puncture is essential for diagnosis. Certainly any demented patient with a history of fever, nuchal rigidity, chronic headaches, or weight loss should have a lumbar puncture as part of the diagnostic evaluation.

Viral encephalitis typically causes acute encephalopathy, headache, fever, seizures, and then stupor or coma. In herpes simplex encephalitis, aphasia is often a prominent finding. Patients who survive the acute illness may be left with permanent intellectual changes amounting to a non-progressive dementia (Hierons *et al.* 1978).

Two other viral causes of dementia are subacute sclerosing panencephalitis (SSPE) and progressive multifocal leukoencephalopathy (PML). The first, a chronic measles encephalitis with immunological inflammatory changes, presents in children or adolescents as a progressive, fatal dementia with seizures and myoclonus (Freeman 1969; Ter Muelen 1973). Its incidence has declined drastically since the introduction of the measles vaccine. The second, PML, is a white matter disease usually developing in patients with lymphoma or other causes of immunological compromise, including AIDS. The disease is associated with multiple areas of white matter demyelination, usually accompanied by obvious neurological signs. It typically progresses to death within several months (Richardson 1961; Narayam *et al.* 1973).

Creutzfeldt–Jakob Disease

One dementia recently moved from the idiopathic to the infectious category is Creutzfeldt–Jakob disease, or spongiform degeneration of the brain. This disease is characterized by a rapidly progressive dementia, often proceeding from first symptoms to death within several months. Myoclonus and an exaggerated startle response are characteristic clinical features (Johnson and Gibbs 1998). The disease occurs at about one case per million per year throughout the world. Most cases are sporadic, though familial forms have also been documented. Numerous clinical variants have been described, including the Heidenhain form with cortical blindness mentioned in Chapter 8. Patients may present with mood changes, memory loss, confusional states, seizures, or even vertigo and ataxia. The disease progresses rapidly, usually over a period of months. Laboratory tests such as CT scanning and standard cerebrospinal fluid (CSF) studies are normal in early stages. Recently, a 14-3-3 protein has been detected in CSF from patients with CJD (Hsich *et al.* 1996; Aksamit *et al.* 2001). The EEG may show periodic spike discharges with suppression of activity between them, though epileptiform discharges are not present in every case or at every stage of the disease.

Pathological specimens from brain biopsy or autopsy show a spongiform change, vacuolation of the cerebral cortex, with loss of neurons and gliosis but no signs of inflammation. These changes are very similar to the disease *kuru*, seen in the Fore tribe of New Guinea, and scrapie, a disease of sheep. The infectious nature of Creutzfeldt–Jakob disease and *kuru* was demonstrated by the pioneering studies of Gajdusek and Gibbs, who successfully transmitted the diseases to chimpanzees by direct intracerebral inoculation of brain tissue from patients (Gajdusek *et al*. 1966). The long latent period for transmission of these spongiform diseases has given rise to the term 'slow virus' encephalopathy. The disease *kuru* was transmitted on New Guinea by ritual cannabalism of deceased family members. In the Western world, transmission of slow virus diseases has occurred with corneal transplants, pituitary extracts used for human growth hormone injections, and depth electrodes (Alter 2000).

The infectious agents that cause the spongiform encephalopathies are not conventional viruses; among their unique properties are passage through the smallest filters, lack of visualization by electron microscopy, and insensitivity to heat, formaldehyde, and agents that destroy nucleic acids (Prusiner 1982). These facts have led to great fear, verging on hysteria, regarding the contagious risk of Creutzfeldt–Jakob disease. In laboratory experiments, however, the disease can be transmitted only by direct tissue inoculation, and the clinical risk of contagion appears small from epidemiological studies (Masters *et al*. 1979; Alter 2000). Furthermore, the agent can readily be inactivated by sodium hypochlorite (ordinary household bleach), autoclaving at 120 °C, and several other chemicals that denature proteins (Brown *et al*. 1982). Scientific interest has focused on this infectious agent because of its very small estimated size, its proteinaceous nature, and the possibility that it replicates without use of nucleic acid, a mechanism unprecedented in biology. Prusiner (1991) has extended the characterization of the infectious particles, proteins that he has called 'prions', or proteinaceous infectious particles. The prion protein itself is called PrP. A naturally occurring protein, PrP^c, is somehow converted to a pathogenetic variant, PrP^{sc}. How this occurs in spontaneously occurring cases of CJD is not known (Alter 2000).

Recently, spongiform encephalopathy has resurfaced in the United Kingdom as bovine spongiform encephalopathy (BSE) or 'mad cow disease', presumably transmitted via infected beef cattle (Anderson *et al*. 1996; Tan *et al*. 1999). Cases in cattle have recently been reported in France. A possible linkage of this disease to 'atypical' cases of Creutzfeldt–Jakob disease has been a major cause of concern in the UK and Europe.

The exciting discoveries about Creutzfeldt–Jakob disease and prions created an expectation that these agents might be the cause of many neurodegenerative diseases. Attempts to find the prion protein in other dementias have failed (Brown *et al*. 1993). Thus far, only rare conditions seem related to this class of agents, and the scientists studying the diseases almost outnumber the patients who suffer from them. Creutzfeldt–Jakob disease, though rare, is dreaded as a rapidly progressive and untreatable dementia.

Vascular Diseases

Vascular diseases were at one time thought to represent the majority of dementia cases; early in the last century, senile dementia was commonly referred to as 'cerebral arteriosclerosis' or 'hardening of the arteries'. In the 1960s, the pendulum of thought about dementing illness shifted towards Alzheimer's disease as a primary neuronal degeneration, with little reference to vascular disease (Wells 1978); this thinking was predominant at the time of the first edition of this book. Over the past few years, the pendulum has shifted back towards vascular diseases as prominent causes of dementia. There are several reasons for this shift. First, in pathological series of dementia cases, vascular diseases are second only to Alzheimer's disease as causes of dementia, and many cases have both cerebral infarcts and changes of AD. Second, a variety of types of cerebrovascular disease, as we shall see, cause dementia. Third, Alzheimer's disease itself includes deposition of amyloid in cerebral vessels, and many patients show on MRI scan and at autopsy deep white-matter ischemic changes. Cerebral amyloidosis also results in brain hemorrhages (Greenberg 1998).

The subject of 'silent' small vessel strokes as a cause of memory and cognitive loss in the elderly has attracted recent attention. Patients with untreated or undertreated hypertension show evidence of cognitive decline even in middle age (Knopman *et al.* 2001). A recent somewhat controversial survey of MRI scans in older people suggested that although the incidence of clinical stroke is only 750,000 per year in the USA, the annual incidence of 'silent' small infarcts may be as high as 22 million (Leary and Saver 2001). The controversy surrounds the question of whether these small white-matter lesions on MRI are truly strokes, and whether they truly correlate with cognitive deterioration (see below, under Binswanger's disease). Preliminary evidence has suggested that cholesterol-lowering agents may prevent cognitive deterioration in older people. Jick and colleagues (2000), in a case–control study from Great Britain, found only 13 patients on 'statin' drugs among 284 newly diagnosed patients with dementia; the relative risk of developing dementia among current statin users was 0.29, a 71% risk reduction. These findings, of course, must be confirmed in a treatment trial before a conclusion can be drawn that cholesterol-lowering drugs prevent dementia. These topics highlight the importance of treatment of cerebrovascular risk factors in preventing both clinical strokes and 'silent strokes' with cognitive deterioration.

Vascular dementia has remained controversial because of differing criteria for diagnosis and the different types of vascular disease included under this category. Nyenhuis and Gorelick (1998) referred to vascular dementia as having 'a rich history, a confusing present, and an uncertain future'. Perhaps the best way to approach the topic is to consider the specific vascular causes of dementia (McPherson and Cummings 1996). Lumping these vascular diseases together under one rubric of 'multi-infarct dementia' only increases the diagnostic confusion.

Multiple, Large Infarcts

There are several distinct patterns of vascular dementia. First, patients with multiple strokes may develop a non-progressive dementia. Hachinski and colleagues (1974) drew attention to this entity under the term 'multi-infarct dementia'. Patients with several large strokes, of course, would be expected to become demented, depending on the location and amount of infarcted tissue. The diagnosis of dementia due to one or several large strokes is usually obvious from the history and the presence of focal neurological signs on examination. Even single strokes may cause confusion and apparent dementia, perhaps because elderly patients already have enough cerebral atrophy to be very susceptible to additional tissue loss. The correlation of single strokes with complex behavioral syndromes is the subject of much of this book. We shall not enumerate all of the syndromes of single strokes here, but left parietal strokes in the area of the angular gyrus may mimic dementia (Benson *et al.* 1982), right temporoparietal strokes may cause acute confusional states (see Chapter 9), and left frontal strokes cause apathy and apparent dementia (see Chapter 10), among others. Patients with strokes frequently become demented, either acutely, or over time (Tatemichi *et al.* 1990, 1994). Reduced cognitive function on bedside testing at the time of the stroke correlates best with the development of dementia, but the location of the stroke is also crucial (Tatemichi *et al.* 1994). In one large survey of 202 acute stroke patients (Henon *et al.* 1999), 24% of patients manifested confusional states. Predictors included pre-existing cognitive decline and other metabolic or infectious disorders. Pohjasvaara and colleagues (2000) analyzed 337 stroke patients and found evidence of dementia in 107 (31.8%), and dementia specifically related to stroke in 87 (25.8%). Volumes of infarcts, specific lesion localization in either superior middle cerebral artery territory or in the left hemisphere interrupting the thalamocortical connections, and left temporal atrophy were associated with increased risk of dementia. Of these factors, infarcts in the left corona radiata interrupting the thalamocortical connections appeared to be the most important factor. Occasionally, infarcts may occur in 'silent' areas of the brain, and the dementia may then be more insidious in its development. Coexistent brain atrophy on CT scan, was also associated with dementia in the series of stroke patients studied by Ladurner *et al.* (1982), suggesting that the combination of stroke and underlying brain degeneration such as Alzheimer's disease may account for many cases of dementia.

Lacunar State

Patients with chronic hypertension are at risk for the development of 'lacunar' strokes, small infarcts deep in the white matter of the cerebral hemispheres, the internal capsule, the basal ganglia, and the brainstem (Fisher 1965; Mohr 1982). These strokes are frequently multiple and in many cases 'silent', though usually there is some history of abrupt or stepwise changes in cognitive status and also in motor signs. By the time multiple lacunar infarcts have occurred (lacunar state, or état lacunaire), the neurological signs may be largely symmetrical, though abnormally increased reflexes, positive Babinski signs, spastic tone, pseudobulbar emotional lability (see Chapters 10, 17, and 21), and frontal release signs are common. The presence of hypertension should be a tip-off to this disorder. Even single lacunar strokes may occasionally cause detectable neuropsychological impairment (Van Zandvoort 2001).

CADASIL

A variant of lacunar state is the genetically inherited disease, CADASIL (Cerebral Autosomal Dominant Arteriopathy with Subcortical Infarcts and

Leukoencephalopathy) (Dichgans *et al.* 1998). Families with multiple members with migraine-like headaches, multiple small territory ischemic strokes, and dementia have been presented, though the reports have come largely from European countries. If CADASIL is as common in the USA as in Europe, then many cases go unrecognized.

Binswanger's Disease

Another variant of multi-infarct dementia is Binswanger's disease, or subcortical arteriosclerotic encephalopathy (Caplan and Schoene 1978; Babikian and Ropper 1987). This rather controversial disease is generally diagnosed in elderly patients with longstanding hypertension and a history of acute strokes. The composer Joseph Haydn may have suffered from Binswanger's disease (Bazner and Hennerici 1997). Examination reveals a non-specific combination of dementia and variable focal neurological signs. The CT scan reveals the identifying characteristic of this disease, showing hydrocephalus and apparent areas of tissue loss in the deep cerebral white matter, without obvious cortical infarcts. Magnetic resonance imaging shows similar areas of abnormal signal intensity in the periventricular white matter of many elderly patients (Bradley *et al.* 1984; Hachinski *et al.* 1987). The pathology of Binswanger's disease includes lacunar infarcts and areas of white matter demyelination with gliosis (Caplan and Schoene 1978). Vascular disease of the white matter secondary to hypertension is presumably the cause. The disease has remained controversial because these changes are often mixed with other vascular lesions and degenerative changes of late life.

Whereas Binswanger's disease has been a rare entity in pathological series, MRI findings of multiple deep white matter hyperintensities are common. Such lesions correlate with age and with vascular disease or hypertension (Awad *et al.* 1987; Hachinski *et al.* 1987). Some series have correlated such lesions with cognitive loss (Steingart *et al.* 1987a, 1987b; Bondareff *et al.* 1990), but others (Hershey *et al.* 1987; Rao *et al.* 1989) have not. A recent study (Moser *et al.* 2001) correlated subcortical hyperintensities on MRI with executive dysfunction. Kertesz and colleagues (1990) compared demented patients with and without periventricular hyperintensity lesions on MRI; those with the periventricular lesions were worse on tests of comprehension and attention, whereas those without the lesions were worse on memory and conceptualization tests. These findings may suggest that patients with pure AD have predominantly memory deficits, whereas vascular dementia patients have other cognitive deficits. Clearly, white matter hyperintensities do not always augur a poor cognitive prognosis; Fein and colleagues (1990) followed patients with severe 'ischemic white matter disease' or 'leukoaraiosis' who had stable cognitive function for several years (Fein *et al.* 1990). The diagnosis of Binswanger's disease should depend on typical clinical features, confirmed at autopsy, and not on MRI features alone (Hachinski *et al.* 1987).

Multiple Cholesterol Emboli

A number of less common vascular disorders can lead to dementia. Patients with advanced atherosclerosis of the great vessels may develop a syndrome of multiple organ involvement from cholesterol emboli. Confusion, transient ischemic attacks, strokes, slowly progressive renal failure, retinal emboli, and ischemia of the distal extremities ('blue toes') are the clinical signs (Beal *et al.* 1981). We encountered one patient in whom a progressive dementia and renal failure were the presenting symptoms of cholesterol embolization.

Sneddon's Syndrome

Sneddon's syndrome (Sneddon 1965) is a combination of multiple ischemic strokes and livedo reticularis. Some but not all cases have had associated anti-cardiolipin antibodies. Wright and Kokmen (1999) reported a 37-year-old male with progressive dementia and livedo reticularis. There was no clinical history of strokes, but imaging studies revealed multiple cortical and white matter infarcts. Anticardiolipin antibody studies were negative.

Collagen Vascular Diseases and Vasculitis

Another relatively uncommon category of dementias related to vascular disease is the family of collagen vascular diseases, many of which produce neurological damage by vascular inflammation, or vasculitis. Most vasculitic illnesses involve inflammation in vessels not only in the brain, but in other organs as well. The neurological syndromes include confusional states, psychosis, affective disorders, seizures, and focal stroke syndromes (Fieschi *et al.* 1998; Moore and Richardson 1998). Some patients may become demented after repeated attacks. The most common collagen vascular disease associated with dementia is systemic lupus erythematosis, which frequently causes neurological symptoms such as psychosis, seizures, stroke-like episodes, and occasionally dementia (Johnson and Richardson 1968; Bluestein 1987; Kirk *et al.* 1991). Only a minority of patients with CNS lupus actually have vasculitis. Antiphospholipid antibodies and non-bacterial endocarditis may underlie the stroke symptoms, and direct immunological attack on the nervous system may produce the psychosis and seizures. Antibodies to ribosomal P protein may be associated with CNS lupus (Bonfa *et al.* 1987).

Other similar diseases include Churg–Strauss vasculitis with eosinophilia (Sehgal *et al.* 1995), mixed connective tissue disease (Bennett *et al.* 1978), periarteritis nodosa (Ford and Sickert 1965), Wegener's granulomatosis (Drachman 1963), Sjogren's syndrome (Mauch *et al.* 1994); giant cell or temporal arteritis (Hollenhorst *et al.* 1960; Cochran *et al.* 1978; Caselli *et al.* 1988), Susac's syndrome (a triad of central nervous system vasculitis, deafness, and retinal infarcts; Susac 1994), and thrombotic thrombocytopenic purpura (TTP) (Lian 1988; Schmidt 1989). These diseases are diagnosed by elevated erythrocyte sedimentation rates and abnormal antibody tests such as ANA, anti-DNA and ANCA (Fieschi *et al.* 1998).

The most difficult diagnosis of all the vasculitic illnesses is the syndrome of isolated cerebral vasculitis, also called granulomatous angiitis (Kolodny *et al.* 1968; Moore and Cupps 1983; Moore 1989). This disease produces multifocal small infarctions in the brain, usually with small lesions on MRI and inflammatory changes in the CSF such as pleocytosis and elevated protein. Systemic antibody tests are typically negative, and diagnosis requires arteriography and, often, brain biopsy. Treatment with corticosteroids and immunosuppressive therapy appears to help in many cases (Moore and Cupps 1983).

Arteriovenous Malformations
Arteriovenous malformations usually present with either bleeding or epileptic seizures. Rarely, an AVM can present with dementia. These lesions may produce cerebral symptoms by mass effect, hemorrhage, production of seizures, and 'stealing' blood from adjacent tissue (Perrett and Nishioka 1966).

Subacute Diencephalic Angioencephalopathy
A final, exceedingly rare, vascular disease associated with dementia is subacute diencephalic angioencephalopathy. This disease, characterized by rapidly progressive memory loss, emotional changes, dementia, and myoclonus, bears a clinical resemblance to Creutzfeldt–Jakob disease. Pathological studies, however, indicate inflammatory vascular degeneration restricted to the thalamus (DeGirolami *et al.* 1974).

Diagnosis of Vascular Dementia
A number of criteria have been developed to aid in the diagnosis of vascular dementia. Hachinski and his colleagues (1975) published an index designed to assess the likelihood of stroke as a cause of dementia. Although designed for research on dementia, the items of the Hachinski index are useful clinically. The criteria are summarized in Table 13.2. Rosen and colleagues (1980) found that

Table 13.2   Hachinski schematic score

Feature	Score
Abrupt onset	2
Stepwise deterioration	1
Fluctuating course	2
Nocturnal confusion	1
Relative preservation of personality	1
Depression	1
Somatic complaints	1
Emotional incontinence	1
History of hypertension	1
History of strokes	2
Evidence of associated atherosclerosis	1
Focal neurological symptoms	2
Focal neurological signs	2

Patients with a total score of 7 or more are considered to have multi-infarct dementia; those scoring ≤4 have primary degenerative dementia (Hachinski *et al.* 1975).

Table 13.3 California criteria for ischemic vascular dementia (IVD) (Chui *et al.* 1992)

1. Dementia established by clinical examination
2. Progressive worsening of cognitive function
3. Evidence of at least two strokes by clinical or neuroradiological criteria
4. Evidence of at least one hemisphere infarct by CT or MRI (T1-weighted)
5. Diagnosis of definite IVD requires neuropathology

the Hachinski ischemic score correctly distinguished vascular dementia from AD, but it was not useful in distinguishing combinations of AD and vascular disease from either disease state alone. Gold and colleagues (1998) have also pointed out the limitations of this distinction, since even patients with pathologically proved AD have deep white matter lesions both at autopsy and on MRI (Englund *et al.* 1988).

Other large consensus groups have attempted to find a better set of criteria to diagnose vascular dementia, using brain imaging as well as clinical criteria. Chui *et al.* (1992) reported the 'California criteria', listed in Table 13.3.

Chui also listed the following factors as 'supporting' the diagnosis of ischemic vascular dementia (IVD): history of transient ischemic attacks, hypertension, or other risk factors for cerebrovascular disease; early gait disorder; extensive deep white matter disease; focal abnormalities on PET or SPECT functional brain imaging. Against IVD, in Chui's scheme, were: absence of focal neurological signs other than cognitive abnormalities; and presence of aphasia, apraxia, or agnosia without appropriate lesions on CT or MRI scans. These factors likely add further to the diagnostic accuracy of the Hachinski ischemic score. The criteria (Roman *et al.* 1993) are quite similar to those of the California criteria (Chui *et al.* 1992), emphasizing impairment of multiple cognitive domains, usual presence of focal neurological signs, gait abnormalities, mood changes, psychomotor slowing, and extrapyramidal signs. Against vascular dementia were: early onset and progressive worsening of a deficit in memory or other cognitive functions, in the absence of focal lesions on CT or MRI scans; absence of focal neurological signs, other than cognitive ones; and absence of infarcts on brain imaging studies.

In summary, several types and patterns of vascular disease can result in dementia, and vascular lesions superimposed on a pre-existing cognitive impairment can tip the patient over into frank dementia (Rockwood *et al.* 1999). The diagnostic criteria of Hachinski (1975), Chui *et al.* (1992), and the NINDS-AIREN group (Roman *et al.* 1993) are all useful in diagnosing vascular dementia. These diagnostic methods have somewhat different sensitivities for diagnosis. In addition, pathological studies have shown that pure vascular dementia is distinguishable from pure Alzheimer's disease by any of the criteria, but the mixed cases of Alzheimer's disease plus vascular disease are very difficult to separate from the pure vascular cases.

Treatment of Vascular Dementia

Very little research has been done on the prevention of dementia in patients with vascular risk factors. In view of the extensive literature on stroke prevention, however, it seems reasonable to assume that control of blood pressure, discontinuation of smoking, moderation of alcohol use, and reduction of cholesterol might all help to reduce the incidence of vascular dementia (Gorelick *et al.* 1999). A number of drug trials for patients with established vascular dementia, including such agents as pentoxyphilline (Trental), donepizil (Aricept), and others, have not established any clear efficacy. Preliminary evidence reported at the 2001 World Congress of Neurology meeting suggested reduced deterioration in patients with vascular dementia treated with the anticholinesterase drug galantamine (Reminyl). Further clinical trials are greatly needed.

Neoplasms and Dementia

Although generally regarded as infrequent causes of the dementia syndrome, neoplasms frequently produce cognitive impairment, and the treatments themselves can contribute to the cognitive loss. First, brain tumors may directly produce dementia by virtue of pressure and mass effect on adjacent tissue, increased intracranial pressure, edema, or hydrocephalus. Brain metastases may be multiple, producing multifocal neurologic deficits. Metastatic carcinomas, lymphomas, and even primary astrocytomas may spread diffusely in the meninges. This 'meningeal carcinomatosis' is associated with mental deterioration, lethargy, headache, and cranial nerve signs (Olson *et al.* 1974). Like meningeal infections, these disorders are diagnosed by lumbar puncture. Cancer patients also undergo a panoply of treatments, including chemotherapy and irradiation, which can produce multifocal or diffuse neurological symptoms and signs. Many chemotherapeutic agents are neurotoxic (Kaplan and Wiernik 1982); methotrexate and irradiation together can produce a multifocal leukoencephalopathy syndrome (Price and Jamieson 1975), and radiation therapy by itself induces vascular hyperplasia, leading to delayed tissue destruction (Rizzoli and Pagnanelli 1984). One follow-up study of patients with focal astrocytomas of the brain showed diffuse cognitive deficits not related to the location of the original tumor and more likely caused by radiation therapy (Hochberg and Slotnick 1980).

A more indirect and uncommon cause of dementia in cancer patients is the syndrome of limbic encephalitis, considered a 'remote effect' of cancer on the nervous system, or a 'paraneoplastic' syndrome. Patients with this disorder develop symptoms of anxiety or depression, memory loss, disorientation, and sometimes seizures, often with supervening dementia. Most patients have had primary lung carcinomas. *Post-mortem* studies have shown inflammatory infiltrates and neuronal loss in the hippocampus, amygdala, mammillary bodies, and cortex of the orbitofrontal and cingulate gyri (Corsellis *et al.* 1968). The resemblance of these changes to herpes simplex encephalitis suggests a viral etiology, but none has been proved, and the exact relationship of the disease to the underlying neoplasm is uncertain. Other paraneoplastic syndromes have been found to be antibody-mediated, but no responsible antibodies have been discovered in limbic encephalitis. Limbic encephalitis has been pathologically proved only in rare instances, although one series of 42 patients with paraneoplastic neurological syndromes secondary to systemic malignancies included 14 cases with significant dementia (Brain and Henson 1958). A malignant tumor should be searched for in demented patients with at least routine tests such as physical examination, chest X-ray films, liver function tests, stool test for occult blood, and possibly mammography in women. Other more specific investigations should be directed by symptoms of dysfunction in specific organ systems.

DEMENTIAS ASSOCIATED WITH NEUROLOGICAL DISEASES

In addition to the medical and systemic diseases discussed up to now, a large number of primary neurological diseases are associated with dementia. We divide these disorders into two groups: (1) those with prominent involvement of other neurological systems as well as cognition; and (2) those with predominant or exclusive involvement of the higher functions.

The first category includes a vast number of degenerative, metabolic, and genetic diseases of the nervous system, many of which are encountered only rarely even by neurologists practicing in large referral centers. Genetic diseases such as the aminoacidurias (e.g. phenylketonuria), lipid storage diseases (e.g. Tay–Sachs disease), leukodystrophies (e.g. metachromatic leukodystrophy), and phakomatoses (e.g. tuberous sclerosis) produce progressive dementia in addition to motor, sensory, and cerebellar signs. These disorders usually present during childhood. If the disease begins early in life, before intellectual function is established, the cognitive dysfunction is properly classed as 'mental retardation'; if dysfunction begins later, the disorder can legitimately be considered a dementia. Occasional cases of cerebral lipofuscinosis (Vercruyssen *et al.* 1982), adrenoleukodystrophy (DeLong and Richardson 1982), and metachromatic leukodystrophy (Percy and Kaback 1971), among others, present with insidious personality change and intellectual deterioration in late childhood, adolescence, or even adult life. None of these diseases typically begins as a progressive dementia of late life. Consideration of the vast array of degenerative neurological diseases that can produce dementia is beyond the scope of this book. A partial summary of these diseases is presented in Table 13.4. Multiple sclerosis, a common neurological disease, is frequently associated with memory loss, mood disturbances, and occasionally with frank dementia. Cognitive changes in multiple sclerosis are discussed in greater detail in Chapter 18. Traumatic brain injury as a cause of confusional states and dementia is described in Chapter 20. Other diseases associated with dementia are the 'subcortical' dementias and normal pressure hydrocephalus.

Subcortical Dementias

Several neurological diseases of adult life, familiar to neurologists because of their prominent motor signs, are important causes of dementia in the elderly.

Table 13.4 Neurological diseases associated with dementia

Diseases with other abnormal neurological signs
  Metabolic diseases
  • Lipid storage diseases
  • Mucopolysaccharidoses
  • Aminoacidurias
  • Leukoencephalopathies
  • Phakomatoses
  • Other heredodegenerative CNS diseases
  'Subcortical' dementias (See Chapter 16)
  • Parkinson's disease, diffuse Lewy Body disease, corticobasal degeneration
  • Huntington's disease
  • Wilson's disease
  • Progressive supranuclear palsy
  • Hallervorden–Spatz disease
  • Striatonigral deneration
  • Spinocerebellar atrophies (olivopontocerebellar degeneration, other systems degenerations)
  Normal-pressure hydrocephalus
  Multiple sclerosis
Diseases with cognitive dysfunction only
  Alzheimer's disease
  Frontotemporal dementia, Pick's disease
  Atypical dementia

These diseases have in common dysfunction of the basal ganglia and related sub-cortical structures; together they have given rise to the concept of 'subcortical dementia' (Mayeux *et al.* 1983; Cummings and Benson 1984). In general, the features of subcortical dementia include psychomotor slowing, impairment of recall memory with intact recognition memory, and associated motor signs. Among the diseases associated with subcortical dementia are Parkinson's disease, Huntington's disease, Wilson's disease, progressive supranuclear palsy, and corticobasal degeneration. A variant of Parkinson's disease termed 'Lewy body dementia' overlaps considerably with Alzheimer's disease. The cognitive aspects of movement disorders are presented in Chapter 16.

Normal pressure hydrocephalus also qualifies as a subcortical dementia and will be discussed here. Finally, some infectious disorders, especially AIDS Dementia Complex, involve prominent subcortical changes. The AIDS Dementia Complex was discussed earlier in this chapter.

In general, the usefulness of the concept of subcortical dementia lies in three prominent features: (1) mental slowing; (2) forgetfulness in which some recollection of the forgotten items remains, as assessed by a recognition test format; and (3) prominent motor signs. In addition, such cortical deficits as aphasia and agnosia are usually lacking, with some exceptions (see especially the section on corticobasal degeneration in Chapter 16). Martin Albert and colleagues (1974) first introduced the term 'subcortical dementia' in a paper on progressive supranuclear palsy. The concept of subcortical dementia has been controversial (Mayeux *et al.* 1983; Cummings and Benson 1984; Whitehouse 1986). Certainly, no pure distinction between cortical and subcortical dementia can be made; Alzheimer's disease, the prototype for all cortical dementias, also produces changes in subcortical structures such as the nucleus basalis of Meynert, and Huntington's and Parkinson's diseases, the prototypes for the subcortical degenerations, have associated cortical changes. For these and other reasons, the very usefulness of the category of subcortical dementia has been questioned (Whitehouse 1986). Despite these problems, the cortical–subcortical distinction remains in use. Disorders characterized by the features of mental slowing, recall but not recognition memory deficits, and prominent motor signs are clinically different from cortical dementias such as Alzheimer's disease.

Normal-Pressure Hydrocephalus

Adams, Hakim, and colleagues introduced the concept of normal pressure hydrocephalus (NPH) to the medical scene in 1965. Considerable excitement resulted from the report of dramatic clinical improvement in several patients with enlarged ventricles following ventriculo-atrial or ventriculo-peritoneal shunt procedures. The clinical syndrome of NPH consists of the triad of progressive mental deterioration, gait difficulty, and urinary incontinence (Adams *et al.* 1965; Greenberg *et al.* 1977). The coexistence of motor signs and dementia, along with the other clinical features, ties this disorder to the 'subcortical' dementias.

The dementia of NPH begins with slowing of thought and movement, apathy, poor concentration, decreased spontaneity, and impairment of memory. Only later does a true cognitive impairment become evident (Benson *et al.* 1970). This pattern resembles both the subcortical dementias and frontal lobe syndromes (see Chapter 10), probably because pressure from the enlarged lateral ventricles affects the deep white matter of the frontal lobes. The gait difficulty, sometimes called 'gait apraxia', is an apparent inability to initiate walking, with the feet appearing to be glued to the floor. The patient takes slow, hesitant, short steps as if he or she has forgotten how to walk. The gait pattern may resemble that of Parkinson's disease, but the Parkinsonian signs of tremor and cogwheel rigidity are absent. Spasticity and increased lower extremity reflexes are sometimes associated, presumably from stretching of the descending motor fibers from the cortical leg areas, which begin medially in the hemispheres and arc around the dilated lateral ventricles. The urinary incontinence may reflect similar stretching of motor fibers from the cortical representation of the urinary bladder. Unawareness of urination and loss of normal self-consciousness may also play a role.

As in the other subcortical dementias, the association of motor findings with mental slowing and dementia distinguish this disorder from Alzheimer's disease, in which gait and bladder function are usually preserved until later stages of the disease. The diagnosis is made by the triad of clinical features, together with the finding of enlarged ventricles, out of proportion to cortical atrophy, on brain imaging studies.

Hydrocephalus is a dilatation of the cerebral ventricles, usually caused by obstruction of flow within the cerebrospinal fluid (CSF) pathway. Fluid is secreted by the choroid plexi of the cerebral ventricles, flows through the ventricular system and then out of the foramena of Luschka and Magendie into the subarachnoid space. CSF moves freely in the subarachnoid space, both down through the spinal canal and up over the cerebral convexities, where it is reabsorbed in the superior sagittal sinus. Obstruction to flow can occur at the level of the lateral ventricles, as in tumors such as choroid plexus papillomas; the third ventricle, as in colloid cysts; the fourth ventricle outflow foramena, as in tumors of the posterior fossa; or at the base of the brain, in the inflammation of the basilar meninges and cisterns seen in chronic meningitis or following subarachnoid hemorrhage. This last type of hydrocephalus is sometimes called 'communicating' hydrocephalus, because all of the ventricles enlarge together and remain in open communication with the spinal subarachnoid space. Presumably, flow is obstructed between the basilar cisterns and the cortical subarachnoid space, and relatively increased pressure within the ventricles leads them to expand, at the expense of the cortical subarachnoid space. In normal pressure hydrocephalus, the pressure measured at lumbar puncture is normal at the time of diagnosis, perhaps because ventricular expansion has allowed the pressure to normalize (Adams *et al.* 1965).

NPH is a communicating hydrocephalus, but the site or cause of the obstruction is not known. A recently proposed theory is that there is a venous obstruction to absorption of CSF at the superior sagittal sinus (Bradley 2000). Obstruction there, however, would not clearly lead to a gradient between the pressures in the intraventricular and subarachnoid CSF spaces, and hence the ventricles might not dilate; the picture would be more akin to that of benign intracranial hypertension or 'pseudotumor cerebri'.

The diagnosis and treatment of idiopathic normal pressure hydrocephalus are controversial. The clinical features of dementia, gait abnormality, and incontinence are critical; generally, if gait abnormality is not present, response to treatment is disappointing (Black 1980). CT and MRI scanning are used to detect ventricular enlargement (Figure 13.1). The presence of a mild degree of cortical atrophy does not exclude the diagnosis or argue against treatment (Jacobs and Kinkel 1976); similarly, the presence of ischemic deep white matter disease does not predict a failure of improvement after shunting (Krauss *et al.* 1996). Isotope cisternography, in which serial scans are performed after injection of isotope into the lumbar subarachnoid space, shows prolonged presence of the isotope in the cerebral ventricles and failure of uptake in the superior sagittal sinus (James *et al.* 1970). Although useful in confirming the physiology of hydrocephalus, the test is cumbersome and has not proved independently predictive of response to shunting (Black 1980; Benzel *et al.* 1990). Monitoring of CSF pressure before shunting has also been useful in some series (Raftopoulos *et al.* 1994). CSF infusion

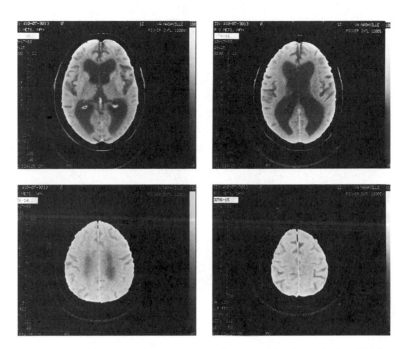

Figure 13.1 CT scan from a patient with normal-pressure hydrocephalus. The lateral ventricles are massively dilated, out of proportion to the mild degree of enlargement of the cortical sulci.

tests have been shown in some studies (Boon *et al.* 1997) to predict which patients will respond to shunting. Infusion tests are cumbersome and are not often used in the USA.

The treatment of NPH involves placement of a shunt tube into a lateral ventricle, with the other end usually tunneled into the abdominal peritoneum. In several large series of cases, shunting has produced improvement in roughly 40–70% of cases, though the presence of the full clinical triad and appropriate CT scan findings may raise this probability to 60–70% (Jacobs and Kinkel 1976; Laws and Mokri 1977; Black 1980; Larsson *et al.* 1991; Benzel *et al.* 1990). The clinical benefit must be weighed against a 30–35% risk of complications, including shunt malfunction, shunt infection, and subdural hematoma. In addition, a recent series from Sweden reported that although two-thirds of patients showed initial improvement after shunting, only 25% showed sustained improvement at the end of 3 years (Malm *et al.* 2000). The decision to perform surgery must include careful discussion of the risks and benefits of the procedure. Although the initial enthusiasm about NPH has been tempered by these variable results, hydrocephalus remains a treatable cause of dementia, and one that should be considered in all demented patients.

DISEASES ASSOCIATED PRIMARILY WITH DEMENTIA

Among diseases associated primarily with dementia are degenerative diseases of the brain that predominantly or exclusively affect the higher cortical functions. Creutzfeldt–Jakob disease, discussed earlier in this chapter, formerly belonged to this group but now has been reclassified as an infectious disease. The remaining disorders to be discussed are Alzheimer's disease (including senile dementia of the Alzheimer type) and frontotemporal dementia, or Pick's disease.

Alzheimer's Disease

Alzheimer's disease is truly the flagship of the fleet of dementing diseases; it is the most common cause of dementia in pathological series, the most difficult to distinguish from the normal aging process, and the most exciting in terms of future research efforts. In the light of the wide attention this disorder is currently receiving in both the medical and popular literature, it is interesting that Alzheimer (1907) first described the entity in a case report of three pages. Alzheimer's disease originally referred only to 'presenile' patients under age 65 at onset, but the disease is clinically and pathologically indistinguishable from cases of senile dementia, now called 'senile dementia of the Alzheimer type' (SDAT). Alzheimer's disease is the disorder on which the general pattern of progressive stages of cognitive deterioration, outlined at the beginning of this chapter, is based. Other diseases may mimic this pattern, but the clear history of progressive cognitive deterioration in an alert patient with no signs of depression, no focal neurological signs, and no history of stroke, head injuries, or medical diseases associated with dementia usually points to Alzheimer's disease. Reisberg (1983) suggested that progression through the successive clinical stages of Alzheimer's disease reliably confirms the diagnosis. Clinical experience, however, suggests a high degree of variability from patient to patient. As discussed earlier, apparently 'focal' presentations of aphasias or visuospatial deficit have been reported in patients who later develop features of a generalized dementia. The rate of progression is also variable, with some patients remaining in the phase of mild forgetfulness for many years, as in the syndrome of mild cognitive impairment discussed earlier.

Although the definition of dementia requires a diffuse or generalized abnormality of cortical function, Alzheimer's disease has strong predilections for specific brain systems and regions. Mental status examinations show short-term memory loss, failure of recall of names, visuoperceptual deficits, and decreased insight and judgment in the early and middle stages. Behavioral disturbances including acute confusional states, hallucinations, delusional thinking including paranoia, and even violent outbursts occur in some patients with Alzheimer's disease. In late stages, severe language, memory, and visuoperceptual deficits abound, and the patient becomes apathetic and incapable of self-care. Primary motor and sensory functions of the brain, including gait, are preserved until the late stages (Koller *et al.* 1984). In one study, measures of motor performance showed only minor differences between normal and demented elderly patients, though decreased rapid alternating movements, abnormal gait, rigidity, and loss of associated movements were all slightly more common in the demented group (Carlen *et al.* 1981). In other studies, extrapyramidal signs (Molsa *et al.* 1984) and myoclonus (Wilkins *et al.* 1984) have been found commonly in Alzheimer's disease, especially in advanced stages.

Many papers on Alzheimer's disease and its treatment divide patients into stages, based on the patterns above. One review (Kraemer *et al.* 1998) pointed out that there is variability not only in the behavioral manifestations in different patients, but also in the criteria that research studies use to measure progression. The authors suggested that cognitive measures such as the Mini Mental State (see Chapter 4) are most sensitive for examining drug treatment at earlier stages of the disease, whereas measures based on home functioning and activities of daily living such as the Global Deterioration Scale might be better for examining drug treatment at more advanced stages.

Diagnosis of Alzheimer's Disease

The diagnosis of Alzheimer's disease should always rest on the clinical features, but laboratory tests are useful in confirming the diagnosis. The clinical diagnosis is based on a multifocal abnormality of memory and other higher functions, as well as the absence of gross motor or sensory signs. A probable diagnosis of AD can be made by NINCDS/ADRDS criteria (McKhann *et al.* 1984); adefinite diagnosis requires pathological confirmation. Table 13.5 lists the NINCDS/ADRDS criteria. These 1984 criteria have stood the test of time for usefulness in the diagnosis of AD and have recently been revalidated as part of an American Academy of Neurology practice parameter (Knopman *et al.* 2001). Autopsy series have shown a correlation of 87–100% in pathological validation of carefully made clinical diagnoses of probable or presumed AD (Joachim *et al.* 1988; Morris *et al.* 1988; Mayeux *et al.* 1998).

Laboratory testing is useful both in confirming the diagnosis of 'probable Alzheimer's disease' and in excluding the treatable causes of dementia. CT or MRI scans typically show ventricular enlargement and dilatation of the cortical sulci consistent with cortical atrophy (Figure 13.2). Many normal elderly patients have some degree of cortical atrophy, however, and this finding on CT scan should not

Table 13.5 MINCDS-ADRDA criteria for probable alzheimer's disease

1. Dementia established by clinical examination and documented by the Mini Mental State or other screening test or neuropsychological testing
2. Deficits in two or more areas of cognition
3. Progressive worsening of memory and other cognitive functions
4. No disturbance of consciousness
5. Onset between ages 40 and 90 years, most often after 65
6. Absence of systemic disorders or other brain diseases that could account for the progressive deficits in memory and cognition

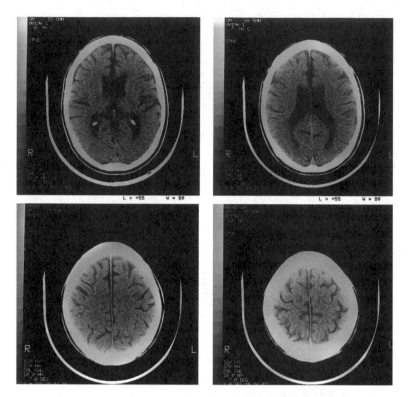

Figure 13.2 CT scan from a patient with Alzheimer's disease. There is a corresponding degree of enlargement of the ventricles and cortical sulci, consistent with diffuse cerebral atrophy.

automatically lead to the diagnosis of dementia or to the assumption that the cause is Alzheimer's disease (Wells and Duncan 1977; Reisberg 1983). Several studies of CT scans and dementia have shown a generally unsatisfactory level of correlation between the degree of cortical atrophy by CT scan and the degree of clinical dementia (Bird 1982; Wilson *et al.* 1982; Bradshaw *et al.* 1983; Laffey *et al.* 1984). Specific measures of medial temporal atrophy (Jobst *et al.* 1992) or ventricular volume (Damasio *et al.* 1983; George *et al.* 1983) or specific CT density readings (Naeser *et al.* 1980; Bondareff *et al.* 1981) may make the CT scan more discriminatory in AD, but these measures have not gained popular acceptance. Increasing atrophy and ventricular enlargement on sequential scans is, of course, more convincing evidence of a degenerative process (Brinkman *et al.* 1984). There remain, however, patients with dementia whose scans appear normal, and normal elderly patients whose CT scans show cortical atrophy. Magnetic resonance imaging (MRI), a magnetic technique based on density and movement of hydrogen atoms in magnetic fields, has advantages over CT in terms of better anatomic resolution, freedom from bone artifacts, and imaging in all three planes (Tanridag and Kirshner 1987), but the technique is still relatively insensitive to the early stages of

Alzheimer's disease and adds only limited discriminative value in the diagnosis of dementia (Erkinjuntti *et al.* 1982; DeCarli *et al.* 1995). Positron emission tomography (PET), a technique by which labeled compounds can be localized in the brain, has the capacity to show levels of metabolic activity and blood flow, rather than just imaging the structure of the brain. PET studies of glucose uptake in demented patients have shown decreased metabolic activity most evident in the parietotemporal and later the frontal regions, sparing the primary sensory and motor areas of the brain (Benson *et al.* 1983; Foster *et al.* 1983; Friedland *et al.* 1984; Mielke *et al.* 1994; Blesa *et al.* 1996). The location of these metabolic changes parallel the clinical symptoms in individual patients (Figure 13.3; Foster

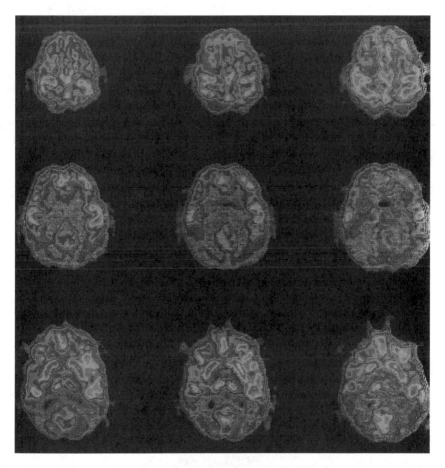

Figure 13.3 PET scan (18 Fluorodeoxyglucose, or FDG PET) from a patient with early Alzheimer's disease. FDG provides a 'metabolic map' of the brain areas where glucose is being taken up and metabolized. This 51-year-old surgeon noted a progressive loss of short-term memory and cognitive function. Note the reduced glucose metabolism in the parietal regions of both cerebral hemispheres.

et al. 1983; Keilp *et al.* 1996). PET remains largely restricted to research institutions, and is also very expensive as a diagnostic test. Single photon emission computed tomography (SPECT) is a similar isotopic technique with somewhat lesser anatomic accuracy, but similar changes in perfusion of the parietal lobes are detectible even in relatively early stages of AD (Hurwitz *et al.* 1991; Bonte *et al.* 1993; Mielke *et al.* 1994; Pickut *et al.* 1997). One or the other of these techniques is helpful in the initial diagnosis of AD.

There is as yet no specific test on blood, urine, or cerebrospinal fluid that can reliably diagnose an individual patient with Alzheimer's disease. The apolipoprotein E typing (see below) can alter risks of developing AD, but it does not permit a reliable diagnosis of AD in an individual patient (Mayeux *et al.* 1998). The neuronal thread protein (Gharnbari *et al.* 1998) in CSF or more recently in urine has a sensitivity of 80–87% and a specificity approaching 90% in the diagnosis of AD (de la Monte *et al.* 1997; Ghanbari *et al.* 1998), but the test does not permit an absolutely definite diagnosis of AD. The test is also expensive, and the added knowledge it provides is not clearly justified by any treatment implication. An eyedrop test for cholinergic abnormalities in the pupil (Scinto *et al.* 1994) was not confirmed in subsequent trials (Gomez-Tortosa *et al.* 1996; Loupe *et al.* 1996; Graff-Radford *et al.* 1997). CSF assays for tau protein have a correlation with AD in groups of patients, but are not reliably diagnostic for the individual patient (Arai *et al.* 1998). CSF assays for both beta-amyloid and tau proteins may offer increased sensitivity to the diagnosis of AD (Andreasen *et al.* 2001). Baskin and colleagues (2000) have presented evidence that the ratios of specific amyloid precursor proteins (APP) decline in platelets from patients with AD; this preliminary finding may provide the basis for a new laboratory test for AD, but larger trials will be needed. In general, the laboratory confirmation of AD remains imperfect, and the clinical criteria for probable AD remain paramount in diagnosis.

Neuropathology of Alzheimer's Disease

The neuropathology of Alzheimer's disease involves diffuse atrophy of the cerebral cortex and enlargement of the ventricles, with sparing of the primary motor and sensory areas. The cortical gyri are narrowed, the sulci are widened, and the overall brain weight is reduced. Microscopic silver stains, as Alzheimer himself described, show loss of neuronal cell bodies and silver-staining 'neurofibrillary tangles' in remaining neurons (Figure 13.4). By electron microscopy these neurofibrillary tangles are seen to be composed of paired helical filaments or double-stranded microtubular structures not present in normal neurons (Wisniewski *et al.* 1976). These structures are now known to be made up of aggregations of the microtubular protein, tau. The intercellular space of the cerebral cortex, or neuropil, also contains silver-staining structures called senile or 'neuritic' plaques. These plaques are difficult to see on routine stains such as hematoxylin and eosin, but stand out prominently on silver stains. The typical plaque is a target-like structure with a central core of amyloid, surrounded by fragments of neural processes or 'neurites' and glial cells (Figure 13.5). The neurites, like the neurofibrillary

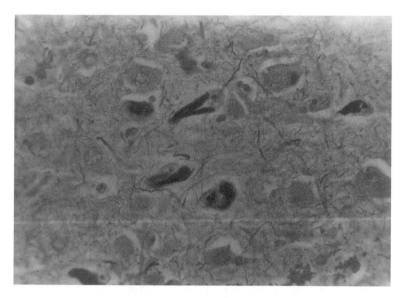

Figure 13.4 Microscopic silver stain preparation from the cerebral cortex patient with Alzheimer's disease. The dense, silver-staining fibers in the two neurons near the center of the picture are neurofibrillary tangles. (Reproduced by courtesy of Dr William O. Whetsell.)

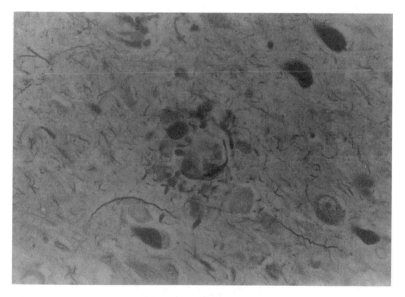

Figure 13.5 Photomicrograph from the same patient as in Figure 13.4. The large structure at the center is a senile plaque. The central amyloid core and surrounding neurites are well seen. (Reproduced by courtesy of Dr William O. Whetsell.)

tangles, contain paired helical filaments. Plaques and tangles are not specific for Alzheimer's disease, occurring in increasing numbers with advancing age in the normal population (Tomlinson *et al.* 1968). Unlike the finding of cortical atrophy on CT scan, however, the number and severity of these changes does appear to correlate closely with the degree of dementia (Blessed *et al.* 1968). In addition to senile plaques and neurofibrillary tangles, hippocampal neurons of patients with Alzheimer's disease may contain 'granulovacuolar degeneration', or combinations of granules and fluid-filled vacuoles.

One of the most exciting developments in our understanding of the pathology of Alzheimer's disease has been the finding of neuronal loss in the nucleus basalis of Meynert, a basal forebrain nucleus known to have extensive cholinergic projections to wide areas of the cerebral cortex (Whitehouse *et al.* 1982; Candy *et al.* 1983). Cholinergic activity of the cerebral cortex, as measured by levels of the synthetic enzyme choline acetyltransferase, is reduced in Alzheimer's disease (Danes 1979), and these depressed enzyme levels correlate with *pre-mortem* behavioral test scores (Perry *et al.* 1978). The primary cause of the degeneration of the nucleus basalis and the loss of cholinergic activity of the cerebral cortex, however, remains unknown.

Etiology of Alzheimer's Disease

Clinical epidemiology is usually the first place to look for clues to the cause of a disease. Alzheimer's disease has had many clues but few solutions. Age is the greatest risk factor; as stated at the beginning of the chapter, the incidence of the disease roughly doubles with each 5 years after age 65. Among acquired risk factors, only head trauma appears to have a predictive effect on development of AD, and only in some studies (Heyman *et al.* 1984). The recently published Rotterdam study found that diabetes (Ott *et al.* 1999) but not head injury (Mehta *et al.* 1999) was associated with the development of AD. Down's syndrome also has an important effect on risk of AD; of Down's patients who die after age 50, virtually all have pathological changes of AD. Diet, toxins, animal contacts, alcohol intake, and smoking all fail to distinguish demented patients from controls (Crapper *et al.* 1980; Heyman *et al.* 1984).

Genetic factors are of greater importance. Three genes have now been conclusively linked to early onset, familial Alzheimer's disease. All appear to follow autosomal dominant transmission; half of offspring of an affected parent are likely to develop the disease. Chromosome 21 was the first discovered gene locus of familial AD. In the context of the known association of AD with Down's syndrome, a trisomy of chromosome 21, this had obvious importance. Virtually 100% of Down's syndrome patients develop AD by their late 40s (Wisniewski *et al.* 1985). The site on chromosome 21 is closely linked with the amyloid precursor protein gene, supporting the amyloid theory of AD. The other two familial, early onset AD genes, on chromosomes 14 and 1, code for proteins called presenilin 1 and 2, respectively (Lendon *et al.* 1997). These proteins are also closely involved with the amyloid precursor protein. We thus have clear evidence that defects in amyloid metabolism are closely related to the pathogenesis of AD, at least in the early onset, familial cases.

For late onset cases of AD, genetics play a lesser role, and most cases appear sporadic. Early studies, however, still implicate a higher incidence of the disease in patients with a positive family history, on the order of 30% (Heston *et al.* 1981; Heyman *et al.* 1984; Breitner 1991). Language disorder and apraxia may be especially common in familial Alzheimer's disease (Folstein and Breitner 1981).

Apolipoproteins have been discovered to play a role in predilection to late onset disease. Patients with at least one apolipoprotein E4 allele have a much greater chance of developing AD than do those with E2 or E3 alleles (Saunders *et al.* 1993). Those rare patients with two E4 alleles have a 90% chance of developing AD by age 70. When combined with the clinical diagnosis, apoE4 testing increases the specificity of the diagnosis (Mayeux *et al.* 1998). Most geneticists feel that presymptomatic testing of persons at genetic risk for AD is not justified, given the lack of specific predictive value and the lack of proved preventive therapies.

A great deal of research has been devoted to the search for the pathogenesis of AD, and new findings are being reported virtually daily. In fact, this chapter has been 'finished' several times, and then newly arrived journals have announced important new findings. The central theory of Alzheimer's disease at present is the deposition of amyloid. Through the pioneering work of Glenner, Selkoe, and others, much has been learned about amyloid metabolism in Alzheimer's disease (Selkoe 1997; Rosenberg, 2000). Amyloid protein is deposited in the cores of the neuritic plaques, and also in small blood vessels in AD. A recent pathological study (Naslund *et al.* 2000) found amyloid deposition very early in the clinical development of the disease in patients who died of other causes, and deposition of the amyloid-beta-peptide preceded the development of tau pathology such as neurofibrillary tangles. The degree of amyloid deposition also correlated with the severity of the cognitive deterioration. Current evidence ties amyloid chemistry to the genetic forms of Alzheimer's disease. Presenilin 1, the defective gene product of the chromosome 14 early onset, autosomal dominant form of AD, may in fact be the secretase enzyme that cleaves amyloid precursor protein (Rosenberg, 2000). Apolipoproteins are also involved in the formation and solubility of amyloid in plaques; E4 has increased affinity for beta-amyloid and may enhance the formation of amyloid fibrils that become incorporated into the senile plaque (Strittmatter *et al.* 1993; Ma *et al.* 1994).

Experimentally, transgenic mice with a mutant APP (amyloid precursor protein) gene also develop neuropathological changes of AD, suggesting that the amyloid deposition is toxic to neurons and is the direct cause of the neuronal degeneration in AD (Hsaio *et al.* 1996; Holcomb *et al.* 1998). The amyloid deposition also occurs in blood vessels and may be the cause of the ischemic white matter lesions frequently seen on MRI in this disease. Studies in mice have also shown that ApoE also influences development of Alzheimer's disease pathology in mice with transgenic amyloid genes (Bales *et al.* 1997). One very exciting research study in mice demonstrated that immunization of the mice with the amyloid beta 42-subunit protein prevented the development of neuritic plaques and other neuropathological changes of Alzheimer's disease in transgenic mice with the amyloid precursor protein gene (Shenk *et al.* 1999; Weiner *et al.* 2000).

Human vaccine trials are anticipated. This type of molecular treatment for AD holds great promise for the future.

Other proposed etiologies of AD have gradually fallen by the wayside. One such finding was an increase in levels of aluminum found in brain tissue of patients with Alzheimer's disease (Trapp *et al.* 1978; Crapper *et al.* 1980). The deposition of aluminum may be a secondary effect of the presence of senile plaques in the cortex of AD brains.

Treatment of Alzheimer's Disease

The treatment of Alzheimer's disease is as yet quite limited. Behavioral therapies have an important role: keeping patients at home in familiar surroundings, with family members nearby, and with frequent orientation cues such as calendars and reminders of the date, is a goal of treatment. The home environment both keeps patients functioning as long as possible and reduces costs for society (Mayeux and Sano 1999).

A second area of therapy is the enhancement of memory function by manipulations of the cholinergic system. Despite clear evidence of loss of cholinergic activity in the cerebral cortex in AD, cholinergic treatments have developed only slowly. As yet, no effective cholinergic agonist drugs have reached the market. An aggressive therapy, the intraventricular infusion of bethanechol, initially appeared promising but later did not prove beneficial (Harbaugh *et al.* 1989). Precursor treatments with choline or lecithin have not shown consistent improvement in the memory loss of AD. Acetylcholinesterase inhibitors have proved to be of modest benefit in improving short-term memory in patients with AD. Tacrine (Cognex) was the first drug used, but its hepatic and gastrointestinal toxicity and four times per day schedule of administration made it impractical. Patients improved in memory at higher doses, but only a minority of patients could tolerate the highest (160 mg/day) doses (Knapp *et al.* 1994). The drug did delay admission to nursing homes in one approximately 3-year study (Knopman *et al.* 1996). Donepezil (Aricept) is a once-a-day acetylcholinesterase inhibitor that has very little toxicity and does not require blood monitoring. The drug has been proved effective in arresting the memory deterioration of AD (Rogers *et al.* 1998; Burns *et al.* 1999). The drug is given initially as a 5 mg bedtime dose, but the dose should be advanced to 10 mg QHS in most patients. The side effects are largely gastrointestinal: abdominal cramps and diarrhea. Many patients fail to show improvement in memory, but at least stabilize for a period of months to a year or two. The newer anticholinesterase drug rivastigmine (Exelon) appears to be efficacious in reducing the memory deterioration of AD (Corey-Bloom *et al.* 1998; Rosler *et al.* 1999). The drug appears to be more potent but also more toxic than donepezil. The drug requires twice daily dosing and an escalation of doses. Rivastigmine promises benefit in patients who have failed donepezil. A fourth anticholinesterase drug, metrifonate, was withdrawn because of unacceptable toxicity (muscle weakness). The most recent anticholinesterase on the market, galantamine (Reminyl), showed significant benefit in two multicenter clinical trials examining memory and behavioral functions in AD patients (Raskind *et al.* 2000; Tariot *et al.* 2000). It appears that anticholinesterase therapy has a definite place in the symptomatic treatment of patients with AD, though these drugs provide at best a delay of the inevitable cognitive deterioration. As one editorial writer put it, we are 'searching for a breakthrough, settling for less' (Drachman and Leber 1997).

Other attempts to modify neurotransmitter systems, stimulate metabolic pathways, or prevent damage have been largely disappointing. In one study, vitamin E (Sano *et al.* 1997) did appear to slow the inexorable progression of the disease, delaying the stage of total dependence or nursing home placement. The dose of vitamin E was large, 2000 iu daily; no smaller doses were tested. Most experts on treatment of AD advise patients to take vitamin E, based on this study. Gingko biloba has been reported to reduce the decline of memory function in patients with Alzheimer's disease (Le Bars 1997), but the effect in this trial was slight, and benefit has not yet been confirmed in US trials. The comparative efficacy of Gingko biloba versus anticholinesterase drugs has not been tested. Vasodilators such as Hydergine have been widely prescribed in AD, but scientific studies have not confirmed any benefit (Hier *et al.* 1980; Thompson *et al.* 1990). Retrospective studies have suggested that estrogen therapy is associated with a reduced risk of development of AD. The one controlled trial of estrogen therapy in patients with diagnosed AD, however, did not show any benefit (Mulnard *et al.* 2000). Likewise, use of non-steroidal anti-inflammatory drugs appears associated with reduced risk of AD, but no controlled trials of either glucocorticoid or non-steroidal drugs have as yet supported a preventive effect in elderly persons or a treatment effect in patients with established AD (Breitner 1996; Flynn and Theesen 1999). A variety of other drugs have been tested in AD with inconsistent results; these will not be discussed, since no practical management implications have yet developed.

Psychotropic medications may aid in the management of the behavioral disturbances, which are not only extremely common in AD, but are frequently the immediate reason for institutionalization (Steele *et al.* 1990; Cohen *et al.* 1993). A comparison study of patients who required nursing home placement versus those who stayed in the home found major differences in behavioral symptoms but none in cognitive measures (Steele *et al.* 1990). The most widely prescribed medications for behavioral disturbances in AD are antidepressants. The SSRI class of antidepressants is usually favored, because of their lack of anticholinergic side effects, which can worsen memory loss, and lack of sedation (Mayeux and Sano 1999). Anxiety and agitation are major problems in AD patients. Benzodiazepine minor tranquilizers sometimes cause paradoxical agitation or worsening of confusion. Buspirone may have some benefit, though the antianxiety effect is less potent. Nightime doses of trazodone or valproic acid (Depakote) may be of some help. Neuroleptics such as haloperidol relieve agitation more effectively, but elderly patients are at high risk of extrapyramidal side effects, and the anticholinergic properties of the drug may worsen cognition (Class *et al.* 1997). The newer, 'atypical' antipsychotic drugs – clozepine (Clozaril), risperidone (Risperdal), olanzepine (Zyprexa), and quetiapine (Seroquel) – all relieve anxiety with only minimal risk of extrapyramidal side effects. These drugs are expensive, but they have aided greatly in the control of abnormal behavior in AD patients.

Aging and Alzheimer's Disease

As stated earlier, the pathological features of Alzheimer's disease, particularly the senile plaques and neurofibrillary tangles, do not differ between presenile and senile cases. These same structural changes, moreover, occur with increasing frequency in older patients, to the extent that they are almost invariable by the ninth or tenth decade (Tomlinson *et al.* 1968). As discussed in the first section of this chapter, memory and speed of cognitive functions are known to decline with age (Burke and McKay 1997). If only quantitative and not qualitative differences in both clinical and pathological findings distinguish Alzheimer's disease from normal aging, the question arises whether Alzheimer's disease represents a disease in its own right, or only an acceleration of the normal aging process. Although it is true that no clinical or pathological feature is specific for Alzheimer's disease, as opposed to normal aging, very large differences exist in clinical patterns and in the degree of the pathological changes. Even clinically, the minor declines in cognitive function that occur with normal aging are strikingly different from the cognitive loss of AD. Similarly, the pathological changes of Alzheimer's disease are of a much greater degree in terms of the widespread distribution and sheer number of plaques and neurofibrillary tangles throughout the cerebral cortex, hippocampus, and other subcortical structures. Most importantly, these changes relate quantitatively with the degree of dementia (Blessed *et al.* 1968).

The lack of specific changes distinguishing normal aging from Alzheimer's disease does not detract from the importance of Alzheimer's as a disease, when one considers the major clinical consequences discussed throughout this chapter. Semantic arguments concerning the status of Alzheimer's as a 'disease' or 'accelerated aging' beg the question of what aging is and why systems fail earlier in some patients than in others. Further understanding of the biology of both aging and Alzheimer's disease should help to clarify the differences between the two.

Pick's Disease, Frontotemporal Dementia, and other Focal Cortical Degenerations

Pick's Disease

Arnold Pick (1892) described the focal, lobar atrophy with dementia that now bears his name 15 years before Alzheimer's famous paper. 'Simple progressive brain atrophy can lead to symptoms of local disturbance through local accentuation of the diffuse process' (Pick 1892, p. 40). Pick saw this disease, like neurosyphilis, as a middle ground between psychiatric disorders and senile dementia, in that the patients first manifest psychiatric symptoms and then develop memory loss, fluent aphasia, and finally progressive dementia. Pick also discussed the contradiction between the 'focal' onset of several of his patients and the presence of a diffuse disease process, a concept which still lies at the crux of current discussions of focal dementing illnesses such as primary progressive aphasia. Although reviews of dementia stress the clinical similarities of Pick's and Alzheimer's diseases (Haase 1977), several reports have documented early and clinically evident dysfunction of the dominant temporal lobe, with fluent aphasia, and sparing of parietal lobe functions such as constructions and calculations (Wechsler *et al.* 1982; Morris *et al.* 1984; Graff-Radford *et al.* 1990). Familial cases are common in Pick's disease (Groen and Endtz 1982; Morris *et al.* 1984). Interestingly, some European series (Sjogren *et al.* 1974; Sulkava *et al.* 1983) have reported Pick's disease nearly as commonly as Alzheimer's disease, although American and British series find it much more rarely.

Classically, Pick's disease is a lobar atrophy affecting the frontal and temporal lobes, either unilaterally or bilaterally. The pattern of selective frontal and temporal atrophy can be detected by CT scan, though the reliability of this lobar atrophy in the diagnosis of Pick's disease is imperfect (McGeachie *et al.* 1979). The microscopic pathology is different from that of Alzheimer's disease, in that neuritic plaques and neurofibrillary tangles are not prominent in most cases, but there are silver-staining intraneuronal inclusions called 'Pick bodies'. There may be loss of neurons in the nucleus basalis of Meynert, as in AD (Uhl *et al.* 1983), and the cholinergic system may show cortical degeneration (Yates *et al.* 1980). Defined by these strict neuropathological rules, Pick's disease is quite rare.

Primary Progressive Aphasia

In the USA, emphasis has been placed on patients who present with progressive aphasia, a syndrome referred to by Mesulam and colleagues (Mesulam 1982; Weintraub *et al.* 1990) as primary progressive aphasia (PPA). Many series of patients with PPA have been reported. Weintraub and colleagues (1990) stressed the progressive nature of the language deficits over a period of over 2 years, in the absence of a generalized dementia. The characteristics of the aphasia are somewhat variable. Weintraub and colleagues (1990) stated that non-fluent aphasia is generally not seen in AD and is a good indicator of a focal, non-Alzheimer pathology. On the other hand, cases of progressive fluent aphasia have been reported with Pick's disease (Holland *et al.* 1985), with non-specific pathology (Kirshner *et al.* 1987), and with Alzheimer's disease (Green *et al.* 1990). Hodges and colleagues (1992) reported a specific degeneration of semantics, referred to as 'semantic dementia', in which patients not only cannot name objects but also cannot define words. Patients can produce only a small number of examples of a category such as animals. In many of these cases, speech remains fluent long into the illness. The largest reported analysis of primary progressive aphasia, by Westbury and Bub (1997), included 112 cases. The average age at onset, 59 years, is considerably younger than the age of onset of typical Alzheimer's disease, and males outnumbered females by nearly two to one. The most common presenting symptom was word-finding difficulty. Progression to frank dementia was variable, and was delayed several years in most cases. The prognosis of PPA is thus more favorable than that of AD, and some patients are able to continue working or to pursue hobbies for years into the illness. A few (Edwards-Lee *et al.* 1997) have even shown new talents for art or other hobbies.

In general, brain-imaging studies in primary progressive aphasia have confirmed the lobar distribution of the atrophy (Tyrell *et al.* 1990). The lobar atrophy in patients with semantic dementia can be detected even on MRI (Chan *et al.* 2001), but PET scans make the changes appear more obvious. In some cases MRI and PET scans suggested bilateral pathology even early in the disease. Figures 13.6 and 13.7 depict MRI and PET findings from a patient with primary progressive aphasia. This 67-year-old retired state trooper presented with progressive anomia and non-fluent speech. Despite his difficulties with communication, he spent his days driving patients to hospitals in Nashville from his hometown in Kentucky, and he never became lost.

This pattern of progressive aphasia is quite distinct from the typical course of AD. Patients with AD also lose memory for names early in the illness, but fluent expression, repetition, reading aloud, and even a degree of comprehension tend to remain intact into later stages of the disease (Appell *et al.* 1982;

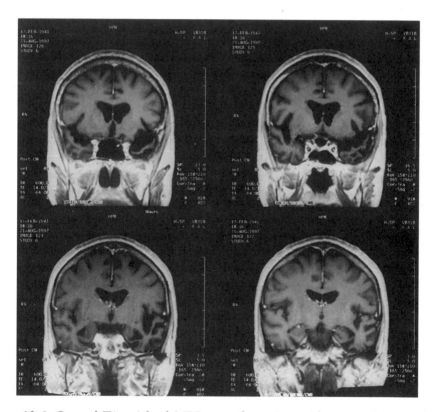

Figure 13.6 Coronal T1-weighted MRI scan of a patient with progressive, non-fluent aphasia. Note the marked atrophy of the left temporal lobe, which is easiest to see in the coronal projection. (Reprinted with permission from WG Bradley, RB Daroff, GM Fenichel, CD Marsden (eds). Neurology in Clinical Practice, Vol. I (3rd edn). Boston: Butterworth-Heinemann, 2000.)

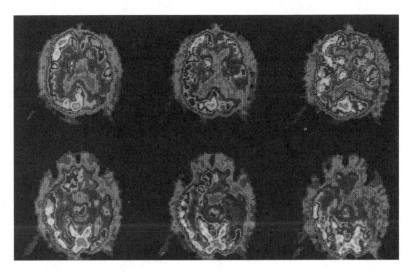

Figure 13.7 Axial fluorine-2-deoxyglucose PET scan from the same patient. Note the extensive hypometabolism of the left temporal region. (Reprinted with permission from WG Bradley, RB Daroff, GM Fenichel, CD Marsden (eds). Neurology in Clinical Practice, Vol. I (3rd edn). Boston: Butterworth-Heinemann, 2000.)

Cummings *et al*. 1985; Price *et al*. 1993). In PPA, early loss of fluency of word list generation (such as animal naming), loss of syntax and fluency, and decreased language comprehension are prominent symptoms and signs. Grossman and colleagues (1996) suggested a useful dissociation between the two disorders: digit span and repetition are more affected early in PPA, whereas short-term memory is more affected early in AD.

Frontotemporal Dementia

Another classification of focal degenerative diseases of the cerebral cortex is the designation frontotemporal dementia (FTD), made popular in England by Neary, Snowden and colleagues (Neary and Snowden 1996; Neary *et al*. 1998). Many cases of PPA would fall under this rubric, and in general the North American and British authors seemed to be using different terminology to describe similar cases. The pathology in frontotemporal dementia includes neuronal loss, gliosis, and sometimes vacuolation of the neuropil, but typically Pick bodies are absent, as are the senile plaques and neurofibrillary tangles of Alzheimer's disease. FTD is thus a non-specific pathology. Neary and Snowden (1996) divide frontotemporal dementia into three subsyndromes: (1) a microvacuolation type; (2) a gliotic type, which is more or less synonymous with Pick's disease; and (3) a variety associated with motor neuron disease. In terms of behavior, Neary and colleagues (1998) provided a set of diagnostic features useful for diagnosing FTD. These are listed in Table 13.6.

Table 13.6 Features of frontotemporal dementia. (Reprinted with permission from D Neary, JS Snowden, L Gustafson *et al.* Frontotemporal lobar degeneration. A consensus on clinical diagnostic criteria. Neurology 1998;51:1546–1554)

I. *Core diagnostic features*
   A. Insidious onset, gradual progression
   B. Early decline in interpersonal conduct
   C. Early impairment in regulation of personal conduct
   D. Early emotional blunting
   E. Early loss of insight

II. *Supportive diagnostic features*
   A. Behavioral disorder
      1. Decline in personal hygiene and grooming
      2. Mental rigidity, inflexibility
      3. Distractibility, impersistence
      4. Hyperorality, dietary changes
      5. Perseverative and stereotyped behavior
      6. Utilization behavior
   B. Speech and language
      1. Altered speech output
         a. Aspontaneity and economy of speech
         b. Press of speech
      2. Stereotypy of speech
      3. Echolalia
      4. Perseveration
      5. Mutism
   C. Physical signs
      1. Primitive reflexes
      2. Incontinence
      3. Akinesia, rigidity, tremor
      4. Low and labile blood pressure
   D. Tests
      1. Frontal and/or temporal atrophy on MRI, PET

These deficits are all suggestive of focal, unilateral or bilateral frontal lobe degeneration, which is the hallmark of this disorder. Figure 13.8 shows a PET scan from a patient clinically diagnosed with this disorder. This patient presented with progressive language and naming difficulty, then became almost mute. Her behavior then progressively deteriorated; she became impatient, fidgety, and agitated and required nursing home placement. The PET scan showed very prominent hypometabolism in both frontal lobes.

Edwards-Lee and colleagues (1997) have also described a temporal variant of frontotemporal dementia. Patients with left temporal degeneration presented with progressive aphasia. Those with right temporal degeneration exhibited a variety of behavioral symptoms, including excessive religiosity, obsessive–compulsive tendencies such as searching for coins on the sidewalk, uninhibited behaviors such as changing

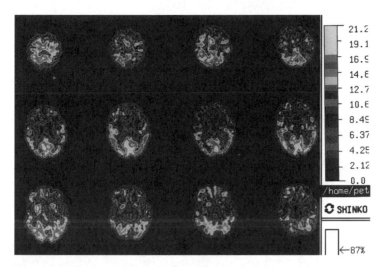

Figure 13.8 PET image showing prominent hypometabolism of glucose in both frontal lobes in a patient clinically diagnosed with frontotemporal dementia.

in public or shoplifting, sexual dysfunction or disinhibition, and alterations in eating. A few developed artistic expression not seen earlier in their lives. Changes in musical tastes have also been reported (Geroldi *et al.* 2000). These case descriptions appear to overlap with those of frontotemporal dementia and those with primary progressive aphasia (see below). MRI and functional brain imaging showed predominantly temporal lobe involvement. Perry and Hodges (2000) studied ten patients with the frontal variant of FTD and five with the temporal variant of FTD, separated by the pattern of atrophy on MRI. Patients with the frontal variant had impaired attention and executive functions, whereas patients with the temporal variant had preserved attention and executive function but severely impaired semantic memory. Patients with early AD also had impaired semantic and other memory functions, but preserved attention and executive function.

Neuropathology of PPA and FTD

The neuropathology underlying primary progressive aphasia and frontotemporal dementia is generally distinct from AD. At autopsy, patients with progressive aphasia have generally had non-Alzheimer's disease pathologies. A small number of cases of autopsy-proved Alzheimer's disease have been described with aphasia as the presenting symptom, but most such cases have had fluent aphasia (Green *et al.* 1990). Progressive, non-fluent aphasia has reliably identified cases with non-Alzheimer pathologies (Weintraub *et al.* 1990; Grossman *et al.* 1996). Cases of classical Pick's disease, a lobar atrophy with intraneuronal silver-staining inclusion bodies, have been described with progressive aphasia (Wechsler *et al.* 1982; Holland 1985; Graff-Radford *et al.* 1990). Kirshner and colleagues (1987) described two cases of progressive aphasia with non-specific changes of neuronal loss, gliosis, and spongiform change in focal areas of the left frontal and temporal lobes. Other cases with similar findings have been reported since then (Westbury and Bub 1997). A variation on this theme is progressive aphasia reported with corticobasal degeneration (Lippa *et al.* 1991). Chapter 16 contains a more complete description of corticobasal degeneration. The frontotemporal dementia literature also includes pathology of mostly the non-specific dementia type: neuronal loss in a localized, lobar pattern; gliosis; microvacuolation or 'spongiform change' of the neuropil (Mann *et al.* 1993; Neary and Snowden 1996). Kertesz *et al.* (1994, 2000) have attempted to unify all of these cases – Pick's disease, non-specific dementia, and corticobasal degeneration – under the term 'Pick complex'.

Molecular Genetics of PPA and FTD

Delineation of the disease processes associated with frontotemporal dementia and progressive aphasia would be greatly aided by genetic or biochemical markers. Recently, families with frontotemporal dementia have been reported with a genetic link to chromosome 17q21-q22, providing the first neurobiological correlate of this behaviorally defined syndrome (Heutink *et al.* 1997). The defective gene appears to affect the tau protein, leading to the new term 'tauopathies' for these conditions (Bird 1998). The family with 'hereditary dysphasic dementia' reported by Morris and colleagues also proved to have this gene locus (Lendon *et al.* 1998). Although tau protein is elevated in CSF in Alzheimer's disease patients, specific abnormalities of tau are more central to the pathological process in frontotemporal dementia. A recent study (Zhukareva *et al.* 2001) found reductions in the tau protein in the brains of patients with frontotemporal dementia; mRNA for tau was present, indicating post-transcriptional abnormality in the expression of the tau protein. Recently, a new gene locus has been discovered on Chromosome 9q for familial ALS associated with frontotemporal dementia (Hosler *et al.* 2000). The other biological marker that distinguishes frontotemporal dementia (or progressive aphasia) from Alzheimer's disease is the increased frequency of apolipoprotein E4 in Alzheimer's disease, which was not found in a series of progressive aphasia patients reported by Mesulam *et al.* (1997). In the future, advances in molecular biology and genetics are likely to permit much more specific diagnostic disease categories.

'Non-specific Dementia', or 'Dementia Lacking Specific Histological Features'

A few reported cases of dementia have shown cerebral atrophy without specific microscopic changes of either Alzheimer's or Pick's disease. Insufficient information is available to distinguish such cases on clinical grounds, except that they show the general clinical evolution of dementia. Such cases have been called atypical presenile dementia or Kraepelin's disease (Schaumburg and Suzuki 1968; Kim *et al.* 1981; Masse *et al.* 1981; Knopman *et al.* 1990). The chief pathological features are the absence of senile plaques, neurofibrillary tangles, and Pick bodies, and the presence of 'non-specific' findings of neuronal loss, gliosis, and spongi-form change in the cortex (Masse *et al.* 1981). Many of these cases, if studied in life, would likely be diagnosed as FTD or PPA. Cases of dementia and motor neu-ron disease (Wikstrom *et al.* 1982; Horoupian *et al.* 1984; Morita *et al.* 1987; Neary *et al.* 1990; Ferrer *et al.* 1991) also fit into this 'non-specific' pathological pattern. Again, most have a lobar pattern of atrophy. Generalized dementing ill-ness with non-specific dementia is rare and diagnosable only at autopsy.

PRACTICAL DIAGNOSIS OF THE DEMENTIAS

When considering the myriad of dementing diseases discussed in this chapter, the behavioral neurologist must have a practical approach to diagnose the common clinical syndromes of dementia. The first step, of course, is the verification of demen-tia, as opposed to the differential diagnoses of delirium, depression, or focal brain lesion. A careful history and physical examination, including the bedside mental sta-tus examination, are essential for this purpose. A careful history of medical symp-toms and diseases, medications, and toxic exposures is recorded. Screening laboratory tests (Table 13.7) should include electrolytes, calcium, liver and renal function tests, blood glucose, thyroid and adrenal function tests, serum vitamin B12 and folate levels, a serological test for syphilis, HIV testing when indicated, ESR, and ANA. Toxic screens for heavy metals, chemical toxins, and drugs are appropriate whenever these factors are suspected clinically. If central nervous system (CNS) infection is suspected, a lumbar puncture should be performed. Nearly all cases should have a CT or MRI scan; these anatomical studies serve to assess the degree of cortical atrophy and to exclude mass lesions and hydrocephalus.

Table 13.7 Laboratory tests for dementia

Tests indicated in all patients:
Electrolytes, calcium, glucose
Renal and hepatic function tests
Vitamin B12 and folate levels
Thyroid and adrenal function tests
Serological test for syphilis, HIV, Lyme
Erythrocyte sedimentation rate, antinuclear antibody
Chest X-ray
CT or MRI scan
EEG

Tests indicated in specific patients:
Toxic, drug screens
24-hour urine for heavy metals
Lumbar puncture
Specific investigations for symptomatic malignancy
Arteriography

The difficult issues of cerebrovascular disease and dementia are best clarified by a careful clinical history and examination, including the Hachinski index and review of the CT or MRI scan for evidence of infarcts. The 'subcortical' dementias are best evaluated clinically, by the combination of motor and cognitive changes. Normal pressure hydrocephalus is diagnosed by the clinical triad of dementia, gait disorder, and urinary incontinence, with confirmation of ventricular enlargement out of proportion to cortical atrophy on neuroradiological studies. Finally, the primary degenerative dementias, Alzheimer's and Pick's diseases, are diagnosed presumptively by the typical clinical evolution, absence of features of the other diseases, and normal laboratory tests except for the neuroradiological finding of cerebral atrophy. Apolipoprotein testing, tau protein in CSF, and neuronal thread protein may be helpful in increasing the likelihood of Alzheimer's disease. Functional brain imaging (PET or SPECT) is also helpful in both Alzheimer's disease and frontotemporal dementia. Definite diagnosis of these diseases requires microscopic pathology. Because brain biopsy is not considered justified by the availability of any specific treatment, the definitive diagnosis usually must await autopsy.

One additional laboratory procedure used routinely by many neurologists in the diagnosis of dementia is the EEG. Patients with Alzheimer's disease tend to show only minor abnormalities, if any, in the EEG, with mild slowing of the background rhythm and intermittent theta and delta activity in the later stages. Patients

Table 13.8   Treatable causes of dementia

Diseases simulating dementia
Depression
Mass lesion
   Tumor
   Subdural hematoma
   Abscess
Delirium
   Metabolic encephalopathy
   Toxic or drug-induced encephalopathy
   Miscellaneous (see Chapter 13)

Dementing diseases
Vitamin B12 deficiency
Endocrinopathies
   Hypothyroidism
   Hyperthyroidism
   Cushing's syndrome
   Hyperparathyroidism
Infections
   Chronic meningitis
   Syphilis
   Cysticercosis
Normal pressure hydrocephalus

with metabolic, toxic, or infectious encephalopathies, on the other hand, typically show profound EEG slowing (Harner 1975). Most of the treatable dementias are more likely to have prominent slowing on EEG than the degenerative dementias.

When both the clinical course, including the NINCDS/ADRDA criteria, and laboratory tests are consistent with a diagnosis of a degenerative dementia, the clinical diagnosis is 'presumed Alzheimer's disease'. As mentioned above, this diagnosis accurately predicts a pathological diagnosis of AD at autopsy. Alzheimer's disease and senile dementia of the Alzheimer type together account for over 50% of all cases of dementia. Table 13.8 lists the treatable causes of dementia. Unfortunately, treatable causes are found in only 15–30% of cases of dementia, and in many fewer of the patients who meet clinical criteria for presumed AD (Piccini *et al.* 1998).

CONCLUSION

The dementias are a complex group of disorders, all having in common the progressive dysfunction of multiple areas of the cerebral neocortex. This chapter is the most expanded topic from the first edition of this book, largely because of advances in the clinical description, neuroimaging, and basic neurochemistry of these diseases. No subject in behavioral neurology has witnessed a greater advance in basic science knowledge. Alzheimer's disease, especially, is a public health problem of major proportions, and one in which a treatment breakthrough is sorely needed.

REFERENCES

Adams RD, Fisher CM, Hakim S, Sweet WH. Symptomatic occult hydrocephalus with 'normal' cerebrospinal fluid pressure: a treatable syndrome. N Engl J Med 1965; 273:117–126.

Aksamit AJ Jr, Preissner CM, Homburger HA. Quantitation of 14-3-3 and neuron-specific enolase proteins in CSF in Creutzfeldt–Jakob disease. Neurology 2001;57: 728–730.

Albert ML. Language in normal and dementing elderly. In LK Obler, ML Albert (eds), Language and Communication in the Elderly: Clinical, Therapeutic, and Experimental Issues. Lexington: DC Heath, 1980;145–150.

Albert ML, Feldman RG, Willis AL. The 'subcortical dementia' of progressive supranuclear palsy. J Neurol Neurosurg Psychiatry 1974;37:121–130.

Alfrey AC, LeGendre GR, Kaehny WD. The dialysis encephalopathy syndrome: possible aluminum intoxication. N Engl J Med 1976:294:184–188.

Alter M. How is Creutzfeldt–Jakob disease acquired? Neuroepidemiology 2000;19:55–61.

Alzheimer A. A unique illness involving the cerebral cortex. In DA Rottenberg, FH Hochberg (eds), Neurological Classics in Modern Translation. New York: Hafner, 1977;41–43 (originally published 1907).

Anderson RM, Donnelly CA, Ferguson NM *et al.* Transmission dynamics and epidemiology of BSE in cattle. Nature 1996;382:779–788.

Andreasen N, Minthon L, Davidsson P *et al.* Evaluation of CSF-tau and CSF-A-B42 as diagnostic markers for Alzheimer disease in clinical practice. Arch Neurol 2001;58: 373–379.

Appell J, Kertesz A, Fisman M. Language functioning in Alzheimer's disease. Brain Lang 1982;17:73–91.

Arai H, Clark CM, Ewbank DC *et al*. Cerebrospinal fluid tau protein as a potential diagnostic marker in Alzheimer's disease. Neurobiol Aging 1998;19:125–126.

Awad IA, Spetzler RF, Hodak JA *et al*. Incidental subcortical lesions identified on magnetic resonance imaging in the elderly. I. Correlation with age and cerebrovascular risk factors. Stroke 1986;17:1084–1089.

Babikian V, Ropper AH. Binswanger's disease: a review. Stroke 1987;18:1–12.

Bales KR, Verina T, Dodel RC *et al*. Lack of apolipoportein E dramatically reduces amyloid beta-peptide deposition. Nat Genet 1997;17:263–264.

Barbizet J, Degos JD, Lejeune A, Leroy A. Syndrome de dysconnection inter-hemispherique avec dyspraxie diagnostique au cours d'une maladie de Marchiafave-Bignami. Rev Neurol (Paris) 1978;134:781–789.

Baskin F, Rosenberg RN, Iyer L *et al*. Platelet APP isoform ratios correlate with declining cognition in AD. Neurology 2000;54:1907–1909.

Bazner HA, Hennerici MG. What was the reason for Joseph Haydn's mental decline and gait disturbance? A case of subcortical vascular encephalopathy in the early 19th century. Cerebrovasc Dis 1997;7:359–366.

Beal MF, Williams RS, Richardson EP, Fisher CM. Cholesterol embolism as a cause of transient ischemic attacks and cerebral infarction. Neurology 1981;31:860–865.

Bennett RM, Bong DM, Spargo BH. Neuropsychiatric problems in mixed connective tissue disease. Am J Med 1978;65:955–962.

Benson DF, LeMay M, Patten DH, Rubens AB. Diagnosis of normal pressure hydrocephalus. N Engl J Med 1970;283:609–615.

Benson DF, Cummings JC, Tsai SI. Angular gyrus syndrome simulating Alzheimer's disease. Arch Neurol 1982;39:616–620.

Benson DF, Kuhl DE, Hawkins RA *et al*. The fluorodeoxyglucose 18F scan in Alzheimer's disease and multi-infarct dementia. Arch Neurol 1983;40:711–714.

Benzel EC, Pelletier AL, Levy PG. Communicating hydrocephalus in adults: prediction of outcome after ventricular shunting procedures. Neurosurgery 1990;26:655–660.

Berchtold NC, Cotman CW. Evolution in the conceptualization of dementia and Alzheimer's disease: Greco-Roman period to the 1960s. Neurobiol Aging 1998;19: 173–189.

Bird, JM. Computerized tomography, atrophy and dementia: a review. Prog Neurobiol 1982;19:91–115.

Bird TD. Genotypes, phenotypes, and frontotemporal dementia. Neurology 1998;50: 1526–1527.

Black, PMcL. Idiopathic normal-pressure hydrocephalus: results of shunting in 62 patients. J Neurosurg 1980;52:371–377.

Blesa R, Mohr E, Miletich RS *et al*. Cerebral metabolic changes in Alzheimer's disease: neurobehavioral patterns. Dementia 1996;7:239–245.

Blessed G, Tomlinson BE, Roth M. The association between quantitative measures of dementia and of senile change in the cerebral grey matter of elderly subjects. Br J Psychiatry 1968;114:797–811.

Bluestein HG. Neuropsychiatric manifestations of systemic lupus erythematosus. New Engl J Med 1987;317:309–310.

Bondareff W, Baldy R, Levy R. Quantitative computed tomography in senile dementia. Arch Gen Psychiatry 1981;38:1365–1368.

Bondareff W, Raval J, Woo B *et al*. Magnetic resonance imaging and the severity of dementia in older adults. Arch Gen Psychiatry 1990;47:47–51.

Bonfa E, Golombek SJJ, Kaufman LD *et al*. Association between lupus psychosis and anti-ribosomal p protein antibodies. N Engl J Med 1987;317:265–271.

Bonte FJ, Tintner R, Weiner MF *et al*. Brain blood flow in the dementias: SPECT with histopathologic correlation. Radiology 1993;186:361–365.

Bonza E, Dreyer IS, Hewitt WL, Meyer RD. Coccidioidal meningitis. Medicine (Baltimore) 1981;60:139–172.

Boon AJW, Tans JTJ, Delwel EJ *et al*. Dutch normal-pressure hydrocephalus study: prediction of outcome after shunting by resistance to outflow of cerebrospinal fluid. J Neurosurg 1997;87:687–693.

Bouwman FH, Skolasky RL, Hes D *et al*. Variable progression of HIV-associated dementia. Neurology 1998;50:1814–1820.

Bradley WG. Normal pressure hydrocephalus: new concepts on etiology and diagnosis. AJNR 2000;21:1586–1590.

Bradley WG, Waluch V, Brant-Zawadski M *et al*. Periventricular white matter lesions in the elderly: a common observation during NMR imaging. Noninvas Med Imag 1984;1:35–41.

Bradshaw JR, Thomson JLG, Campbell MJ. Computed tomography in the investigation of dementia. Br Med J 1983;286:277–280.

Brain R, Henson RA. Neurological syndromes associated with carcinoma. Lancet 1958; 2:971–975.

Breitner JCS. Clinical genetics and genetic counseling in Alzheimer disease. Ann Int Med 1991;115:601–606.

Breitner JC. The role of anti-inflammatory drugs in the prevention and treatment of Alzheimer's disease. Annu Rev Med 1996;47:401–411.

Brinkman SD, Largen JW. Changes in brain ventricular size with repeated CAT scans in suspected Alzheimer's disease. Am J Psychiatry 1984;141:81–83.

Brown P, Gibbs CJ, Amyx HL *et al*. Chemical disinfection of Creutzfeldt–Jakob virus. N Eng J Med 1982;306:1279–1282.

Brown P, Kaur P, Sulima MP *et al*. Real and imagined clinicopathological limits of 'prion dementia'. Lancet 1993;341:127–129.

Burke DM, McKay DG. Memory, language, and aging. Phil Trans R Soc London B 1997;352:1845–1856.

Burns A, Rossor M, Hecker J *et al*. The effects of donepezil in Alzheimer's disease – results from a multinational trial. Dement Geriatr Cogn Disord 1999;10:237–244.

Candy JM, Perry RH, Perry EK *et al*. Pathological changes in the nucleus of Meynert in Alzheimer's and Parkinson's disease. J Neurol Sci 1983;54:277–289.

Caplan LR, Schoene WC. Clinical features of subcortical arteriosclerotic encephalopathy (Binswanger disease). Neurology 1978;28:1206–1215.

Carlen PL, Wilkinson A, Wortzman G *et al*. Cerebral atrophy and functional deficits in alcoholics without clinically apparent liver disease. Neurology (NY) 1981;31:377–385.

Caselli RJ, Hunder GG, Whisnant JP. Neurologic disease in biopsy-proven giant cell (temporal) arteritis. Neurology 1988;38:352–359.

Chan D, Fox NC, Scahill RI *et al*. Patterns of temporal lobe atrophy in semantic dementia and Alzheimer's disease. Ann Neurol 2001;49:433–442.

Chen P, Ratcliff G, Bnelle SH *et al*. Cognitive tests that best discriminate between presymptomatic AD and those who remain undemented. Neurology 2000;55:1847–1853.

Chui HC, Victoroff JI, Margolin D *et al*. Criteria for the diagnosis of ischemic vascular dementia proposed by the State of California Alzheimer's Disease Diagnostic and Treatment Centers. Neurology 1992;42:473–480.

Class CA, Schneider L, Farlow MR. Optimal management of behavioural disorders associated with dementia. Drugs Aging 1997;10:95–106.

Cochran JW, Fox JH, Kelly MB. Reversible mental symptoms in temporal arteritis. J Nerv Ment Dis 1978;166:446–447.

Cockburn J, Smith PT. The relative influence of intelligence and age on everyday memory. J Geront 1991;46:31–36.

Cogan MG, Covey CM, Arieff AI *et al*. Central nervous system manifestations of hyperparathyroidism. Am J Med 1978;65:963–970.

Cohen D, Eisdorfer C, Gorelick P et al. Psychopathology associated with Alzheimer's disease and related disorders. J Geront Med Sci 1993;48:M255–M260.

Corey-Bloom J, Anand R, Veach J. A randomized trial evaluating the efficacy and safety of ENA 713 (rivastigmine tartrate). A new acetylcholinesterase inhibitor, in patients with mild to moderately severe Alzheimer's disease. J Geriatr Psychopharmacol 1998; 1:55–65.

Corsellis JAN, Goldberg GJ, Norton, AR. 'Limbic encephalitis' and its association with carcinoma. Brain 1968;91:481–496.

Crapper DR, Quittkat S, Krishnan SS et al. Intranuclear aluminum content in Alzheimer's disease, dialysis encephalopathy, and experimental aluminum encephalopathy. Acta Neuropathol (Berl) 1980;50:19–24.

Critchley M. The neurology of psychotic speech. Br J Psychiatry 1964;110:353–364.

Crystal HA, Horoupian DS, Katzman R, Jotkowitz S. Biopsy proved Alzheimer disease presenting as a right parietal lobe syndrome. Ann Neurol 1982;12:186–188.

Cullum CM, Rosenberg RN. Memory loss – when is it Alzheimer disease? JAMA 1998;279:1689–1690.

Cummings JL, Benson DF. Subcortical dementia: review of an emerging concept. Arch Neurol 1984;41:874–879.

Cummings JL, Benson DF, Hill MA, Read S. Aphasia in dementia of the Alzheimer type. Neurology 1985;35:394–397.

Damasio H, Eslinger P, Damasio AR et al. Quantitative computed tomographic analysis in the diagnosis of dementia. Arch Neurol 1983;40:715–719.

Danes P. Neurotransmitter-related enzymes in senile dementia of the Alzheimer type. Brain Res 1979;138:385–392.

DeCarli C, Murphy DGM, McIntosh AR et al. Discriminant analysis of MRI measures as a method to determine the presence of dementia of the Alzheimer type. Psychiatry Res 1995;57:119–130.

DeGirolami V, Haas ML, Richardson EP Jr. Subacute diencephalic angioencephalopathy: a clinicopathological case study. J Neurol Sci 1974;22:197–210.

de la Monte SM, Ghanbari K, Grey WH et al. Characterization of the AD7C-NTP cDNA expression in Alzheimer's disease and measurement of a 41-kD protein in cerebrospinal fluid. J Clin Invest 1997;100:3093–3104.

Delaney P. Neurologic manifestations in sarcoidosis: review of the literature, with report of 23 cases. Ann Intern Med 1977;87:336–345.

DeLong GR, Richardson EP Jr. Case records of the Massachusetts General Hospital. N Engl J Med 1982;306:286–293.

Dewberry FL, McKinney TD, Stone WJ. The dialysis dementia syndrome: report of fourteen cases and review of the literature. Am Soc Artif Intern Organs J 1980;3:102–108.

Dichgans M, Mayer M, Uttner I et al. The phenotypic spectrum of CADASIL: clinical findings in 102 cases. Neurology 1998;44:731–739.

Drachman DA. Neurological complications of Wegener's granulomatosus. Arch Neurol 1963;8:145–155.

Drachman DA, Leber P. Treatment of Alzheimer's disease – searching for a breakthrough, settling for less. New Engl J Med 1997;336:1245–1247.

Ellner JJ, Bennett JE. Chronic meningitis. Medicine (Baltimore) 1976;55:341–369.

Englund E, Brun A, Alling C. White matter changes in dementia of Alzheimer's type. Brain 1988;111:1425–1439.

Erkinjuntti T, Sipponen JT, Iivanainen M et al. Cerebral NMR and CT imaging in dementia. J Comput Assist Tomogr 1984;8:614–618.

Ernst RL, Hay JW. The US economic and social costs of Alzheimer's disease revisited. Am J Public Health 1994;84:1261–1264.

Fein G, Van Dyke C, Davenport L et al. Preservation of normal cognitive functioning in elderly subjects with extensive white-matter lesions of long duration. Arch Gen Psychaatry 1990;47:220–223.

Ferm L. Behavioral activities in demented geriatric patients. Gerontol Clin 1974;16: 185–194.

Ferrer I, Roig C, Espino A *et al.* Dementia of frontal lobe type and motor neuron disease. A Golgi study of the frontal cortex. J Neurol Neurosurg Psychiatry 1991;54:932–934.

Fieschi C, Rasura M, Anzini A, Beccia. Central nervous system vasculitis. J Neurol Sci 1998;153:159–171.

Fisher CM. Lacunes: small, deep cerebral infarcts. Neurology 1965;15:774–784.

Flynn BL, Theesen KA. Pharmacologic management of Alzheimer disease Part III: nonsteroidal anti-inflammatory drugs – emerging protective evidence? Ann Pharmacother 1999;33:840–849.

Folstein MF, Breitner JCS. Language disorder predicts familial Alzheimer's disease. John Hopkins Med J 1981;149:145–147.

Ford RG, Siekert RG. Central nervous system manifestations of periarteritis nodosa. Neurology 1965;15:114–122.

Foster NL, Chase TN, Fedio P *et al.* Alzheimer's disease: focal cortical changes shown by positron emission tomography. Neurology 1983;33:961–954.

Freeman JM: The clinical spectrum and early diagnosis of Dawson's encephalitis. J Pediatr 1969;75:590–603.

Freemon FR. Evaluation of patients with progressive intellectual deterioration. Arch Neurol 1976;33:658–659.

Friedland RP, Budinger TF, Brant-Zawadzki M, Jagust WJ. The diagnosis of Alzheimer-type dementia: a preliminary comparison of positron emission tomography and proton magnetic resonance. JAMA 1984;252:2750–2752.

Gajdusek DC, Gibbs CJ, Alpers M. Experimental transmission of a kuru-like syndrome to chimpanzees. Nature 1966;209:794–796.

Gaudino EA, Coyle PK, Krupp LB. Post-Lyme syndrome and chronic fatigue syndrome. Neuropsychiatric similarities and differences. Arch Neurol 1997;54:1372–1376.

George AE, deLeon MJ, Rosenbloom S *et al.* Ventricular volume and cognitive deficit: a computed tomographic study. Radiology 1983;149:493–498.

Geroldi E, Metitieri T, Binetti G *et al.* Pop music and frontotemporal dementia. Neurology 2000;55:1935–1936.

Ghanbari H, Ghanbari K, Beheshti I *et al.* Biochemical assay for AD7-C-NTP in urine as an Alzheimer's disease marker. J Clin Lab Anal 1998;12:285–288.

Go RCP, Todorov AB, Elston RC, Constantinidis I. The malignancy of dementias. Ann Neurol 1978;3:559–561.

Gold G, Giannakopoulos P, Bouras C. Re-evaluating the role of vascular changes in the differential diagnosis of Alzheimer's disease and vascular dementia. Eur Neurol 1998;40:121–129.

Goldman WP, Price JL, Storandt M *et al.* Absence of cognitive impairment or decline in preclinical Alzheimer's disease. Neurology 2001;56:361–367.

Gomez-Tortosa E, del Barrio A, Jimenez-Alfaro I. Pupil response to tropicamide in Alzheimer's disease and other neurodegenerative disorders. Acta Neurol Scand 1996;94:104–109.

Gorelick PB, Erkinjuntti T, Hofman A *et al.* Prevention of vascular dementia. Alzheimer Disease Associated Disorders 1999;13(Suppl. 3):S131–S139.

Graff-Radford NR, Damasio AR, Hyman BT *et al.* Progressive aphasia in a patient with Pick's disease: a neuropsychological, radiologic, and anatomic study. Neurology 1990; 40:620–626.

Graff-Radford NR, Lin S-C, Brazis PW *et al.* Tropicamide eyedrops cannot be used for reliable diagnosis of Alzheimer's disease. Mayo Clin Proc 1997;72:495–504.

Green J, Morris JC, Sandson J *et al.* Progressive aphasia; a precursor of global dementia? Neurology 1990;40:423–429.

Greenberg SM. Cerebral amyloid angiopathy: prospects for clinical diagnosis and treatment. Neurology 1998;51:690–694.

Greenberg JO, Shenkin HA, Adam R: Idiopathic normal-pressure hydrocephalus – a report of 73 patients. J Neurol Neurosurg Psychiatry 1977;40:336–341.

Groen JJ, Endtz LJ. Hereditary Pick's disease. Brain 1982;105:443–459.

Grossman M, Mickanin J, Onishi K et al. Progressive non-fluent aphasia: language, cognitive, and PET measures contrasted with probable Alzheimer's disease. J Cog Neurosci 1996;8:135–154.

Haase GR. Diseases presenting as dementia. In CE Wells (ed.), Dementia (2nd edn). Philadelphia: FA Davis, 1977;27–67.

Hachinski VC, Lassen NA, Marshall J. Multi-infarct dementia: a cause of mental deterioration in the elderly. Lancet 1974;3:207–210.

Hachinski VC, Iliff LD, Zilkha E et al. Cerebral blood flow in dementia. Arch Neurol 1975;32:632–637.

Hachinski VC, Potter P, Merskey H. Leuko-araiosis. Arch Neurol 1987;44:21–23.

Hanninen T, Soininen H. Age-associated memory impairment. Normal aging or warning of dementia? Drugs Aging 1997;11:480–489.

Harner RH. EEG evaluation of the patient with dementia. In DF Benson, D Blumer (eds), Psychiatric Aspects of Neurologic Disease. New York: Grune & Stratton, 1975;63–82.

Harrington CR, Wischik CM, McArthur FK et al. Alzheimer's disease-like changes in tau protein processing; association with aluminium accumulation in brains of renal dialysis patients. Lancet 1994;343:993–997.

Henon H, Lebert F, Durieu I et al. Confusional state in stroke. Relation to pre-existing dementia, patient characteristics, and outcome. Stroke 1999;30:773–779.

Hershey LA, Modic MT, Greenough PG, Jaffe DF. Magnetic resonance imaging in vascular dementia. Neurology 1987;37:29–36.

Heston LL, Mastri AR, Anderson VE, White J. Dementia of the Alzheimer type. Arch Gen Psychiatry 1981;38:1085–1090.

Heutink P, Stevens M, Rizzu P et al. Hereditary frontotemporal dementia is linked to Chromosome 17q21-q22: a genetic and clinicopathological study of three Dutch families. Ann Neurol 1997;41:150–159.

Heyman A, Wilkinson WE, Stafford JA et al. Alzheimer's disease: a study of epidemiological aspects. Ann Neurol 1984;15:335–341.

Hierons, R, Janota I, Corsellis JAN. The late effects of necrotizing encephalitis of the temporal lobes and limbic areas: a clinico-pathological study of 10 cases. Psychol Med 1978;8:21–42.

Hochberg FH, Slotnick B. Neuropsychologic impairment in astrocytoma survivors. Neurology 1980;30:172–177.

Hodges JR, Patterson K, Oxbury S, Funnell E. Semantic dementia. Progressive fluent aphasia with temporal lobe atrophy. Brain 1992;115:1783–1806.

Holcomb L, Gordon MN, McGowan E et al. Accelerated Alzheimer-type phenotype in transgenic mice carrying both mutant amyloid precursor protein and presenilin 1 transgenes. Nature Med 1998;4:97–100.

Holland AL, McBurney DH, Moosy J, Reinmuth OM. The dissolution of language in Pick's disease with neurofibrillary tangles: a case study. Brain Lang 1985;24:36–58.

Hollenhorst RW, Brown JR, Wagener HP, Shick RM. Neurologic aspects of temporal arteritis. Neurology 1960;10:490–498.

Hooshmand H, Escobar MR, Kopf SW. Neurosyphilis: a study of 241 patients. JAMA 1972;219:726–729.

Horoupian DS, Thal L, Katzman R et al. Dementia and motor neuron disease: morphometric, biochemical, and Golgi studies. Ann Neurol 1984;16:305–313.

Hosler BA. Linkage of familial amyotrophic lateral sclerosis with frontotemporal dementia to Chromosome 9q21-q22. JAMA 2000;284:1664–1669.

Hsaio K, Chapman P, Nilsen S et al. Correlative memory deficits, AB elevation, and myeloid plaques in transgenic mice. Science 1996;274:99–102.

Hsich G, Kenney K, Gibbs CJ *et al*. The 14-3-3 brain protein in cerebrospinal fluid as a marker for transmissible spongiform encephalopathies. N Engl J Med 1996;335:924–930.

Hurwitz TA, Ammann W, Chu D *et al*. Single photon emission computed tomography using ^{99m}Tc-HM-PAO in the routine evaluation of Alzheimer's disease. Can J Neurol Sci 1991;18:59–62.

Ironside R, Bosanquet FD, McMenemey WH. Central demyelination of the corpus callosum (Marchiafava–Bignami disease). Brain 1961;84:212–233.

Jacobs L, Kinkel W. Computerized axial tomography in normal pressure hydrocephalus. Neurology 1976;26:501–507.

James AE, Deland FH, Hodges FJ, Wagner HN. Normal-pressure hydrocephalus: role of cisternography in diagnosis. JAMA 1970;213:1615–1622.

Jick H, Zornberg GL, Jick SS *et al*. Statins and the risk of dementia. Lancet 2000;356:1627–1631.

Joachim CL, Morris JH, Selkoe DJ. Clinically diagnosed Alzheimer's disease: autopsy results in 150 cases. Ann Neurol 1988;24:50–56.

Jobst KA, Smith AD, Szatmari M *et al*. Detection in life of confirmed Alzheimer's disease using a simple measurement of medial temporal lobe atrophy by computed tomography. Lancet 1992;340:1179–1183.

Johns DR, Tierney M, Felsenstein D. Alteration in the natural history of neurosyphilis by concurrent infection with the human immunodeficiency virus. New Engl J Med 1987;316:1569–1572.

Johnson RT, Gibbs CJ Jr. Creutzfeldt–Jakob disease and related transmissible spongiform encephalopathies. New Engl J Med 1998;339:1994–2004.

Johnson RT, Richardson EP. The neurological manifestations of systemic lupus erythematosus. Medicine (Baltimore) 1968;47:337–369.

Jones BN, Reifler BV. Depression coexisting with dementia. Evaluation and treatment. Med Clin NA 1994;78:823–840.

Kaplan RS, Wiernik PH. Neurotoxicity of antineoplastic drugs. Semin Oncol 1982; 9:103–130.

Katzman R. The prevalence and malignancy of Alzheimer disease: a major killer. Arch Neurol 1976;33:217–218.

Katzman R, Terry RD. Normal aging of the nervous system. In R Katzman, RD Terry (eds), The Neurology of Aging. Philadelphia: FA Davis, 1983;15–50.

Keilp JG, Alexander GE, Stern Y, Prohovnik I. Inferior parietal perfusion, lateralization, and neuropsychological dysfunction in Alzheimer's disease. Brain Cogn 1996; 32:365–383.

Kennedy DH, Fallon RJ. Tuberculous meningitis. JAMA 1979;241:264–268.

Kertesz A, Polk M, Carr T. Cognition and white matter changes on magnetic resonance imaging in dementia. Arch Neurol 1990;47:387–391.

Kertesz A, Hudson L, MacKenzie I. The pathology and nosology of primary progressive aphasia. Neurology 1994;44:2065–2072.

Kertesz A, Martinez-Lage P, Davidson W, Munoz DG. The corticobasal degeneration syndrome overlaps progressive aphasia and frontotemporal dementia. Neurology 2000;55:1368–1375.

Kiloh LG. Pseudodementia. Acta Psychiatr Scand 1961;37:336–351.

Kim RC, Collins GH, Parisi JE *et al*. Familial dementia of adult onset with pathological findings of a 'non-specific' nature. Brain 1981;104:61–78.

Kirk A, Kertesz A, Polk MJI. Dementia with leukoencephalopathy in systemic lupus erythematosus. Can J Neurol Sci 1991;18:344–348.

Kirshner, HS. Language disorders in dementia. In HS Kirshner, FR Freemon (eds), The Neurology of Aphasia. Amsterdam: Swets, 1982;187–196.

Kirshner HS, Webb WG, Kelly MP. The naming disorder of dementia. Neuropsychologia 1984a;22:23–30.

Kirshner HS, Webb WG, Kelly MP, Wells CE. Language disturbance: an initial symptom of cortical degenerations and dementia. Arch Neurol 1984b;491–496.

Kirshner HS, Tanridag O, Thurman L, Whetsell WO Jr. Progressive aphasia without dementia: two cases with focal spongiform degeneration. Ann Neurol 1987;22:527–532.

Knapp MJ, Knopman DS, Solomon PR et al. A 30-week randomized controlled trial of high-dose tacrine in patients with Alzheimer's disease. JAMA 1994;271:985–991.

Knopman DS, Mastri AR, Frey WH et al. Dementia lacking distinctive histologic features: a common non-Alzheimer degenerative dementia. Neurology 1990;40:251–256.

Knopman D, Schnieder L, Davis K et al. Long-term tacrine (Cognex) treatment: effects on nursing home placement and mortality. Neurology 1996;47:166–177.

Knopman D, Boland LL, Mosley T et al., for the Atherosclerosis Risk in Communities (ARIC) study investigators. Cardiovascular risk factors and cognitive decline in middle-aged adults. Neurology 2001;56:42–48.

Knopman DS, DeKosky ST, Cummings JL et al. Practice parameter: Diagnosis of dementia (an evidence-based review). Report of the Quality Standards Subcommittee of the American Academy of Neurology. Neurology 2001;56:1143–1153.

Koller WC, Wilson RS, Glatt SL, Fox JH. Motor signs are infrequent in dementia of the Alzheimer type. Ann Neurol 1984;16:514–516.

Kolodny EH, Rebeiz JJ, Caviness VS, Richardson EP. Granulomatous angiitis of the central nervous system. Arch Neurol 1968;19:510–524.

Kraemer HC, Taylor JL, Tinklenberg JR, Yesavage JA. The stages of Alzheimer's disease: a reappraisal. Dement Geriatr Cogn Disord 1998;9:299–308.

Kral VA. Senescent forgetfulness: benign and malignant. Can Med Assoc J 1962; 86:257–260.

Krauss JK, Droste DW, Vach W et al. Cerebrospinal fluid shunting in idiopathic normal-pressure hydrocephalus of the elderly: effect of periventricular and deep white matter lesions. Neurosurgery 1996;39:292–300.

Ladurner G, Iliff LD, Lechner H. Clinical factors associated with dementia in ischemic stroke. J Neurol Neurosurg Psychiatry 1982;45:97–101.

Laffey PA, Peyster RG, Nathan JR et al. Computed tomography and aging: results in a normal elderly population. Neuroradiology 1984;26:273–278.

Larbrisseau A, Maravi E, Aguilera F, Martinez-Lage JM. The neurological complications of brucellosis. Can J Neurol Sci 1978;5:369–376.

Larsson A, Wikkelso C, Bilting M, Stephensen H. Clinical parameters in 74 consecutive patients shunt operated for normal pressure hydrocephalus. Acta Neurol Scand 1991;84:475–482.

Laws ER, Mokri B. Occult hydrocephalus: results of shunting correlated with diagnostic tests. Clin Neurosurg 1977;24:316–333.

Leary MC, Saver JL. Incidence of silent stroke in the United States. Poster presented at the 26th American Heart Association Stroke Meetings, Fort Lauderdale, Florida, February 2001.

Le Bars PL, Katz MM, Berman N et al. A placebo-controlled, double-blind, randomized trial of an extract of Ginkgo biloba for dementia. JAMA 1997;278:1327–1332.

Lederman RJ, Henry CE. Progressive dialysis encephalopathy. Ann Neurol 1978; 4:199–204.

Lendon CL, Ashall F, Goate AM. Exploring the etiology of Alzheimer disease using molecular genetics. JAMA 1997;277:825–831.

Lendon CL, Lynch T, Norton J et al. Hereditary dysphasic disinhibition dementia: a frontotemporal dementia linked to 17q21-22. Neurology 1998;50:1526–1527.

Lewis JL, Rabinovich S. The wide spectrum of cryptococcal infections. Am J Med 1972; 53:315–322.

Lian EC-Y. Thrombotic thrombocytopenic purpura. Ann Rev Med 1988;39:203–212.

Lippa CF, Cohen R, Smith TW, Drachman DA. Primary progressive aphasia with focal neuronal achromasia. Neurology 1991;41:882–886.

Lopez OL, Becker JT, Somsak D *et al*. Awareness of cognitive deficits and anosognosia in probable Alzheimer's disease. Eur Neurol 1994;34:277–282.

Loupe DN, Newman NJ, Green RC *et al*. Pupillary response to tropicamide in patients with Alzheimer disease. Ophthalmology 1996;103:495–503.

Luxon L, Lees AJ, Greenwood RJ. Neurosyphilis today. Lancet 1979;1:90–93.

Ma J, Tee A, Brewer HB Jr *et al*. Amyloid-associated proteins alpha 1-antichymotrypsin and apolipoprotein E promote assembly of Alzheimer beta-protein into filaments. Nature 1994;375:92–94.

Madison DP, Baehr ET, Bazell M *et al*. Communicative and cognitive deterioration in dialysis dementia: two case studies. J Speech Hearing Disord 1977;42:238–246.

Maj M, Satz P, Janssen R *et al*. WHO neuropsychiatric AIDS study, Cross-sectional Phase II. Neuropsychological and neurological findings. Arch Gen Psychiatry 1994;51:51–61.

Malm J, Kristensen B, Stegmayr B *et al*. Three-year survival and functional outcome of patients with idiopathic adult hydrocephalus syndrome. Neurology 2000;55:576–578.

Masse G, Mikol J, Brion S. Atypical presenile dementia: report of an anatomo-clinical case and review of the literature. J Neurol Sci 1981;52:245–267.

Masters CL, Harris JO, Gajdusek DC *et al*. Creutzfeldt–Jakob disease: patterns of worldwide occurrence and the significance of familial and sporadic clustering. Ann Neurol 1979;5:177–188.

Mauch E, Volk C, Krapf H *et al*. Neurological and neuropsychiatric dysfunction in primary Sjogren's syndrome. Acta Neurol Scand 1994;89:31–35.

Mayeux R, Sano M. Treatment of Alzheimer's disease. New Engl J Med 1999; 341:1670–1679.

Mayeux R, Stern Y, Rosen I, Benson DF. Is 'subcortical dementia' a recognizable clinical entity? Ann Neurol 1983;14:278–283.

Mayeux R, Saunders AM, Shea S *et al*. Utility of the apolipoprotein E genotype in the diagnosis of Alzheimer's disease. N Engl J Med 1998;338:506–511.

McAllister TW. Overview: pseudodementia. Am J Psychiatry 1983;140:528.

McCormick GF, Zee CS, Heiden I. Cysticercosis cerebri: review of 127 cases. Arch Neurol 1982;39:534–539.

McGeachie RE, Fleming JO, Sharer LR, Hyman RA. Diagnosis of Pick's disease by computed tomography. J Comput Asst Tomogr 1979;3:113–115.

McKhann G, Drachman D, Folstein M *et al*. Clinical diagnosis of Alzheimer's disease: report of the NINCDS–ADRDA Work Group under the auspices of the Department of Health and Human Services Task Force on Alzheimer's Disease. Neurology 1984; 34:939–944.

McPherson SE, Cummings JL. Neuropsychological aspects of vascular dementia. Brain and Cognition 1996;31:269–282.

Mehta KM, Ott A, Kalmijn S *et al*. Head trauma and risk of dementia and AD: The Rotterdam Study. Neurology 1999;53:1959–1962.

Mesulam M-M. Slowly progressive aphasia without generalized dementia. Ann Neurol 1982;11:592–598.

Mesulam M-M, Johnson N, Grujic Z, Weintraub S. Apolipoprotein E genotypes in primary progressive aphasia. Neurology 1997;49:51–55.

Mielke R, Pietrzyk U, Jacobs A *et al*. Eur J Nucl Med 1994;21:1052–1060.

Mohr JP. Lacunes. Stroke 1982;13:3–10.

Molsa PK, Marttila RJ, Rinne, UK. Extrapyramidal signs in Alzheimer's disease. Neurology 1984;34:1114–1116.

Moore PM. Diagnosis and management of isolated angiitis of the central nervous system. Neurology 1989;39:167–173.

Moore PM, Cupps TR. Neurological complications of vasculitis. Ann Neurol 1983;14:155–167.

Moore PM, Richardson B. Neurology of the vasculitides and connective tissue diseases. J Neurol Neurosurg Psychiatry 1998;65:10–22.

Morita K, Kaiya H, Ikeda T, Namba M. Presenile dementia combined with amyotrophy: a review of 34 Japanese cases. Arch Gerontol Geriatr 1987;6:263–277.

Morris JC, Cole M, Banker BQ, Wright D. Hereditary dysphasic dementia and the Pick–Alzheimer spectrum. Ann Neurol 1984;16:455–466.

Morris JC, McKeel DW, Fulling K et al. Validation of clinical diagnostic criteria for Alzheimer's disease. Ann Neurol 1988;24:17–22.

Morris JC, Storandt M, Miller JP et al. Mild cognitive impairment represents early-stage Alzheimer disease. Arch Neurol 2001;58:397–405.

Moser DJ, Cohen RA, Paul RH et al. Executive function and magnetic resonance imaging subcortical hyperintensities in vascular dementia. Neuropsychiatry, Neuropsychology, and Behavioral Neurology 2001;14:89–92.

Mulnard RA, Cotman CW, Kawas C et al. Estrogen replacement therapy for treatment of mild to moderate Alzheimer disease: a randomized controlled trial. Alzheimer's Disease Cooperative Study. JAMA 2000;283:1007–1115.

Naeser MA, Gebhardt C, Levine HL. Decreased computerized tomography numbers in patients with presenile dementia: detection in patients with otherwise normal scans. Arch Neurol 1980;37:401–409.

Narayan O, Penney JB, Johnson RT et al. Etiology of progressive multifocal leukoencephalopathy: identification of papovavirus. N Engl J Med 1973;289:1278–1282.

Neary D, Snowden J. Fronto-temporal dementia: nosology, neuropsychology, and neuropathology. Brain Cogn 1996;31:176–187.

Neary D, Snowden JS, Mann DMA et al. Frontal lobe dementia and motor neuron disease. J Neurol Neurosurg Psychiatry 1990;53:23–32.

Neary D, Snowden JS, Gustafson L et al. Frontotemporal lobar degeneration. A consensus on clinical diagnostic criteria. Neurology 1998;51:1546–1554.

Olson ME, Chernik NL, Posner JB. Infiltration of the leptomeninges by systemic cancer: a clinical and pathologic study. Arch Neurol 1974;30:122–137.

Nyenhuis DL, Gorelick PB. Vascular dementia: a contemporary review of epidemiology, diagnosis, prevention, and treatment. J Am Geriatr Soc 1998;46:1437–1448.

Ott A, Stolk RP, van Harskamp F et al. Diabetes mellitus and the risk of dementia: The Rotterdam Study. Neurology 1999;53:1937–1941.

Paulsen JS, Salmon DP, Thal LJ et al. Incidence and risk factors for hallucinations and delusions in patients with probable AD. Neurology 2000;54:1965–1971.

Percy AK, Kaback MM. Infantile and adult onset metachromatic leukodystrophy: biochemical comparisons and predictive diagnosis. N Engl J Med 1971;285:785–788.

Perret G, Nishioka H. Report on the cooperative study of intracranial aneurysms and subarachnoid hemorrhage. Section VI. Arteriovenous malformations. J Neurosurg 1966;25:467–490.

Perry RJ, Hodges JR. Differentiating frontal and temporal variant frontotemporal from Alzheimer's disease. Neurology 2000;54:2277–2284.

Perry EK, Tomlinson BE, Blessed G et al. Correlation of cholinergic abnormalities with senile plaques and mental test scores in senile dementia. Br Med J 1978;2:1457–1459.

Petersen RC, Smith GE, Waring SC et al. Mild cognitive impairment. Clinical characterization and outcome. Arch Neurol 1999;56:303–308.

Petersen RC, Stevens JC, Ganguli M et al. Practice parameter: Early detection of dementia: Mild cognitive impairment (an evidence-based review). Neurology 2001;56:1133–1142.

Piccini C, Bracco L, Amaducci L. Treatable and reversible dementias: an update. J Neurol Sci 1998;153:172–181.

Pick A: On the relation between aphasia and senile atrophy of the brain. In DA Rottenberg, FH Hochberg (eds), Neurological Classics in Modern Translation. New York: Hafner, 1977;35–40 (originally published 1892).

Pickut BA, Saerens J, Marien P et al. Discriminative use of SPECT in frontal lobe-type dementia versus (senile) dementia of the Alzheimer's type. J Nucl Med 1997;38:929–934.

Pohjasvaara T, Mantyla R, Salonen O *et al.* How complex interactions of ischemic brain infarcts, white matter lesions, and atrophy relate to poststroke dementia. Arch Neurol 2000;57:1295–1300.

Price BH, Gurvit H, Weintraub S *et al.* Neuropsychological patterns and language deficits in 20 consecutive cases of autopsy-confirmed Alzheimer's disease. Arch Neurol 1993;50:931–937.

Price RA, Jamieson PA. The central nervous system in childhood leukemia. II. Subacute leukoencephalopathy. Cancer 1975;35:306–318.

Prusiner SB. Novel proteinaceous infectious particles cause scrapie. Science 1982;216:136–144.

Prusiner SB. Molecular biology of prion diseases. Science 1991;252:1515–1522.

Raftopoulos C, Deleval J, Chaskis C *et al.* Cognitive recovery in idiopathic normal pressure hydrocephalus: a prospective study. Neurosurgery 1994;35:397–405.

Rao SM, Mittenberg W, Bernardin L *et al.* Neuropsychological test findings in subjects with leukoaraiosis. Arch Neurol 1989;46:40–44.

Raskind MA, Peskind ER, Wessel T, Yuan W. Galantamine in AD: a 6-month randomized, placebo-controlled trial with a 6-month extension. Neurology 2000;54:2261–2268.

Reisberg B. Clinical presentation, diagnosis, and symptomatology of age-associated cognitive decline and Alzheimer's disease. In B Reisberg (ed.), Alzheimer's Disease. The Standard Reference. New York: Free Press, 1983;173–187.

Richardson EP. Progressive multifocal leukoencephalopathy. N Engl J Med 1961;265: 815–823.

Ritchie K, Artero S, Touchon J. Classification criteria for mild cognitive impairment. A population-based validation study. Neurology 2001;56:37–42.

Richler M. Barney's Version. New York: AA Knopf, 1998, 93.

Rizzoli HV, Pagnanelli DM. Treatment of delayed radiation necrosis of the brain: a clinical observation. J Neurosurg 1984;60:589–594.

Rockwood K, Bowler J, Erkinjuntti T *et al.* Subtypes of vascular dementia. Alzheimer Disease Associated Disorders 1999;13(Suppl. 3)S59–S65.

Rogers SL, Farlow MR, Doody RS *et al.* Donepizil Study Group. A 24-week, double-blind, placebo-controlled trial of donepezil in patients with Alzheimer's disease. Neurology 1998;50:136–145.

Roman GC, Tatemichi TK, Erkinjuntti T *et al.* Vascular dementia: diagnostic criteria for research studies. Report of the NINDS–AIREN International Work Group. Neurology 1993;43:250–260.

Rosen WG, Terry RD, Fuld PA *et al.* Pathological verification of ischemic score in differentiation of dementias. Ann Neurol 1980;7:486–488.

Rosenberg RN. The molecular and genetic basis of AD: the end of the beginning. The 2000 Wartenberg lecture. Neurology 2000;54:2045–2054.

Rosler M, Anand R, Cicin-Sain A *et al.* Efficacy and safety of rivastigmine in patients with Alzheimer's disease: international randomized controlled trial. BMJ 1999; 318:633–638.

Ron MA. Brain damage in chronic alcoholism: a neuroradiological and psychological review. Psychol Med 1977;7:103–112.

Rozas V, Port FK, Rutt WM. Progressive dialysis encephalopathy from dialysate aluminum. Arch Intern Med 1978;138:1375–1377.

Russouw HG, Roberts MC, Emsley RA, Truter R. Psychiatric manifestations and magnetic resonance imaging in HIV–negative neurosyphilis. Biol Psychiatry 1997; 41:467–473.

Sacks O. A neurologist's perspective on the aging brain. Arch Neurol 1997;54:1211–1214.

Sano M, Ernesto C, Thomas RG *et al.* A controlled trial of selegiline, alpha-tocopherol, or both as treatment for Alzheimer's disease. N Engl J Med 1997;336:1216–1222.

Saunders AM, Strittmatter WJ, Schmechel D *et al.* Association of apolipoprotein E allele e4 with late-onset familial and sporadic Alzheimer's disease. Neurology 1993;43: 1467–1472.

Schacter DL, Buckner RL. Priming and the brain. Neuron 1998;20:185–195.

Schaumburg HH, Suzuki K. Non-specific familial presenile dementia. J Neurol Neurosurg Psychiatry 1968;31:479–486.

Schmidt JL. Thrombotic thrombocytopenic purpura: successful treatment unlocks etiologic secrets. Mayo Clin Proc 1989;64:956–961.

Schwartz MP, Marin OSM, Saffran EM. Dissociations of language in dementia: a case study. Brain Lang 1977;7:277–306.

Scinto LFM, Daffner KR, Dressler D et al. A potential non-invasive neurobiological test for Alzheimer's disease. Science 1994;266:1051–1054.

Sehgal M, Swanson JW, DeRemee RA, Colby TV. Neurologic manifestations of Churg–Strauss syndrome. Mayo Clin Proc 1995;70:337–341.

Seipelt M, Zerr I, Nau R et al. Hashimoto's encephalitis as a differential diagnosis of Creutzfeldt–Jakob disease. J Neurol Neurosurg Psychiatry 1999;66:172–176.

Selkoe DJ. Alzheimer's disease: genotypes, phenotypes and treatments. Science 1997;275:630–631.

Shaw PJ, Walls TJ, Newman PK et al. Hashimoto's encephalopathy: a steroid-responsive disorder associated with high anti-thyroid antibody titers – report of five cases. Neurology 1991;41:228–233.

Shenk D, Barbour R, Junn W et al. Immunization with amyloid-beta attenuates Alzheimer's disease-like pathology in the PDAPP mouse. Nature 1999;400:173–177.

Shimamura AP, Berry JM, Mangels JA et al. Memory and cognitive abilities in university professors. Psychol Sci 1995;6:387–394.

Shraberg D. The myth of pseudodementia: depression and the aging brain. Am J Psychiatry 1978;135:601–603.

Sim M, Sussman I. Alzheimer's disease: its natural history and differential diagnosis. J Nerv Ment Dis 1962;135:489–499.

Simpson DM, Berger JR. Neurologic manifestations of HIV infection. Med Clin NA 1966;80:1363–1394.

Singer R. Diagnosis and treatment of Whipple's disease. Drugs 1998;55:699–704.

Sjogren T, Sjogren H, Lindgren AGH. Morbus Alzheimer and morbus Pick: a genetic, clinical, and pathoanatomic study. Acta Psychiatr Neurol Scand 1974;82(Suppl.): 185–194.

Slooter AJC, van Duijn CM. Genetic epidemiology of Alzheimer disease. Epidemiologic Reviews 1997;19:107–119.

Smith, ADM. Megaloblastic madness. Br Med J 1960;1:1840–1845.

Sneddon IB. Cerebro-vascular lesions and livedo reticularis. Br J Dermatol 1965;77:180–185.

Snow SS, Wells CE. Case studies in neuropsychiatry: diagnosis and treatment of coexistent dementia and depression. J Clin Psychiatry 1981;42:439–441.

Starkman MN, Schteingart DE. Neuropsychiatric manifestations of patients with Cushing's syndrome: relationship to cortical and adrenocorticotrophic hormone levels. Arch Intern Med 1981;141:215–219.

Steele C, Rovner B, Chase GA, Folstein M. Psychiatric symptoms and nursing home placement of patients with Alzheimer's disease. Am J Psychiatry 1990;147:1049–1051.

Steingart A, Hachinski VC, Lau C et al. Cognitive and neurologic findings in subjects with diffuse white matter lucencies on computed tomographic scan (leuko-araiosis). Arch Neurol 1987;44:32–35.

Sternberg DE, Jarvik ME. Memory function in depression: improvement with antidepressant medication. Arch Gen Psychiatry 1976;33:219–224.

Strittmatter WJ, Weisgraber KH, Hanng D et al. Binding of human apolipoprotein E to synthetic amyloid beta peptide: isoform-specific effects and implications for late-onset alzheimer's disease. Proc Natl Acad Sci USA 1993;90:8098–8102.

Sulkava R, Haltia M, Paetau A et al. Accuracy of clinical diagnosis in primary degenerative dementia: correlation with neuropathological findings. J Neurol Neurosurg Psychiatry 1983;46:9–13.

Susac J. Susac's syndrome. The triad of microangiopathy of the brain and retina with hearing loss in young women. Neurology 1994;44:591–593.

Swanson JW, Kelly JJ, McConahey WM. Neurological aspects of thyroid dysfunction. Mayo Clin Proc 1981;56:504–512.

Tan L, Williams MA, Khan MK *et al.* Risk of transmission of bovine spongiform encephalopathy to humans in the United States. Report of the council on scientific affairs. JAMA 1999;281:2330–2339.

Tanridag O, Kirshner HS (1987). Magnetic resonance and CT scan imaging in neurobehavioral syndromes. Psychosomatics 1987;28:517–528.

Tariot PN, Solomon PR, Morris JC *et al.* A 5-month, randomized, placebo-controlled trial of galantamine in AD. Neurology 2000;54:2269–2276.

Tatemichi TK, Foulkes MA, Mohr JP *et al.* Dementia in stroke survivors in the Stroke Data Bank cohort: prevalence, incidence, risk factors, and computed tomographic findings. Stroke 1990;21:858–866.

Tatemichi TK, Paik M, Bagiella E *et al.* Risk of dementia after stroke in a hospitalized cohort: results of a longitudinal study. Neurology 1994;44:1885–1891.

Ter Muelen V. SSPE and measles virus: current state of our knowledge. Neuropodiatrie 1973;4:347–349.

Terry RD. Senile dementia. Fed Proc 1978;37:2837–2840.

Thompson TL, Filley CM, Mitchell WD *et al.* Lack of efficacy of hydergine in patients with Alzheimer's disease. N Engl J Med 1990;323:455–458.

Tomlinson BE, Blessed G, Roth, M. Observations on the brains of old people. J Neurol Sci 1968;7:331–356.

Trapp GA, Miner GD, Zimmerman RL *et al.* Aluminum levels in brain in Alzheimer's disease. Biol Psychiatry 1978;13:709–718.

Tyrrell PJ, Warrington EK, Frackowiak RSJ, Rossor MN. Heterogeneity in progressive aphasia due to focal cortical atrophy. Brain 1990;113:1321–1336.

Uhl GR, Hilt DC, Hedreen JC *et al.* Pick's disease (lobar sclerosis): depletion of neurons in the nucleus basalis of Meynert. Neurology 1983;33:1470–1473.

Van Zandvoort MJE, De Haan EHF, Kappelle LJ. Chronic cognitive disturbances after a single supratentorial lacunar infarct. Neuropsychiatry, neuropsychology, and behavioral neurology 2001;14:98–102.

Vercruyssen A, Martin JJ, Ceuterick C *et al.* Adult ceroid-lipofuscinosis: diagnostic value of biopsies and of neurophysiological investigations. J Neurol Neurosurg Psychiatry 1982;45:1056–1059.

Wang HS. Dementia of old age. In WL Smith, M Kinsbourne (eds), Dementia. New York: Spectrum, 1977;1–24.

Wechsler AF, Verity MA, Rosenschein S *et al.* Pick's disease: a clinical, computed tomographic, and histologic study with Golgi impregnation observations. Arch Neurol 1982;39:287–290.

Weiner HL, Lemere CA, Maron R *et al.* Nasal administration of amyloid-beta peptide decreases cerebral amyloid burden in a mouse model of Alzheimer's disease. Ann Neurol 2000;48:567–579.

Weintraub S, Rubin NP, Mesulam M-M. Primary progressive aphasia: longitudinal course, neuropsychological profile, and language features. Arch Neurol 1990;47:1329–1335.

Wells CE. Dementia: definitions and description. In CE Wells, Dementia (2nd edn). Philadelphia: Davis, 1977;1–14.

Wells CE. Role of stroke in dementia. Stroke 1978;9:1–3.

Wells CE. Pseudodementia. Am J Psychiatry 1979;136:895–900.

Wells CE, Duncan GW. Danger of over-reliance on computerized tomography. Am J Psychiatry 1977;134:811–813.

Westbury C, Bub D. Primary progressive aphasia: a review of 112 cases. Brain Lang 1997;60:381–406.

Whitehouse PJ, Price DL, Struble RG *et al.* Alzheimer's disease and senile dementia: loss of neurons in the basal forebrain. Science 1982;215:1237–1239.

Wikstrom J, Paetau A, Palo J *et al.* Classic amyotrophic lateral sclerosis with dementia. Arch Neurol 1982;39:681–683.

Wilkins DE, Hallett M, Berardelli A *et al.* Physiologic analysis of myoclonus in Alzheimer's disease. Neurology 1984;34:898–903.

Wilson RS, Fox JH, Hickman MS *et al.* Computed tomography in dementia. Neurology 1982;32:1054–1057.

Wisniewski HM, Narang HK, Terry RD. Neurofibrillary tangles of paired helical filaments. J Neurol Sci 1976;27:173–181.

Wisniewski KE, Wisniewski HM, Wen GY. Occurrence of neuropathological changes and dementia of Alzheimer's disease in Down's syndrome. Ann Neurol 1985;17:278–282.

Wright RA, Kokmen E. Gradually progressive dementia without discrete cerebrovascular events in a patient with Sneddon's syndrome. Mayo Clin Proc 1999;74:57–61.

Yates CM, Simpson J, Maloney AFJ, Gordon A: Neurochemical observations in a case of Pick's disease. J Neurol Sci 1980;48:257–263.

Zhukareva V, Vogelsberg-Ragaglia V, Van Deerlin V *et al.* Loss of brain tau defines novel sporadic and familial tauopathies with frontotemporal dementia. Ann Neurol 2001;49:165–175.

14

Delirium and Acute Confusional States

When they came, he was already awake and showed bizarre behaviour, yelling and stabbing, as wide awake as if he had never slept.

And they found him with the sword in one hand, stabbing everything as if he were fighting, and it was of note that he had his eyes closed, for he was sleeping and dreaming that he was in battle against the giants.

(Cervantes, *Don Quixote*, quoted by Garcia Ruiz and Gulliksen 1999)

No disorder in behavioral neurology is more striking or more distressing to patients, families, and medical personnel than delirium, also called acute encephalopathy or confusional state. 'Confusion' is one of the most commonly used terms in behavioral neurology, and one of the most difficult to define; in general it means 'an inability to think with customary speed, clarity, and coherence' (Adams and Victor 1993). Encephalopathy or delirium is defined as 'a transient disorder of cognition and attention, one accompanied by disturbances of the sleep–wake cycle and psychomotor behavior' (Lipowski 1987). As in dementia, multiple cognitive functions are affected, in multiple areas of the brain. In comparison to dementia, however, delirium usually involves alterations in the level of consciousness (somnolence or hypervigilance, agitation), disturbed perception (hallucinations, illusions, delusions), psychomotor abnormalities (restlessness, agitation, disturbed sleep–wake cycle), and autonomic nervous system hyperactivity (tachycardia, hypertension, fever, diaphoresis, tremor). Synonyms include delirium, encephalopathy, acute confusional state, acute brain syndrome, and toxic psychosis.

Although some authorities reserve the term 'delirium' for an agitated encephalopathy (Adams and Victor 1993), most use the above terms interchangeably. Those who diagnose delirium only in the agitated patient will miss many cases of delirium, and there is some evidence that hypoactive delirium patients may have a poorer prognosis than the hyperactive ones (Meagher and Trzepacz, 2000).

Delirium is an extremely common behavioral syndrome. Acute encephalopathies occur in 30–50% of hospitalized patients over the age of 70 years. Since as many as 48% of hospitalized patients are elderly, it is estimated that as many as 10% of hospitalized medical and surgical patients are encephalopathic at any given time (Millar 1981; Lipowski 1987; Lawlor *et al.* 2000). Six-month mortality in hospitalized patients with delirium is over 25% (Cole *et al.* 1998). Encephalopathies affect as many as 2.3 million persons annually in the USA, and the hospital cost is in excess of $4 billion. Yet, compared to dementias, encephalopathies have been relatively little studied.

A number of specific risk factors for delirium have been discovered. These include: age >80 years; prior cognitive impairment or institutionalization; any prior brain disorder; hearing loss; vision loss; fracture on admission; symptomatic infection; stress; environmental change; neuroleptic medications, and possibly narcotic analgesics, sedatives, and anticholinergic drugs; and medical procedures including use of restraints, bladder catheterization, and any surgery during the admission (Schor *et al.* 1992; Inouye and Charpentier 1996; Inouye *et al.* 1999).

DIFFERENTIAL DIAGNOSIS OF DELIRIUM

The differential diagnosis of delirium includes: (1) psychosis; (2) dementia; and (3) focal brain lesions.

Delirium Versus Psychosis

The distinction between delirium and psychosis is made primarily by evidence for 'organic' or physical causes of delirium, and by the prominent cognitive dysfunction: disorientation, reduced attention, memory loss, and focal neurological disturbances. Acute psychoses will be discussed in Chapter 15. Briefly, they include the manic phase of bipolar affective disorder, acute schizophrenia, and dissociative states. In general, psychoses begin before age 40 and are less likely to involve frank disorientation and abnormal memory for simple items such as those of the bedside mental status examination. The incoherence of thought in both psychosis and delirium may appear somewhat similar, and symptoms such as anxiety, agitation, and combativeness can occur in both disorders. Frank autonomic hyperactivity (tachycardia, hypertension, tremor, diaphoresis) always favors delirium. Hallucinations occur in both disorders, but in psychosis they are more likely to be auditory, whereas in delirium they are more often visual. Both syndromes can involve delusional thinking, but the delusions of psychosis tend to be more organized and more consistent.

Whenever an acute psychosis begins in a middle-aged or elderly patient, an organic disorder should be suspected and actively looked for before a diagnosis of functional psychosis is made. Dubin and colleagues (1983) found that four screening criteria accurately distinguished patients with organic disorders from those with functional disorders in an emergency room setting; these were:

(1) disorientation; (2) abnormal vital signs; (3) 'clouded consciousness' or decreased level of alertness; and (4) age greater than 40 years without prior psychiatric history. Rarely, a patient with a very acute psychosis related to schizophrenia or mania (bipolar affective disorder) may suffer apparent cognitive disturbance and disorientation. Such syndromes, sometimes called 'pseudodelirium' (Lipowski 1983), are difficult to diagnose, and laboratory tests to exclude an organic etiology are usually necessary.

Delirium Versus Dementia

The distinction between delirium and dementia is made by the time course, which is slow and gradual in dementia versus more abrupt and fluctuating in delirium. In addition, dementia is characterized by the 'negative' symptoms of cognitive loss, whereas delirium has prominent 'positive' symptoms of sleep/wake abnormality, psychomotor agitation, and the autonomic hyperactivity. Delirium and dementia, however, frequently overlap. Acute delirium may later evolve into chronic dementia. Dementia, on the other hand, may 'decompensate' into delirium under the stress of a metabolic imbalance, subdural hematoma, lack of environmental stimulation ('sundowning'), or even a move to unfamiliar surroundings. One way of looking at this phenomenon is that patients with pre-existing dementia may be tipped into delirium by relatively minor metabolic stresses, whereas a normal patient requires much more potent stimuli to develop delirium (Inouye and Charpentier 1996).

Delirium and Focal Brain Lesions

Focal lesions of the brain can either mimic or produce the full syndrome of delirium. The distinction between syndromes caused by focal lesions and delirium is difficult, since there is such a large overlap. Patients with acute right hemisphere strokes, left temporal infarcts with Wernicke's aphasia, posterior cerebral artery territory strokes, and frontal lesions, for example, often have symptoms and signs that fully justify a diagnosis of delirium. We shall consider this subject further later in the chapter, under 'anatomic substrates of delirium'.

CLINICAL FEATURES OF DELIRIUM

Norman Geschwind (1982), a pioneer of behavioral neurology in general, called the acute confusional states 'a frontier in neuropsychology' on the basis of their common occurrence, frequent misdiagnosis, and distinctive clinical features. The clinical features of delirium are distinctive yet variable. Some patients manifest a prodrome of anxiety, restlessness, drowsiness or insomnia, and vivid dreams. There follows a cognitive/attentional disorder, disruption of the sleep–wake cycle, increased or decreased activity, and fluctuations in mental status, usually with nocturnal exacerbation. The cognitive disturbances involve perception, thinking, memory, orientation, and attention. Subtle changes in language, especially written language, are common. Other clinical features of delirium include emotional changes (fear, anger), altered insight and judgment, disruption of the sleep–wake cycle with either hyper- or hyposomnolence, psychomotor changes that can involve either agitation or lethargy, and autonomic disturbances such as tachycardia and arrhythmias, hypertension, diaphoresis, flushing, dilated pupils, piloerection, and tremor. Table 14.1 lists the common cognitive and behavioral manifestations of delirium.

Attention

Disruption of attention is one of the foremost characteristics of the acute encephalopathies; in fact, Geschwind (1982) termed these syndromes 'disorders of attention'. As summarized by Geschwind, attention is a complex process requiring:

1. 'Selectivity' of focusing on specific features of the external environment
2. 'Coherence' of continued concentration on a succession of relevant stimuli
3. 'Distractibility', or the ability to shift the focus of attention when a more important, novel stimulus appears
4. 'Universality,' or the ability to monitor and screen for relevance, either consciously or unconsciously, the myriad of external events
5. 'Sensitivity,' or the ability to perceive one low-intensity stimulus of importance to the individual among the relevant stimuli (Geschwind 1982).

A mother, for example, attending to housework, can ignore the noise of passing cars and fire sirens but respond immediately to the cry of her infant. In delirium, the patient cannot focus selective attention, becoming distracted by every environmental stimulus, whether trivial or important. The patient is thus rendered incapable of maintaining a coherent sequence in thought, conversation, or action. During the clinical history, the patient is unable to stick to the topic of a question and is continually distracted by intervening stimuli. Tasks such as digit span become totally impossible. Attentional disorders, a prime characteristic of acute

Table 14.1 Clinical features of delirium

Reduced attention, distractibility
Impaired memory, paramnesias
Disorientation to place, time
Abnormal language content, agraphia
Calculation impairment
Misperceptions, hallucinations, delusions
Reduced abstract reasoning, insight, judgment
Labile moods, facetiousness

confusional states, are also seen in frontal lobe syndromes (see Chapter 10) and in other focal encephalopathies.

Memory

Impaired memory is also an invariable feature of acute confusional states. Patients usually manifest both retrograde and anterograde amnesia (Lipowski 1983). They may repetitively ask the same questions in the manner described in Chapter 11 for the syndrome of transient global amnesia. Patients usually recall little of the period of acute encephalopathy after they recover. In comparison to the syndrome of transient global amnesia, delirium usually involves a more global disturbance of cognitive functions.

Geschwind (1982) stressed in addition to amnesia the common occurrence of 'paramnesia', distortion rather than total loss of memory. An example is the Ganser syndrome, in which patients give approximate answers, incorrect but only slightly off target and within the correct category, in response to questions. The Ganser syndrome includes the following features (Catchan *et al.* 1978):

1. Approximate answers
2. Clouding of consciousness, with disorientation
3. 'Hysterical' stigmata
4. Recent history of head injury, infection, or severe emotional stress
5. Hallucinations
6. Amnesia for the period of symptoms.

A tendency to approximate answers, however, can occur in both functional and organic disorders. Related paramnestic disorders are 'reduplicative paramnesia', referred to in Chapters 9 and 10, in which a patient may claim to be at once in the hospital and in his home town (Benson *et al.* 1976; Staton *et al.* 1982) and the Capgras syndrome, in which a patient denies the identity of his spouse or other familiar persons (Alexander *et al.* 1979). These paramnesias may represent a form of confabulation in which the patient tries to fit the current, unfamiliar surroundings into a former, more familiar environment (Staton *et al.* 1982). After misinterpreting a person or place, the patient may then construct an internally logical story around it. A patient who mistakes the hospital for a hotel, for example, may call the doctor a concierge and the nurse a maid. Such stories resemble the delusional systems of psychotic patients, except that they are usually more transitory and changeable.

Disorientation

Disorientation to place and time is the inevitable result of disordered attention and memory in delirium. The degree of disorientation may vary with the time of day, usually worsening at night or in response to other medical factors, e.g. fever or medication use. Orientation to personal identity is usually preserved; patients who claim to be Jesus Christ or George Washington are more likely to suffer from a functional psychosis than from delirium, and most such patients can also state their actual name. As mentioned in Chapter 11, isolated amnesias in which patients claim no memory of their name or identity are also usually not organic. Disorientation to place and time, on the other hand, is much more common in delirium than in psychosis. This feature of disorientation is of great practical importance, as nurses and physicians routinely test orientation in hospitalized patients, and the presence of an encephalopathy is often detected in this way.

Language

Language is usually not grossly disrupted in delirium. As in dementia, the mechanics of language and speech are intact, though the content is often abnormal. More complex language tasks that require memory, close attention, or abstract reasoning are likely to be impaired. Visual language modalities are generally more affected than auditory ones (Wertz 1978). Patients occasionally make bizarre errors on naming tests, substituting names of misperceived items or terms that are part of a reduplicated or confabulated concept of the environment. These naming errors have been termed 'non-aphasic misnaming' by Weinstein and Kahn (1952), indicating that they arise from generalized cognitive dysfunction rather than from a focal aphasic disturbance. Often items relating to the patient's illness are selectively misnamed, as in right hemisphere syndromes of neglect of illness (see Chapter 9, also Weinstein and Keller 1973). Reduced attention and memory may limit performance in tasks of repetition and comprehension of complex spoken or written language. Writing often appears to be selectively disrupted in acute confusional states; patients typically make spelling errors, word substitutions, spatial aberrations when orienting the writing on the paper, and alterations and perseverations of letter forms, with added loops and twists (Chedru and Geschwind 1972a, 1972b).

Calculations

Patients with delirium often cannot attend to tasks, such as calculations, that require sustained concentration. Digit span and serial sevens are especially sensitive to acute encephalopathy, as are all complex calculations.

Perceptual and Visuospatial Functions

Altered perception is a hallmark of the acute confusional state. In the altered consciousness of these patients, perceptions easily became admixed with dream images and hallucinations. Many of the distortions of visual perception discussed in Chapter 8, e.g. metamorphopsia or distortion of shape, occur in delirium (Willanger and Klee 1966). Visual hallucinations occur more commonly than auditory ones in delirium, whereas the reverse is true in functional psychosis (Lipowski 1983). Most clinicians are familiar with the vivid visual hallucinations of animals and insects in delirium tremens, a syndrome of alcohol withdrawal.

Similar hallucinations are frequent in drug-induced and toxic encephalopathies. Such hallucinations frequently provoke fear and agitation, also characteristics of delirium. Altered perceptions, as well, play a role in the 'paramnestic' responses referred to previously. Geschwind's (1982) patient, for example, stated that the hospital was her living room, then misidentified the intravenous apparatus as a Christmas tree and all of the other items in the room as her own furniture.

Anosognosia, or neglect of illness, is also a feature of delirium, as it is in right hemisphere disorders (see Chapter 9). Patients may have knowledge of many of the facts of their illness, yet they seem unconcerned or even deny being ill. The importance of the right hemisphere in attentional alerting functions, reviewed in Chapter 9, may account for the common occurrence of these symptoms in right hemisphere syndromes and diffuse encephalopathies.

Abstraction, Insight, and Judgment

Any thought process requiring sequential or logical analysis, sustained concentration, problem solving, or abstract reasoning becomes difficult for the delirious patient. Artificial tasks such as similarities or proverb interpretation are performed poorly. The deficit is even more obvious in the patient's impaired insight and judgment regarding his or her own personal situation. Patients often develop frankly paranoid delusions, resembling those of schizophrenia but typically fragmented, less organized, and more fleeting (Lipowski 1983). Hospitalized patients may express paranoid delusions concerning the reasons for their incarceration, but these may change from day to day.

Personality and Mood

As in dementia, the affective states of delirium tend to be labile, with rapid fluctuations between elated and depressed moods. The mood states of delirium, however, tend to be more powerful, deeply felt, and persistent than the labile moods of demented patients.

One unusual feature of the mood of patients with delirium is a tendency to witty remarks or playfulness. This playful wit, characterized by silly puns and 'clang' associations, is related to the 'facetiousness', or *Witzelsucht*, discussed in Chapter 10 with regard to frontal lobe disorders. Geschwind (1982) attributed the wittiness of delirious patients not to deliberate humor but rather to the incoherent stream of thought that randomly throws together incongruous elements.

ANATOMIC SUBSTRATES OF DELIRIUM

The clinical picture of delirium, involving a diffuse or multifocal cognitive abnormality, suggests diffuse or bihemispheral pathology similar to that of dementia. Delirium, however, occurs with a much wider distribution of lesions and pathologies than dementia. The numerous metabolic and toxic etiologies of delirium have no structural abnormality in the brain; these syndromes presumably reflect diffuse dysfunction in widespread areas of the brain. Even sensory and motor centers participate, as evidenced by perceptual distortions, restlessness, and tremor. Focal lesions, however, more commonly masquerade as generalized disorders in delirium than in dementia.

Four focal syndromes most commonly cause delirium:

1. Acute right temporoparietal lesions (usually strokes in the right middle cerebral artery territory)
2. Unilateral or bilateral infarctions in the posterior cerebral artery territory
3. Left temporoparietal lesions with acute Wernicke's aphasia
4. Unilateral or bilateral frontal lesions.

Right hemisphere lesions involving the temporoparietal region can cause a true delirium (Mesulam *et al.* 1976; Schmidley and Messing 1984), with hallucinations, impaired attention, spatial disorientation, reduplicative phenomena, and neglect or denial of deficit (see Chapter 9). Caplan and colleagues (1986) called the confusional syndrome of right temporal infarctions the right hemisphere 'analogue of Wernicke's aphasia'. Levine and colleagues (Levine and Finklestein 1982; Levine and Grek 1984) found such syndromes more commonly in elderly right-hemisphere stroke patients with cortical atrophy, suggesting pre-existing dementia, or in association with seizures. Other associated syndromes include prosopagnosia, a failure to recognize familiar persons usually secondary to bilateral posterior hemisphere lesions, and the Capgras syndrome (Lewis *et al.* 1987), a disorder in which patients deny that their relatives are really their relatives, claiming that they are imposters. This condition may occur in psychotic disorders, but it has been reported with right hemisphere or bilateral posterior hemisphere damage (Carney *et al.* 1987). The important role of the right hemisphere in attention was discussed in Chapter 9.

Occasionally, an acute posterior cerebral artery territory stroke, either unilateral or bilateral, produces a confusional state with profound amnesia, and sometimes even agitation and combativeness (Horenstein *et al.* 1967; Benson *et al.* 1974; Medina *et al.* 1974; Devinsky *et al.* 1988). Patients with posterior cerebral artery strokes usually also manifest the 'focal' sign of contralateral hemianopia, but only occasionally motor or sensory abnormalities. In left PCA strokes, alexia is also usually present (see Chapter 6). With recovery, the confusional state usually improves, but memory loss often remains. Patients with bilateral PCA territory infarctions may have cortical blindness or Anton's syndrome (see Chapter 8).

Acute Wernicke's aphasia may be associated with agitation and behavioral evidence of 'confusion'. It is often very difficult to evaluate the patient's thought process, since verbal expression is paraphasic, and auditory comprehension is impaired. Patients who recover from Wernicke's aphasia often have little memory of the acute period. Patients who have limited recovery may develop paranoid ideation (see Chapter 5).

Frontal lesions encompass a large variety of clinical syndromes, as reviewed in Chapter 10. Aneurysms of the anterior communicating artery, involving medial frontal structures such as the septal nuclei, can produce a severe confabulatory amnesia akin to Wernicke–Korsakoff syndrome (see Chapter 11). Other frontal lesions can produce abulia or akinetic mutism, flat or labile moods, inappropriate or 'sick' humor (*Witzelsucht*), and the syndrome of approximate answers (Ganser syndrome, Carney *et al.* 1987). The Ganser syndrome, seen in patients with organic frontal damage, psychosis, and hysteria/malingering, involves approximate answers (e.g. Question: 'how many legs does a horse have?' Answer: 'five'), with or without clouding of consciousness and hallucinations. The syndrome involves impaired memory; in the acute phase there can be agitation or somnolence.

Finally, seizures arising in the temporal or frontal lobes can cause an ictal or postictal encephalopathy. Combined frontal and temporal lesions, as in herpes simplex encephalitis, cause profound amnesia, but acutely a delirium is almost always present (see Chapter 11).

It should be apparent from this discussion that focal lesions in widespread areas of the brain substance can cause delirium. If the focal lesion causes obvious neurological symptoms and signs the diagnosis is relatively straightforward. If the focal signs are subtle or absent, the distinction from a metabolic delirium is difficult. Multifocal lesions can also cause delirium. This topic will be explored further in the next section.

ETIOLOGY OF DELIRIUM

The etiologies of delirium are legion, and a careful search must be made in each patient. Most of the numerous medical diseases associated with dementia, reviewed in Chapter 13, also produce delirium when the onset is more acute. Etiologies of delirium, however, are even more numerous than those of dementia. In many cases, more than one etiology is present. Extreme disturbances of many metabolites and vital signs affect the brain in a diffuse manner, with the common end result of delirium. A partial listing of medical causes of delirium is shown in Table 14.2.

Metabolic disturbances associated with delirium include all of the metabolic, nutritional, endocrine, and toxic conditions discussed in Chapter 13. Among metabolic disorders, abnormalities of glucose metabolism such as hypoglycemia, non-ketotic hyperglycemia, and diabetic ketoacidosis are especially common. Electrolyte imbalances involving an excess or deficiency of sodium, calcium, magnesium, and phosphate all cause delirium. Nutritional disorders include pellagra, thiamine or vitamin B12 deficiency, and accompanying general malnutrition and dehydration, likely contribute to the delirium. Organ failure syndromes such as uremia, hepatic encephalopathy, and chronic pulmonary insufficiency all produce confusional states. Another factor is anoxia secondary to congestive heart failure, pulmonary emboli, hypotension, or cardiac arrhythmia. An additional metabolic disorder is acute intermittent porphyria, a hereditary disease associated with accumulation of porphyrins, precursors of hemoglobin. The disease is characterized by episodes of confusion, seizures, abdominal pain, and peripheral neuropathy

Table 14.2 Etiologies of delirium

Metabolic disorders
  Metabolic imbalances
    • Sodium, calcium, magnesium, phosphate
    • Glucose (hypoglycemia, hyperglycemia), acidosis
    • Anoxia, hypotension, arrhythmias
    • Organ failure (hepatic, renal, pulmonary)
    • Metabolic diseases (porphyria)
  Nutritional disorders (pellagra, vitamin B12 deficiency)
  Endocrine disorders (thyroid, adrenal, parathyroid)
  Toxic encephalopathies
    • Heavy metals
    • Chemical toxins
    • Medications
    • Alcohol, abuse of drugs
    • Withdrawal syndromes
Infections
  CNS infections (meningitis, encephalitis, abscess)
  Systemic infections
    • Bacterial endocarditis
    • Septicemia
    • Focal systemic infections
Neoplasms
  Focal brain lesions, hydrocephalus, edema
  'Paraneoplastic' delirium
  Effects of chemotherapy, irradiation, infections
Vascular diseases
  Stroke syndromes (right parietal, frontal, temporooccipital)
  Multiple emboli (platelets-fibrin, septic, air, fat)
  Hypertensive encephalopathy
  Cerebral hemorrhage (hypertension, aneurysm, arteriovenous malformation)
Head trauma
Seizures
Postoperative delirium

(Santosh and Malhotra 1994; Regan *et al.* 1999; Estrov *et al.* 2000). A large number of other rare hereditary metabolic diseases, such as disorders of the urea cycle and aminoacidurias, produce episodes of confusion, lethargy, and abnormal neurological signs in children (Msall *et al.* 1984; Prensky 1984). Discussion of these childhood encephalopathies is beyond the scope of this book.

    Endocrine disturbances associated with delirium include hypothyroidism, thyrotoxicosis, Addison's disease (adrenal insufficiency), Cushing's syndrome (adrenal excess), hyperparathyroidism, and the complications of diabetes alluded to earlier. References concerning many of these disorders were cited in Chapter 13.

Toxic syndromes are very common causes of delirium. Medications are the most common culprits, including sedatives, tranquilizers, anticholinergics, antihypertensives (alpha-methyldopa), and histamine blockers (cimetidine). In earlier times bromide toxicity was a common cause of both delirium and dementia (Hurst and Hurst 1984). Drugs of abuse such as cocaine, amphetamines, and 'psychedelic drugs' such as phencyclidine and LSD are important to consider in the appropriate populations. Withdrawal states from alcohol, barbiturates, and benzodiazepines are also frequent causes of delirium. Alcoholic intoxication is a form of acute encephalopathy, and alcohol-related nutritional deficiencies underlie the Wernicke–Korsakoff syndrome (see Chapter 11), which features an acute delirium followed by a selective amnestic syndrome (Nakada and Knight 1984). Withdrawal from alcohol may produce tremulousness, seizures ('rum fits'), hallucinosis, or the full-blown syndrome of delirium tremens. Alcoholic hallucinosis can be associated with days or weeks of visual hallucinations in an otherwise clear sensorium. Delirium tremens is one of the most dramatic and classical examples of acute delirium in medicine, associated with restlessness, hyperactivity, visual hallucinations, delusions, tachycardia, diaphoresis, and fever. The illness can run a course of several days and has a significant mortality from cardiac arrhythmias and hypotension (Sellers and Kalant 1976). As in dementia, polypharmacy and the sensitivity of the aging nervous system to either the acute effects of or withdrawal from medications are important factors in delirium.

Chemical toxins, insecticides, and heavy metals all produce delirium. The acute encephalopathy of lead poisoning in children is well known (Needleman 1982), but studies suggest that a milder, more chronic lead encephalopathy can occur in adults, either from industrial exposure (Valciukas *et al.* 1978) or from such home sources as 'moonshine' liquor (Whitfield *et al.* 1972). X-ray contrast materials such as metrizamide are occasionally the cause of delirium (Killebrew *et al.* 1983); newer, ionic contrast agents that are less toxic to the brain have largely replaced metrizamide in radiology.

Infectious diseases are much more common as causes of delirium than of dementia. Primary central nervous system (CNS) infections such as meningitis, encephalitis, and brain abscess typically present with confusion, seizures, headache, and fever, sometimes associated with focal neurological signs. In addition, severe infections anywhere in the body can cause delirium, especially in elderly patients. Delirium is a common presenting picture of septicemia, or bloodstream infection. Bacterial endocarditis, with its tendency to septic emboli, frequently presents to the neurologist as delirium in a chronically or subacutely ill patient (Pruitt *et al.* 1978).

Neoplasms are frequently related to delirium. Both primary and metastatic brain tumors, especially those associated with edema, intracranial hypertension, or hydrocephalus, can cause apparently diffuse encephalopathies. The rare paraneoplastic syndromes and the more common complications of cancer therapy are causes of delirium as well as dementia (see Chapter 13). These complications include radiation damage, effects of chemotherapy, steroid psychosis, nutritional disorders, and opportunistic infections.

Among vascular diseases, focal stroke syndromes are frequent sources of delirium in the elderly (see above). Acute hypertensive encephalopathy is a medical emergency in which delirium can be the most prominent presenting symptom. This syndrome is defined by severely elevated blood pressure (usually above 200/120 mmHg), retinal hemorrhages, renal failure, and multifocal or diffuse neurological deficits. Cerebral symptoms relate to combinations of intracranial vasospasm, small vessel occlusions, and punctate intracerebral hemorrhages (Chester *et al.* 1978).

Delirium can be caused by multiple cerebral emboli from numerous sources including valvular, myocardial, or atherosclerotic heart disease; endocarditis with septic emboli; atherosclerosis of the great vessels with cholesterol emboli; trauma to long bones with fat emboli; air or fibrin-platelet emboli during arteriography or surgery; and toxic emboli related to intravenous drug use.

Intracranial hemorrhages related to hypertension, aneurysms, and arteriovenous malformations can cause delirium. In the case of ruptured aneurysms, focal neurological signs are frequently absent. Cerebral vasculitis results in an acute confusional state more commonly than in dementia (see Chapter 13). In sum, virtually any stroke or cerebrovascular disorder can be associated with delirium.

Traumatic brain injury is an especially common cause of acute confusional states. Major head injuries typically produce initial somnolence or coma, often followed by a prolonged agitated delirium. Minor head injuries produce transient amnesia (see Chapter 11), often followed by a subtle 'postconcussive syndrome' characterized by reduced attention and concentration, irritability, forgetfulness, headache, insomnia, and depressive symptoms (Symonds 1962; Alexander 1995). These mild confusional states cause major loss of work and are the subject of numerous lawsuits. Although some of the symptoms suggest a functional etiology, studies have documented slowing of mental activities and difficulty in the processing of new information in patients with concussions (Gronwall and Wrightson 1974; Alexander 1995). Finally, multiple concussions can result in the 'punch drunk' syndrome, or 'dementia pugilistica', seen regularly in boxers. This syndrome includes memory loss, poor attention, slurred speech, cerebellar signs, extrapyramidal dysfunction resembling Parkinson's disease, and ultimately dementia (Mawdsley and Ferguson 1963). Pathological changes include cerebral and cerebellar atrophy and neurofibrillary tangles (Lampert and Hardman 1984). These post-traumatic syndromes are discussed in Chapter 20.

Epileptic seizures are frequently accompanied or followed by confusional states. This subject is discussed in Chapter 19.

Postoperative Delirium

The postoperative period is an especially common time for the onset of delirium. Neurologists are frequently called on to assess confused patients in surgical intensive care units. Such syndromes are especially frequent after open-heart surgery, presumably because of intraoperative hypoxia or cerebral emboli (Kornfeld *et al.* 1965). Addition of better filters and cardiopulmonary bypass techniques have reduced the incidence of these complications, but postoperative delirium continues to be seen, including after the frequently performed coronary bypass operations (Gonzalez-Scariano and Hurtig 1981; Bojar *et al.* 1983; Furlan and Breuer 1984). Multiple microemboli are almost universally present, and cognitive deficits are detectable in a large proportion of patients. In one recent study (Toner *et al.* 1998), 48% of first-time coronary artery bypass graft (CABG) patients had detectable neuropsychological deficits at 1 week post-operatively, 34% at 2 months. The encephalopathy did not correlate with age, duration of bypass, or the type of oxygenator used (bubble versus membrane). Preoperative cognitive impairment did correlate with postoperative EEG abnormality, suggesting that cognitive impairment makes the brain more vulnerable to ischemic changes during CABG. Another study (Newman *et al.* 2001) found cognitive deficits in 53% of coronary bypass surgery patients at discharge, 36% at 6 weeks, 24% at 6 months, and, surprisingly, 42% at 5 years. Recently, transcranial doppler (TCD) has been used to detect microemboli, referred to as 'high intensity transients', or 'HITS'. One study (Jacobs *et al.* 1998) found between 90 and 1710 HITS per hemisphere during CABG. HITS occurred predominantly during the bypass, but another peak occurred during the cross-clamping of the aorta. The overall number of HITS did not correlate with the degree of neuropsychological deficits, but they did correlate with the regions of most marked decrease in CMRglu (regional cerebral glucose metabolism measured by PET scan). The neuropsychogical deficits in this series were mild and tended to resolve by 3 months. The authors concluded that not all neuropsychological dysfunction appeared to relate to microemboli; other factors such as hypotension and hypoxia during surgery also play a role. The location rather than the number of emboli also appears more important in determining the postoperative deficits. In addition to intraoperative factors such as emboli and hypoxia, the intensive care unit, with its attendant stress/fear, sleep deprivation, environmental change, and constant extraneous stimulation, may contribute to the development of encephalopathy.

Surgical procedures elsewhere in the body also result in delirium, especially in elderly patients (Millar 1981). Multiple factors may contribute to postoperative delirium, including drug toxicity, electrolyte imbalance, metabolic disturbances, infections, withdrawal from alcohol and drugs, and secondary complications such as stroke. A recent paper on patients with alcohol abuse undergoing surgery found increased postoperative ICU admissions, mainly because of alcohol withdrawal symptoms such as agitation and restlessness, but no increase in other complications (Maxson *et al.* 1999).

Even environmental factors such as prolonged sleep loss, the lack of a day–night cycle, reduced sensory stimulation, and fear provoked by the illness and by the intensive care unit itself contribute to the development of delirium in this setting. The neurologist must assess all of these factors, as well as the more serious possibilities of anoxia, cerebral emboli, or sepsis, in order to determine proper treatment. A checklist of the etiologic factors in Table 14.2 should be considered in each case of postoperative delirium.

MANAGEMENT OF DELIRIUM

The treatment of patients with delirium is an important topic in behavioral neurology. Most of these syndromes develop acutely, disrupt behavior in serious ways, and yet are most often reversible and compatible with complete recovery. The first step in the management of delirium, as in any other disorder, is the proper etiological diagnosis. Historical factors such as toxin or drug exposures, symptoms of infection, recent medical problems or surgical procedures, and prior behavioral disorders deserve careful attention. The presence of other neurological signs may help to localize lesions in the brain. Finally, laboratory investigation is needed to exclude electrolyte or metabolic disturbances, infections, seizures, and other specific etiologies. A battery of suggested laboratory tests is shown in Table 14.3. Computed tomography (CT) or magnetic resonance imaging (MRI) scans are useful in excluding focal brain lesions such as infarcts or tumors. Lumbar puncture is important for central nervous system infections. The electroencephalogram (EEG) is more useful in the diagnosis of delirium than dementia. First, active seizure states such as partial complex status epilepticus are readily diagnosed. Second, most metabolic imbalances are associated with marked slowing of the background rhythm. Third, focal slowing may be a clue to the presence of brain lesions.

Once treatable factors in delirium are identified and corrected, a few general principles should guide further management. The patient should be kept on

Table 14.3 Laboratory testing in delirium

Metabolic screening
- Blood chemistries (electrolytes, BUN, blood glucose, liver function tests, Ca, Mg, PO_4)
- Arterial blood gases
- Complete blood count
- Vitamin B12, folate levels
- Sedimentation rate, antinuclear antibody
- Thyroid, adrenal functions
- Plasma drug screen, drug levels
- Urine for porphobilinogen
- Infectious screening
- Chest X-ray
- Urinalysis
- Blood cultures
- Serological test for syphilis, Lyme, HIV
- Lumbar puncture
Electroencephalogram
CT or MRI scan

bed rest, with cautious sedation administered as needed. With delirium tremens, benzodiazepines such as lorazepam (Ativan) should be given by a regular schedule unless oversedation develops. Major tranquilizers may be dangerous in patients with marked autonomic nervous system disorders, as these drugs can induce hypotension. On the other hand, benzodiazepines can lead to increased confusion and even paradoxical agitation in some delirious patients. Some experts use miniscule doses of traditional neuroleptics such as haloperidol; the author's preference is to use one of the atypical antipsychotic agents, especially in elderly patients. Olanzepine (Zyprexa) is helpful in agitated patients because of its sedative effect. Behavioral measures such as the presence of family members or familiar nursing staff, bright lighting, and frequent orientation cues help to reassure and calm the patient. With removal of the causative factors and the passage of time, normal cognitive function gradually returns in most cases.

One encouraging development is a recent study on prevention of encephalopathy by a series of behavioral techniques (Inouye *et al.* 1999), in which 852 patients over age 70, hospitalized on a general medical service, were randomized into active treatment and control groups. Six risk factors were manipulated: cognitive impairment, sleep deprivation, immobility, visual impairment, hearing impairment, and dehydration. The interventions, called the 'Elder Life Program', included orientation boards and frequent cognitive therapy sessions, non-pharmacologic sleep-inducing methods such as warm milk and relaxation techniques, early mobilization protocols and removal of restraints and bladder catheters, visual aids such as glasses and magnifying glasses, hearing amplification devices, and encouragement of fluid intake. The active treatment group had a 9.9% incidence of delirium, whereas the control group had a 15.0% incidence ($P = 0.02$). The only significant predictive factor for delirium was Mini Mental State score <24 ($P<0.01$). The cost of the program was $327 per patient, or $6341 per case of delirium prevented. While this cost may be beyond the means of most hospitals, attention to the six factors studied and adoption of some of the nursing strategies would likely be well worth the expense.

CONCLUSION

Delirium, like dementia, is an extremely common manifestation of bihemispheral (multifocal or diffuse) dysfunction. Delirium presents more acutely than dementia, and features active psychological symptoms such as hallucinations and delusions and active autonomic signs such as restlessness, agitation, tremor, tachycardia, hypertension, and sweating. Delirium represents one of the most dramatic clinical syndromes in neurology. Increased recognition of delirium in recent years has led to the realization that these syndromes are reversible but often associated with serious complications and even fatal outcomes in hospitalized patients. Early identification of causative factors, avoidance of metabolic abnormalities and excessive drugs, and prompt corrective measures are necessary to prevent and treat these important disorders.

REFERENCES

Adams RD, Victor M. Delirium and other acute confusional states. In Principles of Neurology (5th edn). New York: McGraw Hill, 1993;353–363.

Alexander MP. Mild traumatic brain injury: pathophysiology, natural history, and clinical management. Neurology 1995;45:1253–1260.

Alexander MP, Stuss DT, Benson DF. Capgras syndrome: a reduplicative phenomenon. Neurology 1979;229:334–339.

Benson DF, Marsden CD, Meadows JC. The amnesic syndrome of posterior cerebral artery occlusion. Acta Neurol Scand 1974;50:133–145.

Benson DF, Gardner H, Meadows JC. Reduplicative paramnesia. Neurology 1976;26: 147–151.

Bojar RM, Najafi H, DeLaria GA et al. Neurological complications of coronary revascularization. Ann Thorac Surg 1983;36:427–432.

Caplan LR, Kelly M, Kase CS et al. Mirror image of Wernicke's aphasia. Neurology 1986;36:1015–1019.

Carney MWP, Chary TKN, Robotis P, Childs A. Ganser syndrome and its management. Br J Psychiat 1987;151:697–700.

Catchan R, White A, Sims A. Ganser syndrome: the aetiological arguments. J Neurol Neurosurg Psychiatry 1978;41:851–854.

Chedru F, Geschwind N. Disorders of higher cortical functions in acute confusional states. Cortex 1972a;8:395–411.

Chedru F, Geschwind N. Writing disturbances in acute confusional states. Neuropsychologia 1972b;10:343–353.

Chester EM, Agamanolis DP, Banker BQ, Victor M. Hypertensive encephalopathy: a clinicopathologic study of 20 cases. Neurology 1978;28:928–939.

Cole MG, Primeau FJ, Elie ML. Delirium: prevention, treatment, and outcome studies. J Geriatr Psychiatry Neurol 1998;11:126–137.

Devinsky O, Bear D, Volpe BT. Confusional states following posterior cerebral artery infarction. Arch Neurol 1988;45:160–163.

Dubin WR, Weiss KI, Zeccardi JA. Organic brain syndrome: the psychiatric imposter. JAMA 1983;249:60–62.

Estrov Y, Scaglia F, Bodara OA. Psychiatric symptoms of inherited metabolic disease. J Inherit Metab Dis 2000;1:2–6.

Furlan AJ, Breuer AC. Central nervous system and complications of open heart surgery. Stroke 1984;19:7–11.

Garcia Ruiz PJ, Gulliksen L. Did Don Quixote have Lewy body disease? J R Soc Med 1999;92:200–201.

Geschwind N. Disorders of attention: a frontier in neuropsychology. Philos Trans R Soc Lond B 1982;298:173–185.

Gonzalez-Scariano F, Hurtig HI. Neurologic complications of coronary artery bypass grafting: case–control study. Neurology 1981;31:1032–1035.

Gronwall D, Wrightson P. Delayed recovery of intellectual function after minor head injury. Lancet 1974;2:605–609.

Horenstein S, Chamberlain W, Conomy J. Infarction of the fusiform and calcarine regions: agitated delirium and hemianopia. Trans Am Neurol Assoc 1967;92:85–89.

Hurst DL, Hurst MJ. Bromide psychosis: a literary case. Clin Neuropharmacol 1984;7:259–264.

Inouye SK, Charpentier PA. Precipitating factors for delirium in hospitalized elderly patients. JAMA 1996;275:852–857.

Inouye SK, Bogardus ST Jr, Charpentier PA et al. A multicomponent intervention to prevent delirium in hospitalized older patients. N Engl J Med 1999;340:669–676.

Jacobs A, Neveling M, Horst M et al. Alterations of neuropsychological function and cerebral glucose metabolism after cardiac surgery are not related only to intraoperative microembolic events. Stroke 1998;29:660–667.

Killebrew K, Whaley RA, Hayward JN, Scatliff JH. Complications of metrizamide myelography. Arch Neurol 1983;40:78–80.

Kornfield DS, Zimberg S, Maim JR. Psychiatric complications of open-heart surgery. N Engl J Med 1965;273:287–292.

Lampert PW, Hardman JM. Morphological changes in brains of boxers. JAMA 1984;251:2676–2679.

Lawlor PG, Fainsinger RL, Bruera ED. Delirium at the end of life. Critical issues in clinical practice and research. JAMA 2000;284:2427–2429.

Levine DN, Finklestein S. Delayed psychosis after right temporoparietal stroke or trauma: relationship to epilepsy. Neurology 1982;32:267–273.

Levine DN, Grek A. The anatomic basis of delusions after right cerebral infarction. Neurology 1984;34:577–582.

Lewis SW. Brain imaging in a case of Capgras' syndrome. Br J Psychiat 1987;150: 117–121.

Lipowski ZJ. Transient cognitive disorders (delirium, acute confusional states) in the elderly. Am J Psychiatry 1983;140:1426–1436.

Lipowski ZJ. Delirium (acute confusional states). JAMA 1987;258:1789–1792.

Maxson PM, Schultz KL, Berge KH *et al.* Probably alcohol abuse or dependence: a risk factor for intensive–care readmission in patients undergoing elective vascular and thoracic surgical procedures. Mayo Clin Proc 1999;74:448–453.

Mawdsley C, Ferguson FR. Neurological disease in boxers. Lancet 1963;2:795–797.

Meagher DJ, Trzepacz PT. Motoric subtypes of delirium. Semin Clin Neuropsychiatry 2000;5:75–85.

Medina JL, Rubino FA, Ross A. Agitated delirium caused by infarction of the hippocampal formation and fusiform and lingual gyri: a case report. Neurology 1974;24:1181–1183.

Mesulam M-M, Waxman SG, Geschwind N, Sabin TD. Acute confusional states in right middle cerebral artery infarctions. J Neurol Neurosurg Psychiat 1976;39:84–89.

Millar HR. Psychiatric morbidity in elderly surgical patients. Br J Psychiatry 1981;138:17–20.

Msall M, Batshaw ML, Suss R *et al.* Neurologic outcome in children with inborn errors of urea synthesis, outcome of urea-cycle enzymopathies. N Engl J Med 1984; 310:1527–1528.

Nakada T, Knight RT. Alcohol and the central nervous system. Med Clin North Am 1984; 68:121–131.

Needleman HL. The neuropsychiatric implications of low level exposure to lead. Psychol Med 1982;12:461–463.

Newman MF, Kirchner JL, Phillips-Bute B *et al.* Longitudinal assessment of neuro-cognitive function after coronary-artery bypass surgery. N Engl J Med 2001; 344:395–402.

Prensky AL. Time – a fourth dimension for encephalopathies. N Engl J Med 1984;310: 1527–1528.

Pruitt AA, Rubin RH, Karchmer AW, Duncan GW. Neurologic complications of bacterial endocarditis. Medicine 1978;57:329–343.

Regan L, Golsalves L, Tesar G. Acute intermittent porphyria. Psychosomatics 1999; 40:521–523.

Santosh PJ, Malhotra S. Varied psychiatric manifestations of acute intermittent porphyria. Biol Psychiatry 1994;36:744–747.

Schmidley JW, Messing R. Agitated confusional states in patients with right hemisphere infarctions. Stroke 1984;15:883–885.

Schor JD, Levkoff SE, Lipsitz LA *et al.* Risk factors for delirium in hospitalized elderly. JAMA 1992;267:827–831.

Sellers EM, Kalant H. Alcohol intoxication and withdrawal. N Engl J Med 1976;294: 757–762.

Staton RD, Brumback RA, Wilson H. Reduplicative paramnesia: a disconnection syndrome of memory. Cortex 1982;18:23–36.

Symonds CP. Concussion and its sequelae. Lancet 1962;1:1–5.

Toner I, Taylor KM, Newman S, Smith PL. Cerebral functional changes following cardiac surgery: neuropsychological and EEG assessment. Eur J Cardiothorac Surg 1998; 13:13–20.

Valciukas JA, Lilis R, Fischbein A *et al*. Central nervous system dysfunction due to lead exposure. Science 1978;201:465–467.

Weinstein EA, Kahn RL. Non-aphasic misnaming (paraphasia) in organic brain disease. Arch Neurol Psychiatry 1952;67:72–79.

Weinstein EA, Keller NJA. Linguistic patterns of misnaming in brain injury. Neuropsychologia 1973;79–90.

Wertz R. Neuropathologies of speech and language: an introduction to patient management. In D Johns (ed.), Clinical Management of Neurogenic Communicative Disorders. Boston: Little, Brown, 1978;45–62.

Whitfield CL, Chien LT, Whitehead JD. Lead encephalopathy in adults. Am J Med 1972;52:289–298.

Willanger R, Klee A. Metamorphopsia and other visual disturbances with latency occurring in patients with diffuse cerebral lesions. Acta Neurol Scand 1966;42:1–18.

15

Psychosis

Oh, let me not be mad, not mad, sweet Heaven! Keep me in temper. I would not be mad.

(Shakespeare, *King Lear*, Act II, scene v)

Lovers and madmen have such seething brains, such shaping fantasies, that apprehend more than cool reason ever comprehends. The lunatic, the lover, and the poet are of imagination all compact.

(Shakespeare, *A Midsummer Night's Dream*)

Throughout human history, psychosis or insanity has been recorded and described as one of the most dreaded of human afflictions. Shakespeare appears to have understood the phenomena of psychosis in their negative, or fearful, and their positive, or creative poles. Psychosis occurs worldwide, in all countries and cultures, and it has occurred in all eras of history (Andreason 1994). Schizophrenia, the most common psychotic illness, tends to strike adolescents just as they reach maturity. The disease is extremely disabling, resulting in formal disability status in approximately 60% of cases within 1 year (Ho *et al.* 1997). The suicide rate is also high.

Although psychoses are generally the province of psychiatrists or 'neuropsychiatrists' rather than behavioral neurologists, there is increasing evidence that many of these disorders have a physical basis in the brain. In addition, many of the phenomena of psychosis overlap those of delirium, dementia, and syndromes of focal brain lesions, and hence the behavioral neurologist should have familiarity with these disorders. Psychosis also provides some of the most dramatic examples in existence of the symptoms of brain dysfunction.

This chapter is written from the standpoint of a behavioral neurologist, not a psychiatrist. The emphasis will be on symptomatology, overlap with organic brain syndromes, and a brief review of the evidence for biological causes of these disorders.

DIAGNOSIS OF PSYCHOTIC SYNDROMES

The key to the diagnosis of psychosis is the presence of abnormal perception and abnormal thought processes, leading to a loss of reality testing. Psychoses are thought disorders, or abnormalities of the content of thinking and reasoning. The resulting abnormal thought content brings the individual out of synchrony with 'real' phenomena in the external world and also with internal, bodily sensations. Such disturbances of thought and of reality testing include delusional thinking, including paranoid ideation; grandiose personal identifications; feelings of a greater significance in one's life or of meanings behind commonplace events; hallucinations of voices speaking to the patient; and feelings that others are broadcasting thoughts into the patient or *vice versa*. These are the 'positive' symptoms of psychosis; the 'negative' symptoms include social withdrawal, lack of spontaneity in speech and action, lack of motivation, and subtle difficulties with cognitive function.

As discussed in Chapters 13 and 14, the positive symptoms of psychosis also occur in patients with delirium and dementia. Both delirium and dementia differ from psychosis in the presence of grossly abnormal cognitive functions such as orientation, attention, and memory. Acutely psychotic patients may think they are others (including Jesus Christ or the President), but they are usually oriented to their actual name and the date and place, able to perform simple attention tasks such as serial sevens or 'spell world backwards', and able to recall three memory items for 5 minutes. At this simple level, psychotic patients do not show organic brain dysfunction, though more subtle tests of cognitive function do show deficits in patients with schizophrenia. Patients with delirium are more likely to have autonomic disturbances such as tachycardia, sweating, tremor, hypertension, and restless agitation. It must be said, however, that any of these features can be present to some extent in a very acute psychotic illness, and that no single factor has complete reliability in discriminating between a psychosis and an organic illness.

Another difficult differential diagnosis is that between psychosis and focal brain lesions. Patients with frontal lobe disease may closely resemble psychiatric patients, especially in the negative symptoms above. Patients with neurological illnesses from syphilis (Chapter 13) to epilepsy (Chapter 19) may have psychotic symptoms of both positive and negative types. In most cases, these organic disorders also produce cognitive and other physiological dysfunctions that make the diagnosis clear. At times, however, these distinctions become difficult. In addition, the subtle cognitive deficits of schizophrenia may resemble those associated with focal lesions, especially those in the frontal and temporal lobes. For all of these reasons, it is important for neurologists to have some knowledge of psychotic disorders.

Schizophrenia

Schizophrenia is the most common of the primary psychotic disorders. The prevalence of the disorder is nearly 1% in all cultures around the world (Carpenter and Buchanan 1994). In the USA, the disease tends to begin in late adolescence or early adult life. The cost was estimated at $33 billion in 1990, accounting for 2.5% of total expenditure for health care (Rupp and Keith 1993). Many patients require psychiatric hospitalization. Since the advent of neuroleptic therapy most patients can be managed at home rather than in the hospital long term, a trend in mental health care called 'deinstitutionalization', but many patients require frequent treatments and occasional hospital admissions. The cost of lost productivity of these young people is enormous. Most patients also deteriorate socially, and many end up among the ranks of the homeless.

The symptoms of schizophrenia are quite variable. Some patients have a very gradual onset, beginning with social withdrawal and lack of interest, and only later culminating in the dramatic symptoms described above. Some patients have premorbid 'schizoid' traits before they develop overt psychosis. These traits correlate better with the negative symptoms of schizophrenia, rather than with the psychotic thought disorder (Cuesta *et al.* 1999). In other patients, the illness begins with the abrupt onset of bizarre behavior or psychotic thinking (the 'acute psychotic break'). No one symptom is pathognomonic of the disease. Exclusion of organic or neurological causes of psychosis is necessary. Psychiatrists use the *Diagnostic and Statistical Manual of Mental Disorders*, 4th edition (DSM-IV 1994), as criteria for diagnosis. These criteria are summarized in simplified form in Table 15.1. In addition, schizophrenia must be distinguished from other psychoses such as bipolar

Table 15.1 Modified DSM-IV criteria for diagnosis of schizophrenia

I. Characteristic symptoms: ≥ 2 of the following, present ≥ 1 month, unless successfully treated:
  A. Delusions
  B. Hallucinations
  C. Disorganized speech
  D. Disorganized or catatonic behavior
  E. Negative symptoms (flattened affect, lack of volition)

II. Social/occupational dysfunction: decline in work, interpersonal relations, or self care, failure to achieve expected occupational or educational level

III. Duration: at least 6 months

IV. Schizoaffective and mood disorder exclusion: no major depressive or manic episodes with active phase symptoms, or brief in duration with respect to the active symptoms

V. Substance/general medical condition exclusion: disorder not due to substance abuse, medication effects, or general medical condition

affective disorder (BAD) or 'manic-depressive psychosis'. In BAD, affective symptoms such as depressed or manic mood predominate. Schizophrenics do have mood disturbances, but they are usually shorter-lived and less consistent, and schizophrenics tend to have more bizarre hallucinations and delusions. An intermediate syndrome is called 'schizoaffective disorder'.

Historically, Kraepelin (1919) referred to this disorder as 'dementia praecox' and distinguished it from manic-depressive disorder. Bleuler (1911) coined the term 'schizophrenia' because patients did not truly become demented, and instead the emphasis was on the separation or splitting among thought, emotion, and behavior (Carpenter and Buchanan 1994). Various authorities have divided schizophrenia into subsyndromes based on the predominant symptoms. Bleuler (1911) subclassified schizophrenia into the paranoid, catatonic, and hebephrenic categories. The DSM-IV preserves some of these distinctions. The paranoid type of schizophrenia occurs more often in males, who have intact early childhood development and normal personalities, but systematic hallucinations and delusions (Carpenter and Buchanan 1994). The 'hebephrenic' type, now called the 'disorganized' type, usually begins earlier, with more disruption of interpersonal relationships and a wider variety of symptoms. Catatonia refers to a mute, largely motionless state in which the patient has a 'waxy flexibility' of the limbs and maintains postures of limbs placed by the examiner for minutes to hours. Catatonia is much less common, probably as a result of neuroleptic treatment. For our purposes in this chapter, these subtypes are useful only as descriptions of predominant symptoms. There is little evidence that they represent biologically different diseases or pathophysiologies. Some recent research has suggested that patients with the negative deficits of schizophrenia may represent a more homogeneous group, whereas the positive symptoms are likely seen in a number of etiologically different disorders (Carpenter et al. 1999).

The course of schizophrenia is highly variable. The cases with acute onset generally have a better prognosis than the insidious cases. They respond well to neuroleptic therapy and often stay in remission with maintenance therapy. All patients with schizophrenia, however, are at high risk of deterioration of social functioning and vocational performance over the early years of the illness, even with treatment. Some studies suggest that the disease often stabilizes after 5 to 10 years, and the positive symptoms of psychosis become less evident. Medications are more effective in preventing or treating the positive psychotic symptoms, but the negative symptoms are extremely refractory to therapy.

Cognitive Deficits in Schizophrenia

In general, psychiatric patients are distinguished from neurological patients with mental status abnormalities by their normal orientation, attention, and memory, despite an abnormal content of thought and language. Detailed studies of schizophrenic patients, however, have made clear that a cognitive deficit is an important aspect of the disorder. Perseverative behaviors on such tests as the Wisconsin Card Sort Test, characteristic of frontal lobe disorders (see Chapter 10), occur regularly in schizophrenics. Such perseverative behaviors correlate with paranoid ideation (Spaulding *et al.* 1999a). Subtle impairments of attention, memory, learning, and executive functions have been reported frequently in schizophrenic patients (Levin *et al.* 1989; Saykin *et al.* 1991). Higher level verbal and visuospatial dysfunction, suggestive of either left or right hemisphere disease, is less consistently seen in schizophrenia. Language in schizophrenia is mainly remarkable for the abnormal thought content. Very occasional patients show 'word salad' or 'clang association' speech, but such overt language problems are rare in this era of pharmacological treatment of schizophrenia. In general, cognitive deficits tend to be at their worst during an acute psychotic illness, and they typically improve after neuroleptic therapy, but many schizophrenics have some chronic residual deficit (Spaulding *et al.* 1999a). Cognitive deficits predict impairments in social and community functioning in schizophrenic patients, and documentation of such deficits is therefore important in planning treatment (Velligan *et al.* 2000). In chronic schizophrenics, cognitive deficits may accumulate, and a significant percentage may qualify for a diagnosis of dementia (Barak *et al.* 1997). In these chronic, mostly institutionalized schizophrenic patients, Kraepelin's original name dementia praecox may not be as incorrect as previously thought.

Etiology of Schizophrenia

The first clue to an etiology of schizophrenia is in the genetic analysis of the cases. Primary relatives of family members with schizophrenia have an approximately 10% risk of acquiring the disease, a risk much higher than that of the general population (Sanders and Gejman 2001). Identical twins are nearly 50% concordant for the disease. As yet, there is little evidence for specific genes relevant to schizophrenia, and environmental factors also likely play an important role. There is some evidence that intrauterine trauma or infection increases the likelihood of later development of schizophrenia (Lewis and Murray 1987). Damage to structures of the brain during development may predispose to schizophrenia (Bracha *et al.* 1992; Raedler *et al.* 1998). While these pieces of evidence are intriguing, it is likely that they only influence risk or trigger the disease in a minority of genetically susceptible patients (Raedler *et al.* 1998).

Closely related to the evidence for an intrauterine insult to the developing brain in schizophrenia are findings of subtle physical or neurological anomalies, neuropathological changes, and abnormalities on MR imaging of the brain in schizophrenic patients. Several studies have reported an increased incidence of minor physical anomalies, especially involving ectodermal structures of the face, in patients with schizophrenia as compared to control groups. In some studies, however, the criteria for abnormalities used included as many as 10% of normal controls (Green *et al.* 1989; McGrath *et al.* 1995; Griffiths *et al.* 1998a). Other, acquired reasons for these physical changes, such as drug use, were not eliminated as confounding factors in all studies.

Griffiths and colleagues (1998b) performed detailed neurological examinations in schizophrenic patients and found an increase in primary neurological abnormalities, such as abnormal reflexes and Babinski signs, abnormal saccadic eye movements, and involuntary movements; the authors referred to these as 'hard' rather than 'soft' neurological signs. These signs occurred with increased incidence in sporadic schizophrenic patients, but not in familial cases, suggesting an association with acquired, developmental insults in the sporadic cases. Some signs, such as tremor and choreoathetosis, could be explained by antipsychotic drug use, but there was poor correlation with either drug dosage or extrapyramidal side effect scales, suggesting that drugs were not the primary cause of the abnormal signs. In addition, the difference between the sporadic and familial schizophrenic patients could not be explained by differences in drug usage. One study (Sanders et al. 1994) found neurological abnormalities even in first-attack, drug-naïve patients. Higher-level integrative abnormalities, such as abnormal graphesthesia, were more common in the hereditary group, suggesting that there may be a genetic 'neurointegrative deficit' in patients at genetic risk for schizophrenia. These studies of neurological signs provide further evidence for a brain-based, organic foundation for schizophrenia.

The next source of evidence for a neurological cause of schizophrenia comes from structural studies of the brain, either at *post-mortem* or in brain imaging studies. *Post-mortem* studies have shown dilatation of the cerebral ventricles in chronic schizophrenics, as well as atrophy of parts of the basal ganglia and limbic or medial temporal lobe structures such as the hippocampus and amygdala (Bogerts et al. 1985; Pakkenberg 1987). One study (Kulynych et al. 1997) has reported reduced cortical folding, or 'gyrification', in the left temporal lobe of schizophrenic patients. Some studies (Barta et al. 1997), but not others (Frangou et al. 1997; Jacobson et al. 1997) have reported abnormal asymmetries of the planum temporale in schizophrenics. Selective atrophy or loss of neuropil connections has also been reported in the prefrontal cortex (Harrison 1999; Selemon and Goldman-Rakic 1999). Microscopic neuronal abnormalities have been inconsistently reported in neuropathological studies of brains from schizophrenics (Raedler et al. 1998). Findings of abnormal brain development or asymmetry between the hemispheres would be important in suggesting a developmental or genetic etiology of schizophrenia, as opposed to a disorder acquired in later life.

Brain imaging studies have extended the findings of neuropathological surveys in schizophrenia. MRI studies have confirmed the findings of enlargement of the ventricles and atrophy of limbic and medial temporal structures (Pearlson and Marsh 1999). Functional brain imaging with PET and SPECT has also revealed abnormalities in schizophrenic patients. One recent study (Crespo-Facorro et al. 2001) correlated reduced changes in cerebral blood flow in limbic areas of the brain, compared to normals, in response to pleasant and unpleasant odors. The authors suggested a neurological basis for the emotional changes in schizophrenia.

Even more than structural changes in the brain, changes in brain chemistry, especially those involving neurotransmitters such as dopamine, appear to be involved in schizophrenia. Excess dopaminergic function has long been suspected in schizophrenia, based on the known psychotic reactions seen with dopaminergic treatments for Parkinson's disease, the effects of hallucinogenic drugs, and the improvement in psychotic symptoms produced by dopamine-blocking drugs. In *post-mortem* studies, striatal D_2 receptors are increased in density in schizophrenic brains (Seeman 1987), though dopamine-blocking medications may be responsible for at least some of this increase.

Recently, brain imaging modalities have permitted the investigation of brain chemistry and abnormalities of neurotransmitter systems, *in vivo* (Soares and Innis 1999). Dopamine-binding ligands have been studied in schizophrenics with either PET or SPECT scanning techniques. The preponderance of the evidence from such studies indicates increased D_2 receptor density in at least a substantial portion of patients with schizophrenia (Laruelle 1998; Zakzanis and Hansen 1998). Increased amphetamine-induced dopamine release has also been demonstrated via SPECT scans in drug-free schizophrenic subjects (Laruelle *et al.* 1996). Dopamine synthesis in the striatum, as measured by uptake of the PET tracer {^{18}F}FDOPA, has also been reported to be increased in schizophrenics (Hietala *et al.* 1999). These studies suggest that dopamine metabolism, both synthesis and turnover, is increased in schizophrenia. These findings support the clinical evidence that dopamine likely plays a role in the genesis of psychotic symptoms in schizophrenia. Some authorities have postulated that excessive mesolimbic dopamine turnover is responsible for the psychotic symptoms in schizophrenia, whereas decreased dopamine turnover in cortical systems may be related to the negative symptoms of schizophrenia (Davis *et al.* 1991).

Other transmitter systems may also be abnormal in schizophrenia. Findings regarding serotonin and GABA have been less consistent than those regarding dopamine (Soares and Innis 1999). Magnetic resonance spectroscopy has recently been applied to studies of schizophrenic patients. Proton MR spectroscopy can detect a signal for N-acetyl aspartate (NAA), thought to be a marker of neuronal degeneration. NAA is decreased in the hippocampus and dorsolateral prefrontal cortex, even in drug-free schizophrenics (Bertolino *et al.* 1998).

Brain imaging techniques, neurochemistry, and neuropathology all appear to be converging on a biological explanation of schizophrenia, based on abnormal genes, possibly intrauterine exposure to infections or toxins, and abnormal development of portions of the frontal and temporal lobes, basal ganglia, and limbic structures. While a unified theory of schizophrenia has not as yet emerged, the neurochemical abnormalities have already produced a major change in the prognosis of schizophrenia, based on neurotransmitter-related therapies.

Treatment of Schizophrenia

In the past, schizophrenia had a poor prognosis, with most patients becoming disabled, and a large proportion confined to custodial institutions. The drug treatment revolution began in the 1950s with the drug chlorpromazine (Thorazine). Neuroleptic, dopamine-blocking drugs help reduce acute hallucinations and psychotic symptoms in schizophrenia, gradually improve thinking, and prevent relapses of psychosis (Carpenter and Buchanan 1994). Many other drugs have followed, including the newer, 'atypical' antipsychotic drugs, which promise relief of psychotic symptoms without intolerable side effects. These include clozapine (Clozaril), risperidone (Risperdal), olanzepine (Zyprexa) and quetiapine (Seroquel). The first available, clozapine, is declining in use because of the risk of leukopenia and requirement for weekly blood monitoring. The others are safe, with relatively less extrapyramidal side effects than with older agents, but the drugs are expensive and require a compliant patient. The use of neuroleptic drugs has permitted the deinstitutionalization of many patients with schizophrenia. Many remain dependent on others for their care, however, and they easily become non-functional, with homelessness and drug addiction major risks. In addition, drugs benefit the positive symptoms of schizophrenia more than the negative ones.

Cognitive behavioral therapies of schizophrenia, long ignored because of the obvious effect of neuroleptic medications, are currently making a comeback (Spaulding et al. 1999b; Dickerson 2000). Patients can learn, through conditioning, to avoid psychotic thoughts and to deny the reality of hallucinations (Dickerson 2000). These treatments are especially helpful in the social functioning of schizophrenics (Huxley et al. 2000). Cognitive behavioral treatments are expensive, however, and limited research on cost effectiveness has appeared (Kuipers et al. 1998). These treatments should likely be combined with pharmacotherapy. In the future, the 'organic' factors in schizophrenia – genetic, neurochemical, structural, or environmental – may be modified by biological treatments to prevent progression of the disease. Until then, we are left with a patchwork of behavioral and pharmacological treatments to palliate the devastating effects of the disease (Pearlson, 2000).

AFFECTIVE DISORDERS

The subject of depression is covered in Chapter 17, but a few introductory comments are appropriate here, before consideration of affective psychosis. Major depression is an extremely common disorder, occurring throughout the world. Recent epidemiological surveys (Weissman et al. 1996) have reported lifetime prevalence of major depression in from 1.5% in Taiwan to 19% in Beirut, or annual incidence rates from 0.8% in Taiwan to 5.8% in New Zealand. DSM-IV criteria for major depression (see Chapter 17) include any history of a depressive episode, including a grief reaction lasting more than 1 year, but excluding any patient with a history of a manic episode. The variability of incidence rates in different countries suggests that cultural factors, war, economic distress, and other environmental factors are important in determining the incidence of depression. Women have generally higher rates of depression than men.

The symptoms of major depression, though variable, frequently include depressed or dysphoric mood, insomnia, loss of energy, difficulty concentrating, slowed thinking, feelings of worthlessness or guilt, and thoughts of death or suicide (Weissman et al. 1996). Appetite changes, weight loss or gain, hypersomnia, psychomotor retardation or agitation, and decreased interest in sex are less consistent symptoms of depression. The prominence of complaints of reduced concentration and slowed thinking as hallmarks of depression make clear why behavioral neurologists should have some knowledge of depression.

Bipolar Affective Disorder

The term 'manic-depressive disorder' or 'bipolar affective disorder' implies a cycling between depressed and hyperactive phases. In the past, classifications divided BAD into several types, depending on whether the disorder involved only manic phases, only rare manic phases, or alternation between the two poles (Klerman 1987). For the purposes of this review, any affective disorder with a history of even one manic episode will be considered to represent bipolar affective disorder.

The symptoms of mania or the 'up' phase of bipolar affective disorder include either elevated (euphoric) or irritable mood, with a pronounced increase in energy, impaired judgment, grandiose ideas, and loose associations or 'flight of ideas.' Patients may make impulsive purchases beyond their means, arrange poorly planned business deals, or engage in uncharacteristic sexual alliances. Moods may shift rapidly from elation to irritability (Larson and Richelson 1988). Some patients develop frankly psychotic symptoms during a manic episode, including delusional thinking, loose associations, and hallucinations. DSM-IV (1994) criteria for bipolar affective disorder are presented in modified form in Table 15.2.

Table 15.2   Modified DSM-IV diagnostic criteria for manic episode

---

I. Distinct period of abnormally and persistently elevated, expansive, or irritable mood

II. Three of the following (four, if mood is only irritable):
   A. Grandiosity or inflated self-esteem
   B. Decreased need for sleep
   C. Pressure of speech
   D. Flight of ideas or thoughts racing
   E. Easy distractibility
   F. Psychomotor agitation or increased activity
   G. Excessive involvement in pleasurable activities despite risk of adverse consequences

III. Symptoms do not meet criteria for a 'mixed' episode

IV. Substantial impairment in occupational, social, or interpersonal functioning (if not present, episode is called 'hypomanic')

V. Symptoms not due to substance abuse, medication effect, or medical condition; effects of antidepressant treatment should not count towards the diagnosis of bipolar disorder

---

In epidemiologic surveys (Weissman *et al.* 1996), bipolar affective disorder has a more consistent incidence and prevalence across different countries and cultures than does major depression; lifetime rates range from 0.3–1.5%. BAD is less common than major depression, but its consistent incidence and prevalence rates across cultures suggest a more biological cause in BAD as compared to major depression. There is also less difference between men and women in BAD than in major depression. The age of onset averaged 6 years younger in BAD than in major depression in the survey of Weissman *et al.* (1996), but this survey did not examine late onset cases. Genetic studies have also suggested a major hereditary factor in BAD; in fact, many families of typical, early onset bipolar affective disorder appear to follow an autosomal dominant inheritance pattern for BAD. Children raised by adoptive parents are more likely to develop both depression and bipolar affective disorder if a biological parent was similarly affected (Mendlewicz and Rainer 1977; Cadoret 1978).

Late onset cases of bipolar affective disorders are not uncommon. These cases pose a challenge to the behavioral neurologist in distinguishing BAD from delirium. Affective disorders with hyperactivity or mania account for 5–10% of psychiatric admissions of patients over age 60 (Young and Klerman 1992). These late onset cases of BAD have a lower family incidence of BAD than early onset cases, suggesting that the etiologic basis of the late onset cases may be more variable (Hays 1976; Young and Klerman 1992). Other evidence has pointed to a higher incidence of organic causes of mania, sometimes called 'secondary mania', in late onset as compared to early onset cases. Stone (1989), for example, found that 24% of late onset manic disorders in their series from Scotland had 'evidence of organic cerebral impairment', and these patients had both later onset and lower incidence of a positive family history as compared to their average late onset cases.

Specific organic causes of late onset bipolar affective disorder or mania are numerous (Larson and Richelson 1988). DSM-IV criteria for organic mania include: (1) prominent and persistent mood elevation; (2) evidence of an organic etiology; and (3) manic symptoms not associated solely in time with delirium. Head injuries (Reiss *et al.* 1987; Nizamie *et al.* 1988) and seizure disorders (Krauthammer and Klerman 1978) are among the most common causes of organic or secondary mania, but many structural lesions have been found. Tumors, especially of the diencephalon or frontal lobes, strokes-in the basal frontal and temporal lobes or basal ganglia (Cummings and Mendez 1984), and herpes simplex encephalitis have been associated with mania (Larson and Richelson 1988). In general, lesions of the right as opposed to left cerebral hemisphere and lesions involving the diencephalon, limbic structures, and the frontal and temporal lobes have been most closely associated with the development of manic symptoms (Cummings and Mendez 1984). In one series of head injury cases, factors associated with mania were a prior history of depression or bipolar affective disorder, right hemisphere involvement, and damage to limbic structures (Starkstein *et al.* 1987). Other, structural causes of mania include viral encephalitis and other CNS infections and neurological diseases such as multiple sclerosis, Parkinson's disease and postencephalitic parkinsonism, Huntington's disease, and Wilson's disease (Larson and Richelson 1988). Systemic illnesses such as hyperthyroidism, uremia, Vitamin B12 deficiency, and postoperative states have all been reported to cause mania; it should be noted that most of these causes are also listed as etiologies of delirium (see Chapter 14), and not all of the descriptions have strictly followed the DSM-IV criteria listed above. Finally, a long list of drugs have been associated with mania, including corticosteroids, cocaine, phencyclidine, dopaminergic drugs such as levodopa and bromocriptine, cimetidine, and antidepressants (Stasiek and Zetin 1985); it should be noted that antidepressants may induce mania in patients with a tendency to bipolar affective disorder. Withdrawal from benzodiazepines and from baclofen can cause mania. Another more recently described drug producing mania is ziduvidine (AZT), used in the treatment of HIV infection (Wright *et al.* 1989). Personally observed cases of organic mania included an elderly man with herpes zoster of the chest, in association with high-dose steroid therapy, and a man who abruptly discontinued use of baclofen after several months of 60–70 mg per day of therapy. This man, a carpenter who was deeply religious, became hyperactive, ceasing to sleep for several days, speaking incessantly, and making sexually inappropriate innuendos to the nursing staff. He appeared to meet DSM-IV criteria for mania (Arnold *et al.* 1980).

These cases of organic mania should make it clear that mania as a 'functional' psychosis should never be diagnosed unless prior episodes have been documented or a detailed evaluation for physical causes has been undertaken. There is a clear age difference: bipolar affective disorder usually has a first episode before the age of 25 years, whereas organic mania usually begins after age 35 (Larson and Richelson 1988). The pathophysiology is not well understood. Serotonergic, noradrenergic and dopaminergic pathways may be involved, judging by the association with such drugs as antidepressants, levodopa, and bromocriptine. The GABA system may also be involved, as evidenced by mania occurring in association with withdrawal from baclofen.

The treatment of organic mania generally involves removal of the offending drug or correction of the abnormal metabolic disorder, if possible, along with symptomatic treatment. Lithium, carbamazepine, and other agents used in bipolar affective disorder have been used successfully in organic cases (Larson and Richelson 1988).

Pharmacotherapy of Manic Disorders

The major breakthrough in the treatment of bipolar affective disorder came with the use of lithium carbonate, first begun in the 1940s (Schou 1988). Lithium appears to prevent not only the manic phases but also the depressive ones, an effect called a 'mood stabilizing effect'. Clinical trials have supported the usefulness of lithium in bipolar affective disorder (Price and Henninger 1994). The dosage of lithium should be titrated, with frequent blood levels. Maintenance doses generally range from 900–1500 mg per day. There are many drug interactions, and care must be taken in patients with renal insufficiency. Toxic effects include tremor, lethargy, speech and language difficulties, hypothroidism, and gastrointestinal side effects (Price and Henninger 1994). Concomitant antidepressant drugs are often used with the 'mood stabilizing' agents such as lithium or an antiepileptic drug. There is a common suspicion that antidepressant agents can precipitate mania in bipolar patients, though the evidence for this effect of antidepressants is controversial (Wehr and Goodwin 1987). More recently, antiepileptic drugs have been used successfully in bipolar affective disorder, especially carbamazepine, valproic acid, oxcarbamazepine, gabapentin, and lamotrigine (Post *et al*. 1996). The applicability of antiepileptic drugs in this 'paroxysmal' mood disorder is of theoretical interest, and supports the organic etiology of bipolar affective disorder.

CONCLUSION

The psychoses, especially schizophrenia and bipolar affective disorder, are fascinating disorders in which the symptoms seem psychiatric, yet the evidence suggests an organic brain disorder. The evidence for brain dysfunction has been much more subtle than in acquired focal brain lesions such as strokes, in which brain imaging modalities such as CT or MRI scans show 'holes' in the brain. The signs on CT and MRI are extremely subtle, usually involving selective atrophy of cerebral structures. For a long period these were considered 'soft science'. Owing to the subtlety of the findings, however, neuroscientists have had to rely on more sophisticated neurochemical methods such as PET scanning with specific ligands, or neurotransmitter receptor studies in pathological tissue. The reward of this 'hard science' has been clear evidence that there are neurochemical changes in these diseases; such changes have not been fully explored in such obviously organic disorders as stroke. What remains is to tie these neurochemical changes back to the dramatic clinical symptomatology of the psychoses. These processes are at the heart of the science of brain and behavior.

REFERENCES

Andreasen NC. Understanding the causes of schizophrenia. New Engl J Med 1994;340:645–647.

Arnold ES, Rudd SM, Kirshner H. Manic psychosis following rapid withdrawal from baclofen. Am J Psychiatry 1980;137:1466–1467.

Barak Y, Swartz M, Davidson M. Dementia in elderly schizophrenic patients: reviewing the reviews. Int Rev Psych 1997;9:459–463.

Barta PE, Pearlson GD, Brill LB *et al*. Planum temporale asymmetry reversal in schizophrenia: replication and relationship to gray matter abnormalities. Am J Psychiatry 1997;154:661–667.

Bertolino A, Callicott JH, Elman I *et al*. Regionally specific neuronal pathology in untreated patients with schizophrenia: a proton magnetic resonance spectroscopic imaging study. Biol Psychiatry 1998;43:641–648.

Bleuler E. Dementia praecox; or, the group of schizophrenias (trans. J Zinkin, 1950; originally published 1911). New York: International Universities Press.

Bogerts B, Meertz E, Schonfeldt-Bausch R. Basal ganglia and limbic system pathology in schizophrenia. A morphometric study of brain volume and shrinkage. Arch Gen Psychiatry 1985;42:784–791.

Bracha HS, Torrey EF, Gottesman II *et al*. Second-trimester markers of fetal size in schizophrenia: a study of monozygotic twins. Am J Psychiatry 1992;149:1355–1361.

Cadoret RJ. Evidence for genetic inheritance of primary affective disorder in adoptees. Am J Psychiatry 1978;135:463–468.

Carpenter WT, Buchanan RW. Schizophrenia. New Engl J Med 1994;330:681–690.

Carpenter WT, Kirkpatrick B, Buchanan RW. Schizophrenia: syndromes and diseases. J Psychiat Res 1999;33:473–475.

Crespo-Facorro B, Paradiso S, Andreasen NC *et al*. Neural mechanisms of anhedonia in schizophrenia. A PET study of response to unpleasant and pleasant odors. JAMA 2001;286:427–435.

Cuesta MJ, Peralta V, Caro F. Premorbid personality in psychoses. Schizophrenia Bull 1999;25:801–811.

Cummings JL, Mendez MF. Secondary mania with focal cerebrovascular lesions. Am J Psychiatry 1984;141:1084–1087.

Davis KL, Kahn RS, Ko G, Davidson M. Dopamine in schizophrenia: a review and reconceptualization. Am J Psychiatry 1991;148:1474–1486.

Diagnostic and Statistical Manual of Mental Disorders (4th edn). Washington, DC: American Psychiatric Association, 1994.

Dickerson F. Cognitive behavioral psychotherapy for schizophrenia: a review of recent empirical studies. Schizophrenia Res 2000;43:71–90.

Frangou S, Sharma T, Sigmudsson T *et al*. Maudsley family study. 4. Normal planum temporale asymmetry in familial schizophrenia. A volumetric MRI study. Br J Psychiatry 1997;41:995–999.

Green MF, Satz P, Gaier DJ *et al*. Minor physical anomalies in adult male schizophrenics. Schizophr Bull 1989;15:91–99.

Griffiths TD, Sigmundsson T, Takei N *et al*. Minor physical anomalies in familial and sporadic schizophrenia: the Maudsley family study. J Neurol Neurosurg Psychiatry 1998a;64:56–60.

Griffiths TD, Sigmundsson T, Takei N *et al*. Neurological abnormalities in familial and sporadic schizophrenia. Brain 1998b;121:191–203.

Harrison PJ. The neuropathology of schizophrenia: a critical review of the data and their interpretation. Brain 1999;122:593–624.

Hays P. Etiological factors in manic depressive psychosis. Arch Gen Psychiatry 1976;33:1187–1188.

Hietala J, Syvalahti E, Vilkman H *et al*. Depressive symptoms and presynaptic dopamine function in neuroleptic-naïve schizophrenia. Schizophr Res 1999;35:41–50.

Ho BC, Andreasen N, Flaum M. Dependence on public financial support early in the course of schizophrenia. Psychiatr Serv 1997;48:948–950.

Huxley NA, Rendall M, Sederer L. Psychosocial treatments in schizophrenia. A review of the past 20 years. J Nerv Ment Dis 2000;188:187–201.

Jacobsen LK, Giedd JN, Tanrikut C *et al*. Three-dimensional cortical morphometry of the planum temporale in childhood-onset schizophrenia. Am J Psychiatry 1997; 154:685–687.

Klerman GL. The classification of bipolar disorders. Psychiatr Annals 1987;17:13–17.

Kraepelin E. Dementia praecox and paraphrenia (trans. RM Barclay, 1919). Edinburgh, Scotland: ES Livingston.

Krauthammer C, Klerman GL. Secondary mania. Manic syndromes associated with antecedent physical illness or drugs. Arch Gen Psychiatry 1978;35:1333–1339.

Kuipers E, Fowler D, Garety P *et al*. London–East Anglia randomized controlled trial of cognitive-behavioural therapy for psychosis. III. Follow-up and economic evaluation at 18 months. Br J Psychiatry 1998;173:61–68.

Kulynych JJ, Luevano LF, Jones DW, Weinberger DR. Cortical abnormality in schizophrenia: an in vivo application of the gyrification index. Biol Psychiatry 1997; 41:995–999.

Laruelle M. Imaging dopamine transmission in schizophrenia – a review and meta-analysis. Q J Nucl Med 1998;42:211–221.

Laruelle M, Abi-Dargham A, Vandyck CH *et al*. Single photon emission computerized tomography imaging of amphetamine-induced dopamine release in drug-free schizophrenic subjects. PNAS 1996;93:9235–9240.

Larson EW, Richelson E. Organic causes of mania. Mayo Clin Proc 1988;63:906–912.

Levin S, Yurgelun-Todd D, Craft S. Contributions of clinical neuropsychology to the study of schizophrenia. J Abnorm Posychol 1989;98:341–356.

Lewis SW, Murray RM. Obstetric complications, neurodevelopmental deviance, and risk of schizoprenia. J Psychiatr Res 1987;21:413–421.

McGrath JJ, Van Os J, Hoyos C *et al*. Minor physical anomalies in psychoses: associations with clinical and putative aetiological variables. Schizophr Res 1995;18:9–20.

Mendlewicz J, Rainer JD. Adoption study supporting genetic transmission in manic-depressive illness. Nature 1977;268:327–329.

Nizamie SH, Nizamie A, Borde M, Sharma S. Mania following head injury: case reports and neuropsychological findings. Acta Psychiatr Scand 1988;77:637–639.

Pakkenberg B. Post-mortem study of chronic schizophrenic brains. Br J Psychiatry 1987;151:744–752.

Pearlson GD. Neurobiology of schizophrenia. Ann Neurol 2000;48:556–566.

Pearlson GD, Marsh L. Structural brain imaging in schizophrenia. Biol Psychiatry 1999;46:627–649.

Post RM, Ketter TA, Denicoff K *et al*. Psychopharmacology 1996;128:115–129.

Price LH, Heninger GR. Lithium in the treatment of mood disorders. New Engl J Med 1994;331:591–598.

Raedler TJ, Knable MB, Weinberger DR. Schizophrenia as a developmental disorder of the cerebral cortex. Curr Opin Neurobiol 1998;8:157–161.

Reiss H, Schwartz CE, Klerman GL. Manic syndrome following head injury: another form of secondary mania. J Clin Psychiatry 1987;48:29–30.

Rupp A, Keith SJ. The costs of schizophrenia: assessing the burden. Psychiatr Clin North Am 1993;16:413–423.

Sanders AR, Gejman PV. Influential ideas and experimental progress in schizophrenia genetics research. JAMA 2001;285:2831–2833.

Sanders RD, Keshaven MS, Schooler NR. Neurological examination abnormalities in neuroleptic-naïve patients with first break schizophrenia: preliminary results. Am J Psych 1994;151:124–131.

Saykin AJ, Gur RC, Gur RE *et al*. Neuropsychological function in schizophrenia: selective impairment in memory and learning. Arch Gen Psychiatry 1991;48: 618–624.

Schou M. Lithium treatment of manic-depressive illness. Past, present, and perspectives. JAMA 1988;259:1834–1836.

Seeman P. Dopamine receptors and the dopamine hypothesis of schizophrenia. Synapse 1987;1:133–152.

Selemon LD, Goldman-Rakic PS. The reduced neuropil hypothesis: a circuit based model of schizophrenia. Biol Psych 1999;45:17–25.

Soarcs JC, Innis RB. Neurochemical brain imaging investigations of schizophrenia. Biol Psychiatry 1999;46:600–615.

Spaulding WD, Fleming SK, Reed D *et al*. Cognitive functioning in schizophrenia: implications for psychiatric rehabilitation. Schizophrenia Bull 1999a;25:275–289.

Spaulding WD, Reed D, Sullivan M *et al*. Effects of cognitive treatment in psychiatric rehabilitation. Schizophrenia Bull 1999b;25:657–676.

Starkstein SE, Pearlson GD, Boston J, Robinson RG. Mania after brain injury. A controlled study of causative factors. Arch Neurol 1987;44:1069–1073.

Stasiek C, Zetin M. Organic manic disorders. Psychosomatics 1985;26:394–402.

Stone K. Mania in the elderly. Br J Psychiatr 1989;155:220–224.

Velligan DI, Bow-Thomas CC, Mahurin RK *et al*. Do specific neurocognitive deficits predict specific domains of community function in schizophrenia? J Nerv Ment Dis 2000;188:518–524.

Wehr TA, Goodwin FK. Can antidepressants cause mania and worsen the course of affective illness? Am J Psychiatry 1987;144:1403–1411.

Weissman MM, Bland RC, Canino GJ *et al*. Cross-national epidemiology of major depression and bipolar disorder. JAMA 1996;276:293–299.

Wright JM, Sachdev PS, Perkins RJ, Rodriguez P. Zidovudine-related mania. Med J Australia 1989;150:339–341.

Young RC, Klerman GL. Mania in late life: focus on age at onset. Am J Psychiatry 1992;149:867–876.

Zakzanis KK, Hansen KT. Dopamine D2 densities and the schizophrenic brain. Schizophr Res 1998;32:301–306.

16

Behavioral Aspects of Movement Disorders

The senses and intellect being uninjured.

(Parkinson 1817)

A relatively new field in behavioral neurology is the exploration of cognitive and emotional changes in the group of neurodegenerative diseases affecting the basal ganglia and the control of movement. The hallmark of all of these diseases is alteration of movement patterns, either a paucity of movement (hypokinetic movement disorders) or an excess of movement (hyperkinetic movement disorders). In many of these diseases, changes in cognitive and behavioral functions are an important aspect of the overall disability caused by the disease. Many can cause dementia; this group of disorders was introduced in Chapter 13 under the heading 'subcortical dementia'. In addition, movement disorders can be associated with delirium, memory loss, depression or elation, psychotic thought disorder, and focal neurobehavioral deficits such as visuospatial dysfunction or language deterioration. In this chapter, we shall consider the more common movement disorders, disease by disease, with respect to cognitive and behavioral function.

PARKINSON'S DISEASE

In his original essay on the 'shaking palsy', James Parkinson (1817) aptly described the characteristic resting tremor, rigidity, and small-stepped gait of the disease that now bears his name. The three cardinal features of Parkinson's disease – tremor, rigidity, and slowed movement (bradykinesia) – are well known to neurologists. Like Alzheimer's disease (AD), Parkinson's disease (PD) becomes more common with advancing age. Speech is often affected, with low voice volume (hypophonia), decreased intonation, and mild dysarthria. Parkinson (1817) regarded mentation in these patients as normal ('the senses and intellect being uninjured'). Subsequent series of patients with PD, however, have documented delirium or dementia in 15–40% of cases (Celesia and Wanamaker 1972; Leiberman *et al.* 1979; Sroka *et al.* 1981; Mindham *et al.* 1982; Brown and Marsden 1984). Some of this difference likely resulted from the introduction of effective medications for PD. When levodopa first became available, patients remained mobile for much longer periods, and the mental status abnormalities became more evident. Acute confusional states with visual hallucinations are common, especially in relation to levodopa-carbidopa (Sinemet) or dopamine agonist therapy. Drug therapy for PD has advanced; in addition to levodopa there are now four dopamine agonists on the market, as well as selegiline (a monoamine oxidase B inhibitor) and entacapone (a catecholamine-O-methyltransferase inhibitor), both of which potentiate the effect of levodopa. The acute confusional states and hallucinosis related to these drugs are usually reversible, but many patients also develop a true dementia (Sroka *et al.* 1981; Mindham *et al.* 1982). In comparison to Alzheimer's disease, Parkinson's disease with dementia is more fluctuating in character, with more symptoms of delirium. Age at onset seems to be more of a risk factor for dementia than duration of disease, and many patients indeed remain mentally intact for many years after diagnosis (Mindham *et al.* 1982).

Detailed neuropsychological studies have clearly shown that the cognitive difficulty of PD patients is not simply a reflection of slowed motor performance or depression (Leiberman *et al.* 1979), which is also frequently seen in PD (see below). Visuoperceptual function (Proctor *et al.* 1964; Mortimer *et al.* 1982; Boller *et al.* 1984) and memory (Warburton 1967; Halgrin *et al.* 1977) seem especially affected in patients with PD. Facial recognition was impaired in PD patients in one study, though verbal memory was not significantly different from that of controls (Dewick *et al.* 1991). Visuospatial working memory may be more affected than verbal memory in PD patients (Bradley *et al.* 1989). Procedural learning, or the ability to recall newly learned motor tasks, is impaired in PD patients, whereas declarative memory is largely intact, a deficit profile exactly opposite to that of amnesic patients (Saint-Cyr *et al.* 1988; see Chapter 11). The aspect of memory related to the temporal sequence of items to be remembered (e.g. recency differences) may be specifically impaired in PD patients, as compared to the content of memory, which is more affected in AD patients (Sagar *et al.* 1988). This aspect of memory function may be related to frontal dysfunction (Sagar *et al.* 1988). More recent neuropsychological testing profiles of patients with PD suggest that both the visuospatial and perceptual deficits may not be primary deficits, but rather an expression of impaired 'executive functions', or more specifically deficits in the ability to devise strategies to manage novel stimuli and adjust one's actions in response to feedback from previous actions (Taylor and Saint-Cyr 1995). These 'frontal' deficits likely reflect dysfunction in the frontal–basal ganglia loops discussed in Chapter 10.

Some authors have suggested that parkinsonian patients with dementia may suffer from a disease different from typical idiopathic Parkinson's disease, based on later age of onset, more rapid progression, poorer response to therapy, and the presence of cognitive deficits early in the course of the disease (Sroka *et al.* 1981; Mindham *et al.* 1982). Studies of cognitive dysfunction in patients with Parkinson's disease have found increased cognitive and memory deficits in patients with later ages of onset (Canavan *et al.* 1989; Dubois *et al.* 1990). This pattern of presentation, late onset and early cognitive deficits, is also suggestive of Lewy body dementia (see below). Mental impairments in Parkinson's disease also appear to correlate with the severity of the bradykinesia but not with tremor or rigidity (Mortimer *et al.* 1982). Two studies have also documented a worsening of cognitive performance during the akinetic phase of the 'on–off effect', a fluctuation between an immobile state and a nearly normal one, in individual patients (Delis *et al.* 1982; Brown *et al.* 1984; Mohr *et al.* 1989). Rafal and colleagues (1984), on the other hand, found that motor responses are more likely to be slowed during the 'off' state than purely cognitive operations; they criticize the concept of 'bradyphrenia', or slowing of mental processes in PD. The active hallucinations and other psychotic features are more likely to occur with dopamine excess secondary to medications than with the 'off' phase of Parkinson's disease.

In recent years, surgical treatments have been developed for patients who fail to respond or lose their response to medications (Follett 2000). These operations began with thalamotomy in the 1950s, a treatment discovered serendipitously when Dr Irving Cooper operated on a patient to clip an aneurysm and sacrificed the anterior choroidal artery. The patient awoke not with the anticipated contralateral hemiparesis, but with disappearance of her tremor from the contralateral limbs. Surgical treatments have advanced during the past decade, both with surgical ablation of the ventrolateral thalamus or globus pallidus, and more recently with placement of electrode stimulators in the thalamus, globus pallidus, or subthalamic nucleus. The most commonly performed procedure currently in the USA is surgical ablation of the posteroventral globus pallidus, or pallidotomy. Unilateral pallidotomy generally produces only minor cognitive impairments (York *et al.* 1999; Fine *et al.* 2000), but neuropsychological testing has shown deficits in frontal lobe or 'frontostriatal' functions such as psychomotor processing speed, executive aspects of working memory, and tests of reasoning (Green and Barnhart 2000; Stebbins *et al.* 2000). Extension of the lesion into the anterior portion of the internal globus pallidus or into the external globus pallidus may result in greater deficits, and bilateral operations leave many patients with reduced cognitive function. Another approach to the surgical treatment of PD, as yet experimental, is the transplantation of fetal neurons into the basal ganglia. The fetal cells survived and produced dopamine; younger patients showed some benefit in terms of movement, but older patients did not, and 15% of the younger patients developed excessive dopaminergic function, with severe dyskinesias (Freed *et al.* 2001). These results indicate that transplanted fetal cells do survive in the adult brain, but their function may need more modulation before such transplants can be used routinely. Transplantation of adrenal cells, an earlier technique, was less successful. The surgical treatment of Parkinson's disease is evolving rapidly, and safer, less cognitively-impairing procedures are likely to develop. The placement of stimulating electrodes into the thalamus, globus pallidus, or subthalamic nucleus (Benabid *et al.* 2000; Follett 2000) should have lower risk of tissue damage than ablative procedures. Bilateral stimulation of the subthalamic nucleus improved motor function with a modest negative effect on verbal memory and on prefrontal and visuospatial functions in one series (Alegret *et al.* 2001) and with no effect on memory or executive functions in another (Ardouin *et al.* 1999). Interestingly, high frequency deep brain stimulation occasionally causes acute mood changes, especially depression (Bejjani *et al.* 1999). Localized ablations or stimulation of subcortical structures should add to our knowledge of the behavioral and cognitive correlates of these areas of the brain.

Depression is also a frequent concomitant of Parkinson's disease (Vogel 1982; Starkstein *et al.* 1989; Brown and McCarthy 1990; Hantz *et al.* 1994). Starkstein and colleagues (1989) found a direct correlation between depression and the degree of cognitive impairment in Parkinson's disease. The biochemical basis for depression in Parkinson's disease is not well delineated, but presumably the dopaminergic deficit seen in this disease may also relate to adrenergic and noradrenergic changes seen in depression. CSF levels of 5-HIAA, a serotonin metabolite, were depressed in a group of PD patients with depression or dementia, suggesting that serotonin may also play a role in the depression associated with PD (Mayeux *et al.* 1988). Patients with PD also have a high incidence of anxiety (Stein *et al.* 1990).

The basis of the cognitive changes in Parkinson's disease is complex. Although the disease primarily affects the basal ganglia, the nature of the cognitive deficits suggests that the cerebral cortex is also affected. CT scans confirm the presence of cortical atrophy in patients with dementia and Parkinson's disease, and these changes are more severe in such patients than in age-matched controls or in Parkinson's disease patients without dementia (Schneider *et al.* 1979; Mindham *et al.* 1982). Pathological studies have shown not only the well-known loss of pigmented neurons in the substantia nigra and other pigmented nuclei but also diffuse cortical changes, including neuronal loss, senile plaques, and neurofibrillary tangles (Hakim and Mathieson 1979; Boller *et al.* 1980). These changes are indistinguishable from those of Alzheimer's disease, are more common in brains of PD patients than in control brains, and bear at least some correlation with the clinical history of dementia (Boller *et al.* 1980). They are also separate from the pattern of Lewy body deposition in cortical neurons seen in Lewy body dementia (see below).

From a practical point of view, the behavioral neurologist should be alert to the presence of mental deterioration or confusion in patients with Parkinson's disease. Medications are often contributing factors, especially anticholinergics, e.g. trihexyphenidyl (Artane) and benztropine (Cogentin), and dopaminergics, e.g. L-DOPA-carbidopa (Sinemet) and direct dopamine agonists such as bromocriptine (Parlodel), pergolide (Permax), pramipexole (Mirapex), and ropinirole (Requip). Reduction or discontinuation of these drugs often helps, albeit with some loss of motor function. In the past, the use of antipsychotic agents such as chlorpromazine (Thorazine) or haloperidol (Haldol) were contraindicated in PD, because of the risk of worsening motor deficits. Occasionally, small doses of less potent phenothiazines such as perphenazine (Trilafon) were tried. The availability of 'atypical' antipsychotic drugs, such as clozapine (Clozaril), risperidol (Risperdal), olanzepine (Zyprexa), and quetiapine (Seroquel) has allowed the treatment of psychotic symptoms without the major extrapyramidal side effects that limit the use of older antipsychotic drugs in PD. Such medications make it possible to continue treatment with levodopa or dopamine agonists and yet keep the psychosis or delirium within manageable bounds (The Parkinson Study Group 1999).

LEWY BODY DEMENTIA

A subgroup of patients with Parkinsonism who become demented show findings at autopsy of diffuse deposition of Lewy bodies in the cerebral cortex (Perry *et al.* 1990; Cummings 1995; Filley 1995; Galasko *et al.* 1996). Lewy bodies are spherical intracytoplasmic inclusions containing neurofilaments. The newly described disease 'Lewy body dementia' is part of a spectrum of disorders between Parkinson's disease with dementia and Alzheimer's disease. Cummings (1995), for example, distinguishes four separate pathologies associated with dementia and Parkinsonism:

1. Parkinson's disease
2. Parkinson's disease with Alzheimer's changes (neuritic plaques, neurofibrillary tangles, and degeneration of the cholinergic system from the nucleus basalis of Meynert)
3. Cortical Lewy bodies with neurofibrillary tangles, referred to by Hansen (1997) as the Lewy body variant of AD
4. Cortical Lewy bodies with no Alzheimer's changes (pure Lewy body disease).

Types 3 and 4 above, with the presence of Lewy bodies, are referred to as 'diffuse Lewy body disease' or 'Lewy body dementia (LBD)'.

Despite the considerable overlap in the four syndromes of Parkinsonism with dementia, several distinguishing features appear useful in distinguishing LBD from AD. Visual hallucinations tend to occur early in the course of LBD, only late in AD (Galasko *et al.* 1996; Ala *et al.* 1997). Garcia Ruiz and Gullikson (1999), as quoted in Chapter 13, suggest that Cervantes' Don Quixote may have suffered from Lewy body disease, based on the descriptions of visual hallucinations of windmills as giants and on his striking confusion and sleep disturbance. Features associated with subcortical dementia, such as psychomotor slowing, impairment of recall more than recognition memory, and perhaps visuospatial dysfunction, are more common in LBD than in AD. The motor slowing and rigidity (parkinsonism) also distinguish LBD from AD at early stages. Patients with any of the Parkinson's with dementia subtypes tend to have more fluctuation in level of confusion than patients with AD, more depression, more dysphagia, and more orthostatic hypotension (Filley 1995).

Table 16.1 Features of Parkinsonian syndromes with dementia

Dementia
Parkinsonism
Early hallucinations, psychosis
Depression
Fluctuating confusional state
Agitation
Myoclonus
Orthostatic hypotension
Dysphagia, weight loss
Recognition memory more affected than recall
Psychomotor slowing
Visuospatial impairment

These features are presented in Table 16.1. Older patients with confusion or dementia at the time of their initial presentation with the motor symptoms of parkinsonism are particularly likely to suffer from LBD. These patients tend to have the usual parkinsonian symptoms of bradycardia, stooped posture, and rigidity, with small-stepped gait, but they are less likely to have resting tremor than patients with typical Parkinson's disease.

CORTICOBASAL DEGENERATION

In 1968, Rebeiz and colleagues described the disorder corticobasal degeneration, also called cortical–basal ganglionic degeneration, in three patients with Parkinson-like stooped posture and gait difficulty, without tremor. Often there is asymmetric weakness of one arm, with motor difficulty out of proportion to weakness, or apraxia (Graham *et al.* 1999). The pathology involved asymmetric cortical atrophy in the frontal and parietal regions, with neuronal loss and gliosis both in the cortex and in the substantia nigra. Swollen, pale neurons, without inclusions, were present in the cortex. The original cases had almost exclusively motor deficits, with no mental deterioration until late in the course of the disease. Since the original description, however, varying patterns of illness have emerged. Motor syndromes also predominated in the patients reported by Gibb and colleagues (1989), Riley *et al.* (1990) and Rinne *et al.* (1994). Other authors, however, have described progressive aphasia or dysarthria in patients with corticobasal degeneration (Lippa *et al.* 1991; Bergeron *et al.* 1996). Patients can present with dementia (Bergeron *et al.* 1996) or behavioral disturbances such as disinhibition, hypersexuality, and irritability (Bergeron *et al.* 1996; Litvan *et al.* 1998). There appears to be an overlap between the syndromes of corticobasal degeneration and frontotemporal dementia (see Chapter 13) (Lippa *et al.* 1991; Mathuranath *et al.* 2000).

HUNTINGTON'S DISEASE

The English physician Huntington described the disease that now bears his name in 1872, in a single family with dominant inheritance. This genetic pattern has been confirmed in cases all over the world. The disease occurs at 5–8 cases per 100,000 of population (Furtado and Suchowersky 1995). Clinically, Huntington's disease is characterized by two principal features: (1) abnormal, involuntary movements; and (2) mental deterioration. The movement disorder often begins with choreiform movements of the fingers and hands, which look like minor restlessness or fidgety behavior to an untrained observer. Later, it progresses to dystonic posturing and uncontrollable, writhing chorea. Affective changes, either depression or hypomania, often herald the onset of cognitive impairment; later, severe progressive dementia supervenes. Either the movement disorder or the mental changes can come first, and in some cases a period of years may separate the two. Charcot (Goetz 1987) described the course of Huntington's disease as follows: "It is most uncommon...to see the abnormal movements persist for long without the associated psychiatric problems also appearing and soon taking on their definitive form – mania, melancholia, etc. – all ending as dementia. At the terminal stage, choreic movements become intense enough to make standing and walking impossible and intellectual function deteriorates to the lowest level, so the unfortunate patient is reduced to a bedridden state, now prone to every destructive force imaginable."

The most tragic aspect of the disease is the appearance of symptoms in most patients during their thirties and forties, when reproduction and transmission of the disease to a new generation have already occurred (Martin 1984). A less common variant of the disease presents during the teens or twenties with rigidity, seizures, dementia, and little if any chorea (Bittenbender and Quadfasel 1962; Oliva *et al.* 1993). This 'juvenile' form of Huntington's disease is more common when the affected parent is the father (Went *et al.* 1984).

The cognitive changes of Huntington's disease may begin as a psychiatric disorder of mood or psychotic thought process, with normal cognition. Personality changes such as irritability and short temper are common. One study of 'presymptomatic' patients (children of parents with HD) found deficits in frontal lobe tests and in visuospatial function in all seven gene-positive patients, and in none of three gene-negative subjects (Jason *et al.* 1988). The theme of deficits in visuospatial and frontal functions is similar to that of PD. Even patients with recently diagnosed disease have abnormal short-term memory function, and this memory loss progresses as the disease worsens (Caine *et al.* 1977; Butters *et al.* 1978). Late in the disease more generalized abnormalities on intelligence testing or bedside examination become evident. Focal cortical syndromes such as aphasia are rare or non-existent in HD, but speech and language dysfunction has been described as part of the disorder. Common speech and language abnormalities include dysarthria, reading and writing difficulty, confrontation naming deficits, a simplified syntactic structure of speech utterances, and reduced discourse organization (Podoll *et al.* 1988). Starkstein and colleagues (1988) found correlations between cognitive abnormalities on simple tests of frontal lobe function such as the Trails A and B test of the Halstead–Reitan battery and caudate atrophy by CT scan. These authors implicate the frontal–caudate loops involved in frontal lobe functioning (see Chapter 10). Visuospatial functioning and recognition of faces or emotional expression on faces are also deficient in HD patients (Sprengelmeyer *et al.* 1996). The cognitive changes in advanced Huntington's disease are diffuse, resembling those of Alzheimer's disease (Caine *et al.* 1977; Taylor and Hansotia 1983).

In Huntington's disease, as in Parkinson's disease, pathological changes are not confined to the basal ganglia. Shrinkage of the caudate nucleus, visible on CT scan in advanced cases, is accompanied by cortical atrophy as well, especially in the frontal regions. Selective loss of spiny neurons in the striatum occurs early in the disease. These spiny neurons project to the globus pallidus, and presumably involve an inhibitory GABA-ergic system for movements. Unlike Parkinson's disease, in which depletion of dopaminergic neurons is clearly involved, in Huntington's disease an apparent overactivity of the dopaminergic system is evident.

The molecular genetics of Huntington's disease have been worked out in great detail over the past two decades. The disease was first linked to the short arm of chromosome 4, and the gene (now called IT15 or HD) has been cloned. Cases of Huntington's disease all have a zone of cytosine–adenine–guanine (CAG) repeats; patients with more than 40 such repeats virtually always manifest the disease, those with less than 36 do not, and patients with 36–39 repeats may or may not manifest the disease (Rubinsztein *et al.* 1996). The age at onset is younger the higher the number of repeats, and the severity of the disease also correlates with the number of repeats. The number of repeats tends to increase in successive generations of a family with HD; clinically, the tendency of the disease to become more severe in successive generations is called 'anticipation'.

The precise mechanism by which the gene product of the Huntington gene, called 'huntingtin', results in cell death is under active investigation. The CAG repeats are translated into multiple repeats of glutamine in the protein, huntingtin. The protein is associated with the cellular cytoskeleton of neurons and interacts with a number of structural proteins and enzymes. The polyglutamine expansions alter these interactions and may lead to huntingtin inclusions, which cause cell death by apoptosis (Martin 1999) or by interference with cellular respiration, perhaps through mitochondrial damage (Wellington *et al.* 1997; Walling *et al.* 1998). The overactivity of glutamatergic neurons may also result in 'excitotoxicity', or cellular damage resulting from the overstimulation of glutamate receptors.

The diagnosis of Huntington's disease is easily accomplished by the onset of characteristic motor or cognitive changes in a patient with a family history of the disease. A genetic test is available, without restriction, for patients who have already developed symptoms, but presymptomatic testing is advisable only in centers with genetic and psychological counseling programs, since the risk of suicide is real (Harper *et al.* 1990).

The treatment of Huntington's disease is limited. From a practical standpoint, treatment with dopamine-blocking drugs such as haloperidol may help both the chorea and the mental agitation, but the memory loss and dementia proceed unabated.

WILSON'S DISEASE

A recessively inherited disease of the basal ganglia and liver, Wilson's disease was described in 1912 by the British neurologist S. A. Kinnier Wilson. The disease is inherited in an autosomal recessive manner and occurs in approximately 1 in 40,000 births (Brewer and Yuzbasiyan-Gurkan 1992). The gene has been localized to the long arm of chromosome 13. The disorder typically presents in adolescents or young adults with a coarse intention tremor, later accompanied by rigidity, dysarthria, dysphagia, and sometimes cerebellar signs. Psychiatric symptoms may be among the earliest features, with depression, pseudobulbar emotional lability, schizophreniform psychosis, and later dementia (Cartwright 1978; Brewer and Yuzbasiyan-Gurkan 1992). Neuropsychological testing reveals memory deficits and reduced verbal and performance IQ in symptomatic patients with Wilson's disease (Medalia *et al.* 1988). Medalia *et al.* (1992) found that the motor, cognitive (memory loss), and emotional symptoms were independent of each other in patients with Wilson's disease.

Wilson's disease is also associated with liver dysfunction, which can manifest either as acute hepatitis with hemolytic anemia or as progressive cirrhosis. Wilson's disease is now known to result from copper deposition, first in the liver and later in the basal ganglia of the brain. Copper deposition can also be detected in the eyes (Kayser–Fleischer rings) and the kidneys (aminoaciduria, uricosuria) (Dobyns *et al.* 1979). High copper levels in serum and urine and low serum ceruloplasmin, a copper-binding protein, are helpful in diagnosis. If these are negative in an asymptomatic sibling of a diagnosed patient, a liver biopsy with quantitative copper assay may be necessary for diagnosis (Cartwright 1978).

Wilson's disease is treatable by copper-binding therapy, usually penicillamine, at an initial dose of 1 gram per day. For patients with hypersensitivity to penicillamine, an alternative chelating agent, trine (triethylene tetramine dihydrochloride), can be used. Zinc, at a dosage of 50 mg three times daily, also helps to block copper absorption. Dramatic improvement in neurological symptoms has resulted from chelation and zinc therapy (Dobyns *et al.* 1979; Deiss 1983; Brewer and Yuzbasiyan-Gurkan 1992). Maintenance therapy must be maintained for life. One study documented nearly normal psychological test results in a group of Wilson's disease patients on penicillamine therapy (Davis and Goldstein 1974). Liver transplantation is also necessary in cases with irreversible liver damage, and the graft appears to treat the disease such that chelation therapy is no longer needed (Yarze *et al.* 1992).

The practical significance of Wilson's disease for the behavioral neurologist is the recognition of the diagnosis so that treatment can be instituted before irreversible neurological damage has occurred. The combination of mood changes, early dementia, and extrapyramidal symptoms should be an important clue, with or without a history of liver disease.

PROGRESSIVE SUPRANUCLEAR PALSY

Progressive supranuclear palsy, or PSP, was delineated in 1964 by the Canadian investigators Steele, Richardson, and Olszewski (Steele et al. 1964; Steele 1972). This disease presents during middle to late life with parkinsonian-like rigidity, progressive loss of voluntary extraocular movements, pseudobulbar palsy, dysarthria, and variable cerebellar and motor signs. The rigidity has a predilection for the neck muscles, which are often held in extension, in contrast to the flexed, kyphotic posture of Parkinson's disease patients. This posture, along with the early loss of vertical eye movements, makes it difficult for patients to walk down steps. The eye movements are characteristically lost in the vertical plane, first downward, then upward, and finally in the horizontal plane, with pre-served reflex oculocephalic ('doll's head') eye movements until very late in the course. The rigidity and bradykinesia bear a strong resemblance to Parkinson's disease, but tremor is typically absent. Some patients manifest psychiatric symp-toms at the onset of the disease, before the neurological signs are evident. Depression, psychomotor retardation, and pseudobulbar emotional lability are common (Janati and Appel 1984). Patients blink infrequently and may have their eyes wide open, a 'look of perpetual astonishment'. Later, dementia develops in most cases. Prominent features include forgetfulness, slowing of thought processes, and difficulty with calculations and abstract reasoning. Language and perceptual functions are largely intact, especially if extra time is given for the patient to respond. Even the forgetfulness may be associated with surprisingly normal memory function if the patient is encouraged and given time to remem-ber, though studies have shown memory impairment in comparison with normal persons (Litvan et al. 1989). Both rapid forgetting and impaired short-term mem-ory storage have been documented in patients with PSP (Litvan et al. 1989; Grafman et al. 1995).

Albert and colleagues (1974) suggested that cortical systems are intact in PSP, but the subcortical centers that activate them function defectively or with delay. In fact, these authors coined the term 'subcortical dementia' to describe the mental deterioration in PSP and related diseases. Recently the disease has received attention because of the announcement that the British musician and actor Dudley Moore has been diagnosed with PSP.

The clinical differentiation of PSP from other movement disorders rests on the characteristic loss of vertical and then horizontal eye movements, the postural abnormalities and falls early in the disease, the absence of tremor, and the lack of response to levodopa (Litvan et al. 1997). The neck posture, extended rather than flexed as in Parkinson's disease, is also a distinguishing feature. There is also a lack of delusions and hallucinations, which separates PSP from diffuse Lewy body disease, and an absence of asymmetric upper limb motor difficulties, which separates PSP from corticobasal degeneration.

The pathology of progressive supranuclear palsy involves neuronal loss, neurofibrillary tangles, and overgrowth of glial cells in the nuclei of the brainstem, thalamus, and cerebellum. Some cases have senile plaques in the cerebral cortex, but these cortical changes are less striking than the subcortical ones (Steele 1972). More recent studies have found cortical changes to be common (Braak *et al.* 1992; Daniel *et al.* 1995; Verny *et al.* 1996). Verny *et al.* (1996), for example, found cortical changes in ten out of ten cases of PSP, with neurofibrillary tangles most prominent in the precentral and angular gyri. These authors pointed to the pedunculopontine nucleus as the source of projections to the cortical areas affected in PSP.

The treatment of progressive supranuclear palsy is very limited. Some patients respond partially to dopaminergic drugs such as Sinemet, but not as dramatically as those with Parkinson's disease.

MULTISYSTEM ATROPHY

Multi-system atrophy (MSA) is a recent clinical designation for a family of disorders including features of autonomic dysfunction (especially orthostatic hypotension), ataxia, and Parkinsonism. Patients presenting with orthostatic hypotension as the primary symptom have previously been diagnosed with Shy–Drager syndrome (Shy and Drager 1960). These are uncommon disorders; a recent survey estimated a prevalence of 4.4 per 100,000 of population in England, compared to 6.4 per 100,000 for PSP (Schrag *et al.* 1999).

Patients with predominantly cerebellar presentations are often diagnosed as sporadic ataxias or 'olivopontocerebellar atrophy (OPCA)'. OPCA is one of a group of multi-systems degenerations in which signs of basal ganglia pathology are mixed with cerebellar signs, autonomic insufficiency (especially orthostatic hypotension), and dementia (van Bogaert 1946).

Finally, cases with predominantly Parkinsonian syndromes have been diagnosed as 'striatonigral deneration'. Striatonigral degeneration is a variant of Parkinson's disease in which cerebellar signs, dysarthria, and pseudobulbar palsy coexist with the typical tremor, rigidity, and bradykinesia. The author has seen one patient with autopsy-proved MSA who presented with dysarthria and speech apraxia, progressing to total anarthria. The disease does not respond to antiparkinsonian medications. The pathology is also different from that of Parkinson's disease, involving atrophy not only of the substantia nigra but also of the caudate and putamen. Lewy bodies, the inclusions seen in pigmented neurons in Parkinson's disease, are absent (Adams *et al.* 1964). All of these variants of multisystem atrophy are associated with mental slowing, but dementia is usually a late feature if present at all.

The diagnosis of multisystem atrophy can be difficult. Wenning and colleagues (2000) found the following features to be more predictive of MSA than Parkinson's disease, in an autopsy-documented study:

1. Autonomic dysfunction
2. Speech or bulbar abnormalities
3. Absence of dementia
4. Absence of levodopa-induced confusion
5. Prominent falls.

CONCLUSION

All of the diseases just discussed – Parkinson's disease, diffuse Lewy body disease, Huntington's disease, Wilson's disease, progressive supranuclear palsy, and multisystem atrophy – have in common the combination of movement disorder and mental changes that together comprise a 'subcortical dementia'. Other less common diseases that affect the basal ganglia or thalamus also produce dementia in at least some cases.

Hallervorden–Spatz disease is a rare hereditary disease of children, with dysarthria, rigidity, athetoid movements, and progressive dementia. The pathology involves iron deposition in the basal ganglia, especially the globus pallidus, and swelling and degeneration of axons in the basal ganglia and cerebellum (Rozdilsky *et al.* 1968).

In all of the basal ganglia diseases, rigidity and impaired volitional movement appear to have correlates in the cognitive sphere in the form of slowed mental processes, apathy, and forgetfulness. Albert and colleagues (1974) suggested that disease of the subcortical structures ('subcortical dementias') produces these changes as well as depressive features, pseudobulbar emotional lability, and difficulty with the manipulation of previously acquired information, as in tasks of calculations and abstract reasoning. 'Cortical' dementias, by this conception, lack the motor signs, depression, and mental slowing of subcortical disease and have in their place disorders of cortical processes such as language and visuoperceptual function.

This simple dichotomy between cortical and subcortical dementias, unfortunately, has several limitations. First, Mayeux and colleagues, in mental status tests of 56 Parkinson's disease, 20 Huntington's disease, and 46 Alzheimer's disease patients, failed to find consistent differences among the groups except for a higher incidence of depression and lower overall cognitive deficit score in the two subcortical groups (Mayeux *et al.* 1983). Second, the subcortical diseases often have associated cortical pathology. As discussed previously, Parkinson's and Huntington's diseases especially are associated with cortical atrophy as well as subcortical disease. 'Cortical' deficits of visual perception are also prominent in Parkinson's disease. Third, cortical degenerations such as Alzheimer's disease have associated changes in subcortical regions, and these diseases are not totally devoid of motor signs. As a practical concept, however, the diagnosis of subcortical dementia has some clinical usefulness, based on the combination of extrapyramidal motor signs, mental slowing, depression, and pseudobulbar emotional lability.

REFERENCES

Albert ML, Feldman RG, Willis AL. The 'subcortical dementia' of progressive supranuclear palsy. J Neurol Neurosurg Psychiatry 1974;37:121–130.

Adams RD, Van Bogaert L, VanderEecken H. Striatonigral degeneration. J Neuropathol Exp Neurol 1964;23:584–608.

Ala TA, Yang K-H, Frey WH. Hallucinations and signs of parkinsonism help distinguish patients with dementia and cortical Lewy bodies from patients with Alzheimer's disease at presentation: a clinicopathological study. J Neurol Neurosurg Psychiatry 1997;62:16–21.

Alegret M, Junque C, Valldeoriola F et al. Effects of bilateral subthalamic stimulation on cognitive function in Parkinson disease. Arch Neurol 2001;58:1223–1227.

Ardouin C, Pillon B, Peiffer E et al. Bilateral subthalamic or pallidal stimulation for Parkinson's disease affects neither memory nor executive functions: A consecutive series of 62 patients. Ann Neurol 1999;46:217–223.

Bejjani BP, Damier P, Arnulf I et al. Transient acute depression induced by high-frequency deep-brain stimulation. New Engl J Med 1999;340:1476–1480.

Benabid AL, Koudsie A, Pollak P et al. Future prospects of brain stimulation. Neurol Res 2000;22:237–246.

Bergeron C, Pollanen MS, Weyer L et al. Unusual clinical presentations of cortical–basal ganglionic degeneration. Ann Neurol 1996;40:893–900.

Bittenbender JB, Quadfasel FA. Rigid and akinetic forms of Huntington's chorea. Arch Neurol 1962;7:37–50.

Boller F, Mizutani T, Roessman U, Gambetti, P. Parkinson disease, dementia, and Alzheimer disease: clinicopathological correlations. Ann Neurol 1980;7:329–335.

Boller F, Passafiume D, Keefe NC et al. Visuospatial impairment in Parkinson's disease. Arch Neurol 1984;41:485–490.

Braak H, Jellinger K, Braak E, Bohl J. Allocortical neurofibrillary changes in progressive supranuclear palsy. Acta Neuropathol (Berl) 1992;84:478–483.

Bradley VA, Welch JL, Dick DJ. Visuospatial working memory in Parkinson's disease. J Neurol Neurosurg Psychiatry 1989;52:1228–1235.

Brewer GJ, Yuzbasiyan-Gurkan V. Wilson's disease. Medicine 1992;71:139–164.

Brown RG, MacCarthy B. Psychiatric morbidity in patients with Parkinson's disease. Psychol Med 1990;20:77–87.

Brown RG, Marsden CD. How common is dementia in Parkinson's disease? Lancet 1984;1:1262–1265.

Brown RG, Marsden CD, Quinn N, Wyke MA. Alterations in cognitive performance and affect–arousal state during fluctuations in motor function in Parkinson's disease. J Neurol Neurosurg Psychiatry 1984;47:454–465.

Butters N, Sax D, Montgomery K, Tarlow S. Comparison of the neuropsychological deficits associated with early and advanced Huntington's disease. Arch Neurol 1978;35:585–589.

Caine ED, Ebert MH, Weingartner H. An outline for the analysis of dementia: the memory disorder of Huntington's disease. Neurology 1977;27:1087–1092.

Canavan AGM, Passingham RE, Marsden CD et al. The performance on learning tasks of patients in the early stages of Parkinson's disease. Neuropsychologia 1989;27:141–156.

Cartwright GE. Diagnosis of treatable Wilson's disease. N Engl J Med 1978;298:1347–1350.

Celesia GO, Wanamaker WM. Psychiatric disturbances in Parkinson's disease. Dis Nerv Sys 1972;33:577–583.

Cummings JL. Lewy body diseases with dementia: Pathophysiology and treatment. Brain Cognition 1995;28:266–280.

Daniel SE, de Bruin VM, Lees AJ. The clinical and pathological spectrum of Steele–Richardson–Olszewski syndrome (progressive supranuclear palsy): a reappraisal. (Review). Brain 1995;118:759–770.

Davis LJ, Goldstein NP. Psychological investigation of Wilson's disease. Mayo Clin Proc 1974;49:409–411.

Deiss A. Treatment of Wilson's disease. Ann Intern Med 1983;99:398–400.

Delis D, Direnfeld L, Alexander MP, Kaplan E. Cognitive fluctuations associated with the on–off phenomenon in Parkinson disease. Neurology 1982;32:1049–1052.

Dewick HC, Hanley JR, Davies ADM et al. Perception and memory for faces in Parkinson's disease. Neuropsychologia 1991;29:785–802.

Dobyns WB, Goldstein NP, Gordon H. Clinical spectrum of Wilson's disease (hepatolenticular degeneration). Mayo Clin Proc 1979;54:35–42.

Dubois B, Pillon B, Sternic N et al. Age-induced cognitive disturbance in Parkinson's disease. Neurology 1990;40:38–41.

Filley CM. Neuropsychiatric features of Lewy body disease. Brain Cogn 1995;28:229–239.

Fine J, Duff J, Chen R et al. Long-term follow-up of unilateral pallidotomy in advanced Parkinson's disease. N Engl J Med 2000;342:1708–1714.

Follett KA. The surgical treatment of Parkinson's disease. Annu Rev Med 2000;51:135–147.

Freed CR, Greene PE, Breeze RE et al. Transplantation of embryonic dopamine neurons for severe Parkinson's disease. N Eng J Med 2001;344:710–719.

Furtado S, Suchowersky O. Huntington's disease: recent advances in diagnosis and management. Can J Neurol Sci 1995;22:5–12.

Galasko D, Katzman R, Salmon DP, Hansen L. Clinical and neuropathological findings in Lewy body dementias. Brain Cogn 1996;31:166–175.

Garcia Ruiz PJ, Gulliksen L. Did Don Quixote have Lewy body disease? J R Soc Med 1999;92:200–201.

Gibb WRG, Luthert PJ, Marsden CD. Corticobasal degeneration. Brain 1989;112:1171–1192.

Goetz CG. Charcot the Clinician. The Tuesday Lectures. New York: Raven Press, 1987;84.

Grafman J, Litvan I, Stark M. Neuropsychological features of progressive supranuclear palsy. Brain Cogn 1995;28:311–320.

Graham NL, Zeman A, Young AW et al. Dyspraxia in a patient with corticobasal degeneration: the role of visual and tactile inputs to action. J Neurol Neurosurg Psychiatry 1999;67:334–344.

Green J, Barnhart H. The impact of lesion laterality on neuropsychological change following posterior pallidotomy: a review of current findings. Brain Cogn 2000;42:379–398.

Hakim AM, Mathieson G. Dementia in Parkinson disease: a neuropathologic study. Neurology 1979;29:1209–1214.

Hale MS, Bellizzi J. Low dose perphenazine and levodopa/carbidopa in a patient with parkinsonism and a psychotic illness. J Nerv Ment Dis 1980;168:312–314.

Halgrin R, Riklan M, Misiak H. Levodopa, parkinsonism and recent memory. J Nerv Ment Dis 1977;164:268–272.

Hansen LA. The Lewy body variant of Alzheimer disease. J Neural Transm 1997;suppl 51:83–93.

Hantz P, Caradoc-Davies G, Caradoc-Davies T et al. Depression in Parkinson's disease. Am J Psychiatry 1994;151:1010–1014.

Harper PS, Morris MJ, Tyler A. Genetic testing for Huntington's disease. Internationally agreed guidelines are being followed. Br Med J 1990;300:1089–1090.

Huntington G. On Chorea. Med Surg Reporter 1872;26:317–321.

Jason GW, Pajurkova EM, Sucholwersky O et al. Presymptomatic neuropsychological impairment in Huntington's disease. Arch Neurol 1988;45:769–773.

Janati A, Appel AR. Psychiatric aspects of progressive supranuclear palsy. J Nerv Ment Dis 1984;172:85–89.

Leiberman A, Dziatolowski M, Kupersmith M *et al*. Dementia in Parkinson's disease. Ann Neurol 1979;6:355–359.

Lippa CF, Cohen R, Smith TW, Drachman DA. Primary progressive aphasia with focal neuronal achromasia. Neurology 1991;41:882–886.

Litvan I, Grafman J, Gomez C, Chase TN. Memory impairment in patients with progressive supranuclear palsy. Arch Neurol 1989;46:765–767.

Litvan I, Campbell G, Mangone CA *et al*. Which clinical features differentiate progressive supranuclear palsy (Steele–Richardson–Olszewski syndrome) from related disorders? A clinicopathological study. Brain 1997;120:65–74.

Litvan I, Cummings JL, Mega M. Neuropsychiatric features of corticobasal degeneration. J Neurol Neurosurg Psychiatry 1998;65:717–721.

Martin JB. Huntington's disease: new approaches to an old problem. Neurology 1984;34:1059–1072.

Martin JB. Molecular basis of the neurodegenerative disorders. New Engl J Med 1999;340:1970–1980.

Mathuranath PS, Xuereb JH, Bak T, Hodges JR. Corticobasal ganglionic degeneration and/or frontotemporal dementia? A report of two overlap cases and review of the literature. J Neurol Neurosurg Psychiatry 2000;68:304–312.

Mayeux R, Stern Y, Rosen J, Benson DF. Is 'subcortical dementia' a recognizable clinical entity? Ann Neurol 1983;14:278–283.

Mayeux R, Stern Y, Sano M *et al*. The relationship of serotonin to depression in Parkinson's disease. Movement Disorders 1988;3:237–244.

Medalia A, Isaacs-Glaberman K, Scheinberg H. Neuropsychological impairment in Wilson's disease. Arch Neurol 1988;45:502–504.

Medalia A, Galynker I, Scheinberg IH. The interaction of motor, memory, and emotional dysfunction in Wilson's disease. Biol Psychiatry 1992;31:823–826.

Mindham RHS, Ahmed SWA, Clough CG. A controlled study of dementia in Parkinson's disease. J Neurol Neurosurg Psychiatry 1982;45:965–974.

Mohr E, Fabbrini G, Williams J *et al*. Dopamine and memory function in Parkinson's disease. Movement Disorders 1989;4:113–120.

Mortimer JA, Pirozzolo FJ, Hansch EC, Webster DD. Relationship of motor symptoms to intellectual deficits in Parkinson's disease. Neurology 1982;32:133–137.

Oliva D, Carella F, Savoiardo M *et al*. Clinical and magnetic resonance features of the classic and akinetic-rigid variants of Huntington's disease. Arch Neurol 1993;50:17–19.

Parkinson J. An Essay on the Shaking Palsy. London: Sherwood, Neely and Jones, 1817.

Perry RH, Irving D, Blessed G *et al*. Senile dementia of Lewy body type. A clinically and neuropathologically distinct form of Lewy body dementia in the elderly. J Neurol Sci 1990;95:119–139.

Podoll K, Caspary P, Lange HW, Noth J. Language functions in Huntington's disease. Brain 1988;111:1475–1503.

Proctor F, Riklan M, Cooper IS, Teuber HL: Judgement of visual and postural vertical by parkinsonian patients. Neurology 1964;14:287–293.

Rafal RD, Posner MI, Walker JA, Friedrich FJ. Cognition and the basal ganglia. Separating mental and motor components of performance in Parkinson's disease. Brain 1984;107:1083–1094.

Rebeiz JJ, Kolodny EH, Richardson EP Jr. Corticodentatonigral degeneration with neuronal achromasia. Arch Neurol 1968;18:20–33.

Riley DE, Lang AE, Lewis A *et al*. Cortical–basal ganglionic degeneration. Neurology 1990;40:1203–1212.

Rinne J, Lee M, Thompson P, Marsden C. Corticobasal degeneration. A clinical study of 36 cases. Brain 1994;117:1183–1196.

Rozdilsky B, Cumings JN, Huston AF. Hallervorden–Spatz disease – late infantile and adult tyupes, report of two cases. Acta Neuropathol (Berl) 1968;10:1–16.

Rubinsztein DC, Leggo J, Coles R *et al*. Phenotypic characterization of individuals with 30–40 CAG repeats in the Huntington disease (HD) gene reveals HD cases with 36 repeats and apparently normal individuals with 36–39 repeats. Am J Hum Genet 1996;59:16–22.

Sagar HJ, Sullivan EV, Gabriele JDE *et al*. Temporal ordering and short-term memory deficits in Parkinson's disease. Brain 1988;111:525–539.

Saint-Cyr JA, Taylor AE, Lang AE. Procedural learning and neostriatal dysfunction in man. Brain 1988;111:941–959.

Schneider E, Fischer P-A, Jacobi P *et al*. The significance of cerebral atrophy for the symptomatology of Parkinson's disease. J Neurol Sci 1979;42:187–197.

Schrag A, Ben-Shlomo Y, Quinn NP. Prevalence of progressive supranuclear palsy and multiple system atrophy: a cross-sectional study. Lancet 1999;354:1771–1775.

Shy GM, Drager GA. A neurological syndrome associated with orthostatic hypotension. Arch Neurol 1960;2:511–527.

Sprengelmeyer R, Young AW, Calder AJ *et al*. Loss of disgust. Perception of faces and emotions in Huntington's disease. Brain 1996;119:1647–1665.

Sroka H, Elizan TS, Yahr MD *et al*. Organic mental syndrome and confusional states in Parkinson's disease: relationship to computerized tomographic signs of cerebral atrophy. Arch Neurol 1981;38:339–342.

Starkstein SE, Brandt J, Folstein S *et al*. Neuropsychological and neuroradiological correlates in Huntington's disease. J Neurol Neurosurg Psychiatry 1988;51:1259–1263.

Starkstein SE, Preziosi TJ, Berthier ML *et al*. Brain 1989;112:1141–1153.

Stebbins GT, Gabrieli JD, Shannon KM *et al*. Impaired frontostriatal cognitive functioning following posteroventral pallidotomy in advanced Parkinson's disease. Brain Cogn 2000;42:348–363.

Steele JC. Progressive supranuclear palsy. Brain 1972; 95:693–704

Steele JC, Richardson JC, Olszewski J. Progressive supranuclear palsy. Arch Neurol 1964;10:353–359.

Stein MB, Heuser IJ, Juncos JL, Uhde TW. Anxiety disorders in patients with Parkinson's disease. Am J Psychiatry 1990;147:217–220.

Taylor HG, Hansotia P. Neuropsychological testing of Huntington's patients: clues to progression. J Nerv Ment Dis 1983;171:492–496.

Taylor AE, Saint-Cyr JA. The neuropsychology of Parkinson's disease. Brain Cogn 1995;28:281–296.

The Parkinson Study Group. Low-dose clozapine for the treatment of drug-induced psychosis in Parkinson's disease. New Engl J Med 1999;340:757–763.

Van Bogaert L. Aspects cliniques et pathologiques des atrophies pallidales et pallido-luysiennes progressives. J Neurol Neurosurg Psychiatry 1946;9:125–157.

Verny M, Duyckaerts C, Agid Y, Hauw J-J. The significance of cortical pathology in progressive supranuclear palsy. Clinico-pathological data in 10 cases. Brain 1996;119:1123–1136.

Vogel H-P. Symptoms of depression in Parkinson's disease. Pharmacopsychiatrica 1982;15:192–196.

Walling HW, Baldassare JJ, Westfall TC. Molecular aspects of Huntington's disease. J Neuroscience Res 1998;54:301–308.

Warburton JW. Memory disturbance and the Parkinson syndrome. Br J Med Psychol 1967;40:169–171.

Wellington CL, Brinkman RR, O'Kusky JR, Hayden MR. Toward understanding the molecular pathology of Huntington's disease. Brain Pathology 1997;7:979–1002.

Wenning GK, Ben-Shlomo Y, Hughes A *et al*. What clinical features are most useful to distinguish definite multiple system atrophy from Parkinson's disease? J Neurol Neurosurg Psychiatry 2000;68:434–440.

Went LN, Vegter-Vander Vlis M, Bruyn GW. Parental transmission of Huntington's disease. Lancet 1984;2:110–1102.

Wilson SAK. Progressive lenticular degeneration: a familial nervous disease associated with cirrhosis of the liver. Brain 1912;34:295–509.

Yarze JC, Martin P, Munoz SJ, Friedman LS. Wilson's disease: current status. Am J Medicine 1992;92:643–654.

York MK, Levin HS, Grossman RG, Hamilton WJ. Neuropsychological outcome following unilateral pallidotomy. Brain 1999;122:2209–2220.

17

Emotion and the Brain

When faced with a task to which he was not equal – even if it were only, as instanced, an elementary arithmetic problem – he invariably fell into a state of violent trembling and finally even into a brief state of uncommunicativeness. In this case, a 'catastrophic reaction', of the severest type, a reaction leading to unconsciousness, could be experimentally produced.

(Goldstein 1948)

The subject of emotion is a complex one. The physiological states associated with our emotions likely evolved from temporary states of motivation in animals related to rewards and punishments. In fact, Rolls (2000) has defined emotions as 'states elicited by rewards or punishments', where rewards are anything an animal or person will work to achieve, and punishments are anything an animal or person will work to avoid. For example, a positive reinforcement or reward may induce a positive emotion called 'happiness', whereas withdrawal of a rewarding stimulus or onset of punishment may cause a negative emotion called 'sadness'. The brain system most involved in reward and punishment is the limbic system, and especially the orbitofrontal cortex (see Chapter 10) and the amygdala; these are centers where sensory inputs are analyzed in terms of their reward/punishment or emotional significance and where behavioral responses are initiated. The amygdala projects to the hypothalamus and brainstem nuclei to activate autonomic responses to emotional stimuli. Frontal cortical areas are essential in motor responses to reward or punishment stimuli (Rolls 2000). One interesting observation during deep brain stimulation for Parkinson's disease and tremor (see Chapter 16) is that high frequency stimulation occasionally induces depression (Bejjani et al. 1999). The fact that depressed mood can be produced by electrical activation of subcortical structures underlines the importance of biological brain processes in depression.

These principles of mood seem simplistic in describing the complexity and richness of emotional states in human beings. In people, pleasure can be derived from cultural experiences, the arts, and music, without any direct reward to the individual. Similarly, empathetic responses to the plight of others can cause sadness, even without any specific punishment or lack of reward to the individual. These phenomena seem to belie the concept of emotion as resulting only from rewards and punishments.

The mood states evoked by environmental reward and punishment stimuli are fleeting, and they come and go frequently in normal persons. When mood states become pervasive over longer periods, we can speak of personality traits such as a 'dysthymic' (or depressed) personality, or a sunny, perpetually happy personality. Abnormal, sustained mood states such as depression are the principal subject of this chapter.

DEPRESSION

Depression is one of the most common worldwide afflictions of mankind. As mentioned in Chapter 15, recent epidemiological surveys (Weissman *et al.* 1996) have reported a lifetime prevalence of major depression in from 1.5–19% of people in different parts of the world. In general, depression correlates with cultural and environmental stress factors; depression rates are higher in war zones, countries afflicted by drought, and geographical areas with less sunshine. Depression is a significant public health problem all over the world. In the USA, 5–12% of men and 10–20% of women have a lifetime incidence of a major depression (Nemeroff 1998). In addition to the burden of lost work, lost enjoyment of life, and lost creativity, the suicide rate in major depression is as high as 15% (Guze and Robins 1970). Suicide is the ninth leading cause of death in the USA. Among medical patients, pessimists had a higher mortality than optimists in a Mayo Clinic study (Maruta *et al.* 2000). Depressed or hopeless cancer patients survive a shorter time than those with positive attitudes (Breitbart *et al.* 2000).

The diagnostic criteria for major depression (DSM-IV, 1994) are shown in Table 17.1. These symptoms must be severe enough to interfere with functioning and must last at least 2 weeks. Minor depression, also called dysthymic disorder, involves depressed mood for most of the day, more days than not, for a period of at least 2 years, with at least two of the following:

1. Poor appetite or overeating
2. Insomnia/hypersomnia
3. Low energy/fatigue
4. Low self-esteem
5. Poor concentration or difficulty making decisions
6. Feelings of hopelessness.

Dysthymic disorder also excludes patients with a major depressive episode during the first 2 years, patients who have had a manic or schizophrenic episode, and those with an organic cause for their depression.

The symptoms of major depression are quite variable. In addition to depressed or dysphoric mood, the most consistent symptoms in the survey of Weissman *et al.* (1996) were insomnia, loss of energy, difficulty concentrating,

Table 17.1 Modified DSM-IV (1994) criteria for major depression

Depressed mood for most of the day, with feelings of depression and hopelessness
Markedly diminished interest or pleasure in activities
Major increase or decrease in appetite
Insomnia or excessive sleeping
Restlessness or slowness of movement
Fatigue or loss of energy
Feelings of worthlessness or guilt
Indecisiveness or inability to think or concentrate
Recurrent thoughts of death or suicide

Note: Five of the nine items must be present, including one of the first two

slowed thinking, feelings of worthlessness or guilt, and thoughts of death or suicide. Appetite changes, weight loss or gain, hypersomnia, retardation or agitation, and decreased interest in sex were less consistent symptoms of depression. For the behavioral neurologist, the prominence of complaints of reduced concentration and slowed thinking as hallmarks of depression should be kept in mind.

Depression versus Grief Reaction

A differential diagnosis that frequently causes problems in diagnosis and treatment is the distinction between normal grief and depression. Patients who lose a loved one go through a three-phase reaction of shock, preoccupation with the deceased, and finally resolution (Brown and Stoudemire 1983). Some cases of grief become pathologically prolonged or disabling, either because of the patient's premorbid psychological functioning or history of losses, or because of other factors coming into play after the loss. A history of depression, a guilt-ridden relationship with the deceased, or poor family support after the loss are all common causes of prolonged grief (Brown and Stoudemire 1983). Clearly, behavioral management is important in helping grieving patients. Antidepressant drug therapy should be considered when the patient begins to meet criteria for major depression in addition to a grief reaction.

This chapter will consider the available knowledge regarding the effects of focal brain lesions on emotion and mood, then attempt to touch on the larger subject of depression without known brain disease. Psychosis and bipolar affective disorder were discussed in Chapter 15; this chapter will consider only non-psychotic emotional states.

FOCAL BRAIN LESIONS AND MOOD
Post-Stroke Emotional Changes

Focal lesions have been associated with depression in several disease states. The first set of data is the literature on post-stroke depression, which is also discussed in Chapter 21. Perhaps the first neuroscientist to associate emotion with focal lesions of the brain was Kurt Goldstein (1948), who described the 'catastrophic reaction' associated with left hemisphere strokes and aphasia (see the quotation at the beginning of this chapter). Patients with aphasia are calm and cooperative when performing tasks of which they are capable, but when faced with a more difficult task they may become anxious, or even distressed to the point of unresponsiveness. Babinski (1914), as discussed in Chapter 9, described indifference or euphoria with right hemisphere strokes, sometimes referred to as the 'indifference reaction', in distinction to the left hemisphere 'catastrophic reaction' (Denny-Brown et al. 1952). In a systematic study of emotional states associated with strokes, Gainotti (1972) found that depression was clearly associated with left hemisphere strokes, whereas indifference was associated with right hemisphere strokes. This difference in side of lesion implies that depression after stroke is not simply a psychological reaction to physical illness, but rather that it is tied to the biological nature of the brain disorder.

Robinson and colleagues (1984) studied 36 stroke patients and found that depressed mood was clearly associated with anterior left hemisphere lesions. Within the right hemisphere group, posterior lesions were more associated with depression than anterior lesions. This anatomic association of depression with left versus right hemisphere has found confirmation in some studies (Starkstein et al. 1984) but not others (Sinyor et al. 1986; Ghika-Schmidt and Bogousslavsky 1997; Kim and Choi-Kwon, 2000). One study even found more depression in right hemisphere than left hemisphere stroke patients (Dam et al. 1989). Astrom and colleagues (1993) and Robinson (2000) have pointed out that some of the apparent association between depression and left hemisphere strokes is a phenomenon of the early post-stroke period; studies carried out at least 4 months post-stroke have found roughly equal incidence of depression in right and left hemisphere stroke patients. In other words, neglect of or indifference to a right hemisphere deficit eventually wears off; the patient becomes aware of the deficits, and depression then ensues. The increased prevalence of depression with anterior as compared to posterior lesions within either hemisphere has largely been confirmed by most series, reinforcing the importance of the frontal lobes to emotion (Kim and Choi-Kwon 2000). Depression has been seen in between 18% (Kim and Choi-Kwon 2000) and 40% of stroke patients (Robinson 2000). It is a major limiting factor in stroke rehabilitation and recovery.

Another mood state associated with structural lesions of the brain is abnormal emotional lability, also referred to as pathological laughter and crying, emotional incontinence, or pseudobulbar affect. These patients may shift abruptly from elation to tears. Some deny any inner thought corresponding to their emotional display, but most describe a fleeting emotion, which they would normally be able to suppress from external expression. Seen in this light, pseudobulbar emotional lability can be considered a failure to control volitionally the expression of internal affective states. If the voluntary nervous system cannot suppress the facial expressions and other displays of emotion, the limbic system directs these expressions in an uninhibited manner. It is said that patients with pseudobulbar palsy cannot play poker again; they reveal their hands with their facial expressions every time. Although pathological laughter and crying are usually attributed to bilateral cerebral lesions (Loeb *et al.* 1990), they are also seen in patients with unilateral (Kim 1997) and even brainstem (Asfora *et al.* 1989) lesions. Kim and Choi-Kwon (2000) found emotional incontinence to be more common than depression in their series of stroke patients, and it correlated more with subcortical strokes.

Treatment of post-stroke depression has largely been similar to treatment of idiopathic depression. Lipsey and colleagues (1984) found that nortriptyline was clearly superior to placebo in treatment of post-stroke depression. Reding and colleagues (1986) reported similar findings with trazodone. Recently, Robinson and colleagues (2000) found that nortriptyline appeared superior to fluoxetine (Prozac) in a controlled trial in post-stroke depression. Pathological laughter and crying may also respond to antidepressant therapy with a selective serotonin reuptake inhibitor (SSRI; Mukand *et al.* 1996).

Mood and Epilepsy

Mood has been studied in patients undergoing the Wada test for determination of cerebral dominance in patients with epilepsy during screening for possible epilepsy surgery. Lee *et al.* (1990) reported that laughter or elation was significantly more frequent after right carotid amobarbital injections, whereas left hemisphere injections were more associated with crying. Similar findings have been reported in patients undergoing excision of cortical tissue for the surgical management of epilepsy. Patients with right hemisphere excisions had difficulty in matching different faces with the same emotional expression, whereas patients with left hemisphere excisions had difficulty matching the name of an emotional state with a paragraph describing a person's emotions (Kolb and Taylor 1981). In addition, patients with left frontal lesions were largely mute in terms of spontaneous spoken emotional expression, whereas patients with right frontal lesions were excessively talkative, often giving spontaneous descriptions of their emotional states (Kolb and Taylor 1981).

A related subject of considerable theoretical interest is the relationship of mood changes to electrical stimulation of the brain. As mentioned earlier, deep brain stimulation, performed for Parkinson's disease and movement disorders (see Chapter 16), occasionally causes an acute mood change (Bejjani *et al.* 1999). Vagus nerve stimulation, used in the treatment of refractory epilepsy, has also been found to be a treatment for depression (Rush *et al.* 2000). The fact that electrical stimulation of the vagus nerve or the brain can produce profound alterations in emotional state again highlights the close relationship between depression and brain disorders.

Mood, Traumatic Brain Injury, and Posttraumatic Stress Disorder

Depression is very common in patients with traumatic brain injury, just as it is after stroke. As compared to strokes, head injuries are likely to affect the frontal lobes; the 'frontal' behavioral deficits discussed in Chapter 10 are much more commonly seen in patients with head injury than in those with stroke. Among the effects of localized head injuries are alterations in mood. Grafman and colleagues (1986) studied Vietnam veterans with penetrating injuries of the frontal lobes. Patients with right orbitofrontal lesions appeared prone to increased anxiety, anger, and depression as compared to patients with left orbitofrontal lesions. Other effects of orbitofrontal lesions included disinhibition and decreased concern for other people. Dorsolateral frontal lesions produced blunted affect, and the left dorsolateral frontal lesion patients had more cognitive deficits and more mood changes – anger and irritability more than depression – than did the right dorsolateral frontal lobe patients. Another study of acute brain injury patients (Fedoroff et al. 1992) found an overall prevalence of major depression in 17 of 66 patients; major depression correlated with CT evidence of lesions in the left dorsolateral frontal lobe and left basal ganglia, but there was also correlation with previous psychiatric disorders and poor premorbid psychological functioning. Robinson and Szetela (1981) emphasized the correlation of depression after head injury with the closeness of the lesion to the frontal pole, a finding similar to that seen in post-stroke depression. Head injuries, with their predilection for the frontal regions, frequently produce apathy and personality change (Kwentus et al. 1985).

Depression is also a part of the 'post-concussive syndrome' discussed in Chapter 20, and part of the post-traumatic stress disorder (PTSD). Post-traumatic stress disorder is sometimes difficult to distinguish from the post-concussive syndrome, but the term is often used when the patient has ongoing psychological symptoms in the absence of evidence of significant traumatic brain injury (Davidson 2001). A large part of the post-traumatic stress disorder is the inappropriate activation of emotional reactions by neutral stimuli, and the frequent re-experiencing of traumatic events, sometimes to the extent of loss of reality testing or 'depersonalization experiences' (Rauch et al. 1998). One study found reduced volume by MRI in the hippocampus and amygdala bilaterally (Bremner et al. 1995). Increased activation of the amygdala has also been reported during readings of narratives of their traumatic events in patients with PTSD, indicating a facilitated fear response (Rauch et al. 1996). Rauch and colleagues (1998) suggest that the amygdala is less inhibited than usual by inputs from the anterior cingulate cortex, a frontal lobe area that may funnel cognitive inputs into the emotional system. An uncontrolled emotional reaction to stimuli is a hallmark of the post-traumatic stress disorder.

Mania is less common than depression after closed head injury. Starkstein and colleagues (1987) reported 11 cases of post-traumatic mania, with lesions involving the right hemisphere limbic system. The subject of 'organic mania' was discussed in Chapter 15.

Mood and Alzheimer's Disease

As discussed in Chapter 13, depression can be either a mimicker of dementia ('depressive pseudodementia') or an accompaniment of dementia (Reifler et al.

1982; Jones and Reifler 1994). Jost and Grossberg (1996) reported that depression frequently predates the onset of Alzheimer's disease, whereas delusional or paranoid thinking develops only after the diagnosis. Rabins and colleagues (1984) found that some patients with cognitive dysfunction and depression improved and maintained normal function after antidepressant treatment, whereas others did not. The importance of the identification of depression in elderly patients with cognitive deterioration is that treatment may result in significant improvement in functioning.

Mood and Parkinson's Disease

As discussed in Chapter 16, depression is a frequent concomitant of Parkinson's disease (Vogel 1982; Starkstein *et al.* 1989; Brown and McCarthy 1990; Hantz *et al.* 1994). Vogel (1982) found that even patients with early PD, who had not received any dopaminergic therapy, were frequently depressed. Depression scores did not correlate with motor disability, though there did appear to be a correlation between depression and akinesia or apathy. Patients with predominant tremor had lesser incidence of depression. Starkstein and colleagues (1989) found a correlation between depression and the degree of cognitive impairment in Parkinson's disease. Only one study (Hantz *et al.* 1994) found that depression seemed no more common in PD than in patients with other disabling conditions. PD and depression share several features both clinically and biochemically: both have prominent psychomotor retardation and bradykinesia, and both involve depletion of catecholamines. Serotonin metabolites such as 5-HIAA may also be diminished in the cerebrospinal fluid and brain in Parkinson's disease (Mayeux *et al.* 1988). Patients with PD also have a high incidence of anxiety (Stein *et al.* 1990). Identification and treatment of depression is important in PD, just as it is in Alzheimer's disease.

PRIMARY DEPRESSION

Patients who have primary depression, or depression without evidence of physical brain disease, have symptoms identical to the depressive syndromes associated with focal or diffuse brain injury. The cause of depression, of course, is unknown. Genetic factors doubtless play a role, as summarized in the discussion of bipolar affective disorder in Chapter 15. There is considerable evidence for neurochemical alterations in depression. Details of the science behind these discoveries will not be presented here. The field of neurotransmitters and depression began with the finding that the catecholamine-depleting agent, reserpine, caused a reversible depression. Both norepinephrine and serotonin are decreased in areas of the brain in major depression (Richelson 1990; Nemeroff 1998). Hormonal changes also play a role, especially chronic hyperactivity of the hypothalamic–pituitary–adrenal axis (Gold *et al.* 1988; Nemeroff 1998). These changes are even reflected in brain imaging. MRI studies have shown white matter and periventricular T2 hyperintensities in chronically depressed patients

(Soares and Mann 1997). Atrophy of the frontal lobes, caudate, and putamen are variably present in unipolar depression (Steffens and Ranga Rama Krishnan 1998). PET scans show relative hypermetabolism in areas of the left prefrontal region and amygdala in depressed patients (Nemeroff 1998); patients who cycle from depressed to manic phases have markedly increased metabolism in frontal and temporal areas during the manic phase and lower metabolism during the depressed phase than patients with unilateral depression (Schwartz *et al.* 1987). The causes of these biochemical, hormonal, structural, and metabolic changes in depression remain largely unknown.

Watson and colleagues (1995) have proposed a 'tripartite model' of depression, in which the syndrome is divided into three symptom groups: (1) symptoms of general distress (including hopelessness, fatigue, tension, crying, worry, pessimism); (2) symptomatic anxiety (tachycardia, sweating, tachypnea); and (3) low affect (lacking in the qualities of happiness, energy, sociability, confidence, and interest). There is some evidence (Shelton, personal communication 2001) that the distress and anxiety symptoms are related to serotonin levels, whereas the positive affect symptoms are related to catecholamine (norepinephrine and dopamine) levels. The prevalence of these three groups of symptoms may help to determine drug therapy.

Cognitive Deficits in Depression

As noted in Chapter 13, depression has in the past been considered a treatable or reversible cause of dementia ('depressive pseudodementia'). Studies have shown that patients with active depression perform abnormally on tests of sustained attention and short-term memory (Lachner and Engel 1994; Williams *et al.* 2000). Depression especially interferes with effortful tasks, whereas automatic tasks remain generally unaffected (Hartlage *et al.* 1993). Schatzberg and colleagues (2000) studied attention and verbal memory in patients with both psychotic and non-psychotic depression; those with psychotic depression had more severe deficits in both areas than those without psychosis. These cognitive deficits are usually mild; in fact, many depressed patients who complain of memory loss actually perform normally on neuropsychological tests (Popkin *et al.* 1982).

Occasionally, depressed patients have such marked cognitive and memory difficulties that they are thought to have dementia. Wells (1979) and Yesavage (1993) have presented clinical criteria for distinguishing depression from dementia. Depression develops over a shorter period, progresses more rapidly, and is more obvious to family members than dementia. Depressed persons complain of cognitive deficits and seek help for them, whereas demented patients usually have to be dragged to the doctor by a family member. Depressed patients make poor effort on tests, give more 'I don't know' than erroneous answers, and have a variable performance on tests, often missing easy items but giving correct answers on difficult ones. Demented patients, by contrast, try to perform, produce many 'near miss' errors, and are generally consistent in performance on different tests. In general, the complaints and behavior are often contradictory in depressed patients – for example, the depressed patient complains bitterly of memory loss yet makes it to every appointment on time. Experimentally, depressed patients can be distinguished from demented patients by performance on delayed recall tests (Lachner and Engel 1994). Language and praxis are more likely to be abnormal in dementia than in depression.

Treatment of Depression

Treatment of depression with antidepressant medications or psychotherapy techniques is beyond the scope of a behavioral neurology text, but a few comments are in order. There is ample evidence that a variety of antidepressant drugs are effective in treating both major and minor depression. Most antidepressant drugs are derived from the known neurochemistry of depression, in terms of depletion of catecholamines and serotonin. The selective serotonin reuptake inhibitors, fluoxetine (Prozac), sertraline (Zoloft), paroxetine (Paxil), and citalopram (Celexa) have increasingly replaced older drugs, such as the tricyclic antidepressants, because of greater efficacy and lesser side effects. Recent reviews have emphasized the safety and tolerability of these drugs, and the important role that all physicians, including primary care physicians and neurologists, can play in identifying and treating depression (Whooley and Simon 2000; Sampson 2001). Buproprion (Wellbutrin) is occasionally used in patients who cannot tolerate the SSRIs because of sexual dysfunction. A few newer agents, including nefazodone (Serzone), venlafaxine (Effexor), and mirtazapine (Remeron), have also become popular in refractory patients. Venlafaxine increases both serotonin and norepinephrine levels. Less commonly, monoamine oxidase inhibitors or stimulants such as methylphenidate are used in refractory depression (Goodwin 1996). When rare patients with depression fail to respond to antidepressant drug therapy, electroconvulsive therapy may occasionally be needed (Crowe 1984); use of this technique has decreased in recent years. As mentioned earlier, vagus nerve stimulation is under investigation as a treatment for refractory depression (Rush *et al.* 2000). Recent studies (e.g. Keller *et al.* 2000) have found that antidepressant drugs such as nefazodone combined with a behavioral psychotherapy program are more effective than either treatment alone; treatment with the drug alone did not differ from behavioral treatment alone. This evidence should pave the way for physicians to recommend combined drug and behavioral therapy for depression, and for insurance companies to pay for it.

ANXIETY AND PANIC DISORDERS

Anxiety is a mood state associated with response to stressors either in the environment or in internal thinking. A variety of psychopathologies feature anxiety as a prominent symptom, including generalized anxiety disorder, acute stress disorder, post-traumatic stress disorder, obsessive-compulsive disorder, various phobias but especially agoraphobia or fear of crowds or public places, and panic disorder (Clement and Chapouthier 1998). Many neurotransmitter systems in the brain are likely related to anxiety, including dopamine, norepinephrine, serotonin, glutamate, and cholecystokinin. Chemicals that induce seizures in animals often induce anxiety at lower doses, and benzodiazepines reduce both anxiety and seizures (Clement and Chapouthier 1998).

There is limited evidence for an effect of focal brain lesions on anxiety. Reiman and colleagues (1986) found PET abnormalities in the right parahippocampal region in patients with panic disorder. Maricle *et al.* (1991) reported a case of right parahippocampal infarction in a woman with panic attacks that began only after the stroke event. Fontaine and colleagues (1990) also reported abnormalities in the temporal lobes, especially the right temporal lobe, in patients with panic disorders. From these reports, it appears that destructive lesions of the right temporal lobe or parahippocampal region may be important to the development of panic attacks.

Panic attacks are dramatic episodes of acute anxiety, often completely unprovoked by any external event. Charles Darwin reportedly suffered such attacks throughout his life (Barloon and Noyes 1997). The symptoms included palpitations, shortness of breath, nausea, tremor, dizziness, and feelings of impending doom. Darwin himself wrote: 'I have awakened in the night being slightly unwell and felt so much afraid though my reason was laughing and told me there was nothing and tried to seize hold of objects to be frightened of' (Barloon and Noyes 1997). Darwin became both hypochondriacal and agoraphobic at various times in his life.

The symptoms of generalized anxiety or panic include shortness of breath, dizziness, palpitations, tremor, sweating, choking, nausea, depersonalization or derealization, numbness and tingling, flushes or chills, chest pain, fear of dying, or fear of going crazy or failing to control behavior (DSM-IV). Occasional patients describe focal neurological symptoms, especially unilateral paresthesias, blurred vision, and dizziness. These symptoms raise diagnostic suspicion of transient ischemic attacks, seizures, or hormonal imbalances . Most of the patients in the series of Coyle and Sterman (1986) were under obvious stress. In 42% of the cases, symptoms could be reproduced with hyperventilation. Neurologists clearly should be aware of the symptoms of panic disorder in order to avoid unnecessary testing and delay of appropriate treatment for these patients. In addition, there is a real risk of suicide in patients with panic disorder, making treatment all the more important (Weissman *et al.* 1989).

The pathophysiology of panic attacks includes biological as well as psychological changes. Cameron and colleagues (1987) found transient increases in prolactin, cortisol, and plasma norepinephrine during panic attacks. A body of experimental evidence indicates that lactate infusion induces panic in patients with anxiety disorders but not in normal controls (Pitts and McClure 1967; Kelly *et al.* 1971; Gaffney *et al.* 1988). The lactate infusions seem to reproduce a spontaneous biochemical change. The patients with panic disorder interpreted these changes as panic, whereas controls did not. This evidence suggests a biochemical basis for panic disorder. Panic may also be associated with cardiovascular disorders such as mitral valve prolapse (Forman *et al.* 1988;

Margraf *et al.* 1988), though this association appears to be weaker than originally thought.

The treatment of anxiety disorders, as in depression, is a combination of psychotherapy, reassurance, and medications. SSRI antidepressants appear effective in panic disorder (Michelson *et al.* 1998). Benzodiazepines and buspirone also relieve symptoms (Shader and Greenblatt 1993).

ALEXITHYMIA

Alexithymia is a syndrome discussed in the psychiatric literature but rarely used by neurologists. It refers to patients who cannot express their emotional states verbally, and who form poor relationships with other people, sometimes alternating between aloof, impersonal and dependent forms of relationships (Miller 1986). Psychosomatic symptoms are common. Alexithymic patients do not report many dreams, and their thought and communication in general are very concrete and practical. Miller (1986) explains alexithymia in terms of a failure of communication between the right hemisphere's emotional centers and the left hemisphere's verbal and reasoning processes. Direct evidence for a hemispheral 'disconnection', however, is lacking.

CONCLUSION

This chapter was a whirlwind tour of emotional and anxiety states and brain pathology. Psychiatrists can point to a richer, more complex literature surrounding most of the topics just discussed. The key points here are that emotions do have important relationships to local brain lesions, as well as to psychological vicissitudes. In either case, the phenomena of depression and anxiety reflect changes in brain chemistry and physiology, and biological treatments such as drugs that affect neurotransmitter levels have important benefits. Interestingly, even in this age of genes and neurotransmitters, behavioral techniques such as psychotherapy are maintaining their usefulness, especially when combined with pharmacological therapy.

REFERENCES

Asfora WT, DeSalles AF, Masamitsu A, Kjellberg RN. Is the syndrome of pathological laughing and crying a manifestation of pseudobulbar palsy? J Neurol Neurosurg Psychiatry 1989;52:523–525.

Astrom M, Adolfsson R, Asplund K. Major depression in stroke patients. Stroke 1993;24: 976–982.

Babinski J. Contribution a l'étude des troubles mentaux dans l'hemiplegie organique cerebrale (Anosognosie). Revue Neurologique 1914;22:845–848. Translated in Rottenberg DA, Hochberg FH, Neurological Classics in Modern Translation. New York: Hafner Press, 1977;131–135.

Barloon TJ, Noyes R. Charles Darwin and panic disorder. JAMA 1997;277:138–141.

Bejjani BP, Damier P, Arnulf I et al. Transient acute depression induced by high-frequency deep-brain stimulation. New Engl J Med 1999;340:1476–1480.

Breitbart W, Rosenfeld B, Pessin H et al. Depression, hopelessness, and desire for hastened death in terminally ill patients with cancer. JAMA 2000;284:2907–2911.

Bremner JD, Randall P, Scott RM et al. MRI-based measurement of hippocampal volume in patients with combat-related post-traumatic stress disorder. Am J Psychiatry 1995;152:973–981.

Brown RG, MacCarthy B. Psychiatric morbidity in patients with Parkinson's disease. Psychol Med 1990;20:77–87.

Brown JT, Stoudemire GA. Normal and pathological grief. JAMA 1983;250:378–382.

Cameron OG, Lee MA, Curtis GC, McCann DS. Endocrine and physiological changes during 'spontaneous' panic attacks. Psychoneuroendocrinology 1987;12:321–331.

Clement Y, Chapouthier G. Biological bases of anxiety. Neurosci Behav Rev 1998;22: 623–633.

Coyle PK, Sterman AB. Focal neurologic symptoms in panic attacks. Am J Psychiatry 1986;143:648–649.

Crowe RR. Electroconvulsive therapy – a current perspective. New Engl J Med 1984;311: 163–167.

Dam H, Pedersen HE, Ahlgren P. Depression among patients with stroke. Acta Psychiatr Scand 1989;80:118–124.

Davidson JRT. Recognition and treatment of posttraumatic stress disorder. JAMA 2001;286:584–588.

Denny-Brown D, Meyer JS, Horenstein S. The significance of perceptual rivalry resulting from parietal lesions. Brain 1952;75:434–471.

Diagnostic and Statistical Manual of Mental Disorders (4th edn). Washington, DC: American Psychiatric Association, 1994.

Fedoroff JP, Starkstein SE, Forrester AW et al. Depression in patients with acute traumatic brain injury. Am J Psychiatry 1992;149:918–923.

Fontaine R, Breton G, Dery R et al. Temporal lobe abnormalities in panic disorder: an MRI study. Biol Psychiatry 1990;27:304–310.

Gaffney FA, Fenton BJ, Lane LD, Lake CR. Hemodynamic, ventilatory, and biochemical responses of panic patients and normal controls with sodium lactate infusion and spontaneous panic attacks. Arch Gen Psychiatry 1988;45:53–60.

Gainotti G. Emotional behavior and hemispheric side of brain. Cortex 1972;8:41–45.

Ghika-Schmid F, Bogousslavsky J. Affective disorders following stroke. Eur Neurol 1997;38:75–81.

Gold PW, Goodwin FK, Chrousos GP. Clinical and biochemical manifestations of depression. Relation to the neurobiology of stress. New Engl J Med 1988;319:348–353, 413–420.

Goldstein K. Language and language disturbances. Aphasic symptom complexes and their significance for medicine and theory of language. New York: Grune & Stratton, 1948; 10–13.

Goodwin F. A 47-year-old man with chronic depression. Clinical crossroads. JAMA 1996;275:479–485.

Gorman JM, Goetz RR, Fyer M et al. The mitral valve prolapse–panic disorder connection. Psychosom Med 1988;50:114–122.

Grafman J, Vance SC, Weingartner H et al. The effects of lateralized frontal lesions on mood regulation. Brain 1986;109:1127–1148.

Guze SB, Robins E. Suicide among primary affective disorders. Br J Psychiatry 1970;117: 437–438.

Hantz P, Caradoc-Davies G, Caradoc-Davies T et al. Depression in Parkinson's disease. Am J Psychiatry 1994;151:1010–1014.

Hartlage S, Alloy LB, Vazquez C, Dykman B. Automatic and effortful processing in depression. Psychol Bull 1993;113:247–278.

Jones BN, Reifler BV. Depression coexisting with dementia. Evaluation and treatment. Med Clin North Am 1994;78:823–840.

Jost BC, Grossberg GT. The evolution of psychiatric symptoms in Alzheimer's disease: a natural history study. J Am Geriatr Soc 1996;44:1078–1081.

Keller MB, McCullough JP, Klein DN *et al*. A comparison of nefazodone, the cognitive behavioral-analysis system of psychotherapy, and their combination for the treatment of chronic depression. New Engl J Med 2000;342:1462–1470.

Kelly D, Mitchell-Heggs N, Sherman D. Anxiety and the effects of sodium lactate assessed clinically and physiologically. Br J Psychiatry 1971;119:129–141.

Kim JS. Pathologic laughter after unilateral stroke. J Neurol Sci 1997;148:121–125.

Kim JS, Choi-Kwon S. Post-stroke depression and emotional incontinence. Correlation with lesion location. Neurology 2000;54:1805–1810.

Kolb B, Taylor L. Affective behavior in patients with localized cortical excisions: role of lesion site and side. Science 1981;214:89–91.

Kwentus JA, Hart RP, Peck ET, Kornstein S. Psychiatric complications of closed head trauma. Psychosomatics 1985;26:8–17.

Lachner G, Engel RR. Differentiation of dementia and depression by memory tests. A meta-analysis. J Nerv Ment Dis 1994;181:34–39.

Lee GP, Loring DW, Meador KJ, Brooks BB. Hemispheric specialization for emotional expression: a re-examination of results from intracarotid administration of sodium amobarbital. Brain Cogn 1990;12:267–280.

Lipsey JR, Robinson RG, Pearlson GD. Nortryptiline treatment for post-stroke depression: a double-blind trial. Lancet 1984;1:297–300.

Loeb C, Gandolfo C, Caponnetto C, Del Sette M. Pseudobulbar palsy: a clinical computed tomography study. Eur Neurol 1990;30:42–46.

Margraf J, Ehlers A, Roth WT. Mitral valve prolapse and panic disorder: a review of their relationship. Psychosom Med 1988;50:93–113.

Maricle RA, Sennhauser S, Burry M. Panic disorder associated with right parahippocampal infarction. J Nerv Ment Dis 1991;179:374–375.

Maruta T, Colligan RC, Malinchoc M, Offord KP. Optimists versus pessimists: survival rate among medical patients over a 30-year period. Mayo Clin Proc 2000;75:140–143.

Mayeux R, Stern Y, Sano M *et al*. The relationship of serotonin to depression in Parkinson's disease. Movement Disorders 1988;3:237–244.

Michelson D, Lydiard RB, Pollack MH *et al*. Outcome assessment and clinical improvement in panic disorder: evidence from a randomized controlled trial of fluoxetine and placebo. Am J Psychiatry 1998;155:1570–1577.

Miller L. Is alexithymia a disconnection syndrome? A neuropsychological perspective. Int J Psychiatry Med 1986;16:199–209.

Mukand J, Kaplan M, Senno RG, Bishop DS. Pathological crying and laughing: treatment with sertraline. Arch Phys Med Rehabil 1996;77:1309–1311.

Nemeroff CB. The neurobiology of depression. Scientific American 1998;42–49.

Pitts FN, McClure JN. Lactate metabolism in anxiety neurosis. New Engl J Med 1967;277:1329–1336.

Popkin SJ, Gallagher D, Thompson LW, Moore M. Memory complaint and performance in normal and depressed older adults. Exp Aging Res 1982;8:141–145.

Rabins PV, Merchant A, Nestadt G. Criteria for diagnosing reversible dementia caused by depression: validation by 2-year follow-up. Br J Psychiatry 1984;144:488–492.

Rauch SL, Van der Kolk BA, Fisler RE *et al*. A symptom provocation study of post-traumatic stress disorder using positron emission tomography and script-driven imagery. Arch Gen Psychiatry 1996;53:380–387.

Rauch SL, Shin LM, Whalen PJ, Pitman RK. Neuroimaging and the neuroanatomy of post-traumatic stress disorder. CNS Spectrums 1998;3(Suppl. 2):31–41.

Reding MJ, Orto LA, Winter SW. Antidepressant therapy after stroke: a double-blind trial. Arch Neurol 1986;43:763–765.

Reifler BV, Larson E, Hanley R. Coexistence of cognitive impairment and depression in geriatric outpatients. Am J Psychiatry 1982;139:5.

Reiman EM, Raichle ME, Robins E *et al.* The application of positron emission tomography to the study of panic disorder. Am J Psychiatry 1986;143:469–477.

Richelson E. Antidepressants and brain neurochemistry. Mayo Clin Proc 1990;65: 1227–1236.

Robinson RG. An 82-year-old woman with mood changes following a stroke. Clinical crossroads. JAMA 2000;283:1607–1614.

Robinson RG, Szetela B. Mood change following left hemisphere brain injury. Ann Neurol 1981;9:447–453.

Robinson RG, Kubos KL, Starr LB *et al.* Mood disorders in stroke patients. Importance of location of lesion. Brain 1984;107:81–93.

Robinson RG, Schultz SK, Castillo C *et al.* Nortriptyline vs. fluoxetine in the treatment of depression and short-term recovery following stroke: a placebo controlled double-blind study. Am J Psychiatry 2000;157:351–359.

Rolls ET. Precis of the brain and emotion. Behav Brain Sci 2000;23:177–234.

Rush AJ, George MS, Sackheim HA *et al.* Vagus nerve stimulation (VNS) for treatment-resistant depression: a multicenter study. Biol Psychiatry 2000;47:276–286.

Sampson SM. Treating depression with selective serotonin reuptake inhibitors: a practical approach. Mayo Clin Proc 2001;76:739–744.

Schatzberg AF, Posener JA, DeBattista C *et al.* Neuropsychological deficits in psychotic versus non-psychotic major depression and no mental illness. Am J Psychiatry 2000;157;1095–1100.

Schwartz JM, Baxter LR, Mazziotta JC *et al.* The differential diagnosis of depression. Relevance of positron emission tomography studies of cerebral glucose metabolism to the bipolar–unipolar dichotomy. JAMA 1987;258:1368–1374.

Shader RI, Greenblatt DJ. Use of benzodiazepines in anxiety disorders. New Engl J Med 1993;328:1398–1405.

Sinyor D, Jacques P, Kaloupek DG *et al.* Post-stroke depression and lesion localization: an attempted replication. Brain 1986;109:537–546.

Soares JC, Mann JJ. The anatomy of mood disorders – review of structural neuroimaging studies. Biol Psychiatry 1997;41:86–106.

Starkstein SE, Kubos KL, Starr LB *et al.* Mood disorders in stroke patients: importance of lesion localization. Brain 1984;107:81–93.

Starkstein SE, Pearlson GD, Boston J, Robinson RG. Mania after brain injury. A controlled study of causative factors. Arch Neurol 1987;44:1069–1073.

Starkstein SE, Preziosi TJ, Berthier ML *et al.* Depression and cognitive impairment in Parkinson's disease. Brain 1989;112:1141–1153.

Steffens DC, Ranga Rama Krishnan K. Structural neuroimaging and mood disorders: recent findings, implications for classification, and future directions. Biol Psychiatry 1998;43:705–712.

Stein MB, Heuser IJ, Juncos JL, Uhde TW. Anxiety disorders in patients with Parkinson's disease. Am J Psychiatry 1990;147:217–220.

Vogel H-P. Symptoms of depression in Parkinson's disease. Pharmacopsychiatry 1982;15:192–196.

Watson D, Clark LA, Weber K *et al.* Testing a tripartite model: II. Exploring the symptom structure of anxiety and depression in student, adult, and patient samples. J Abnorm Psychol 1995;104:15–25.

Weissman MM, Klerman GL, Markowitz JS, Ouellette R. Suicidal ideation and suicide attempts in panic disorder and attacks. New Engl J Med 1989;321:1209–1214.

Weissman MM, Bland RC, Canino GJ *et al.* Cross-national epidemiology of major depression and bipolar disorder. JAMA 1996;276:293–299.

Wells CE. Pseudodementia. Am J Psychiatry 1979;136:895–900.

Whooley MA, Simon GE. Managing depression in medical outpatients. New Engl J Med 2000;343:1942–1950.

Williams RQ, Hagerty BM, Cimprich B *et al*. Changes in directed attention and short-term memory in depression. J Psychiat Res 2000;34:227–238.

Yesavage J. Differential diagnosis between depression and dementia. Am J Medicine 1993;94(Suppl. 5A):23S–28S.

PART IV

Neurobehavioral Aspects of Specific Diseases

18

Cognitive Aspects of Multiple Sclerosis

Marked enfeeblement of the memory.

(Charcot 1877)

Multiple sclerosis (MS) is known as the 'crippler of young adults', an inflammatory or autoimmune disease of the central nervous system white matter that afflicts 250,000–300,000 persons in the USA (Noseworthy *et al.* 2000). The disease is divided into relapsing–remitting MS, which represents approximately 80% of the cases, and primary progressive MS, which accounts for about 20%. Most patients develop first symptoms between the ages of 20 and 40 years. Multiple sclerosis has a female to male preponderance of nearly 2 to 1, especially in relapsing–remitting patients. Patients with relapsing–remitting MS improve during the remissions, sometimes back to their previous baseline, but sometimes with a new plateau of disability. Over many years, a majority of such patients develop a chronic, progressive form of the disease now called 'secondary progressive MS'. About 10% of cases never develop disabling disease ('benign MS'). The pathology of the disease involves inflammatory, demyelinating plaques in the central nervous system white matter, including optic nerves, cerebral hemispheres, brainstem, cerebellum, and spinal cord. Other characteristic features of MS are the worsening of neurological deficits and symptoms with increased temperature (Uhtoff's symptom), the complaint of fatigue, often in the afternoon hours, and the tendency of exacerbations to occur during the post-partum period. The precise cause and pathophysiology of the disease remain unknown; the immune activation in the nervous system is strongly influenced by genetic factors, but there are likely triggering factors in the environment such as viral and other infections (Noseworthy *et al.* 2000).

The clinical diagnosis of multiple sclerosis is more difficult than the pathological diagnosis. The exacerbations consist of episodic symptoms involving vision, sensation, motor power, or coordination, with periods of improvement in between. Paresthesias, especially on flexing the neck (Lhermitte's symptom), are especially common. The diagnosis of multiple sclerosis is divided into clinically definite, probable, and possible categories (Poser *et al.* 1983). Clinically definite MS is diagnosed when an individual has separate attacks of symptoms, with objective signs attributable to distinct areas of the central nervous system white matter, without another disease process to explain the symptoms. Probable MS would include cases with a single, progressive history but separate lesion localizations, or multiple attacks but with objective abnormalities pointing to a single CNS lesion. Possible MS would include patients with a single attack of symptoms, or progressive symptoms involving one area of the nervous system. These clinical classifications are aided in turn by laboratory tests. MRI scanning has been very helpful in detecting characteristic demyelinating lesions in the white matter of the brain and spinal cord in approximately 90% of cases (Miller *et al.* 1998). Enhancement of MS plaque lesions with gadolinium also indicates acute or recent lesions and indicates that the disease process is active. Lumbar puncture and CSF analysis provide evidence of immune activity in the nervous system, including increased synthesis of immunoglobulin and the presence of oligoclonal bands in the cerebrospinal fluid. Finally, evoked potential tests (visual, auditory, and somatosensory evoked potentials) can provide evidence of clinically undetected lesions. These laboratory findings can be combined with the clinical classification to yield a 'laboratory supported' diagnosis of definite multiple sclerosis (Poser *et al.* 1983). The classification of multiple sclerosis is currently under revision, without a clear consensus as yet.

COGNITIVE IMPAIRMENT IN MULTIPLE SCLEROSIS

Most accounts of multiple sclerosis emphasize the physical and neurological disabilities of the disease: vision loss, double vision, weakness, spasticity, incoordination, and bowel and bladder impairment. As in epilepsy, discussion of cognitive and mood disturbances has been less prominent, perhaps to avoid prejudicing the public about the ability of patients with multiple sclerosis to function. Charcot (1877), however, mentioned both 'marked enfeeblement of the memory' and 'conceptions...formed slowly' in his initial description of the disease. McKhann (1982), in a more modern review of the disease, mentioned cognitive deterioration only in chronic, disabled patients. Over the past 15 years, however, a considerable literature on cognitive and emotional disorders in multiple sclerosis has developed (Rao 1986; Rao *et al.* 1991a; Hamalainen and Ruutiainen 1999). Informal surveys based on obvious mental impairment have suggested that fewer than 5% of MS patients have cognitive deficits, but more formal neuropsychological studies have found a much higher prevalence of such deficits. Ron and colleagues (1991) found that over 50% of hospital-ascertained MS patients had cognitive deficits. Rao and colleagues (1991a) reported that 43% of 100 community-based patients with MS had cognitive impairment; these patients were chosen to avoid the biases of patients who seek out treatment in MS clinics. Of course, many patients with MS, even chronically disabled patients, have relatively normal cognitive functions. These patients should not be treated as if they are cognitively impaired, but it would be equally wrong to ignore the cognitive and emotional problems which many MS patients have, and which cause them considerable disability in their daily lives (Rao *et al.* 1991b).

Multiple sclerosis can be seen as the prototypic disease of the cerebral white matter and as a focus for the study of the cognitive effects of white matter lesions (Filley 1998). Investigations of cognitive impairments in multiple sclerosis have shown common patterns of deficit. The principal abnormalities involve short-term or recent memory (Rao *et al.* 1986; Beatty *et al.* 1988; Litvan *et al.* 1988; Grigsby *et al.* 1994), abstract reasoning (Rao *et al.* 1991a), sustained attention, frontal lobe 'executive functions' (Arnett *et al.* 1994; Foong *et al.* 1997), speed of processing (Litvan *et al.* 1988), higher level visuospatial functions (Heaton *et al.* 1985; Rao *et al.* 1991a), and verbal fluency (Beatty *et al.* 1988). Within memory testing, recall of items is much more affected than recognition memory (Rao *et al.* 1986). Litvan and colleagues (1988) suggested that slowing of information processing in MS leads to reduced memory. Grigsby *et al.* (1994) found deficits in both immediate or working memory and short-term memory, but it should be noted that these deficits were fairly mild; MMSE scores, for example, did not differ between patients and controls. In comparison to normal controls, MS patients show abnormal 'cognitive fatigue' or decline in performance on tasks during a single test session (Krupp and Elkins 2000). Fatigue is a common symptom in MS, and it is likely related to the cognitive effects of the disease (Comi *et al.* 2001). Most studies have shown that other cognitive functions, such as immediate memory, simple attention, language, and general intellectual functioning, are relatively preserved in most patients with MS (Litvan *et al.* 1988; Rao *et al.* 1991). Rare reports have described aphasia (Olmos-Lau *et al.* 1977; Achiron *et al.* 1992; Arnett *et al.* 1996) and agnosia (Okuda *et al.* 1996) in patients with MS, but these deficits are much less frequent than the disorders of memory, attention, and cognitive processing speed, discussed above. One study did find mild language deficits, such as naming and verbal fluency, in patients with MS (Friend *et al.* 1999). One case report of a callosal disconnection syndrome in a patient with multiple sclerosis failed to find similar deficits in all but one of a series of 15 patients with definite MS (Schnider *et al.* 1993). In comparing this pattern of deficits to the dementias (Chapter 13), the cognitive disorders in MS resemble the 'subcortical dementias' such as Parkinson's disease and AIDS dementia complex more than cortical dementias such as Alzheimer's disease. Filley (1998) has also coined the term 'white matter dementia' to reflect the slowing of cognitive processing, deficits in sustained attention, short-term memory, and executive functioning, with preservation of language and other 'cortical' functions. Clearly, the concepts of 'subcortical' and 'white matter dementia' overlap. What is most important, however, is the presence of cognitive deficits in this white matter disease; most of the time, the severity of the deficits does not reach the level of dementia.

Correlation of Cognitive Deficits with Disability and Brain Imaging in MS

In general, the degree of cognitive impairment in MS patients has little correlation with measures of physical disability such as the EDSS (Kurtzke 1983), which emphasize motor deficits, and especially ambulation. Cognitive deficits also have little correlation with duration of disease. Jennekens-Schinkel and Sanders (1986), for example, reported three patients with progressive cognitive difficulties at a time when they had only mild physical disability. Correlation of cognitive deficits with demyelinating lesion burden, measured by MRI, has been more positive. Figure 18.1 depicts MRI findings in a typical case of multiple sclerosis. Deficits of executive function and other frontal lobe processes, such as performance on the Wisconsin Card Sorting Test (See Chapter 8), correlate to some extent with frontal lobe white matter lesions (Ron *et al.* 1991; Arnett *et al.* 1994). In another study (Brainin *et al.* 1988), memory deficits showed correlation with temporal white matter lesions, especially when bilateral. More general cognitive deficits have shown a correlation with the number and volume of cerebral white matter lesions on MRI (Franklin *et al.* 1988; Rao *et al.* 1989; Swirsky-Sacchetti *et al.* 1992; Sperling *et al.* 2001); in the study of Rao and colleagues (1989), periventricular white matter lesions in the brain in excess of 30 square centimeters of lesion area predicted cognitive deficits. Not all studies have confirmed these findings (Huber *et al.* 1987; Foong *et al.* 2000); Fulton *et al.* (1999) found that only a few specific functions correlated with MRI lesion burden, whereas most of the others did not. Other findings on brain imaging that have correlated in some studies with cognitive deficits are atrophy of the corpus callosum (Huber *et al.* 1987; Rao *et al.* 1989) and increased ventricular size (Clark

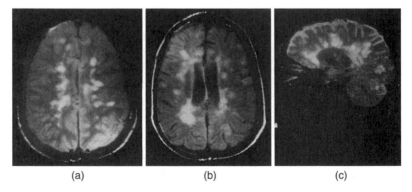

(a)   (b)   (c)

Figure 18.1 MRI photographs in the axial (a and b) and sagittal (c) planes in a patient with typical lesions of multiple sclerosis. The axial images are proton density images, the sagittal image is t2-weighted. Reprinted courtesy of Dr Michael J. Olek and David M. Dawson, Multiple sclerosis and other inflammatory demyelinating diseases of the central nervous system. In WG Bradley, RB Daroff, GM Fenichel, CD Marsden (eds). Neurology in Clinical Practice, Vol. I (3rd edn). Boston: Butterworth-Heinemann, 2000.)

et al. 1992; Swirsky-Sacchetti *et al.* 1992; Miller *et al.* 1998; Berg *et al.* 2000). Sperling and colleagues (2001) suggested that the frontal and parietal white matter lesions that are so common in MS affect sustained attention and verbal memory by disrupting frontoparietal subcortical networks.

Temporal Course of Cognitive Deficits in MS

Another controversy has surrounded the course of cognitive deficits over time in MS patients. Several studies (Jennekins-Schinkel *et al.* 1990; Mariani *et al.* 1991) have suggested that the deficits remain stable over time, a few have shown progressive worsening (Amato *et al.* 1995), and one showed that cognitively normal MS patients tend to remain normal, while cognitively impaired patients tend to worsen progressively (Kujala *et al.* 1997). One study has pointed to the extreme variability of cognitive testing in individual subjects who are having active relapsing–remitting disease, even over short periods of time (Feinstein *et al.* 1993).

Treatment of Cognitive Deficits in MS

Relatively little has been written about the treatment of cognitive deficits in MS patients. Presumably, medical treatments that reduce formation of cerebral white matter plaques would reduce the accumulation of cognitive disability. A trial of interferon beta-1a (Avonex) in relapsing–remitting MS did show a reduced accumulation of deficits on a neuropsychological test battery (Fischer *et al.* 2000). It is likely that the other interferon drug, interferon beta-1b (Betaseron), and the amino acid polymer glatiramer (Copaxone) would have similar benefit, though a trial of glatiramer versus placebo for 2 years did not demonstrate any effect on cognitive function (Weinstein *et al.* 1999), and a similar trial involving Betaseron did not show a change in verbal memory (Selby *et al.* 1998). Memory enhancing, anticholinesterase drugs such as donepizil (Aricept), rivastigmine (Exelon), and galantamine (Reminyl) may have promise in patients with MS-related memory loss, but their use is based on only anecdotal evidence at present. Rehabilitation programs have been developed for cognitive deficits in MS, but little evidence of efficacy has been presented.

EMOTIONAL CHANGES IN MULTIPLE SCLEROSIS

Like cognitive changes, emotional changes are extremely common in patients with multiple sclerosis. Early studies (Cottrell and Wilson 1926; Surridge 1969) emphasized euphoria as the predominant mood in patients with MS, but more recent studies have shown that depression is much more common. One study reported a point incidence of 40% of major depression in 45 recently diagnosed patients with multiple sclerosis (Sullivan *et al.* 1995). A study in more chronic MS patients found a correlation between depression and physical disability (Millefiorini *et al.* 1992), but several studies have shown that MS patients are more likely to be depressed than other patients with chronic disabilities from other illnesses (Surridge 1969; Whitlock and Siskind 1980; Rabins *et al.* 1986). Depression in MS patients is also associated with an increased risk of suicide (Sadovnik *et al.* 1991; Stenager *et al.* 1992). Filippi and colleagues (1994) reported that cognitive deficits and depression also correlated with each other. Euphoria, in the present era, is recognized mainly in patients with such extreme frontal lobe lesion burdens as to be grossly demented, or in patients with bipolar affective disorder (Rabins *et al.* 1986). A few studies have suggested a correlation between depression and the presence of temporal lobe white matter lesions (Rabins *et al.* 1986; Honer *et al.* 1987), but other studies have failed to confirm a clear relationship between affective symptoms and white matter lesions ascertained by MRI (Millefiorini *et al.* 1992).

The treatment of depression in patients with multiple sclerosis generally involves drug therapy and psychotherapy. One study showed desipramine to be superior to placebo in MS patients, but side effects were dose-limiting (Schiffer and Wineman 1990). Most MS specialists now use the SSRI antidepressants (see Chapter 16). Another problem in the treatment of depressed MS patients is that interferon therapies, and particularly the drug Betaseron (Neilley *et al.* 1996), can cause depression, and combined treatment with an interferon and an antidepressant is often indicated.

Although depression is the most common psychiatric complication of multiple sclerosis, rare cases have been described with psychotic illness (Feinstein *et al.* 1992). In the ten cases studied by these authors, there appeared to be a correlation between psychosis and periventricular white matter lesions, particularly involving the periventricular white matter of the temporal lobe. The patients most often had a persecutory delusional system but relatively preserved affect; these patients thus resembled psychotic patients with epilepsy (see Chapter 19) more than patients with schizophrenia. Mania or bipolar affective disorder has also been described in patients with multiple sclerosis (Peselow *et al.* 1981; Kellner *et al.* 1984; Joffe *et al.* 1987). Finally, conversion symptoms and hysterical neurological deficits have been commonly observed in patients with documented multiple sclerosis (Caplan and Nadelson 1980; Petersen and Kokmen 1989).

CONCLUSION

Multiple sclerosis, the prototypic disease of the cerebral white matter, is a good example of the cognitive and behavioral effects of cerebral white matter lesions. Although only a small minority of patients with MS have such marked cognitive deficits as to be functionally demented, nearly half of patients with MS have detectable deficits on neuropsychological testing. These deficits affect memory, sustained attention, speed of processing, verbal fluency, frontal lobe 'executive' functions, and other cognitive and behavioral processes. Depression is also extremely common in MS patients, and current therapies to prevent progression of the disease may increase the risk of depression. Treatment of depression in MS patients is important to the overall therapy of the condition. Far from leading to prejudice against patients with MS, recognition of these disorders should make the MS patient adjust better to society and to family and friends.

REFERENCES

Achiron AI, Ziv I, Djaldetti R *et al*. Aphasia in multiple sclerosis: clinical and radiological correlations. Neurology 1992;42:2195–2197.

Amato MP, Ponziani G, Pracucci G *et al*. Cognitive impairment in early-onset multiple sclerosis. Pattern, predictors, and impact on everyday life in 4-year follow-up. Arch Neurol 1995;52:168–172.

Arnett PA, Rao SM, Bernardin L *et al*. Relationship between frontal lobe lesions and Wisconsin Card Sorting Test performance in patients with multiple sclerosis. Neurology 1994;44:420–425.

Arnett PA, Rao SM, Hussain M *et al*. Conduction aphasia in multiple sclerosis: a case report with MRI findings. Neurology 1996;47:576–578.

Beatty WW, Goodkin DE, Monson N *et al*. Anterograde and retrograde amnesia in patients with chronic progressive multiple sclerosis. Arch Neurol 1988;45:611–619.

Berg D, Maurer M, Warmuth-Metz M *et al*. The correlation between ventricular diameter measured by transcranial sonography and clinical disability and cognitive dysfunction in patients with multiple sclerosis. Arch Neurol 2000;57:1289–1292.

Brainin M, Goldenberg G, Ahlers C *et al*. Structural brain correlates of anterograde memory deficits in multiple sclerosis. J Neurol 1988;235:362–365.

Caplan LR, Nadelson T. Multiple sclerosis and hysteria. Lessons learned from their association. JAMA 1980;243:2418–2421.

Charcot JM. Lectures on the Diseases of the Nervous System delivered at La Salpetriere. London: New Sydenham Society, 1877;194–195.

Clark CM, James G, Li D *et al*. Ventricular size, cognitive function and depression in patients with multiple sclerosis. Can J Neurol Sci 1992;19:352–356.

Comi G, Leocani L, Rossi P, Colombo B. Physiopathology and treatment of fatigue in multiple sclerosis. J Neurol 2001;248:174–179.

Cottrell SS, Wilson SAK. The affective symptomatology of disseminated sclerosis: a study of 100 cases. J Neurol Psychopathol 1926: 7:1–30.

Feinstein A, du Boulay G, Ron MA. Psychotic illness in multiple sclerosis. A clinical and magnetic resonance imaging study. Br J Psychiat 1992;161:680–685.

Feinstein A, Ron M, Thompson A. A serial study of psychometric and magnetic resonance imaging changes in multiple sclerosis. Brain 1993;116:569–602.

Filippi M, Alberoni M, Martinelli V *et al*. Influence of clinical variables on neuropsychological performance in multiple sclerosis. Eur Neurol 1994;34:324–328.

Filley CM. The behavioral neurology of cerebral white matter. Neurology 1998;50:1535–1540.

Fischer JS, Priore RL, Jacobs LD *et al*. Neuropsychological effects of interferon beta-1a in relapsing multiple sclerosis. Ann Neurol 2000;48:885–892.

Foong J, Rozewicz L, Quaghebeur G *et al*. Executive function in multiple sclerosis. The role of frontal lobe pathology. Brain 1997;120:15–26.

Foong J, Rozewicz L, Chong WK *et al*. A comparison of neuropsychological deficits in primary and secondary progressive multiple sclerosis. J Neurol 2000;247:97–101.

Franklin GM, Heaton RK, Nelson LM *et al*. Correlation of neuropsychological and MRI findings in chronic/progressive multiple sclerosis. Neurology 1988;38:1826–1829.

Friend KB, Rabin BM, Groninger L *et al*. Language functions in patients with multiple sclerosis. Clin Neuropsychol 1999;1:78–94.

Fulton JC, Grossman RI, Udupa J *et al*. MR lesion load and cognitive function in patients with relapsing–remitting multiple sclerosis. Am J Neuroradiol 1999;20: 1951–1955.

Grigsby J, Ayarbe SD, Kravcisin N, Busenbark D. Working memory impairment among persons with chronic progressive multiple sclerosis. J Neurol 1994;241:125–131.

Hamalainen P, Ruutiainen J. Cognitive decline in multiple sclerosis. Int MSJ 1999;6: 51–57.

Heaton RK, Nelson LM, Thompson DS et al. Neuropsychological findings in relapsing–remitting and chronic progressive multiple sclerosis. J Consul Clin Psychol 1985; 53:103–110.

Honer WG, Hurwitz T, Li DKB et al. Temporal lobe involvement in multiple sclerosis patients with psychiatric disorders. Arch Neurol 1987;44:187–190.

Huber SJ, Paulson GW, Shuttleworth EC et al. Magnetic resonance imaging correlates of dementia in multiple sclerosis. Arch Neurol 1987;44:732–736.

Jennekens-Schinkel A, Sanders EACM. Decline of cognition in multiple sclerosis: dissociable deficits. J Neurol Neurosurg Psychiatry 1986;49:1354–1360.

Jennekens-Schinkel A, La Boyrie PM, Lanser JBK, Van der Velde EA. Cognition in patients with multiple sclerosis after four years. J Neurol Sci 1990;99:229–247.

Joffe RT, Lippert GP, Gray TA et al. Mood disorder and multiple sclerosis. Arch Neurol 1987;44:376–378.

Kellner CH, Davenport Y, Post RM et al. Rapidly cycling bipolar disorder and multiple sclerosis. Am J Psychiat 1984;141:112–113.

Krupp LB, Elkins LE. Fatigue and declines in cognitive functioning in multiple sclerosis. Neurology 2000;55:934–939.

Kujala P, Portin R, Ruutiainen J. The progress of cognitive decline in multiple sclerosis. A controlled 3-year follow-up. Brain 1997;120:289–297.

Kurtzke JF. Rating neurologic impairment in multiple sclerosis: an Expanded Disability Status Scale (EDSS). Neurology 1983; 33:1444–1452.

Litvan I, Grafman J, Vendrell P, Martinez JM. Slowed information processing in multiple sclerosis. Arch Neurol 1988;45:281–285.

Mariani C, Farina E, Cappa SF et al. Neuropsychological assessment in multiple sclerosis: a follow-up study with magnetic resonance imaging. J Neurol 1991;238:395–400.

McKhann GM. Multiple sclerosis. Ann Rev Neurosci 1982;5:219–239.

Millefiorini E, Padovani A, Pozzilli C et al. Depression in the early phase of MS: influence of functional disability, cognitive impairment and brain abnormalities. Acta Neurol Scand 1992;86:354–358.

Miller DH, Grossman JI, Reingold SC, McFarland HF. The role of magnetic resonance techniques in understanding and managing multiple sclerosis. Brain 1998;121:3–24.

Neilly LK, Goodin DS, Goodkin DE, Hauser SL. Side effect profile of interferon beta-1b in MS: results of an open trial. Neurology 1996;46:552–554.

Noseworthy JH, Lucchinetti C, Rodriguez M, Weinshenker BG. Multiple sclerosis. New Engl J Med 2000;343:938–952.

Okuda B, Tanaka H, Tachibana H et al. Visual form agnosia in multiple sclerosis. Acta Neurol Scand 1996;94:38–44.

Olmos-Lau N, Ginsberg MD, Geller JB. Aphasia in multiple sclerosis. Neurology 1977;27: 623–626.

Peselow ED, Deutsch SI, Fieve RR et al. Coexistent manic symptoms and multiple sclerosis. Psychosomatics 1981;22:824–825.

Petersen RC, Kokmen E. Cognitive and psychiatric abnormalities in multiple sclerosis. Mayo Clin Proc 1989;64:657–663.

Poser CM, Paty DW, Scheinberg L et al. New diagnostic criteria for multiple sclerosis: guidelines for research protocols. Ann Neurol 1983;13:227–231.

Rabins PV, Brooks BR, O'Donnell P et al. Structural brain correlates of emotional disorder in multiple sclerosis. Brain 1986;109:585–597.

Rao SM. Neuropsychology of multiple sclerosis: a critical review. J Clin Exp Neuropsychol 1986;8:503–542.

Rao SM Leo GJ, Haughton VM et al. Correlation of magnetic resonance imaging with neuropsychological testing in multiple sclerosis. Neurology 1989;39:161–166.

Rao SM, Leo GJ, Bernardin L, Unverzagt F. Cognitive dysfunction in multiple sclerosis. I. Frequency, patterns, and prediction. Neurology 1991a;41:685–691.

Rao SM, Leo GJ, Ellington L et al. Cognitive dysfunction in multiple sclerosis. II. Impact on employment and social functioning. Neurology 1991b;41:692–696.

Ron MA, Callanan MM, Warrington EK. Cognitive abnormalities in multiple sclerosis: a psychometric and MRI study. Psychol Med 1991;21:59–68.

Sadovnik AD, Eisen K, Ebers GC, Paty DW. Cause of death in patients attending multiple sclerosis clinics. Neurology 1991;41:1193–1196.

Schiffer RB, Wineman NM. Antidepressant pharmacotherapy of depression associated with multiple sclerosis. Am J Psychiatry 1990; 147:1493–1497.

Schnider A, Benson DF, Rosner LJ. Callosal disconnection in multiple sclerosis. Neurology 1993;43:1243–1245.

Selby MJ, Ling N, Williams JM, Dawson A. Interferon beta 1-b in verbal memory functioning of patients with relapsing–remitting multiple sclerosis. Percept Motor Skills 1998;86:1099–1106.

Sperling RA, Guttmann CRG, Hohol MJ et al. Regional magnetic resonance imaging lesion burden and cognitive function in multiple sclerosis. Arch Neurol 2001;58: 115–121.

Stenager EN, Stenager E, Koch-Henrikson N et al. Suicide and multiple sclerosis: an epidemiological investigation. J Neurol Neurosurg Psychiatry 1992;55:542–545.

Surridge D. An investigation into some psychiatric aspects of multiple sclerosis. Br J Psychiatry 1969;115:749–764.

Swirsky-Sacchetti T, Mitchell DR. Seward J et al. Neuropsychological and structural brain lesions in multiple sclerosis: a regional analysis. Neurology 1992;42:1291–1295.

Sullivan MJL, Weinshenker B, Mikail S, Edgley K. Depression before and after diagnosis of multiple sclerosis. Multiple Sclerosis 1995;1:104–108.

Weinstein A, Schwid SIL, Schiffer RB et al. Neuropsychological status in multiple sclerosis after treatment with glatiramer. Arch Neurol 1999;56:319–324.

Whitlock FA, Siskind NM. Depression as a major symptom of multiple sclerosis. J Neurol Neurosurg Psychiatry 1980;43:861–865.

19

Behavioral Aspects of Epilepsy

The epilepsy itself comes on instantaneously. At this moment the face is suddenly horribly distorted, especially the eyes. Convulsions and spasms seize the whole body and the features of the face. A terrible, incredible scream, unlike anything imaginable, breaks forth; and with this cry all resemblance to a human being seems suddenly to disappear...It is actually as if someone else was screaming, inside the person.

(Dostoevsky, *The Idiot*)

The behavioral manifestations of seizures and epilepsy are increasingly important to behavioral neurology. First, epilepsy is one of the most common afflictions of mankind, affecting as many as 3% of the population (Epilepsy Foundation of America 1975; Hauser and Kurland 1975). The cumulative incidence of seizures in the population is 1.2% by age 24, 3.1% by age 74, and 4.4% by age 85 (Hauser *et al.* 1993). Second, seizures and their associated clinical phenomena are dramatic occurrences, terrifying to patients and families, fascinating and thought provoking to students of the nervous system, as Dostoevsky's description makes clear. Defined clinically, a seizure is a temporary change in function of the nervous system associated with an electrical discharge of brain cells. Normal behavior is interrupted during seizures, with rare exceptions. The higher cortical functions and behavior are altered not only during seizures, but also after and between seizures. Third, the mechanisms of the behavioral manifestations of epilepsy are of great theoretical interest. Epilepsy provides a unique opportunity to study the effects of hyperactivity of brain structures, as opposed to the effects of destructive lesions of the brain, either focal or diffuse, as in most of the other disorders discussed throughout this book.

Seizures can also be defined as surges of electrical activity in the brain, with many cells discharging in synchronized or rhythmic patterns not seen during normal brain activity (McNamara 1999). A recurring tendency to have seizures is

387

called epilepsy. The brain can be mapped electrically, by electroencephalography (EEG), either during brief periods of monitoring or over days. Specialized EEG procedures, used to increase the sensitivity for detecting epileptiform discharges, include intracranial electrodes such as 'depth electrodes' or subdural grid electrodes, placed during surgery. Brain imaging modalities such as ictal single photon emission tomography (SPECT) or PET also help to map the site of the seizure focus. Some epileptic patients undergo surgical procedures to ablate seizure foci or to disconnect areas of seizure spread. The outcome of patients undergoing ablative surgery provides another window into the functions of focal areas of the brain, and the results have shown surprising differences from information based on patients with destructive brain lesions such as strokes. Behavioral manifestations of epilepsy are active disorders, fluctuating with the occurrence of seizures, the use of medications, and simply the passage of time. These disorders exemplify the difficulty of teasing out the complex interrelationships of mind and brain.

The changes in cognition and personality associated with epilepsy are highly controversial. From ancient conceptions of possession by demons to nineteenth century ideas of epileptic insanity (Berrios 1984), and even to the present day, these disorders have been enshrouded in mystery and fear. Victims of epilepsy have been subjected to an undeserved stigma, often more difficult to bear than the disease itself. Partly as a reaction to this stigma, physicians and lay organizations have emphasized that people with epilepsy are normal and can lead normal lives. Attempts to deny the existence of personality and cognitive changes in epilepsy, however, ignore the facts and deny epileptic patients much-needed understanding and treatment.

When assessing the objective facts concerning epilepsy and behavior, the effects of acute seizures, medications, and long-term epilepsy must be distinguished. The long-term behavioral manifestations of epilepsy, generally the least understood, may relate to:

1. The cumulative effects of seizures
2. Electrical activity occurring between clinical seizures
3. Underlying brain diseases that produce both seizures and behavioral changes
4. Medication effects
5. Psychological reactions to seizures and to the presence of a chronic disease, epilepsy (Kwan and Brodie 2001).

Much of the controversy surrounding epilepsy and behavior results from differing interpretations of these factors.

CLINICAL FORMS

An epileptic seizure, simply stated, is a temporary change in behavior or of consciousness resulting from an abnormal electrical discharge of nerve cells (Lennox and Lennox 1960). The relation of the clinical phenomena to the electrical discharges is greatly aided by the electroencephalogram (EEG), a recording of surface electrical potentials from the scalp. The clinical manifestations of a seizure are divided into four stages:

1. The 'aura', a group of symptoms that are the earliest subjective manifestations of a seizure, preceding altered consciousness or abnormal motor activity
2. The 'ictus', or clinical seizure itself
3. The 'postictal' period, symptoms that follow the clinical seizures and are usually associated with slowing of the EEG
4. 'Interictal' manifestations, or symptoms occurring between seizures but related in some way to the seizure disorder.

Seizures and related manifestations are defined by subjective or objective clinical phenomena; the EEG provides confirmation only. An abnormal EEG does not automatically mean that the patient has epilepsy, and a normal interictal EEG does not exclude epilepsy (Scheuer and Pedley 1990).

Epilepsy represents a family of disorders that have in common the recurrent tendency to seizures. Children with single febrile seizures and adults with seizures resulting from such temporary metabolic disturbances as hyponatremia or alcohol withdrawal are not regarded as having epilepsy. Among epilepsies, behavioral disturbances both during and between seizures vary greatly. Table 19.1 lists a few common forms of seizures, modified and greatly abbreviated, from the classification of the International League Against Epilepsy (Commission on Classification and Terminology 1981, 1989). Note that epileptologists stress the distinction between seizures, which are single events, and epilepsy, a condition that may include multiple seizure types. Terminology referring to seizure types has evolved; a few of the more common, older clinical terms are also shown in Table 19.1. In addition to seizure types, epilepsy syndromes have been described, some of which are hereditary; discussion of these syndromes is outside of the scope of this chapter. For the purpose of this discussion, we consider only partial seizures of simple and complex varieties, partial seizures with secondary generalization, and generalized seizures of the absence and tonic-clonic types.

Table 19.1 Major forms of seizures

Partial seizures
Simple partial
Complex partial (psychomotor, temporal lobe)
Partial with secondary generalization

Generalized seizures
Absence (petit mal)
Generalized tonic–clonic (grand mal)
Myoclonic

Simple Partial Seizures

The first type of seizures, partial seizures with simple symptomatology, refers to seizures that occur in one part of the brain and do not 'generalize', or spread to other brain regions, either clinically or electroencephalographically. The symptoms must involve elementary motor, sensory, psychic, or autonomic phenomena without alteration of consciousness. Examples are focal motor seizures, e.g. clonic twitching of one thumb or hand, and focal sensory seizures, e.g. recurrent dysesthesias of the hand or face. The postictal period involves only motor or sensory deficits ('Todd's paralysis') similar to the ictal manifestations, with no cognitive changes. A high correlation exists between seizures of this type and a structural lesion in the appropriate brain region. Interictal personality changes are rare in individuals who have only this form of seizures (Blumer 1975).

Complex Partial Seizures

The complex partial form of seizures comprises those spells that are partial, in the sense that only part of the brain is involved, but that involve complex symptoms, with alteration of consciousness. Older synonyms for partial complex seizures include 'psychomotor', 'temporal lobe', and 'limbic' seizures. Many of these seizures do originate in temporal lobe structures, but others arise from frontal lobe or other sites; technically, the term 'temporal lobe epilepsy' is correct only if the seizure focus has been documented to arise in the temporal lobe. Without such documentation, the clinical term 'complex partial seizure' is more correct. The symptoms of the aura of a complex partial seizure are many and varied, often involving very peculiar and ineffable experiences. Abdominal sensations of 'something rising' are common. Sensory symptoms include olfactory, gustatory or, less commonly, auditory or visual hallucinations. Vertigo or lightheadedness may also occur. Alterations of memory, such as inappropriate feelings of familiarity (*déja vu*) or unfamiliarity (*jamais vu*), may be accompanied by dreamy states such as depersonalization and derealization, or emotions such as fear, anxiety, elation, or even sexual arousal (Blumer 1975; Schomer 1983). Many patients find it impossible to describe these behavioral states, and refer to them simply as 'funny feelings'. The ictus itself is manifested by staring and by a variety of automatic motor phenomena, or 'automatisms'. These movements prominently involve the mouth and face, with chewing, lip-smacking, and swallowing. Patients may also make stereotyped, repetitive movements of the extremities and trunk, such as picking repetitively at the bedclothes. Speech arrest is frequently associated with partial complex seizures, but occasionally repetitive utterances and even aphasic speech may occur (Lecours and Joanette 1980; Gilmore and Heilman 1981; Kirshner *et al.* 1996). The postictal period is characterized by mild confusion and somnolence; many patients fall asleep after the episode. Some patients appear to be awake throughout the seizure, but often only partial awareness is present, and most patients are amnestic for at least the ictal period. Occasionally more prolonged dreamy states continue, as in the fugue states or prolonged confusional episodes of 'complex partial status epilepticus'. These patients may stare, perform automatic motor acts, smack their lips, and intermittently even respond verbally (Goldensohn and Gold 1960; Markand *et al.* 1978; Mayeux and Luders 1978). Prolonged episodes of aphasia secondary to partial complex status have been described (Racy *et al.* 1980; Kirshner *et al.* 1996). The diagnosis of such seizure-related states is difficult, especially if a history of epileptic seizures is not available. An EEG taken during such a period reveals diagnostic seizure discharges, and a small dose of intravenous diazepam or lorazepam may temporarily restore the patient to lucidity. Prolonged ictal or postictal episodes of aimless wandering, with amnesia for the episodes, have been called 'poriomania' (Mayeux *et al.* 1979). These prolonged manifestations of complex partial seizures may bear a close resemblance to psychogenic fugue states, or hysterical dissociative reactions. With such predominantly psychic manifestations accompanying complex partial seizures, it should not be surprising that long-term behavioral effects have been most commonly recognized in this variety of seizures.

The interictal EEG in patients with complex partial seizures may be entirely normal, or it may show interictal spike or slow wave discharges. These discharges are most common in the temporal lobe leads and are best seen during light sleep. Like simple partial seizures, complex partial seizures are often associated with focal lesions, in this case in the deep temporal and orbital frontal regions. When complex partial seizures begin during childhood, a common pathological correlate is 'mesial temporal sclerosis', or scarring of the limbic areas of the deep temporal lobes secondary to anoxia either at birth or during seizures. When complex partial seizures begin during adult life, other structural lesions become more likely. These include tumors, hamartomas, vascular malformations, scars from head injuries, and cerebral infarcts (Blumer 1975).

Partial Seizures with Secondary Generalization

A partial seizure of either the simple or complex type may spread over the brain to produce a generalized, tonic-clonic seizure. Unless the focal onset of such a seizure is witnessed, there may be no clinical evidence to suggest partial epilepsy. The patient is frequently amnestic for the partial seizure at the onset, and only the sequelae of the generalized seizure may be detected. Focal abnormalities in the interictal EEG may be helpful, but such findings may be absent. At least part of the controversy surrounding the association of behavioral changes with complex partial as opposed to generalized tonic-clonic seizures may result from the failure to diagnose the focal or partial origin of these secondarily generalized seizures.

Absence Seizures

Absence seizures, also called 'petit mal', typically begin in children aged 5–10 years, with occasional persistence into adult life. Clinically, the absence seizure consists of a brief staring spell, beginning and ending abruptly, lasting only a few seconds, and generally associated with no aura and no postictal state.

Briefer spells may involve simply staring or a lapse of consciousness, and longer episodes may be accompanied by lip-smacking, chewing, blinking, and partial loss of postural tone (Penry *et al.* 1975). Clinical distinction between absence seizures and complex partial seizures may thus be difficult. Very occasionally, prolonged episodes of 'absence status' resemble complex partial status epilepticus, with prolonged staring behavior and intermittent failure to respond to stimuli (D'Agostino *et al.* 1999). The EEG in absence seizures shows characteristic generalized, three-per-second spike and wave discharges brought out by hyperventilation. These spells occur frequently, often with multiple episodes during one routine EEG. These discharges are quite different from the EEG findings of complex partial seizures. Most cases of absence epilepsy have no identifiable structural brain abnormality, and many appear to be hereditary. Long-term behavioral consequences are probably not seen unless other neurological disease is present or other types of seizures develop.

Generalized Tonic-Clonic Seizures

Tonic-clonic seizures are convulsions, or generalized, tonic-clonic, 'grand mal' seizures. These dramatic occurrences are what the general public generally thinks of as epileptic seizures. Several distinct patterns exist, but the most common sequence of events is a 'tonic' phase, with apnea, a 'cry' (or inspiration through a partially closed glottis), and stiffening of the extremities, followed by a 'clonic' phase, with repetitive jerking of the extremities. Tongue-biting, foaming at the mouth, and urinary incontinence frequently accompany these seizures, and a postictal phase of drowsiness, confusion, and headache typically follows. The presence of an aura or a focal postictal deficit ('Todd's paralysis') suggests a partial epileptic focus with secondary generalization. The interictal EEG in patients with primary, generalized tonic-clonic seizures may be normal or may show brief spike- and wave discharges; in cases of secondarily generalized seizures, focal abnormalities may be seen. Tonic-clonic seizures may be hereditary; may result from metabolic disturbances such as uremia, alcohol withdrawal, and hyponatremia; or may be associated with focal lesions, in the case of partial seizures with secondary generalization.

LONG-TERM BEHAVIORAL EFFECTS OF EPILEPSY

Since the work of Gibbs (1951), Pond and Bidwell (1959) and others, neurologists have had the general impression that people with epilepsy, particularly those with complex partial seizures, are at increased risk for the development of psychopathology. Epidemiological surveys of psychopathology in epilepsy have tended to confirm this impression (Gudmundsson 1966; Trimble 1983; Hermann and Whitman 1984), and follow-up studies of children with epilepsy have found a high incidence of personality changes and psychiatric disorders during maturation (Lindsay *et al.* 1979; Hoare 1984).

The psychopathological consequences of epilepsy may be divided into four areas:

1. Personality changes
2. Psychoses
3. Affective disorders
4. Violence.

In each of these areas, the relationship of behavioral changes to epilepsy must be considered in terms of the type and site of seizures, the presence of underlying neuropathology, the use of medications, and the psychosocial consequences of seizures and epilepsy.

Personality Changes

Subtle alterations in personality are probably the most common long-term behavioral effects of epilepsy, though documentation and characterization of these changes have been difficult and controversial. Personality traits should not be considered either normal or abnormal, referring simply to trends or patterns in cognitive and emotional functions that characterize a given individual over extended periods of time. Waxman and Geschwind (1976), in case studies, described a series of personality traits that appeared to be associated with complex partial seizures in some patients. These traits included: (1) preoccupation with philosophical and religious concerns; (2) increased writing or diary keeping ('hypergraphia'); (3) decreased or altered sexual interests; and (4) aggressiveness. The preoccupation with philosophical and religious concerns may take the form of exploration of the meaning of life, either through traditional religions or other transcendental philosophies. These patients seem humorless, viewing their lives as entirely devoted to the service of a greater purpose, beyond their own control. Minor, routine personal or public events take on added significance. Dewhurst and Beard (1970) reported frequent religious conversions in patients with complex partial seizures. On the other hand, Tucker and colleagues (1987) failed to confirm a greater religiosity in 76 temporal lobe epileptics as compared to 31 patients with primary generalized epilepsy and 27 patients with pseudoepileptic seizures. Religious preoccupation is common in psychoses of numerous types and etiologies (Brewerton 1994).

The second trait, hypergraphia, is typified by the epileptic patient who presents his or her physician with long, handwritten lists of seizures and other symptoms, often meticulous, ritualistic, and interposed with elaborate interpretations. These writings may include religious or sexual themes, and may take the form of diaries or even original poetry (Waxman and Geschwind 1976; Roberts *et al.* 1982). In one study, hypergraphia appeared to correlate with right temporal EEG foci (Roberts *et al.* 1982). Okamura and colleagues found that hypergraphia in epileptics correlated with prior history of psychiatric symptoms and with abnormalities on CT scans, but not with the side of the epileptic focus. These authors considered hypergraphia to represent a deepening of emotions associated with the seizure phenomena, and possibly with organic lesions in the temporal lobe (Okamura *et al.* 1993).

The third personality trait, altered sexual behavior, usually comprises a global reduction in sexual interest activity, or hyposexuality (Blumer and Walker 1967; Shukla *et al.* 1979). This interictal hyposexuality is in contradistinction to the ictal undressing behavior (Hooshmand and Brawley 1969) and postictal sexual arousal (Blumer 1970) occasionally seen in relation to complex partial seizures. Much less common than hyposexuality are cases of deviant sexual behavior, e.g. homosexuality or fetishism, in patients with complex partial seizures (Mitchell *et al.* 1954; Blumer 1975). Interestingly, these alterations in sexuality are sometimes reversed by treatment of seizures or by temporal lobectomy (Mitchell *et al.* 1954; Blumer and Walker 1967; Blumer 1975).

The fourth character trait, aggressiveness, is discussed later in this chapter with respect to the problem of violence and epilepsy.

A large number of systematic analyses of personality traits in patients with seizure disorders, compared to various control groups, have been published. In general, personality studies using the standard Minnesota Multiphasic Personality Inventory (MMPI) have shown slight if any differences in overall personality ratings (Stevens 1975; Hermann and Whitman 1984; Reynolds 1983a; Trimble 1983; Whitman *et al.* 1984) among patients with complex partial seizures, all epileptic patients, and patients with various other chronic illnesses. These studies have not lent support to the concept of an 'epileptic personality'.

Other investigators have abandoned the MMPI in favor of personality inventories specifically devised to assess the characteristics described in patients with long-term complex partial or temporal lobe epilepsy. In a landmark but much criticized study of personality and epilepsy, Bear and Fedio (1977) presented questionnaires reflecting 18 personality traits to normals, patients with complex partial seizures, and patients with other neuromuscular disorders. The traits were rated by the patients themselves and also by spouses, family members, or friends. All 18 traits, listed in Table 19.2, distinguished the patients with epilepsy from the two control groups.

Table 19.2 Personality traits of the Bear–Fedio personal inventory and personal behavioral survey (Bear and Fedio 1977)

Humorlessness	Dependence
Circumstantiality	Personal destiny
Obsessionalism	Viscosity
Emotionality	Guilt
Philosophical interest	Anger
Religiosity	Hypermoralism
Paranoia	Sadness
Hyperg raphia	Elation
Aggression	Altered sexuality

The traits of humorlessness, dependence, sense of personal destiny, philosophical interest, religiosity, and hypermoralism all relate to the philosophical and religious concerns discussed previously by Waxman and Geschwind (1976). Dependence, as a personality trait, refers to the related feelings of passivity, helplessness, or being at the mercy of a predetermined fate. Circumstantiality, viscosity, obsessionalism, and hypergraphia relate to the tendency of these patients to stick obsessively to a topic of conversation or of writing, giving detailed and repetitive descriptions of their experiences. These traits make history taking from these patients a prolonged and frustrating task.

Altered sexuality as a feature of temporal lobe or complex partial epilepsy has already been discussed. Paranoia is related to the sense of personal destiny experienced by these patients, but is best seen in the psychoses associated with complex partial epilepsy, to be discussed later. The affective traits of emotionality, guilt, anger, sadness, elation, and aggression relate to the mood changes and violent behavior associated with epilepsy, also discussed later.

Some traits in the Bear and Fedio study appeared to distinguish patients with left from right temporal lobe EEG foci. Patients with right temporal lobe foci ranked highest on the characteristics of emotionality, sadness, and elation, as well as on viscosity and hypermoralism. Patients with left temporal foci scored higher on the ruminative, intellectual qualities of religiosity, philosophical interest, and sense of personal destiny.

The 18 personality traits did not appear to correlate with seizure frequency, but the duration of epilepsy did seem important. The authors postulated that repeated activation of limbic structures by a temporal lobe focus produces enhanced emotional reactions to stimuli that would normally be affectively neutral. In the authors' words, 'experiencing objects and events shot through with affective coloration engenders a mystically religious world view;...the result is an augmented sense of personal destiny'. Bear (1979) later termed this limbic activation a 'hyperconnection' of sensory inputs to the limbic system, in contradistinction to the 'disconnection' syndromes caused by destructive brain lesions.

The Bear-Fedio study has met with several criticisms of its methodology and interpretations. Perhaps the most important limitation is the selection of two control groups not characterized by behavioral disturbances. Mungas (1982) and Rodin and Schmaltz (1984) applied the Bear-Fedio questionnaires to patients with psychiatric symptoms secondary to neurological or primary psychiatric diseases and found high scores on the 18 personality traits, similar to or greater than those of patients with complex partial seizures. These authors suggested that the character traits are associated with psychopathology of any etiology and are not specific for complex partial epilepsy.

A second objection to the Bear–Fedio analysis has been the absence of control groups with other types of epilepsy. Rodin and Schmaltz (1984) found only minor differences between epileptic patients with temporal lobe EEG foci and those with only generalized spike-wave discharges. Hermann and Riel (1981) found differences between patients with complex partial epilepsy and primary generalized epilepsy in only four traits: sense of personal destiny, dependence, paranoia, and philosophical interest. Another study by the same group also found that hypergraphia distinguished patients with complex partial seizures from other epileptic patients (Hermann *et al.* 1983). As mentioned earlier, Tucker *et al.* (1987) did not find a greater incidence of hyperreligiosity in patients with temporal lobe epilepsy as compared with those with primary generalized epilepsy or even those with pseudoepileptic seizures, nor did they find a difference in religiosity between complex partial seizure patients with left or right foci. Hyperreligiosity is also a frequent manifestation of psychoses in general, not just those associated with epilepsy (Brewerton 1994).

Other objections to the Bear-Fedio study have included the lack of close control for possible medication effects or underlying neuropathology, which could produce psychopathology independent of seizures. Patients with complex partial or temporal lobe epilepsy often have poorly controlled seizures over periods of years, requiring numerous medications and possibly taking a greater toll on psychological well-being than other types of epilepsy. Hermann and Whitman (1984) raised the more fundamental issue of validity with regard to the personality inventories themselves; the relationship of personality trait scores to behavior outside the artificial test setting has not been systematically explored. Bear and colleagues (1982) attempted to answer some of these criticisms with a study of psychiatric inpatients with complex partial seizures, other types of epilepsy, character disorders, affective disease, and schizophrenia. In this study, 14 personality traits were assessed by means of a coded interview technique. In comparison to the combined groups with primary psychiatric disorders, the patients with complex partial seizures scored higher on viscosity, circumstantiality, religiosity, philosophical interests, humorlessness, paranoia, and hypermoralism. Compared to other epileptics, patients with complex partial seizures scored higher on religiosity, philosophical interests, sadness, and emotionality. Although these differences are impressive, Rodin and Schmaltz (1984) pointed out that no single trait or group of traits was specific or pathognomonic for patients with complex partial seizures.

In conclusion, considerable evidence suggests that long-term complex partial seizures are associated with alterations in personality. These personality traits involve thought processes (philosophical interests, religiosity, sense of personal destiny), emotion (anger, sadness, elation), external behavior (viscosity, obsessiveness, circumstantiality), and sexuality. These personality traits, however, may develop only over years of seizures and only in a minority of patients. Many of the same traits are seen in patients with other chronic illnesses, either medical or psychiatric (Hermann and Whitman 1984). In individual cases, consideration must be given to underlying brain lesions such as tumors, medication effects, and prolonged stress, any of which may predispose to changes in personality. The intriguing possibility remains, however, that either the peculiar ictal experiences of complex partial seizures or the electrical effects of interictal spike activity in limbic structures produce unique, long-term changes in brain physiology, which in turn lead to changes in personality and behavior.

Psychosis and Epilepsy

Although overt psychosis occurs less commonly than subtle changes in personality in epileptic patients, these more dramatic behavioral manifestations have attracted great attention. The British psychiatrist Eliot Slater and colleagues (1963) established an association between paranoid psychosis and epilepsy in a study of 69 patients, more than the authors could have expected to encounter by a chance association of the two conditions. Most cases of psychosis and epilepsy had complex partial seizures, with the psychosis beginning an average of 14.1 years after the onset of seizures. There appeared to be no relationship between seizure frequency and psychosis; in fact, several patients developed psychosis after periods of reduced frequency or total cessation of seizures. This phenomenon of increased thought disorder occurring with reduced seizure frequency is related to a decrease in EEG abnormalities, referred to as 'forced normalization' of the EEG (Pakalnis *et al.* 1987; Krishnamoorthy and Trimble 1999). The association between psychosis and epilepsy has been controversial, but a recent epidemiological survey (Mendez *et al.* 1993a) found that only 1% of migraine patients had psychosis, in contrast with a 9% incidence in an age-matched group of epileptic patients.

In many cases reported by Slater and colleagues (1963), chronic psychosis appeared after a long history of epileptic confusional states or as a 'culmination' of personality traits of suspiciousness obsessionalism, and depression. Auditory hallucinations were common, as were delusional systems with mystical or religious themes, ideas of persecution, or attachment of special significance to common events. Many patients claimed special powers to communicate with God, influence the thought or actions of others, or foretell the future. Many patients manifested a thought disorder characterized by circumstantiality, perseverative thought, concreteness, and illogical associations. Depression, irritability, and aggressiveness typified the affective states of these patients, rather than the 'flat' affect of schizophrenia. In follow-up studies, the acute psychoses tended to resolve, but many patients remained disabled by chronic mood disorders, obsessiveness, and suspiciousness.

In general, the epileptic psychoses described by Slater and colleagues resembled schizophrenia, but several features distinguished this group from typical, idiopathic schizophrenia:

1. Absence of a family history of schizophrenia
2. A premorbid personality structure that was either normal or associated with 'epileptic' but not 'schizoid' personality traits
3. Later age of onset
4. History of seizures
5. Preservation of affective responsiveness and ability to maintain close, personal relationships with family members or friends
6. A tendency toward paranoid, mystical, and religious content to the hallucinations and delusions.

When considering the pathogenesis of the psychoses of epilepsy, Slater and colleagues discussed a psychological theory, in which repeated mystical clouded states of consciousness become integrated into the patient's psychic life and personality, and a physiological theory, in which abnormal activity in the temporal lobes produces both the seizures and the psychosis. These authors favored the second explanation, which resembles Bear's (1979) later concept of' 'limbic hyperconnectivity'. They also speculated that other psychotic states, such as amphetamine psychosis and schizophrenia, might also reflect abnormal functioning of the temporal lobes. Stevens (1988) also amplified this theory in terms of 'microseizures', or electrical hyperactivity occurring in limbic structures, as the basis of the psychosis associated with complex partial seizures. 'Kindling' of epileptic pathways may also be involved in the pathogenesis of psychosis in epileptic patients (Smith and Darlington 1996).

Other studies have confirmed an association between psychosis and complex partial seizures (Flor-Henry 1969, 1983; Kristensen and Sindrup 1979; Lindsay et al. 1979; Perez and Trimble 1980; Pritchard et al. 1980; Parnas and Korsgaard 1982; Sherwin et al. 1982; Sachdev 1998; Adachi et al. 2000a); temporal lobe foci are usually seen in epileptic patients with psychosis, but Adachi and colleagues (Adachi et al. 2000b) reported that frontal lobe epilepsy was also associated with both interictal and postictal psychoses, though less commonly in their series than in patients with temporal lobe foci.

Postictal psychoses are likely more common than interictal psychoses. In one study (Kanemoto et al. 1996), these psychoses were characterized by grandiose and religious delusions, elevated moods, and feelings of mystic fusion of the body with the universe. These positive experiences were not as often seen in interictal psychoses. In addition, the schizophreniform psychotic traits, such as hallucinations of voices and chronic paranoid delusions, were less often seen in postictal than interictal psychoses.

The prevalence of psychosis in patients with long-term complex partial seizures approximates 10–15% (Lindsay et al. 1979; Pritchard et al. 1980; Sherwin et al. 1982), whereas overall psychopathology may occur two to three times as frequently (Pritchard et al. 1980). Whitman and colleagues (1984) failed to find any correlation of overall psychopathology or personality disorder with complex partial seizures, but even in this series psychosis did occur more frequently in patients with complex partial seizures than in other patients with chronic neurological diseases. Hence although psychosis is less frequent than alterations of personality and affect in epilepsy, the specific association of psychosis to complex partial seizures is more definite. Adachi et al. (2000a) reported the following correlations with interictal psychosis: family history of psychosis; early age of onset of seizures; complex partial or generalized, tonic-clonic seizures, and borderline intelligence. In Sachdev's 1998 review of psychosis and epilepsy, risk factors for psychosis included severe or intractable epilepsy, early onset of seizures, secondary generalization of seizures, use of specific drugs, and temporal lobectomy.

The general features of the psychosis have remained much as Slater and colleagues (1967) described them: late onset psychosis developing years after the onset of seizures, characterized by paranoid delusions and auditory hallucinations, associated with deepening rather than flattening of affective states and preservation of the ability to relate to other people (Kristensen and Sindrup 1979; Perez and Trimble 1980; Parnas and Korsgaard 1982; Sherwin *et al.* 1982; Toone *et al.* 1982; Sachdev 1998).

Other studies have confirmed the trend for psychosis to develop at times of decreased seizure frequency (Flor-Henry 1969) or reduced interictal EEG abnormality ('forced normalization of the EEG'; Flor-Henry 1983; Pakalnis *et al.* 1987; Krishnamoorthy and Trimble 1999). Studies of the lateralization of the EEG focus have suggested that the typical paranoid psychosis is more frequent in patients with left temporal foci (Flor-Henry 1969, 1983; Parnas and Korsgaard 1982; Sherwin *et al.* 1982), whereas affective disturbances are more often associated with right temporal foci (Flor-Henry 1969, 1983). Affective changes are common in patients with complex partial seizures (see the next section), but the common, traditional affective psychoses such as depressive psychosis or manic-depressive disorder are uncommon (Toone *et al.* 1982).

The pathogenesis of psychosis in patients with complex partial seizures has remained controversial. As discussed earlier in this chapter, psychopathology in epilepsy could relate to:

1. Seizures themselves
2. Interictal electrical activity
3. Underlying brain lesions
4. Medication effects
5. Psychological reactions to having seizures or epilepsy.

Seizures are unlikely to be a direct cause of psychosis, since in some series psychosis has had an inverse correlation to seizure frequency (Slater *et al.* 1963; Flor-Henry 1969). Seizures may even act in a manner similar to electroconvulsive therapy in relieving psychosis. Interictal electrical activity, as suggested by the theories of Bear and Fedio (1977) and Slater and colleagues (1963), may be related to psychosis by way of enhanced activity of limbic system connections. The occasional occurrence of psychosis in patients with tumors of the temporal lobes and limbic areas suggests that brain lesions involving these areas, even without seizures, may lead to psychosis (Malamud 1967). Lesions in limbic areas of the brain may repetitively activate circuits involved in emotion and related functions and may thereby engender long-term psychiatric changes in a manner similar to that of the interictal spike activity in temporal lobe epilepsy. Even surgical removal of the brain lesion may leave the psychosis relatively unchanged (Falconer 1973). The two factors of pathological lesions of the limbic system and interictal activation of these same structures thus appear intertwined and impossible to separate as causes of psychosis.

The last two factors cited as possible causes of psychosis in patients with epilepsy are medication effects and psychological reactions. Medications such as anticholinergic agents and psychedelic drugs can cause confusion and psychosis, and it is possible that even antiepileptic medications can contribute to psychosis. Psychological reactions to the strange experiences of seizures may also play a role in the pathogenesis of chronic personality changes and even psychosis. Attention to these factors, as well as to the seizures themselves, is therefore important in the treatment of individual patients. We shall return to these issues in the section on treatment at the end of this chapter.

Depression and Epilepsy

Patients with epilepsy have a high incidence of affective disorders, especially depression (Dominian *et al.* 1963; Robertson and Trimble 1983; Kanner and Nieto 1999; Lambert and Robertson 1999). Personality inventories such as the MMPI (Rodin *et al.* 1976; Robertson and Trimble 1983) and the Bear–Fedio questionnaire (Bear and Fedio 1977) have yielded elevated depression scores. Depression is one of the most important behavioral concomitants of epilepsy in terms of effect on the quality of life of the individual, potential for serious consequences such as suicide, and availability of treatment. Deaths by suicide occur more frequently than would be predicted by chance in epileptic patients (Hawton *et al.* 1980; Barraclough 1981; Matthews and Barabas 1981). Depression seems common in epilepsy generally, without a specific association to any single type of epilepsy (Perez and Trimble 1980; Robertson and Trimble 1983), but patients with complex partial seizures may be at especially high risk of suicide (Barraclough 1981). Although depression as a character trait or neurosis is common in epilepsy, depressive psychosis and bipolar affective disorder or mania are distinctly uncommon (Toone *et al.* 1982; Robertson and Trimble 1983).

As discussed with reference to both personality changes and psychosis, the laterality of a temporal lobe focus of epilepsy may influence the behavioral changes that emerge. Personality traits related to emotionality and depression appear more common in patients with right temporal foci, whereas patients with left temporal foci are more likely to develop personality traits of religiosity and sense of personal destiny (Bear and Fedio 1977), as well as paranoid psychoses (Flor-Henry 1969, 1983; Sherwin *et al.* 1982). These affective accompaniments of complex partial seizures are opposite to those of destructive brain lesions; patients with left hemisphere strokes and aphasia are more likely to manifest depression, whereas those with right hemisphere strokes frequently seem unconcerned or even euphoric (see Chapters 4, 7, and 16). These differences between epilepsy and stroke are consistent with the concept of epileptogenic lesions as manifesting increases in function or metabolic activity in a brain region, whereas strokes and other destructive lesions manifest decreases in activity. Not all studies of depression and epilepsy, however, have agreed on a laterality effect. Robertson and Trimble (1983) found no correlation between depression and side of focus, and Perini and Mendius (1984) reported self-ratings of depression more commonly in patients with left than right temporal EEG foci.

The entire concept of epileptic foci as hyperactive as contrasted to the hypoactivity of structural lesions may be an oversimplification. Perini and Mendius (1984) pointed out that epileptigenic lesions are not always 'overactive'; in fact, studies of brain metabolic activity by positron emission tomography

(PET) with labeled deoxyglucose (Engle *et al.* 1982) have shown that many epileptogenic lesions are actually hypometabolic, suggesting that epileptic foci act like 'destructive' lesions, at least interictally. In addition, as noted by Bear and Fedio (1977), patients with left temporal lobe foci tend to over-report their own state of depression or their own limitations; they tend to 'tarnish' their self-images.

The subject of depression and epilepsy has been less studied than the topics of personality changes or psychosis in epileptic patients, and perhaps there is even less agreement in the area of depression. The pathogenesis of depression in epileptic patients is likely multifactorial. In addition to the biological effects of brain lesions and of interictal electrical activity in limbic structures, 'reactive' depression undoubtedly plays some role. Seizures themselves are frightening and embarrassing, and patients with epilepsy have difficulty finding employment, maintaining the right to drive a motor vehicle, and being treated as normal persons. These stressors lead to a loss of dignity and self-esteem, and take a cumulative emotional toll on persons with epilepsy (Robertson and Trimble 1983). Drug effects, especially those of the older, sedative drugs such as barbiturates, probably also contribute to depression (Reynolds 1983b; Robertson *et al.* 1987). The mood states of patients with epilepsy are thus much more complex than can be predicted by biological factors such as side or site of epileptic focus.

Aggression and Epilepsy

Aggressive or violent behavior among epileptic patients has generated considerably more attention than the other behavioral effects of epilepsy, more than seems justified by the rare occurrence of violent acts in this population. Historically, epileptic patients were thought to have violent behavior after seizures. Charcot (Goetz 1987) said in one of his 'Tuesday lectures': 'An individual has a fit and in the aftermath, in the midst of postictal nightmares, becomes violent and breaks everything about him...These epileptics can kill people, even commit suicide'. Public fear has been aroused by publicity surrounding the use of epilepsy as a defense in cases involving criminal acts, sometimes including senseless violence or murder. In the aftermath of such publicity, studies of incarcerated prisoners have revealed an increased prevalence of clinical epilepsy and of abnormal EEGs compared to normal populations (Gunn and Fenton 1971; King and Young 1978). These reports have kindled public fear of persons with epilepsy. Analysis of the facts is thus essential. Specific, objective studies analyzing the relationship of violent behavior to epilepsy have been relatively few.

As with the personality changes, psychoses, and affective disorders associated with epilepsy, a distinction must first be made between ictal behavior and long-term interictal tendencies. Several reports of ictal violence have appeared. Pincus (1980) noted symptoms suggestive of complex partial seizures in juvenile delinquents with a history of violent behavior; these included memory lapses, dreamy states, hallucinations, and drowsiness after the event. Mark and Ervin (1970) recorded seizure discharges from depth electrodes in the temporal lobes during ictal violent behavior, sometimes even in patients whose surface EEGs failed to detect the discharge. These studies, combined with the population studies of prisoners suggesting a high incidence of epilepsy, have fueled a fear of epileptics.

In one of the best-documented reports, Ashford and colleagues (1980) described a 29-year-old epileptic male whose seizures, recorded on videotape, repetitively involved aggressive behavior. The patient screamed, appeared frightened, and then committed primitive, violent acts such as pulling drapes, flailing with his arms, striking bedrails, and kicking objects in his path. Similar ictal outbursts have been described by Saint-Hilaire and associates (1981) and Delgado-Escueta and colleagues (1981).

Delgado-Escueta and an international panel of epilepsy experts (1981) convened to review videotapes of violent, ictal behavior culled from epilepsy centers around the world. Ictal violence was extremely rare and typically involved non-directed, stereotyped aggressive movements. Violence to property was much more common than violence to persons, except when the patient was restrained or held down by others during a seizure. Most episodes were associated with partial complex seizures, usually involving focal temporal lobe spike activity. Aggressive behavior typically lasted less than 1 minute during a seizure similar to others experienced by the same patient. Amnesia was present for the aggressive acts in all cases. Most importantly, these stereotyped automatisms never involved the sort of consecutive, purposeful movements required to accomplish criminal acts such as murder, manslaughter, or robbery. The authors also stressed that none of the acts involved weapons, though access to weapons in the EEG/video-monitoring laboratory would have been difficult. As noted by Pincus (1981), however, such videotape studies do not absolutely exclude the possibility that an epileptic patient could commit an assault on another person or use a deadly weapon if the right combination of circumstances came together during a seizure. Subsequent studies have largely confirmed the findings of Delgado-Escueta and colleagues. Patients with partial complex seizures should be treated with caution and not forcibly restrained during the seizure itself or during the postictal confusional period. The evidence suggests, however, that acts of criminal violence are exceedingly rare in patients with epilepsy, and that ictal violence can rarely if ever be the true explanation of a complex criminal act. Legal testimony regarding patients who allegedly committed violent offenses while in the midst of a seizure is discussed by Treiman (1999).

Recent studies have documented the occasional occurrence of a violent outburst during the postictal period, as described in the quotation cited earlier by Charcot. In the series of Mendez and colleagues (1993b, 1998), these outbursts correlated better with the presence of a postictal psychosis than with the type or frequency of seizures, date of onset of epilepsy, or EEG findings. Kanemoto and colleagues (1999) also found a close correlation between both violent outbursts and suicide attempts and the presence of postictal psychosis. Borum and Appelbaum (1996) also reported on a patient who committed violent actions during the postictal state.

The differential diagnosis of ictal violence includes alcoholic blackouts, hysterical dissociative states, malingering, and the 'episodic dyscontrol syndrome'. Alcoholic blackouts are especially likely in persons accused of criminal acts, who claim no memory of the event. As mentioned in Chapter 10, amnesia for a period of alcoholic inebriation is quite common in alcoholic patients (Goodwin *et al.* 1969). Psychogenic causes of violent acts with loss of memory for the event include hysterical dissociative states, or 'fugues', voluntary violent acts with repression of the conscious memory for the events, and outright malingering, or feigning of amnesia. The distinction of these syndromes of psychogenic amnesia is the province of forensic psychiatry.

A last consideration in the differential diagnosis of ictal violence is the 'episodic dyscontrol syndrome', an entity that raises fundamental questions concerning the behavioral neurology of violence and aggression in general. 'Episodic dyscontrol' refers to episodes of violent behavior, often directed against family members or friends and frequently occurring without much provocation. The episodes are brief, lasting from minutes to a few hours. Some are heralded by an 'aura' of anxiety, fear of losing control, or occasionally nausea or paresthesias. After these events, the patient may have symptoms of headache, exhaustion, or need for sleep. Many patients claim amnesia for the episode. They typically show great remorse for their actions. Many such patients have a history of violent acts including arrests, imprisonment, divorce, and firings from jobs (Bach-Y-Rita *et al.* 1971; Maletsky 1973).

Although the characteristics of episodes of 'episodic dyscontrol' are reminiscent of partial complex seizures, only a minority of individuals with this disorder have definite evidence of epilepsy. A larger number have other evidence of pre-existing brain damage, such as a history of hyperactivity during childhood, head injuries with loss of consciousness, prior seizures, or a family history of epilepsy. 'Soft' neurological signs are common in these patients (Bach-Y-Rita *et al.* 1971; Maletsky 1973). Environmental or psychological factors, however, also seem important. Episodes often occur in normally dependent males who are placed in a situation of stress, with feelings of inability to control the situation. The violent behavior then occurs in the context of a 'breakdown' or disorganization of thought processes (Maletsky 1973). Both a background of organic brain dysfunction and environmental factors may thus be involved in the poor impulse control seen in this syndrome (Maletsky 1973; Leicester 1982).

Despite the lack of a clear association with epilepsy in the episodic dyscontrol syndrome, anticonvulsant therapy has been found helpful in preventing violent outbursts in some cases (Maletsky 1973). The drug carbamazepine (Tegretol) has seemed especially helpful (Tunks and Dermer 1977). Currently, several new antiepileptic drugs are being tested in psychiatric syndromes such as bipolar affective disorder and patients with poor impulse control.

The neurological basis of ictal violence presumably lies in the limbic structures responsible for partial complex seizures. Abundant evidence from experimental animals indicates that stimulation of the hypothalmus and related limbic areas, including the fornix, preoptic region, or amygdala, can induce 'rage' reactions (Goldstein 1974). Tumors of the hypothalamus and deep, temporal lobe limbic areas have been associated with violent behavior in human patients (Alpers 1937; Malamud 1967). Based on the animal and human experience, surgical procedures such as amygdalectomy have been advocated for patients with violent behavior (Mark and Ervin 1970). At present, however, the entire concept of 'psychosurgery', or ablation of brain structures to alter behavior, is highly controversial. Temporal lobectomy is generally reserved for removal of pathological tissue, such as tumors or arteriovenous malformations, and for control of intractable seizures.

Interictal violence in patients with epilepsy is an entirely different subject from violence associated with the ictal or immediate postictal period. Anger and aggression are two of the traits associated with temporal lobe epilepsy in the Bear and Fedio (1977) study. Descriptions of the 'temporal lobe' personality have noted irritability, temper outbursts, and rage, often alternating with a friendlier, good-natured demeanor (Blumer 1975). Interictal violent outbursts in these patients are usually more verbal than physical, directed typically against family members or friends. Some provocation, albeit trivial, is usually present, and there is no amnesia for the outburst. The patient remembers the event, is remorseful afterward, and is usually forgiven. This aspect of complex partial seizures does not usually lead to criminal cases. All of these characteristics distinguish interictal violence in epilepsy from the unprovoked, primitive physical actions carried out during seizures, with amnesia for the events. Irritability, anger, and aggressive outbursts can be seen as a reflection of the deepening of emotions and the humorlessness described in patients with complex partial seizures (Bear and Fedio 1977; Blumer and Benson 1982).

TREATMENT ISSUES
Antiepileptic Medications

The management of patients with epilepsy and behavioral alterations is a challenging task. The foremost fact to be kept in mind is that most epileptic patients can and do adjust to their illness and lead relatively normal lives. The first task of the physician is to control the seizures as completely as possible with anticonvulsant medications, avoiding at the same time the toxic effects of excessive medication. Lennox (1942) first brought attention to the cognitive effects of antiepileptic drugs: 'many physicians, in attempting to extinguish seizures, only succeed in drowning the finer intellectual processes of their patients'. In recent years the depressant effects of the barbiturates, e.g. phenobarbital and primidone (Mysoline), have been increasingly recognized (Reynolds 1983b). Phenytoin (Dilantin) is less sedating, and carbamazepine (Tegretol) appears even less so in long-term use. There is evidence, however, that even these drugs produce some cognitive impairment. Dikmen et al. (1991) studied 244 head injury patients randomized to phenytoin or placebo; they found that phenytoin slowed cognitive functions, and removal of phenytoin was associated with more rapid improvement. Pullianen and Jokelainen (1994) compared newly diagnosed epileptic patients treated with either phenytoin or carbamazepine and found more cognitive slowing with phenytoin. Dodrill and Troupin (1977) initially reported similar findings, but in 1991 (Dodrill and Troupin, 1991) they reported that if patients with elevated phenytoin levels were excluded, the differences largely disappeared. Meador and colleagues also reported a detailed neuropsychological study of 15 patients with complex partial seizures treated for 3 months with carbamazepine, phenobarbital, and phenytoin. With drugs used in therapeutic amounts, differences among the three drugs were minor, though phenobarbital was the most sedating and produced the most cognitive slowing.

Carbamazepine, its newer cousin oxcarbazepine (Trileptal), and valproic acid (Depakote) are popular in the management of both partial complex and generalized, tonic–clonic seizures (Brodie and Dichter 1996). In general these drugs are about equally effective in controlling seizures, and the differences have more to do with side effects.

Multiple drug regimens ('polypharmacy') are especially likely to take a toll on mental efficiency without appreciably improving the level of seizure control. In the 1980s, epilepsy experts (Lesser *et al.* 1984) and manufacturers of newer antiepileptic drugs recommended 'monotherapy' whenever possible. Several studies reported improvement in cognitive functions when patients were switched from polytherapy to monotherapy regimens (Shorvon and Reynolds 1979; Thompson and Trimble 1982; Prevey *et al.* 1989). When possible, patients should be managed on one antiepileptic drug; when one drug fails, it should be withdrawn and another single drug added (Scheuer and Pedley 1990; Devinsky 1999). Only when multiple drugs have failed are combinations recommended. This recommendation has changed somewhat in the last few years, however, with the introduction of several new antiepileptic drugs that are effective in reducing seizure frequency without major side effects; some of these drugs are not approved for monotherapy. These agents include gabapentin (Neurontin), lamotrigine (Lamictal), topiramate (Topamax), levitiracetam (Keppra), oxcarbazepine (Trileptal), tiagabine (Gabatril), and zonisamide (Zonegran) (Dichter and Brodie 1996; Meador 1998; Kwan and Brodie, 2001). These newer drugs are generally not associated with cognitive side effects, with the exception of topiramate, which does cause somnolence, psychomotor slowing, and difficulty thinking of words (Rosenfeld 1997; Meador 1998). One of these drugs may be added to a first-line drug (usually phenytoin, carbamazepine, or valproic acid), and the combination is called 'rational polypharmacy'. Oxcarbazepine is often substituted for carbamazepine because it is metabolized via a different pathway from that of carbamazepine; the 11-epoxide that produces many of the side effects of carbamazepine is not produced. Monotherapy applications of these newer drugs are growing. The monitoring of compliance and of toxicity with blood anticonvulsant levels is important in the management of epileptic patients. Elimination of barbiturates and simplification of anticonvulsant regimens in patients with refractory seizures can lead to improvement in neuropsychological functioning (Reynolds 1982; Giordani *et al.* 1983; Devinsky 1999).

Surgical Management of Epilepsy

For those patients not controlled by antiepileptic medications, a variety of surgical techniques are available to improve seizure control. Many partial complex seizures arise from deep temporal structures such as the amygdala and hippocampus, and resections of epileptogenic cortex from the medial temporal lobe have been very successful in reducing or eliminating seizures (Dam 1996; Engel 1996; Sperling *et al.* 1996; Wass *et al.* 1996). Up to two-thirds of such refractory seizure patients have had complete control after surgery, and many others are improved. Recently, the first randomized clinical trial comparing temporal lobe resection against optimal medical therapy clearly supported the superior efficacy of surgery (Wiebe *et al.* 2001). Centers offering this surgery must assemble a multidisciplinary team to offer preoperative neuropsychological testing and Wada testing to ensure that cortex crucial to memory or language is not resected (Wyllie *et al.* 1990), subdural grid and depth electrode monitoring to ensure correct identification of the epileptogenic focus, often ictal SPECT or PET for confirming seizure onset, and neurosurgical expertise in the procedures. Even then, as discussed in Chapter 11 on memory disorders, memory dysfunction can often be detected after epilepsy surgery. Other techniques used to suppress refractory seizures include hemispherectomy and subpial transections to prevent spread of seizures when the primary focus involves 'eloquent' cortex that cannot be resected (Engel 1996). Another, more palliative surgical approach to reduce seizures is section of the corpus callosum, discussed in Chapter 12.

One other procedure now used for control of refractory partial seizures is the vagus nerve stimulator, implanted with wires on the left vagus nerve. Up to 30% of patients show greater than 50% reduction in seizure frequency (The Vagus Nerve Stimulation Study Group 1995).

A byproduct of these procedures, which have helped to control seizures in thousands of individuals, has been the study of cortical functions in patients whose epileptogenic foci have been elaborately studied by neurophysiological and neuropsychological techniques, and then the effects of resection have been studied. As mentioned in Chapter 5, mapping of cortical areas involved in language in surgical patients with epilepsy has led to an independent body of information about language and the brain, as compared to the traditional studies of stroke patients. Work by Ojemann (Ojemann and Mateer 1979; Ojemann 1990, 1991) and others has indicated that the traditional Broca's and Wernicke's areas are both less consistent and less large than anticipated from stroke patients, though in general the traditional principles of localization of language have been supported. Studies on epilepsy patients have led to the identification of the basal temporal language area (Luders *et al.* 1986, 1991; Kirshner *et al.* 1996). The contribution of studies of language mechanisms in patients undergoing evaluation and treatment of epilepsy has been reviewed by Abou-Khalil (1995). Figure 19.1 shows cortical stimulation maps from four patients with epilepsy. The variability of language area localization in the brains of patients with epilepsy is strikingly different from the traditional teaching, derived from the long experience with stroke patients, that the size and location of Broca's and Wernicke's areas are uniform and stereotyped from one brain to another. Occasional patients do not appear to have a Broca's area (Ojemann 1991). The precision of localization of cortical function by this method has contributed greatly to our understanding of both localized functions of the brain and the interconnection of these areas into cortical networks. Studies on stimulation of the inferior parietal area have served to confirm the association of the four elements of the Gerstmann syndrome (agraphia, acalculia, right–left confusion, and finger agnosia, see Chapter 6). In the area of memory, studies of patients with medial temporal resections first led to the confirmation of the hippocampus as the seat of memory (see Chapter 11), as well as the importance of the left hippocampus for verbal memory and the right hippocampus for non-verbal memory. Finally, studies of patients with corpus callosum section (see Chapter 12) have taught us most of the lessons about the importance of this connecting structure between the two hemispheres and the evidence for separate consciousnesses of the two, divided hemispheres.

Management of Emotional and Behavioral Disorders in Epileptic Patients

In addition to anticonvulsant drugs, psychotropic medications are occasionally needed in patients with behavioral manifestations of epilepsy. Carbamazepine appears to have a beneficial effect for affective disorders and aggressive behavior in patients with epilepsy and those with primary psychiatric disorders (Tunks and Dermer 1977; Folks *et al.* 1982). Other antiepileptic drugs are also used in bipolar affective disorder, including valproic acid, gabapentin, lamotrigine, and topiramate. When a severe depression develops in an epileptic patient, antidepressant therapy is appropriate. Tricyclic antidepressants were problematic because of sedative effect and lowering of the seizure threshold (Reynolds 1982; Mendez *et al.* 1984), but the selective serotonin reuptake inhibitor (SSRI) antidepressants have been much better tolerated in patients with epilepsy, with only rare reports of seizures induced by SSRIs. Psychosis presents a greater therapeutic dilemma, as neuroleptic, antipsychotic drugs have an even greater tendency to provoke seizures. The newer 'atypical' antipsychotic agents (see Chapter 14) appear to be safer in epileptic patients than the older, dopamine-blocking drugs such as chlorpromazine or haloperidol.

The psychosocial management of patients with epilepsy requires an understanding physician and often a 'team' approach, with social workers and counselors available to provide emotional support and practical advice. The affective disorders and psychoses associated with epilepsy can be treated with drugs, but the personality changes must generally be treated by an understanding, supportive attitude. Appreciation of the behavioral manifestations discussed in this chapter is a necessary prerequisite for the psychosocial management of patients with epilepsy (Rodin 1975).

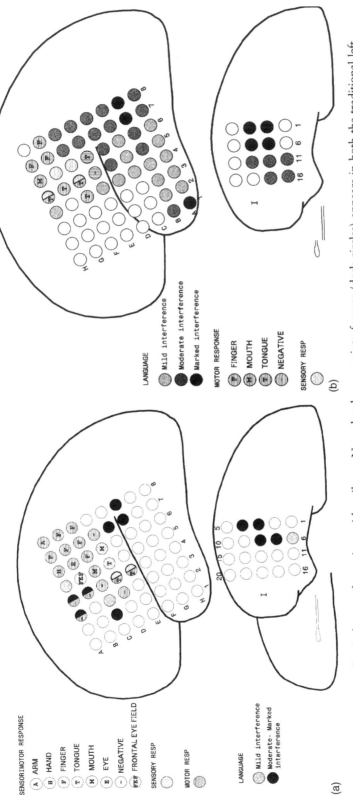

Figure 19.1 (a) Cortical map of a patient with epilepsy. Note that language interference (dark circles) appears in both the traditional left frontal (Broca's) area and the left temporal (Wernicke's) area. Sites from which motor activity was elicited are also shown for the arm, hand, finger, tongue, mouth, and eyes. This cortical stimulation map represents the 'normal', or most common distribution of function seen in mapping of patients with epilepsy; (b) Cortical map of another epileptic patient. In this case, only mild or moderate language interference was noted with stimulation of frontal lobe sites. This patient represents an 'atypical' functional map, in this case possibly related to cortical reorganization after a traumatic brain injury.

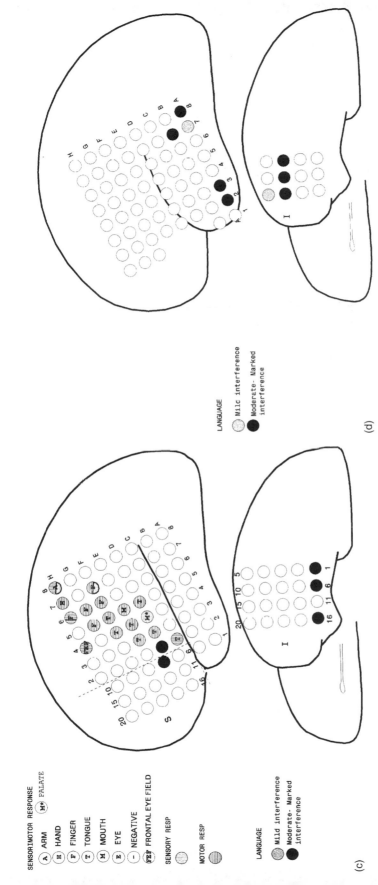

Figure 19.1 (c) Cortical map from another 'atypical' patient, in this case a woman with epilepsy following resection of an arachnoid cyst. This patient was atypical in the apparent absence of a temporal language area, a very rare pattern; (d) Cortical map showing the presence of a language area in the left anterior temporal lobe. This is the most common 'atypical' language organization pattern seen in the Vanderbilt Epilepsy Service experience. Of course, surgical resection of the anterior temporal lobe in such a patient could result in permanent aphasia. This figure was kindly provided by Dr Bassel Abou-Khalil.

REFERENCES

Abou-Khalil B. Insights into language mechanisms derived from the evaluation of epilepsy. In HS Kirshner (ed.), Handbook of Neurological Speech and Language Disorders. New York: Marcel Dekker Inc., 1995;213–275.

Adachi N, Matsuura M, Okubo Y et al. Predictive variables of interictal psychosis in epilepsy. Neurology 2000a;55:1310–1314.

Adachi N, Onuma T, Nishiwaki S et al. Inter-ictal and post-ictal psychosis in frontal lobe epilepsy: a retrospective comparison with psychoses in temporal lobe epilepsy. Seizure 2000b;9:328–335.

Alpers BJ. Relation of the hypothalamus to disorders of personality: report of a case. Arch Neurol Psychiatry 1937;38:291–303.

Ashford JW, Schulz, SC, Walsh, GO. Violent automatism in a partial complex seizure: report of a case. Arch Neurol 1980;37:120–122.

Bach-Y-Rita G, Lion JR, Climent CE, Ervin FR. Episodic dyscontrol: a study of 130 violent patients. Am J Psychiatry 1971;127:1473–1478.

Barraclough B. Suicide and epilepsy. In EG Reynolds, MR Trimble (eds), Epilepsy and Psychiatry. Edinburgh: Churchill Livingstone, 1981;72–76.

Bear DM. Temporal lobe epilepsy: a syndrome of sensory-limbic hyperconnection. Cortex 1979;15:357–384.

Bear DM, Fedio P. Quantitative analysis of interictal behavior in temporal epilepsy. Arch Neurol 1977;34:454–467.

Bear D, Levin K, Blumer D et al. Interictal behavior in hospitalized temporal lobe epileptics: relationship to idiopathic psychiatric syndromes. J Neurol Neurosurg Psychiatry 1982;45:481–488.

Berrios GE. Epilepsy and insanity during the 19th century: a conceptual history. Arch Neurol 1984;41:978–981.

Blumer D. Hypersexual episodes in temporal lobe epilepsy. Am J Psychiatry 1970;126:1099–1106.

Blumer D. Temporal lobe epilepsy and its psychiatric significance. In DF Benson, D Blumer (eds), Psychiatric Aspects of Neurologic Disease. New York: Grune & Stratton, 1975;171–198.

Blumer D, Benson DF. Psychiatric manifestations of epilepsy. In DF Benson, D Blumer (eds), Psychiatric Aspects of Neurological Disease, Vol. II. New York: Grune & Stratton, 1982;25–48.

Blumer D, Walker AE. Sexual behavior in temporal lobe epilepsy. Arch Neurol 1967;16:37–43.

Borum R, Appelbaum EL. Epilepsy, aggression, and criminal responsibility. Psychiatr Ser 1996;47:762–763.

Brewerton TD. Hyperreligiosity in psychotic disorders. J Nerv Ment Dis 1994;182:302–304.

Brodie MJ, Dichter MA. Antiepileptic drugs. New Engl J Med 1996;334:167–175.

Commission on Classification and Terminology of the International League Against Epilepsy: Proposal for revised clinical and electroencephalographic classification of epileptic seizures. Epilepsia 1981;22:489–501.

Commission on Classification and Terminology of the International League Against Epilepsy. Proposal for revised clinical and electroencephalographic classification of epilepsies and epileptic syndromes. Epilepsia 1989;30:389–399.

D'Agostino MD, Andermann F, Dubeau F et al. Exceptionally long absence status: multifactorial etiology, drug interactions, and complications. Epileptic Disord 1999;1:229–232.

Dam M. Epilepsy surgery. Acta Neurol Scand 1996;94:81–87.

Delgado-Escueta AV, Mattson RH, King L et al. The nature of aggression during epileptic seizures. N Engl J Med 1981;305:696–698.

Devinsky O. Patients with refractory seizures. New Engl J Med 1999;340:1565–1570.

Dewhurst K, Beard AW. Sudden religious conversion in temporal lobe epilepsy. Br J Psychiatry 1970;117:497–507.

Dichter MA, Brodie MJ. New antiepileptic drugs. New Engl J Med 1996;334:1583–1590.

Dikmen SS, Temkin NR, Miller B *et al.* Neurobehavioral effects of phenytoin prophylaxis of post-traumatic seizures. JAMA 1991;265:1271–1277.

Dodrill CB, Troupin AS. Psychotropic effects of carbamazepine in epilepsy: a double-blind comparison with phenytoin. Neurology 1977;27:1023–1028.

Dodrill CB, Troupin AS. Neuropsychological effects of carbamazepine and phenytoin: a reanalysis. Neurology 1991;41:141–143.

Dominian J, Serfetinides EA, Dewhurst M. A follow-up study of late onset epilepsy. II. Psychiatric and social findings. Br Med J 1963;1:431–435.

Engel J. Surgery for seizures. New Engl J Med 1996;334:647–653.

Engle J, Kuhl DE, Phelps ME, Mazziota JC. Interictal cerebral glucose metabolism in partial epilepsy and its relation to EEG changes. Ann Neurol 1982;12:510–517.

Epilepsy Foundation of America. Basic Statistics on the Epilepsies, Philadelphia: Davis, 1975.

Falconer MA. Reversibility by temporal-lobe resection of the behavioral abnormalities of temporal-lobe epilepsy. N Engl J Med 1973;289:451–455.

Flor-Henry P. Psychosis and temporal lobe epilepsy. Epilepsia 1969;10:363–395.

Flor-Henry P. Determinants of psychosis in epilepsy: laterality and forced normalization. Biol Psychiatry 1983;18:1045–1057.

Folks DG, King LD, Dowdy SB *et al.* Carbamazepine treatment of selected affectively disordered inpatients. Am J Psychiatry 1982;139:115–117.

Gibbs FA. Ictal and non-ictal psychiatric disorders in temporal lobe epilepsy. J Nerv Ment Dis 1951;113:522–528.

Gilmore RL, Heilman KM. Speech arrest in partial seizures: evidence of an associated language disorder. Neurology 1981;31:1016–1019.

Giordani B, Sackellares JC, Miller S *et al.* Improvement in neuropsychological performance in patients with refractory seizures after intensive diagnostic and therapeutic intervention. Neurology 1983;33:489–493.

Goetz CG. Charcot, the Clinician, The Tuesday Lessons. New York: Raven Press, 1987;36.

Goldensohn E, Gold A. Prolonged behavioral disturbances as ictal phenomena. Neurology 1960;10:1–9.

Goldstein M. Brain research and violent behavior. Arch Neurol 1974;30:1–35.

Goodwin DW, Crane JP, Guze SB. Phenomenological aspects of the alcoholic 'blackout'. Br J Psychiatry 1969;115:1033–1038.

Gudmundsson G. Epilepsy in Iceland. Acta Neurol Scand 1966;43(Suppl. 25):1–124.

Gunn J, Fenton G. Epilepsy, automatism and crime. Lancet 1971;1:1173–1176.

Hauser WA, Kurland LT. The epidemiology of epilepsy in Rochester, Minnesota. Epilepsia 1975;16:1–66.

Hauser WA, Annegers JF, Kurland LT. Incidence of epilepsy and unprovoked seizures in Rochester, Minnesota: 1935–1984. Epilepsia 1993;34:453–468.

Hawton K, Fagg J, Marsack P. Association between epilepsy and attempted suicide. J Neurol Neurosurg Psychiatry 1980;43:168–170.

Hermann BP, Riel P. Interictal personality and behavioral traits in temporal and generalized epilepsy. Cortex 1981;17:125–128.

Hermann BP, Whitman S, Arntson P. Hypergraphia in epilepsy: is there a specificity to temporal lobe epilepsy? J Neurol Neurosurg Psychiatry 1983;46:848–853.

Hermann BP, Whitman S. Behavioral and personality correlates of epilepsy: a review, methodological critique, and conceptual model. Psychol Bull 1984;95:451–497.

Hoare P. The development of psychiatric disorder among school children with epilepsy. Dev Med Child Neurol 1984;26:3–13.

Hooshmand H, Brawley B. Temporal lobe seizures and exhibitionism. Neurology 1969;19:1119–1124.

Kanemoto K, Kawasaki J, Kawai I. Postictal psychosis: a comparison with acute interictal and chronic psychoses. Epilepsia 1996;37:551–556.

Kanemoto K, Kawasaki J, Mori E. Violence and epilepsy: a close relation between violence and postictal psychosis. Epilepsia 1999;40:107–109.

Kanner AM, Nieto JC. Depressive disorders in epilepsy. Neurology 1999;53(Suppl. 2):S26–S32.

King LN, Young Q. Increased prevalence of seizure disorders among prisoners. JAMA 1978;239:2674–2675.

Kirshner HS, Hughes T, Fakhoury T, Abou-Khalil B. Aphasia secondary to partial status epilepticus of the basal temporal language area. Neurology 1995;45:1616–1618.

Krishnamoorthy ES, Trimble MR. Forced normalization: clinical and therapeutic relevance. Epilepsia 1999;10:S57–S64.

Kristensen O, Sindrup EH. Psychomotor epilepsy and psychosis. III. Social and psychological correlates. Acta Neurol Scand 1979;59:1–9.

Kwan P, Brodie MJ. Neuropsychological effects of epilepsy and antiepileptic drugs. Lancet 2001;357:216–222.

Lambert MV, Robertson MM. Depression in epilepsy: etiology, phenomenology, and treatment. Epilepsia 1999;40, suppl 10:S21–S47.

Lecours AR, Joanette Y. Linguistic and other psychological aspects of paroxysmal aphasia. Brain Lang 1980;10:1–23.

Leicester J. Temper tantrums, epilepsy, and episodic dyscontrol. Br J Psychiatry 1982;141:262–266.

Lennox WG. Brain injury, drugs and environment as causes of mental decay in epilepsy. Am J Psychiatry 1942;99:174–180.

Lennox WG, Lennox MA. Epilepsy and Related Disorders. Boston: Little, Brown, 1960;39–46.

Lesser RP, Pippenger CE, Luders H, Dinner DS. High-dose monotherapy in treatment of intractable seizures. Neurology 1984;34:707–711.

Lindsay J, Ounsted C, Richards P. Long-term outcome in children with temporal lobe seizures. III. Psychiatric aspects in childhood and adult life. Dev Med Child Neurol 1979;21:630–636.

Luders H, Lesser RP, Hahn J et al. Basal temporal language area demonstrated by electrical stimulation. Neurology 1986;36:505–510.

Luders H, Lesser RP, Hahn J et al. Basal temporal language area. Brain 1991;114:743–754.

Malamud N: Psychiatric disorder with intracranial tumors of the limbic system. Arch Neurol 1967;17:113–123.

Maletsky B. The episodic dyscontrol syndrome. Dis Nerv Syst 1973;34:178–185.

Mark VH, Ervin FR. Violence and the Brain. New York: Harper & Row, 1970.

Markand ON, Wheeler GL, Pollack SL. Complex partial status epilepticus (psychomotor status). Neurology 1978;28:189–196.

Matthews WS, Barabas G. Suicide and epilepsy: a review of the literature. Psychosomatics 1981;22:515–524.

Mayeux R, Alexander MP, Benson DF et al. Poriomania. Neurology 1979;29:1616–1619.

Mayeux R, Luders H. Complex partial status epilepticus: case report and proposal for diagnostic criteria. Neurology 1978;28:957–961.

McNamara JO. Reviews: emerging insights into the genesis of epilepsy. Nature 1999;399:A15–22.

Meador KJ. Cognitive effects of the new antiepileptic drugs. Neurologist 1998;4:S35–39.

Meador KJ, Loring DW, Huh K et al. Comparative cognitive effects of anticonvulsants. Neurology 1990;40:391–394.

Mendez MF. Postictal violence and epilepsy. Psychosomatics 1998;39:478–480.

Mendez MF, Cummings JL, Benson DF. Epilepsy: psychiatric aspects and use of psychotropics. Psychosomatics 1984;25:883–894.

Mendez MF, Grau R, Doss RC, Taylor JL. Schizophrenia in epilepsy: seizures and psychosis variables. Neurology 1993a;43:1073–1077.

Mendez MF, Doss RC, Taylor JL. Interictal violence in epilepsy. Relationship to behavior and seizure characteristics. J Nerv Ment Dis 1993b;181:566–569.

Mitchell W, Falconer MA, Hill D. Epilepsy with fetishism relieved by temporal lobectomy. Lancet 1954;2:626–630.

Mungas D. Interictal behavior abnormality in temporal lobe epilepsy: a specific syndrome or non-specific psychopathology? Arch Gen Psychiatry 1982;39:108–111.

Ojemann G. Organization of language cortex derived from investigations during neuro-surgery. Semin Neurosci 1990;2:297–305.

Ojemann G. Cortical organization of language. J Neurosci 1991;11:2281–2287.

Ojemann GA, Mateer C. Human language cortex: localization of memory, syntax and sequential motor–phoneme identification systems. Science 1979;205:1401–1403.

Okamura T, Fukai M, Yamadori A *et al*. A clinical study of hypergraphia in epilepsy. J Neurol Neurosurg Psychiatry 1993;56:556–559.

Pakalnis A, Drake ME Jr, John K, Kellum JB. Forced normalization. Acute psychosis after seizure control in seven patients. Arch Neurol 1987;44:289–292.

Parnas J, Korsgaard S. Epilepsy and psychosis. Acta Psychiatr Scand 1982;66:89–99.

Penry JK, Porter RK, Dreifuss FE. Simultaneous recordings of absence seizures with videotape and EEG. Brain 1975;98:427–440.

Perez MM, Trimble MR. Epileptic psychoses: diagnostic comparisons with process schizophrenia. Br J Psychiatry 1980;137:245–249.

Perini G, Mendius R. Depression and anxiety in complex partial seizures. J Nerv Ment Dis 1984;172:287–290.

Pincus JH. Can violence be a manifestation of epilepsy? Neurology 1980;30:304– 307.

Pincus JH. Violence and epilepsy. N Engl J Med 1981;305:696–698.

Pond DA, Bidwell BH. A survey of epilepsy in 14 general practices. Epilepsia 1959;1:285–299.

Prevey ML, Mattson RH, Cramer JA. Improvement in cognitive functioning and mood state after conversion to valproate monotherapy. Neurology 1989;39:1640–1641.

Pritchard PB, Lombroso CT, McIntyre M. Psychological complications of temporal lobe epilepsy. Neurology 1980;30:227–232.

Racy A, Osborn MA, Vern BA, Molinari GF. Epileptic aphasia: first onset of prolonged monosymptomatic status epilepticus in adults. Arch Neurol 1980;37:419–422.

Reynolds EG. The pharmacological management of epilepsy associated with psychological disorders. Br J Psychiatry 1982;141:549–557.

Reynolds EG. Interictal behavior in temporal lobe epilepsy. Br Med J 1983a;286:918–919.

Reynolds EH. Mental effects of antiepileptic medication: a review. Epilepsia 1983b;24 (Suppl. 2):585–595.

Roberts, JKA, Robertson, MM. Trimble MR. The lateralizing significance of hypergraphia in temporal lobe epilepsy. J Neurol Neurosurg Psychiatry 1982;45:131–138.

Robertson MM, Trimble MR. Depressive illness in patients with epilepsy: a review. Epilepsia 1983; 24(Suppl. 2):5109–5116.

Robertson MM, Trimble MR, Townsend HRA. Phenomenology of depression in epilepsy. Epilepsia 1987;28:364–372.

Rodin EA. Psychosocial management of patients with complex partial seizures. Adv Neurol 1975;11:383–414.

Rodin E, Schmaltz S. The Bear–Fedio personality inventory and temporal epilepsy. Neuro-logy 1984;34:591–596.

Rodin EA, Katz M, Lennox K. Difference between patients with temporal lobe seizures and those with other forms of epileptic attacks. Epilepsia 1976;17:313–320.

Rosenfeld WE. Topiramate: a review of preclinical, pharmacokinetic, and clinical data. Clin Therapeutics 1997;19:1294–1308.

Sachdev P. Schizophrenia-like psychosis and epilepsy: the status of the association. Am J Psychiatry 1998;155:325–336.

Saint-Hilaire JM, Gilbert M, Bouvier G, Barbeau A. Epilepsie avec manifestations aggressives: deux cas étudies avec electrodes en profoundeur. Rev Neurol (Paris) 1981; 137:161–179.

Scheuer ML, Pedley TA. The evaluation and treatment of seizures. New Engl J Med 1990;323:1468–1474.

Schomer DL. Partial epilepsy. N Engl J Med 1983;309:536–539.

Sherwin I, Peron-Magnan P, Bancaud J et al. Prevalence of psychosis in epilepsy as a function of the laterality of the epileptogenic lesion. Arch Neurol 1982;39:621–625.

Shorvon SD, Reynolds EH. Reduction in polypharmacy for epilepsy. Br Med J 1979;2: 1023–1025.

Shukla GD, Srivastava ON, Katiyar BC. Sexual disturbances in temporal lobe epilepsy: a controlled study. Br J Psychiatry 1979;134:288–292.

Slater E, Beard AW, Glithero E. The schizophrenia-like psychoses of epilepsy. Br J Psychiatry 1963;109:95–150.

Smith PF, Darlington CL. The development of psychosis in epilepsy: a re-examination of the kindling hypothesis. Behav Brain Res 1996;75:59–66.

Sperling MR, O'Connor MJ, Saykin AJ, Plummer C. Temporal lobectomy for refractory epilepsy. JAMA 1996;276:470–475.

Stevens JR. Interictal clinical manifestations of complex partial seizures. Adv Neurol 1975; 11:85–112.

Stevens JR. Epilepsy, psychosis, and schizophrenia. Schizophrenia Res 1988;1:79–89.

The Vagus Nerve Study Group. A randomized controlled trial of chronic vagus nerve stimulation for treatment of medically intractable seizures. Neurology 1995;45:224–230.

Thompson PJ, Trimble MR. Anticonvulsant drugs and cognitive functions. Epilepsia 1982;23:531–544.

Toone BK, Garralda ME, Ron MA. The psychoses of epilepsy and the functional psychoses: a clinical and phenomenological comparison. Br J Psychiatry 1982;141:256–261.

Treiman DM. Violence and the epilepsy defense. Neurol Clin 1999;17:245–255.

Trimble MR. Personality disturbances in epilepsy. Neurology 1983;33:1332–1334.

Tucker DM, Novelly RA, Walker PJ. Hyperreligiosity in temporal lobe epilepsy: redefining the relationship. J Nerv Ment Dis 1987;175:181–184.

Tunks EP, Dermer SW. Carbamazepine in the dyscontrol syndrome associated with limbic dysfunction. J Nerv Ment Dis 1977;164:156–162.

Wass CT, Rajala MM, Hughes JM et al. Long-term follow-up of patients treated surgically for medically intractable epilepsy: results in 291 patients treated at Mayo Clinic Rochester between July 1972 and March 1985. Mayo Clin Proc 1996;71:1105–1113.

Waxman SG, Geschwind N. The interictal behavior syndrome of temporal lobe epilepsy. Arch Gen Psychiatry 1976;32:1580–1586.

Whitman S, Hermann BP, Gordon A. Psychopathology in epilepsy: how great is the risk? Biol Psychiatry 1984;19:213–236.

Wiebe S, Blume WT, Girvin JP et al. A randomized, controlled trial of surgery for temporal-lobe epilepsy. New Engl J Med 2001;345:311–318.

Wyllie E, Luders H, Murphy D et al. Intracarotid amobarbital (Wada) test for language dominance: correlation with results of cortical stimulation. Epilepsia 1990;31:156–161.

20

Behavioral Aspects of Traumatic Brain Injury

Concussion has been recognized throughout history and possibly was recognized by our primate ancestors... Most of our knowledge of concussion comes from observations on the human model, and down through the ages he has been a most obliging model... He has waged almost continual warfare, and even in current peacetime North America he goes aggressively to and from work in a high-powered vehicle, usually just a little faster than he should. He goes forth to compete at the various rings, and rinks, and fields, and arenas, and for other forms of amusement he attends bars and political rallies... The combined world neurosurgical experience down through the years must total many, many millions of well-documented concussions. But from all of this we possess few facts.

(Parkinson 1977)

Traumatic brain injury (TBI) is one of the most common afflictions of mankind. It was estimated in 1990 that two million people suffer head injuries each year in the USA, of whom 500,000 require hospitalization, 70,000–90,000 have permanent, severe disabilities, and up to 50,000 die (Goldstein 1990; Thurman and Guerrero 1999). Head injury is also the leading cause of death in persons under the age of 24 years (White and Likavec 1992). Traumatic brain injuries are more common than breast cancer, AIDS, and multiple sclerosis.

Head injuries are often divided into severe, moderate, and mild, based on the Glasgow Coma Scale (Teasdale and Jennett 1974; Table 20.1). Severe head injuries are those with initial Glasgow Coma Scale (GCS) scores of 3–8, moderate head injuries are those with scores of 9–12, and mild head injuries are those GCS scores of 13–15. The severe and moderate injuries are all treated in the hospital, whereas patients with minor head injuries frequently present to a physician days or weeks after the initial injury.

415

Table 20.1 Glasgow Coma Scale (Teasdale and Jennett 1974)

Category	Score
Eyes open	
Never	1
To pain	2
To verbal stimuli	3
Spontaneously	4
Best verbal response	
None	1
Incomprehensible sounds	2
Inappropriate words	3
Patient disoriented and converses	4
Patient oriented and converses	5
Best motor response	
None	1
Extension (decerebrate rigidity)	2
Flexion (decorticate rigidity)	3
Flexion withdrawal	4
Patient localizes pain	5
Patient obeys commands	6
Total	3–15

SEVERE TRAUMATIC BRAIN INJURY

This chapter will emphasize the milder head injuries, since they are the most controversial in diagnosis and treatment, and they involve almost exclusively the higher functions, behavior, and mood, as has been known since the important contributions of Sir Charles Symonds (1962). A brief discussion of the pathophysiology and treatment of moderate and severe head injuries follows.

The brain is suspended in spinal fluid, covered by a thick membrane, the dura, and encased by a hard yet pliable skull, all of which render the brain relatively resistant to trauma. When the head is struck on one side, however, the brain may move to the opposite direction and strike the inside of the skull, causing a *contrecoup* injury. The hard surfaces of the inner skull base, particularly the jagged bony contours of the frontal and temporal areas, can contuse and injure the brain. Hemorrhages occur into the epidural, subdural, or subarachnoid spaces, or into the brain parenchyma. In addition to hemorrhage, there are shear injuries of the brain tissue itself, sometimes referred to as 'diffuse axonal injury'. The combination of focal and diffuse injury is at the heart of the presentation of patients with traumatic brain injury. Axonal injury and edema in the hemispheres or brainstem causes initial stupor or coma. Hypotension or hypoxia after the initial trauma can also increase the degree of injury to the brain (Miller 1981). Subarachnoid bleeding may obstruct the cerebrospinal fluid pathways and lead to hydrocephalus. Scars from brain injury also lead to post-traumatic seizures.

Initial management of the patient with severe traumatic brain injury involves the use of CT scanning to look for hematomas or edematous contusions. Medical treatment of brain edema with hyperventilation and osmotic agents such as mannitol begins immediately. Surgical intervention may be needed to drain an epidural, subdural, or occasionally intracerebral hematoma, or to place a shunt or ventricular drain for hydrocephalus. Many patients undergo intracranial pressure monitoring, in order to optimize the use of other medical management such as hyperventilation, which can constrict cerebral arteries excessively and reduce perfusion to the brain (White and Likavec 1992). Occasionally, portions of the skull are removed to allow room for the brain to expand (Ghajar 2000). The management of acute traumatic brain injuries has become much more aggressive in recent years, with improved outcomes in major trauma centers.

Patients who survive major head injuries are usually impaired in clinically obvious ways. Frontal lobe signs such as excessive passivity, or alternatively a disinhibited or agitated state, are prominent. Some patients also have focal signs of brain injury, such as hemiparesis, hemianopsia, and aphasia or neglect resembling stroke deficits. Patients with severe closed head injuries had a 36% mortality in one large series of 1030 patients, ranging from 76% for patients with a GCS score of 3 to 18% for those with GCS scores of 6–8 (Marshall *et al.* 1991). Most patients who survive such injuries need intensive rehabilitation and are left with significant neurobehavioral deficits. The types of behavioral deficits seen after severe head injury with diffuse axonal injury are captured in the Rancho Los Amigos Scale of Cognitive Functioning (Hagen *et al.* 1972). This scale is summarized in Table 20.2.

Language disorders are frequent in patients who recover from severe and moderate TBI. Frank aphasia is seen when the left hemisphere language cortex is injured. The more common frontal lobe injuries result in diminished spontaneous speech as well as diminished behavior; the aphasia syndrome of 'transcortical aphasia' (see Chapter 5) and the general cognitive syndromes of abulia or akinetic mutism are frequent accompaniments. Language deficits such as reduced verbal fluency, deficient naming, and difficulty with complex comprehension are common in patients with moderate or severe traumatic brain injury (Sarno *et al.* 1986). Finally, reduced ability to produce organized, meaningful discourse is almost universally found in patients tested after head injury (Chapman *et al.* 1992).

As in stroke (see Chapter 21), considerable effort goes into the rehabilitation of patients with traumatic brain injury. An NIH conference publication (NIH Consensus Statement 1998) discussed the common occurrence and severe economic impact of severe head injury. Rehabilitative therapies are considered a standard of care. Patients still in coma or at Rancho Los Amigos Scales 1–2 (see Table 20.2) are usually admitted to nursing facilities for care, and transferred later to rehabilitation hospitals if they improve. A controversial approach called 'coma stimulation' attempts to reach the comatose patient through tactile, visual,

Table 20.2 Rancho Los Amigos Scale of Cognitive Functioning (abbreviated from Hagen *et al.* 1972)

I. No response Complete lack of response to stimuli	*V. Confused, inappropriate, non-agitated response* Alert, responds to simple commands, but non-purposeful to complex commands. Agitation. Distractibility, unable to focus on specific tasks. Inappropriate verbalization. Severe memory impairment. Lack of initiation of tasks, inappropriate use of objects, inability to learn new information. Wandering. Responds to family members. Performs self-care with assistance
II. Generalized response Reaction to stimuli inconsistent, non-purposeful. Responses often same, regardless of stimuli. Responses may include physiological changes, gross body movements, or vocalizations. Responses often delayed	*VI. Confused, appropriate response* Goal-directed behavior, but needs direction. Consistently follows simple commands, recalls relearned tasks such as self-care, responses appropriate
III. Localized response Reaction to stimuli specific but inconstant, directionally related to stimulus (turning towards sound). May follow simple commands. Responds to discomfort. May respond to some persons	*VII. Automatic, appropriate response* More goal-directed and self-initiated everyday behavior
IV. Confused, agitated response Heightened activity, decreased information processing. Bizarre, non-purposeful behavior. Verbalization incoherent or inappropriate, sometimes confabulation. Mood hostile to euphoric. Reduced attention. Inability to perform self-care	*VIII. Purposeful, appropriate response* Self-directed behavior, accomplishes basic and skilled tasks. Supervision still sometimes necessary

and auditory stimuli. As in stroke, rehabilitation may take place in inpatient rehabilitation hospitals, skilled nursing facilities or subacute units, and in outpatient therapy programs.

MODERATE TRAUMATIC BRAIN INJURY

Moderate head injuries, or patients with GCS scores of 9–12, should also be admitted to hospital, and all should be imaged with CT or MRI scanning. One series of 341 patients with initial GCS scores of 9–12 (Stein and Ross 1992) found that 40% had abnormal CT scans, 8% required neurosurgical intervention, and four patients died of their head injuries. Half of the patients either recovered more slowly than expected or deteriorated after admission; the authors advocated repeat CT scans for these patients. They also found that patients with GCS scores on admission of 13, who qualified for the 'mild head injury' category, had a very similar rate of abnormal CT scans, 44%; they recommended reclassification of such patients into the 'moderate head injury' group and routine admission to hospital and brain imaging. MRI scanning is more sensitive in detecting lesions in patients with moderate and mild head injuries, but only rarely detects surgically important lesions missed on CT scan (Levin *et al.* 1987a). Lesions on MRI do correlate with deficits in memory and frontal lobe functioning (Levin *et al.* 1987a). Another study (Wilson *et al.* 1988), confirmed a correlation between MRI lesion burden and memory impairment, but only for the delayed MRI study.

In general, the literature on traumatic brain injury suggests that the length of coma, the length of post-traumatic amnesia, and the severity of memory loss all correlate with the severity of a closed head injury (Dikmen *et al.* 1987). The severity of the memory impairment in this series was proportional to the time until the patient could follow commands, the duration of the post-traumatic amnesia, and the GCS score. Many of the memory deficits in this series, however, recovered by 1 year; only those with greater than 1 day of coma, a GCS score of 8 or less, and post-traumatic amnesia of 2 weeks or greater had memory scores significantly different from those of control subjects (Dikmen *et al.* 1987).

MILD HEAD INJURY

The most controversial area in head injury management is the assessment of deficits and the rehabilitation of patients with minor head injury. These patients are usually not admitted to hospital, or are observed only overnight, yet they later return to physicians and attorneys frequently with the post-concussive syndrome. This disorder was brought to medical attention by Sir Charles Symonds (1962): 'Prominent among (the sequelae of concussion) are anxiety, irritability, difficulty in sustaining mental concentration, impaired memory, and excessive liability to fatigue'. To these, contemporary neurologists would add headache, dizziness, irritability, and depressed mood. Lezak (1978) conceptualized the subtle neurobehavioral effects of minor head injury under the three categories of 'perplexity', 'distractibility', and 'fatigue'. Alexander (1995) pointed out that mild head injury is one of the most common neurological disorders, yet neither the training of neurologists nor the neurological literature affords this disorder the attention it deserves. Of the 180 cases per 100,000 of population per year, approximately 15% are still disabled at 1 year (Alexander 1995).

Mild head injury is defined by an initial GCS score of 13–15. Loss of consciousness after the impact is brief or partial; a brief period of being 'dazed' or 'seeing stars' may be sufficient for the injury to qualify as a minor head injury or concussion. Retrograde amnesia is always present, but may be as brief as a few minutes or as long as a few hours. Patients virtually always have normal, nonfocal neurological examinations. Brain imaging studies are usually normal. CT scans should be done not only immediately, but also during follow-up if symptoms appear to worsen; subdural hematoma can be absent on a scan done immediately after injury but present days or weeks later (Deitch and Kirshner 1989).

The causes of mild head injury are the same as those of moderate and severe head injury, except that personal assaults and whiplash injuries are more commonly the cause of minor than severe head injuries (Alexander 1995). More forceful blows to the cranium, such as from a fall from a height or a windshield striking the head in a motor vehicle accident, are more likely to be associated with moderate or severe head injury. Linear fractures may not carry an increased risk of long-term disability, but cortical contusions likely do (Williams *et al.* 1990). The pathology of mild traumatic brain injury is likely the same as in severe head injury – diffuse axonal injury, shear hemorrhages, and edema – the degree is simply less (Alexander 1995). The general principles of the correlation of the severity of head injury with the length of unresponsiveness and the length of post-traumatic amnesia apply to all levels of head injury. Young people who have a brief loss of consciousness, post-traumatic amnesia of 1 hour or less, and GCS scores of 15 generally recover within a few weeks (Levin *et al.* 1987b). Older patients (Binder 1986; Mazzuchi *et al.* 1992; Goldstein *et al.* 1994), or those with more severe trauma, loss of consciousness for more than 10 minutes, and longer post-traumatic amnesia periods (Rimel *et al.* 1981; Hugenholtz *et al.* 1988) are likely to take much longer to recover, or not to recover completely.

Persistent Post-Concussive Syndrome

About 15% overall of minor head injury patients have persistent disability at 1 year following injury (Alexander 1995). These patients are diagnosed with 'persistent post-concussive syndrome'. They have prominent neurobehavioral complaints, such as forgetfulness, poor concentration, inability to stick to tasks, a tendency to misplace items, and reduced initiation of routine activities. In addition, emotional symptoms, such as irritability, depressed mood, and anxiety, are common (Alexander 1995). Predictors for the persistent post-concussive syndrome include (Alexander 1995):

1. Ongoing litigation
2. Low socioeconomic status
3. History of prior head injuries
4. Persistent headache
5. Other significant injuries
6. Possibly female gender
7. Prior history of psychological disorders.

The emotional symptoms are particularly prominent in the persistent post-concussive syndrome patients (Schoenhuber and Gentilini 1988; Bohnen *et al.* 1992). Alexander (1992) compared patients with mild traumatic brain injury and severe TBI at 6 months post-onset; headaches and depression were much more common in the mild than the severe group. This observation is familiar to physicians and therapists who work with TBI patients; mild head injury patients typically complain of chronic headaches and appear depressed, whereas severe patients complain little despite their much more obvious cognitive and often motor deficits. Chronic headaches may represent, at least in part (see below), an effect of anxiety and depression.

The diagnosis of 'post-traumatic stress disorder' (Davidson 2001) clearly overlaps with that of post-concussive syndrome, particularly in cases with prominent psychological factors and little evidence of physical injury, such as loss of consciousness or a mechanical blow to the head sufficient to produce a concussion. Another feature of the psychological component of minor head injury is the tendency for emotional distress to worsen over weeks to months, perhaps related to loss of income, family stress, changes in relationships, and loss of self-image. This pattern of deteriorating function is characteristic of the stress-related persistent post-concussive syndrome; organic deficits following head injury tend to stabilize or improve, rarely to worsen progressively. The slow pace of litigation may also reinforce the patterns of the persistent post-concussive syndrome ('accident neurosis'; Miller 1961). On the other hand, skeptics who accuse these patients of simply performing a role to obtain a favorable legal settlement are probably wrong in most cases; in fact, legal settlements do not usually bring an end to these persistent symptoms (McKinlay and Kilfedder 1992).

Post-Traumatic Headaches

Headaches following minor head injury are a frequent problem. The International Headache Society (1988) classification of headache includes both acute and chronic post-traumatic headaches, as well as aggravation of pre-existing migraine or tension headache following trauma. Packard (1992) discussed headaches as a disabling feature of the post-concussive syndrome and stressed that legal settlements do not usually end the headaches. As mentioned above, headaches are common in minor head injury but relatively rare in patients with severe TBI.

An additional factor common in the mild head injury population is the presence of 'rebound headaches' related to the use of daily analgesics (Warner and Fenichel 1996). Many patients are started on analgesics soon after their traumatic injuries, and they supplement these with over-the-counter analgesics such as acetaminophen, aspirin, and non-steroidal anti-inflammatory drugs. All of these agents have the potential to transform occasional severe headaches into chronic daily headaches. As a corollary of the theory of rebound headaches, the headaches fail to respond to agents that would usually be effective in the treatment of acute headaches (Mathew 1993). If the patient stops taking analgesics, the headaches tend to worsen acutely, then to resolve gradually, over weeks to months. The headaches may then disappear completely or be replaced by occasional migraine-like episodes, which will then respond to either acute agents such as triptan drugs or prophylactic agents such as beta blockers, calcium channel blockers, or valproic acid.

Mood and Psychiatric Changes after Closed Head Injury

Depressed mood is extremely common in the early months following minor head injuries (Kwentus *et al.* 1985). Robinson and Szetela (1981) and Fedoroff and colleagues (1992) reported the correlation of post-traumatic depression with lesions near the frontal pole, a finding analogous to the same group's studies of post-stroke depression (see Chapter 21). Jorge and colleagues (1993) found that subjective mood changes of depression were reliable in indicating depression in head injured patients; 'masked' or hidden depression was an infrequent problem. Just as right hemisphere strokes and frontal lobe syndromes are associated with a flat affect, head injuries may also produce apathy as a part of the mood change. Personality changes are particularly common with frontal lobe injury (Kwentus *et al.* 1985).

Mania is less common than depression after closed head injury, but it has been reported. Starkstein and colleagues (1987) found a correlation in their 11 cases with lesions involving the right hemisphere limbic system. Shukla and colleagues (1987) reported a correlation with severe head injury and also with post-traumatic seizures. The mania was more often irritable than euphoric.

Treatment of Patients with Minor Head Injury

Alexander (1995) presented several specific recommendations for physicians treating patients with mild head injuries. First, the examiner should obtain as complete a history as possible about the injury itself; was there a fall of more than 6 feet (1.8 meters) or a severe impact such as a motor vehicle accident? Second, what was the duration of loss of consciousness? This cannot be obtained accurately unless records from emergency rooms and emergency medical technicians are reviewed. Third, how long was the period of post-traumatic amnesia? This, too, cannot be obtained from the patient, though patients' recollection of how long they were 'out' may be a crude estimate of the duration of post-traumatic amnesia. Fourth, the treatment plan depends critically on the time post-onset at which the patient is evaluated. Acute patients need only be examined for any unexpected neurological deficits and counseled about the mild head injury syndrome. Delayed patients may already have developed many of the psychosocial problems associated with the persistent post-concussive syndrome. Fifth, patients with persistent post-concussive syndrome require treatment of several, separate symptoms and problems, such as headaches, dizziness, and depressed mood. In general, patients with persistent post-concussive syndrome defy successful treatment by an individual physician; a 'rehabilitation team' is usually required, consisting of physician, psychologist, cognitive therapists, and social workers.

Boxing Injuries

The sport of boxing involves repetitive, minor traumatic brain injuries. A 'knockout' in a boxing match is essentially a concussion (Council on Scientific

Affairs 1983). Even healthy young boxers have reduced verbal learning as compared to control subjects (Levin *et al.* 1987c). Pathological studies of the brains of boxers have shown contusions, old hemorrhages, and evidence of axonal injury (Lampert and Hardman 1984). Depigmentation of the substantia nigra is seen pathologically, as might be predicted from the frequent occurrence of Parkinsonism in boxers (Corsellis *et al.* 1973). The example of Mohammed Ali readily comes to mind. Finally, widespread neurofibrillary tangles are also found in boxers who have had many knockouts. These are usually unaccompanied by senile plaques, distinguishing 'dementia pugilistica' from Alzheimer's disease (Lampert and Hardman 1984). Approximately 15% of chronic boxers suffer memory loss, slurred speech, tremor, abnormal gait, and eventually dementia (Council on Scientific Affairs 1983). The occurrence of dementia in boxers should be a warning to young people who choose this career; the movement to ban boxing in the USA, however, has met with little success.

Concussion in Athletes

Although considered less dangerous than boxing, many sports carry a risk of concussion. As many as 300,000 concussions occur in sports and recreation; the most common offender is football (Powell and Barber-Foss 1999). Professional sports announcers often treat such minor 'headers' as inconsequential. Neuropsychological studies have shown, however, that repeated minor head injuries in college athletes result in detectable deficits in attention, memory, and planning (Macciocchi *et al.* 1996; Collins *et al.* 1999; Matser *et al.* 1999). Many of these injuries, especially those in non-contact sports such as soccer (Matser *et al.* 1999), do not involve complete loss of consciousness. High school and college athletes who have sustained a definite concussion should be counseled carefully before being permitted to return to competitive sports (Report of the Quality Standards Subcommittee, American Academy of Neurology 1997). Cases of second concussions occurring before complete recovery from the first ('second impact syndrome') have occasionally led to malignant brain swelling and even death (Saunders and Harbaugh 1984; Kelly and Rosenberg 1997). Even minor concussions should therefore keep an athlete out of competition for at least a week, or until the symptoms have completely resolved. If the athlete has a definite loss of consciousness, and if a CT or MRI scan is abnormal, the guidelines suggest keeping the athlete out of competition for the season, and possibly for life.

CONCLUSION

Traumatic brain injury is an extremely common cause of neurological deficits in our society. The two areas of greatest change over the past few years are in the acute, medical management of moderate and severe traumatic brain injuries, and in the identification and treatment of persistent symptoms and disability related to minor head injuries. Minor head injury is a very common problem for behavioral neurologists and rehabilitation specialists, and a good understanding of the syndrome is crucial for the proper management of the patient.

REFERENCES

Alexander MP. Neuropsychiatric correlates of persistent post-concussive syndrome. J Head Trauma Rehabil 1992;7:60–69.

Alexander MP. Mild traumatic brain injury: pathophysiology, natural history, and clinical management. Neurology 1995;45:1253–1260.

Binder LM. Persisting symptoms after mild head injury: a review of the post-concussive syndrome. J Clin Exp Neuropsychol 1986;8:323–346.

Bohnen N, Twijnstra A, Jolles J. Post-traumatic and emotional symptoms in different subgroups of patients with mild head injury. Brain Inj 1992;6:481–487.

Chapman SB, Culhane KA, Levin HS et al. Narrative discourse after closed head injury in children and adolescents. Brain Lang 1992;43:42–65.

Collins MW, Grindel SH, Lovell MR et al. Relationship between concussion and neuropsychological performance in college football players. JAMA 1999;282:964–970.

Corsellis JAN, Bruton CJ, Freeman-Browne D. The aftermath of boxing. Psychol Med 1973;3:270–277.

Council on Scientific Affairs. Brain injury in boxing. JAMA 1983;249:254–257.

Davidson JRT. Recognition and treatment of posttraumatic stress disorder. JAMA 2001;286:584–588.

Deitch D, Kirshner HS. Subdural hematoma after normal CT. Neurology 1989;39:985–987.

Dikmen S, Temkin N, McLean A et al. Memory and head injury severity. J Neurol Neurosurg Psychiatry 1987;50:1613–1618.

Fedoroff JP, Starkstein SE, Forrester AW et al. Depression in patients with acute traumatic brain injury. Am J Psychiatry 1992;149:918–923.

Ghajar J. Traumatic brain injury. Lancet 2000;356:923–929.

Goldstein M. Traumatic brain injury: a silent epidemic (editorial). Ann Neurol 1990;27:327.

Goldstein F, Levin H, Presley R et al. Neurobehavioral consequences of closed head injury in older adults. J Neurol Neurosurg Psychiatry 1994;57:961–966.

Hagen C, Malkmus D, Durham P. Levels of Cognitive Functioning. Downey, CA: Rancho Los Amigos Hospital, 1972.

International Headache Society, Headache Classification Committee. Classification and diagnostic criteria for headache disorders, cranial neuralgias and facial pain. Cephalalgia 1988;8(Suppl. 7):44–45.

Hugenholtz H, Stuss DT, Stethem LL, Richard MT. How long does it take to recover from a mild concussion? Neurosurgery 1988;22:853–858.

Jorge RE, Robinson RG, Arndt S. Are there symptoms that are specific for depressed mood in patients with traumatic brain injury? J Nerv Ment Dis 1993;181:91–99.

Kelly JP, Rosenberg JH. Diagnosis and management of concussion in sports. Neurology 1997;48:575–580.

Kwentus JA, Hart RP, Peck ET, Kornstein S. Psychiatric complications of closed head trauma. Psychosomatics 1985;26:8–17.

Lampert PW, Hardman JM. Morphological changes in brains of boxers. JAMA 1984;251:2676–2679.

Levin HS, Amparo E, Eisenberg HM et al. Magnetic resonance imaging and computerized tomography in relation to the neurobehavioral sequelae of mild and moderate head injuries. J Neurosurg 1987a;66:706–713.

Levin HS, Mattis S, Ruff RM *et al*. Neurobehavioral outcome following minor head injury: a three-center study. J Neurosurg 1987b;66:234–243.

Levin HS, Lippold SC, Goldman A *et al*. Neurobehavioral functioning and magnetic resonance imaging findings in young boxers. J Neurosurg 1987c;67:657–667.

Lezak MD. Subtle sequelae of brain damage. Perplexity, distractibility, and fatigue. Am J Physical Medicine 1978;57:9–15.

Macciocchi SN, Barth JT, Alves W *et al*. Neuropsychological functioning and recovery after mild head injury in college athletes. Neurosurgery 1996;39:510–514.

Marshall LF, Gautille T, Klauber MR *et al*. The outcome of severe closed head injury. J Neurosurg 1991;75:S28–S36.

Mathew NT. Chronic refractory headache. Neurology 1993;43(Suppl. 3):S26–S33.

Matser EJT, Kessels AG, Lezak MD *et al*. Neuropsychological impairment in amateur soccer players. JAMA 1999;282:971–973.

Mazzuchi A, Cattelani R, Missale G *et al*. Head-injured subjects aged over 50 years: correlations between variables of trauma and neuropsychological follow-up. J Neurol 1992;239:256–260.

McKinlay WW, Kilfedder C. Financial compensation and head injury. Brain Injury 1992; 6:387–389.

Miller DJ. Physiology of trauma. Clin Neurosurg 1981;29:103–130.

Miller H. Accident neurosis. Br Med J 1961;1:919–925, 992–998.

NIH Consensus Statement. Rehabilitation of persons with traumatic brain injury. NIH Consensus Statement 1998;16:1–41.

Packard RC. Posttraumatic headache: permanency and relationship to legal settlement. Headache 1992;32:496–500.

Parkinson D. Concussion. Mayo Clin Proc 1977;52:492–496.

Powell JW, Barber-Foss KD. Traumatic brain injury in high school athletes. JAMA 1999;282:958–963.

Report of the Quality Standards Subcommittee, American Academy of Neurology. Practice parameter: the management of concussion in sports (summary statement). Neurology 1997;48:581–585.

Rimel RW, Giordani B, Barth JT *et al*. Disability caused by minor head injury. Neurosurgery 1981;9:221–228.

Robinson RG, Szetela B. Mood change following left hemisphere brain injury. Ann Neurol 1981;9:447–453.

Sarno MT, Buonaguro A, Levita E. Characteristics of verbal impairment in closed head injury. Arch Phys Med Rehabil 1986;67:400–405.

Saunders RL, Harbaugh RE. The second impact in catastrophic contact-sports head trauma. JAMA 1984;252:538–539.

Schoenhuber R, Gentilini M. Anxiety and depression after mild head injury: a case–control study. J Neurol Neurosurg Psychiatry 1988;51:722–724.

Shukla S, Cook BL, Mukherjee S *et al*. Mania following head trauma. Am J Psychiatry 1987;144:93–96.

Starkstein SE, Pearlson GD, Boston J, Robinson RG. Mania after brain injury. A controlled study of causative factors. Arch Neurol 1987;44:1069–1073.

Stein SC, Ross SE. Moderate head injury: a guide to initial management. J Neurosurg 1992;77:562–564.

Symonds C. Concussion and its sequelae. Lancet 1962;1:1–5.

Teasdale G, Jennett B. Assessment of coma and impaired consciousness: a practical scale. Lancet 1974;2:81–84.

Thurman D, Guerrero J. Trends in hospitalization associated with traumatic brain injury. JAMA 1999;282:954–957.

Warner JS, Fenichel GM. Chronic post-traumatic headache often a myth? Neurology 1996;46:915–916.

White RJ, Likavec MJ. The diagnosis and initial management of head injury. New Engl J Med 1992;327:1507–1511.

Williams DH, Levin HS, Eisenberg HM. Mild head injury classification. Neurosurgery 1990;27:422–428.

Wilson JTL, Wiedmann KD, Hadley DM *et al*. Early and late magnetic resonance imaging and neuropsychological outcome after head injury. J Neurol Neurosurg Psychiatry 1988;51:391–396.

21

Neurorehabilitation and Recovery from Behavioral Effects of Stroke

> Rehabilitation implies the restoration of patients to their fullest physical, mental, and social capability... in the shortest possible time.

> (Illis *et al.* 1982)

Stroke is of obvious practical importance as the most common of serious neurological diseases, and as the leading cause of neurological disability in adults. The statistics on stroke are staggering. Of the approximately 700,000 strokes per year in the USA, 150,000 prove fatal, making stroke the third leading cause of death. Most patients, however, survive their strokes, albeit with disability. An estimated four million persons in the USA have residual disability from stroke. Of every 100 stroke survivors, only 10 return to work with no disability; 40 suffer mild disability, 40 have moderate or severe disability, and 10 require care in a long-term nursing facility (Gresham *et al.* 1975). Stroke accounts for 31% of the patients in rehabilitation facilities, and nearly half of the $43 billion annual cost of stroke is spent for inpatient and nursing facility rehabilitation (Hoenig *et al.* 1999).

There is not a separate chapter in this book on the behavioral neurology of stroke, for the obvious reason that stroke accounts for much of our knowledge of the behavioral syndromes discussed throughout this book. To a behavioral neurologist, stroke is an 'experiment of nature' in which one part of the nervous system is selectively damaged, while the rest continues to function. Stroke teaches neurologists how to correlate functions with focal lesions in the brain; in the words of C. Miller Fisher, 'we learn neurology stroke by stroke'. Stroke is the classical source of information on focal behavioral syndromes, from the aphasias to the alexias and agraphias, apraxias, agnosias, and frontal lobe syndromes, to the more generalized memory loss syndromes, encephalopathies, and dementias. To recount all of these topics would be to repeat most of this volume. The recovery

427

of these neurobehavioral deficits is a somewhat separate subject, and in this area as well, stroke has been a fount of knowledge. We shall therefore undertake a brief, mostly conceptual review of brain plasticity and neurorehabilitation, drawing heavily on the stroke rehabilitation literature.

NEUROPLASTICITY AND THE SCIENTIFIC BASIS OF REHABILITATION

For years, rehabilitation therapists have developed exercise and training methods to try to enhance the recovery of neurological deficits. Most of these approaches were developed empirically, without specific scientific evidence. A considerable literature has accumulated, however, indicating that even the adult brain has plasticity, and that the functional organization of brain systems can change in response to rehabilitation after injuries. Brain plasticity is the scientific rationale for rehabilitation. The early recovery after a stroke is likely mediated by three factors: (1) the revival of ischemic cells that are not yet necrotic; (2) the resolution of edema; and (3) the disappearance of diaschisis, a poorly understood depression of blood flow and metabolism in synaptically connected but structurally undamaged areas of the brain after stroke. These processes take place without active rehabilitative efforts and are likely complete within days or a few weeks. Later recovery requires reorganization or remodeling of functional brain anatomy. Cramer and Chopp (2000) review the evidence that the cortical reorganization after a stroke is similar to the events in the initial development of a specialized area of cortex; just as a pleuripotential cortical area becomes specialized for one function, so can this specialization change during recovery from brain injury. The growth factors and other biochemical actors in the process of development are likely important also in the cortical remodeling after brain injury.

Paul Bach-Y-Rita has been one of the major contributors to the concept of brain plasticity as the basis for rehabilitation. Bach-Y-Rita (1990) defined plasticity as 'the adaptive capacities of the central nervous system...to modify its own organization and function'. Plasticity, along with excitability, is one of the key functions of the nervous system. He pointed out that since Broca's 1861 contribution to localization of higher functions with localized areas of the brain, functions carried out by damaged areas were thought to be permanently lost; later experiments, however, make clear that in animals, and potentially in humans, rehabilitation can enhance cortical reorganization and plasticity after strokes (Bach-Y-Rita 1990; Seitz and Freund 1997).

Reorganization of the Motor Cortex following Stroke

The best-studied example of brain plasticity is the motor cortex. Nudo and colleagues (Nudo and Milliken 1996; Nudo et al. 1996) created an animal model of stroke in squirrel monkeys by electrocauterization of portions of the motor cortex, producing small cortical infarcts. They mapped the motor cortex by electrical stimulation and left the electrodes in place, so that they could compare the cortical distribution for specific movements before and after experimental interventions. After injury, the areas from which they could elicit hand (forepaw) movement decreased in size. Active training of the limb in an exercise program, however, resulted in an increase in the size of the cortical hand area, almost to the pre-stroke level. This change in the motor cortical map clearly indicated motor reorganization. In addition, restraint of the unaffected limb produced even greater increases in the function of the paralyzed limb and in the area of the cortex devoted to movement of the affected limb. Most importantly for rehabilitation research, if the unaffected upper limb was restrained, but the exercise training was withheld, the hand area failed to increase in size. These studies provide unequivocal evidence, at least in monkeys, that rehabilitative exercise actually facilitates the remodeling of the motor cortex.

In human stroke patients, positron emission tomography (PET) scanning can be used to map the motor cortex during exercise of the paretic limb (Dettmers *et al.* 1997). After stroke, the motor cortex for the affected limb appeared smaller on PET studies, just as it did in the squirrel monkey model. By PET measures, attempts at exercise produced less activation of the motor cortex in stroke patients than in normal people. Other areas of the same hemisphere, such as the parietal cortex and the dorsal prefrontal cortex, lit up during movements that did not activate these areas in normal subjects, suggesting that the motor cortex can reorganize and integrate adjacent cortical areas not normally devoted to arm or hand movement. Similar findings have been reported with passive elbow movement as the activation condition, with reorganization of the motor system occurring within 6 weeks of a stroke with major hemiplegia (Nelles *et al.* 1999). From these experiments, it is evident that cortical remodeling of the motor system in response to exercise occurs in human stroke patients, as well as in experimental animals. Restraint of the unaffected upper limb has also been reported to improve motor recovery of the weak limb in human stroke patients (Taub *et al.* 1993; Liepert *et al.* 2000). Liepert and colleagues (2000) utilized transcranial magnetic stimulation (TMS) to map the motor cortex of stroke patients, all more than 1 year post-stroke, all with some movement of the paretic upper limb. As in the squirrel monkey experiments, intensive therapy for the weak arm and restraint of the good arm ('constraint-induced therapy') not only facilitated increased movement of the arm, but also appeared to increase the area of the brain from which contractions of the contralateral hand could be produced by magnetic stimulation. Critics have pointed out that these stroke patients may have had potential to improve, since most had small, subcortical infarcts, and since their motor paralysis had already partially recovered, but they had not been receiving active therapy. These studies also involved small numbers of carefully chosen patients. The program of constraint-induced therapy is now being tested in a large, multicenter study. The important message, however, is that these experiments demonstrate convincingly that the motor cortex can reorganize after stroke, and that rehabilitation techniques and patterns of motor use can influence the reorganization of the cortex and the functional recovery from deficits.

This experimental work on remodeling of the motor cortex with stroke rehabilitation is not the only evidence of motor reorganization. String musicians, for example, have much larger areas of right hemisphere motor cortex devoted to the left hand than do average, control subjects (Elbert *et al.* 1995). Likewise, blind subjects who learn to read Braille show increases in motor cortical activation of the fingers of both hands (Pascual-Leone *et al.* 1995; Sterr *et al.* 1998). Rehabilitative therapy can thus be seen as just an example of a general phenomenon, the enlargement of cortical areas in response to training in fine motor use of a limb. That such changes can take place even after a stroke damages the motor cortex suggests that the paralysis caused by a stroke is not irreversibly lost, but that some of the deficit can be attributed to a 'learned non-use' of the affected limb (Taub *et al.* 1998). The program of constraint-induced therapy at the University of Alabama has received considerable media attention, and has kindled hope for improved recovery of disability in stroke victims.

Reorganization of the Language Cortex following Stroke

The evidence that the motor cortex can reorganize after stroke suggests that other cortical areas, involved in higher functions and behavior, may also have a capacity for reorganization with rehabilitative therapies. In acute stroke, language deficits change dramatically with changes in perfusion of the language cortex. Hillis and colleagues (Hillis *et al.* 2000, 2001) at Johns Hopkins have shown that both aphasia and visuospatial deficits correlate with hypoperfusion of the cortex, as imaged by perfusion-weighted MRI (PWI). These authors have demonstrated in several patients that increases in perfusion induced by pressor drugs or by carotid endarterectomy improve behavioral functioning (Hillis *et al.* 2000). They have also shown (Hillis *et al.* 2001) that the delay in peak perfusion of Wernicke's area (see Chapter 5), as measured by PWI, correlates quantitatively with the comprehension of single words on a word–picture matching test. Acute stroke represents an opportunity to study the localization of brain functions before compensatory mechanisms, via recruitment of other parts of brain networks and reorganization of the brain, can come into play. These correlations between brain imaging and behavioral function in acute stroke also represent a striking example of the practical usefulness of behavioral neurology in the management of patients (Kirshner 2001).

As language function recovers, patterns of activation also change. Some investigators have emphasized the activation of right hemisphere cortical sites (Cappa *et al.* 1997) not normally activated during the same language tasks in normal subjects. These findings would suggest that the right hemisphere might mediate the recovery of language function after stroke. Weiller and colleagues (1995) also found that recovery of language comprehension in six patients with Wernicke's aphasia involved activation of the right temporal lobe, the analogue of the left hemisphere Wernicke's area, an area not activated in normal controls. The work of Heiss and colleagues (1999), however, suggests that a major abnormality in PET activation of the left temporal area precludes recovery, and that only cases with reactivation of adjacent left hemisphere cortex achieve high levels of recovery. Activation of right hemisphere areas, in Heiss's studies (1997, 1999), may be a 'second best' effort, associated with incomplete recovery of function.

Speech and language therapy is widely used to facilitate improvement in language function after stroke. The specific techniques of speech/language therapy are beyond the scope of this book; the reader can find more information in the Continuum volume by Kirshner and colleagues (1999) or in Wertz (1995). Rehabilitation specialists would like to think that speech and language therapy techniques facilitate the reorganization of the language cortex, just as physical rehabilitation techniques facilitate remodeling in the motor cortex. Direct evidence of therapy-induced brain reorganization for the higher cortical functions does not yet exist, but there is considerable clinical evidence that speech and language therapy bring about more than spontaneous clinical recovery.

Among the literature on aphasia rehabilitation are three randomized trials of speech/language therapy. The first, by Wertz and colleagues (1986), involved 8–10 hours of therapy per week for 12 weeks in one group of aphasic stroke patients, while a control group did not receive therapy during the first 12 weeks. From 12–24 weeks, the two groups crossed over. The patients who received speech therapy showed much greater improvement during the first 12 weeks than did the control group, but the control group made up much of the difference during the second 12 weeks. In a second study, Katz and Wertz (1997) compared groups of aphasic patients treated with computer language therapy, computer stimulation without active manipulation of language deficits, and no treatment. The computer language therapy group clearly exceeded the progress of the other two groups over a 6-month study period. The only randomized study to fail to document improvement in aphasia recovery with therapy was the study of Lincoln *et al.* (1984), in which patients received only 2 hours of therapy per week for 24 weeks; there was no difference at the end of the 24 weeks between treated patients and non-treated controls, but few of the treated patients actually received 48 hours of therapy. Two meta-analyses of aphasia therapy (Whurr *et al.* 1992; Robey 1998) reported increased recovery in patients receiving active speech/language therapy. These studies provide little guidance in the selection of what type of therapy to recommend, whether individual or group therapy is needed, and whether the expensive use of trained therapists can be reduced, without loss of effectiveness, by use of computer therapy techniques or therapy sessions by trained volunteers (Hartman and Landau 1987). They do strongly suggest, however, that the language cortex, like the motor cortex, can reorganize, and that speech and language therapy are useful in facilitating this reorganization.

Reorganization of Right Hemisphere Association Cortex following Stroke

An area even less studied is the use of rehabilitation techniques to facilitate recovery of right hemisphere stroke syndromes of neglect and visual–spatial dysfunction. Neglect usually shows a gradual pattern of recovery; by 1 year post-onset, very few patients with right hemisphere strokes still manifest hemispatial neglect (Ferro *et al.* 1999). There is some evidence from PET studies that the early disappearance of neglect correlates with the resolution of diaschisis affecting non-infarcted areas of the right hemisphere (Perani *et al.* 1993). The cognitive rehabilitation of right hemisphere deficits has been studied less than has speech therapy for aphasia, but several studies do suggest efficacy of therapy methods such as training of visual scanning, trunk rotation, and use of ocular prisms (Weinberg *et al.* 1977; Pizzamiglio *et al.* 1992; Robertson *et al.* 1995; Wiart *et al.* 1997; Rossetti *et al.* 1998). Ferro and colleagues (1999) have provided an excellent review of the studies on both aphasia and neglect rehabilitation.

Hyperbaric Oxygen in Stroke Rehabilitation

A therapy yet to be proved as a stroke rehabilitation technique is hyperbaric oxygen. This treatment showed initial promise in acute stroke (Nighoghossian and Trouillas 1997), but two randomized pilot trials of hyperbaric oxygen versus air in acute stroke patients appeared to show no difference (Anderson *et al.* 1991; Nighoghossian *et al.* 1995). Hyperbaric oxygen facilities have claimed some success in treating patients in the chronic period following stroke, with advertisements and Internet websites recounting positive results in series of treated patients. No scientifically adequate randomized trials, however, have as yet supported the use of hyperbaric oxygen therapy in either acute stroke or stroke rehabilitation.

Neural Transplants in Stroke Rehabilitation

Another breakthrough in the rehabilitation of patients with brain injury may be the use of cell transplants into areas damaged by strokes. At the University of Pittsburgh, 12 patients who suffered major strokes more than 1 year prior to surgery received cell transplants into the area of damage. The cells used were 'stem' neuronal cells originally derived from a testicular tumor (Kondziolka *et al.* 2000). In a brief follow-up report, 11 of 12 transplant patients showed increased glucose uptake by PET scan after transplant, and modest clinical improvement by the NIH Stroke Scale was reported in 8 of 12 patients; 1 showed no change, and 3 patients deteriorated (Kondziolka *et al.* 2000). Although the follow-up has been too short to demonstrate definite recovery of function, these early results show promise for the use of stem cells in the treatment of neurobehavioral deficits after stroke. Larger studies of stem cell implantation in stroke patients are planned.

Transcranial Magnetic Stimulation in Neurorehabilitation

Transcranial magnetic stimulation has been used to map the motor cortex, as cited above. In addition, there is some evidence that repetitive trains of magnetic stimulation can excite cortical tissue and potentially facilitate performance of cognitive tasks. Facilitation of picture naming after repetitive stimulation of the left hemisphere Wernicke's area (Mottaghy *et al.* 1999) and shortening of response time in an analogical reasoning task after left prefrontal magnetic stimulation (Boroojerdi *et al.* 2001) have been reported. These studies have involved only normal subjects, and both reported results in terms of reduced response times rather than improvement in actual error rates. These applications of magnetic stimulation are in their infancy, but repetitive transcranial magnetic stimulation appears to have promise in neurorehabilitation (Triggs and Kirshner 2001).

Pharmacotherapy in Rehabilitation

Another new area of stroke rehabilitation is the use of drugs to facilitate neurologic recovery. Bromocriptine has been used with some success in patients with non-fluent aphasia (Albert *et al.* 1988), though randomized clinical trials have failed to support its efficacy (Gupta 1995). Amphetamines have been used experimentally in stroke rehabilitation patients to improve motor recovery (Davis *et al.* 1987; Walker-Batson *et al.* 1995), hemineglect (Crisostomo *et al.* 1988), and aphasia (Walker-Batson, 2000). A clinical trial is currently underway testing the use of amphetamines in stroke patients undergoing rehabilitation (Goldstein L, personal communication). Milder stimulants such as amantadine have been used in patients with traumatic brain injury (Gualtieri *et al.* 1989; Nickels *et al.* 1994). Routine use of stimulants such as amphetamines in stroke patients is probably not warranted at present, but patients who are somnolent to the point of interference with therapy can be tried on amphetamine regimens. An experimental drug, piracetam, a gamma aminobytyric acid (GABA)-like compound used extensively in Europe as a 'nootropic' agent or stimulant of cognitive reorganization, has been applied to stroke rehabilitation (Enderby *et al.* 1994) and as an adjunct to aphasia therapy (Huber *et al.* 1997). The drug is not available in the USA, but is related to the antiepileptic drug leviteracetam (Keppra).

Attention should also be paid to avoidance of medications that impede recovery. One randomized study of an experimental agent in stroke rehabilitation also examined concurrent drug use. This study found that four classes of medication were associated with reduced or delayed recovery: (1) benzodiazepines; (2) antiepileptic drugs, particularly phenytoin, carbamazepine, and phenobarbital; (3) antihypertensive agents such as clonidine or prazocin; and (4) neuroleptics (Goldstein *et al.* 1995). Avoidance of these drugs as much as clinically feasible is advised. Other medications interfere with bladder function in stroke patients, and should likewise be avoided. These include diuretics that overfill the bladder, anticholinergics and narcotics that inhibit detrusor contraction, alpha adrenergic antihypertensive agents that increase internal sphincter tone, and alpha blockers that decrease sphincter tone (Staskin 1991). Some of the same agents interfere with sexual function, as do the selective serotonin reuptake inhibitors used to treat depression. In summary, close attention to medication use in stroke, for both positive and negative effects, is important in the overall planning of rehabilitation for stroke patients.

REHABILITATION THERAPIES

The traditional modalities of physical, occupational, and speech therapy provide the meat of rehabilitation programs. Physical therapists work to strengthen weak muscles through exercise and to increase mobility, beginning with changes in position in bed ('bed mobility'), proceeding to transfers from bed to chair and chair to commode, then to wheelchair propulsion, and finally to walking. Occupational therapists deal with independence in activities of daily living, including dressing, grooming, bathing, feeding, and higher level activities such as cooking, shopping, and making financial decisions. Occupational therapists also work with upper limb weakness and incoordination, and they assist physical therapists in transfers and gait training. Speech pathologists address not only speech and language disorders, but also cognitive function and swallowing. Speech pathologists, along with occupational therapists and psychologists, provide 'cognitive rehabilitation' for patients with behavioral or cognitive disorders. Recreational therapists help not only with leisure activities but also with the application of newly learned skills to the 'real world' setting, on outings and community re-entry programs. Rehabilitation nurses are important members of the rehabilitation team, providing continuity between therapy sessions and the hospital ward in terms of the patient's increasing functional independence in bathing, dressing, grooming, toileting, feeding, and taking medications. Nurses, psychologists, and social workers or case managers all help the physician with patient care and with discharge planning. The physician leads the team, educates and cheers on the patient and family, and also melds therapy goals to the patient's disease and prognosis. In short, all members of the multidisciplinary team contribute to the rehabilitation of the patient (Kirshner 1997).

REHABILITATION GOALS

Although the scientific evidence for efficacy of specific rehabilitation techniques is limited, rehabilitative therapies have become a standard of care for the rehabilitation of stroke patients (Gresham *et al.* 1995). Rehabilitative therapies in inpatient units, home health services, and outpatient facilities all have the same goals: (1) to facilitate spontaneous recovery of lost functions; (2) to provide compensatory strategies to deal with remaining deficits; and (3) to help the patient achieve independence in activities of daily living (ADLs) and, if possible, in return to work.

Where independence is not feasible, family training is important to permit home discharge. Treatment of the stroke patient in a rehabilitation setting requires the physician to ensure that measures have been taken to prevent stroke extension or recurrence, to avoid or treat complications of stroke, to provide psychological support, and to supervise the rehabilitative therapists, including prescription of adaptive equipment such as canes, walkers, wheelchairs, hospital beds, and bathroom equipment.

MEDICAL COMPLICATIONS OF STROKE

One of the major roles of the rehabilitation physician is the prevention and treatment of medical complications following stroke. Medical complications include:

1. Dysphagia and aspiration pneumonia
2. Deep vein thrombophlebitis (DVT) and pulmonary embolism
3. Incontinence, urinary tract infections, constipation, and sexual dysfunction
4. Skin breakdown
5. Orthopedic complications such as shoulder–hand syndrome and falls
6. Post-stroke pain
7. Spasticity
7. Seizures
8. Post-stroke depression.

Since this review emphasizes the rehabilitation of neurobehavioral deficits related to stroke, we shall consider here only the issues of post-stroke sexual dysfunction and post-stroke depression. Three recent reviews have provided information on other medical complications of stroke (Kalra *et al.* 1995; Johnston *et al.* 1998; Van der Worp and Kappelle 1998).

Sexual Dysfunction after Stroke

Sexual dysfunction is very common after stroke. In general, most stroke patients of both genders remain interested in sex, but the ability to perform declines (Mongra *et al.* 1986). In one study, male stroke patients' ability to achieve erection declined from 75% to 46% after stroke, ejaculation decreased from 88% to 29%, and female orgasms dropped from 45% to 9% (Bray 1981). It is not clear what portion of the reduced sexual dysfunction is related to the focal brain injury, the physical impairments caused by the stroke, or psychological factors such as depression and altered personal relationships. Erection in males requires the functioning of limbic and thalamic regions that may be damaged by strokes, but erection also involves psychological attitudes, including the ability to use the imagination and to conceptualize sexual arousal (Krane *et al.* 1989). Korpelainen and colleagues (1999) found that, while erectile function and vaginal lubrication were diminished after stroke, behavioral factors were also highly correlated with sexual dissatisfaction; these factors included disturbed attitude towards sexuality and inability to discuss it with spouses. After a stroke in one spouse, 33% of stroke patients and 27% of spouses reported total cessation of sexual activity. Many stroke patients fear that sexual activity will be harmful, or that the spouse will not desire it.

As the Pfizer commercial states, diagnosis of sexual or erectile dysfunction does not require sophisticated laboratory tests, but only a conversation. Physicians often fail to bring up the subject of sexuality in their discussions with stroke patients. Freud considered the goals of psychotherapy to be 'arbeit und liebe' (to work and to make love); perhaps these would be worthy goals for the rehabilitation physician as well. Physicians should try to eliminate medications that interfere with sexual functioning, including specific antihypertensive and antidepressant medications. Counseling, teaching of behavioral techniques or positioning techniques (Boldrini et al. 1991), and use of sildenafil (Viagra; Goldstein et al. 1998) or referral to a urologist for penile injections or implants should be offered (Murray et al. 1995).

Post-stroke Emotional Changes

Post-stroke depression is a major impediment to successful stroke rehabilitation. As discussed in Chapter 17, studies have shown an increased incidence of depression in patients with left as opposed to right hemisphere strokes, and anterior more than posterior hemisphere strokes (Starkstein et al. 1984; Robinson 1997). Not all studies have confirmed these findings, especially the left versus right dimension (Sinyor et al. 1986; Ghika-Schmid and Bogousslavsky 1997). Right hemisphere stroke patients may have indifference rather than depression in the early period after stroke, but later they become dysphoric and depressed. Studies conducted 4 months or more after stroke show little difference in overall incidence of depression between left and right hemisphere strokes (Robinson 2000). Hence the apparent association of depression with left hemisphere, and especially left anterior, damage may be an artifact of the early testing period. Over time, patients with strokes on either side are likely to suffer from depression. Early identification of post-stroke depression and treatment with antidepressant medications and supportive counseling is essential. The newer selective serotonin reuptake inhibitors such as fluoxetine, sertraline, paroxetine, and citalopram are better tolerated than traditional tricyclic antidepressant drugs, though a recent study by Robinson and colleagues (2000) found that nortriptyline was more effective than fluoxetine in the treatment of post-stroke depression.

A related topic is the emotional lability seen after stroke, or 'pathological laughter and crying' (see also Chapter 17). Many stroke patients have this symptom either with or without depression. Robinson and colleagues (1993) did not find the same association with left frontal lesions that they found with depression. Brainstem and subcortical strokes, especially when bilateral, are commonly associated with emotional lability (Robinson et al. 1993, Kim and Choi-Kwan 2000). Easy crying is also seen in many patients with unilateral right hemisphere strokes, though those with bilateral lesions are especially likely to show this phenomenon. Antidepressants may also be of some use in blunting the affective displays in emotionally labile stroke patients.

Mania is a rather rare emotional consequence of stroke. Starkstein and colleagues (1987) reported mania in approximately 1% of 300 stroke patients. Lesions were usually in the right hemisphere or bilateral (Starkstein *et al.* 1988). Further consideration of 'organic mania' may be found in Chapter 15 (psychosis).

PRACTICAL AND ECONOMIC ASPECTS OF STROKE REHABILITATION

In practical terms, third-party payers dictate early discharge of stroke patients from the acute hospital, and the inpatient rehabilitation unit provides an interim placement for the patient and family to prepare for care at home. In the UK and Europe, many hospitals have combined acute stroke and stroke rehabilitation units; the evidence for improved outcome in patients treated in such units as compared to general hospital wards will be discussed later. In the USA, subacute units and skilled nursing facilities compete with inpatient rehabilitation hospitals as sites for rehabilitation therapies. These facilities offer rehabilitation in less intensive formats that are less expensive and may be more suitable for low-level, elderly stroke patients who cannot tolerate a full schedule of inpatient rehabilitation. An ideal rehabilitation plan might be to transfer a low-level patient from the acute hospital to a subacute or skilled nursing facility, then on to inpatient rehabilitation when progress justifies more intensive therapy. Though it has been traditional to provide intensive therapy immediately, even in patients with severe deficits, there is some evidence that severely impaired patients may benefit more from intensive rehabilitation after a period of recuperation. Studies of global aphasia, for example, have suggested that some patients actually recover more during the second 6 months after a stroke than during the first 6 months (Sarno and Levita 1971).

Selection of Patients for Stroke Rehabilitation and Prediction of Outcome

The first task of any rehabilitation program is the proper selection of patients. Patients with mild deficits can usually be discharged home and receive outpatient therapies, while those with severe deficits may not benefit from intensive inpatient rehabilitation and may be more appropriate for subacute or skilled nursing units. Too often, undue rehabilitative efforts are expended on the most severely ill patients, who can benefit least. The best candidates for inpatient rehabilitation are the moderately impaired, who are unable to return home initially but have a good chance of eventual independence. From a variety of studies on outcome following stroke, the following factors have been identified as poor prognostic indicators:

1. Initial coma
2. Urinary incontinence (Wade and Hewer 1985)
3. Complete hemiplegia, especially when accompanied by sensory loss

4. Severe unilateral neglect, global aphasia with inability to follow commands, or general confusion
5. History of multiple strokes
6. Severe cardiac or medical disease with lack of endurance
7. Lack of a caregiver (Jongbloed 1986; Galski *et al.* 1993; Taub *et al.* 1994).

Any one of these factors, however, can be misleading in individual cases. Advanced age by itself should not exclude a patient from rehabilitation, but it does influence endurance, medical stability, and ability to benefit from therapy. Dobkin (1996) listed the following criteria for admission to an inpatient rehabilitation hospital after stroke: the patient must (1) be medically stable enough to tolerate 3 hours of therapy per day; (2) need more than minimal assistance for ambulation and self-care; (3) be motivated and have adequate cognition and language function to participate in treatments; and (4) have adequate social supports to anticipate a return home. Gresham *et al.* (1995) provide similar recommendations on behalf of the US Public Health Service.

A closely related subject to the eligibility of patients for stroke rehabilitation is the prediction of functional outcomes. Multivariate models (Barer 1989; Alexander 1994) have largely echoed the prognostic factors for individual patients, as cited above. One simple factor is the number of deficits a stroke patient manifests. Reding and Potes (1988) reported that patients with pure motor hemiparesis walked with assistance at 12 weeks, and 65% were independent in ADLs at 12 weeks. Patients who had both hemiparesis and either hemisensory loss or hemianopsia did not walk until 22 weeks. Patients who had motor, sensory, and visual field deficits did not walk until 28 weeks, and only 10 % regained independence in ADLs. These simple gradations of deficit do not take into account cognitive or language deficits, which surely influence recovery (Novack *et al.* 1987; Galski *et al.* 1993). Gompertz and colleagues (1994) also compiled a G-score (see Table 21.1) for outcome prediction; scores of 1–2 were associated with good, 3–4 intermediate, and 5–7 poor outcome.

Table 21.1 The G-score (Gompertz *et al.* 1994)

Criterion	Point scores
Complete paralysis of any limb	1 point
Motor + sensory + cortical deficit	1 point
Initial loss of consciousness	1 point
Drowsiness at 24 hours	1 point
Age <50	1 point
Age 50–75	2 points
Age >75	3 points
Isolated (pure motor) hemiparesis	−1 point

Evidence for Efficacy of Stroke Rehabilitation

Although many studies have examined the efficacy of rehabilitative therapies, few are truly randomized or placebo controlled. Nonetheless, considerable
evidence points to a beneficial effect of rehabilitation. Several studies have compared patients given therapy on specialized stroke or rehabilitation units to those
treated on traditional wards, and all indicate a better outcome in the specialized
units, usually in a shorter time (Garraway *et al.* 1980; Strand *et al.* 1985;
Indredavik *et al.* 1991; Kalra *et al.* 1996). In the UK and Europe, care on such
stroke units combines the acute stroke units and stroke rehabilitation units as
organized in the USA. Specialists trained in prevention and treatment of medical
complications of stroke and in the utilization of interdisciplinary therapy programs
likely make the stroke care more efficient and effective. A meta-analysis by
Ottenbacher and Jannell (1993) of 3,717 stroke patients in 36 studies indicated
that patients treated in rehabilitation programs fared better in measures of gait,
upper limb function, independence in ADLs, and visuospatial function than those
not referred to such programs, and the treatment effect was especially strong
in younger patients treated soon after stroke onset. These studies also indicate
a higher percentage of home discharge and return to work in patients undergoing intensive rehabilitation programs. While evidence is limited for specific rehabilitation techniques, these studies clearly indicate that patients recover better
when provided with an intensive exposure to rehabilitative therapies in a hospital setting, as compared to routine hospital care followed by discharge to home
or nursing facility.

A currently controversial issue is the selection of inpatient rehabilitation
hospital versus subacute units or skilled nursing facilities for rehabilitation of
stroke patients. Such units provide rehabilitative therapies, though usually only
one of each therapy per day, or less than half the therapy provided on the typical
inpatient rehabilitation unit. One comparative study found that patients in inpatient rehabilitation improved faster than subacute patients, but the overall cost
was twice as high, and the relative cost per gain in functional independence measures (FIM) was 1.5 (Keith *et al.* 1995). A more recent study found that inpatient
rehabilitation resulted in better outcome as compared to subacute rehabilitation
in stroke patients, but not in hip fracture patients (Kramer 1997). The intensity
of rehabilitation therapies may be a predictor of outcome (Kwakkel *et al.* 1997).
Since rehabilitation is so costly, further studies are clearly needed.

CONCLUSION

More than 500,000 patients survive strokes each year in the USA, and
increasing resources are being devoted to stroke rehabilitation. Scientific evidence
has supported the importance of rehabilitative therapies in facilitating the remodeling of the cerebral cortex following a stroke or brain injury. Practical evidence
favors intensive rehabilitation programs for patients who are alert and able to
cooperate but have moderate stroke deficits. More severely affected patients are

more appropriately treated in subacute or skilled nursing facilities until their progress justifies transfer to an acute rehabilitation unit. Studies of the efficacy of specific therapy techniques and of intensive versus subacute therapy programs are increasingly needed.

REFERENCES

Albert ML, Bachman DL, Morgan A, Helm-Estabrooks N. Pharmacotherapy for aphasia. Neurology 1988;38:877–879.

Alexander MP. Stroke rehabilitation outcome. A potential use of predictive variables to establish levels of care. Stroke 1994;25:128–134.

Anderson DC, Bottini AG, Jagiella WM et al. A pilot study of hyperbaric oxygen in the treatment of human stroke. Stroke 1991;22:1137–1142.

Bach-Y-Rita P. Brain plasticity as a basis for recovery of function in humans. Neuropsychologia 1990;28:547–554.

Barer DH, Mitchell JRA. Predicting the outcome of acute stroke: do multivariate models help? Q J Med 1989;70:27–40.

Boldrini P, Basaglia N, Calanca M. Sexual changes in hemiparetic patients. Arch Phys Med Rehabil 1991;72:202–207.

Boroojerdi B, Phipps M, Kopylev L et al. Enhancing analogical reasoning with rTMS over the left prefrontal cortex. Neurology 2001; 56:526–528.

Bray GP, DeFrank RS, Wolfe TL. Sexual functioning in stroke survivors. Arch Phys Med Rehabil 1981;62:286–288.

Broca P. Remarques sur le siege de la faculte du langage articule, suivies d'une observation d'aphemie (perte de la parole). Bull Soc Anat Paris 1861;6:330–357.

Cappa SF, Perani D, Grassi F, et al. A PET follow-up study of recovery after stroke in acute aphasics. Brain Lang 1997;56:55–67.

Cramer SC, Chopp M. Recovery recapitulates ontogeny. Trends Neurosci 2000;28: 265–271.

Crisostomo EA, Duncan PW, Propst MA et al. Evidence that amphetamine with physical therapy promotes recovery of motor function in stroke patients. Ann Neurol 1988;23:94–97.

Davis JN, Crisostomo EA, Duncan P et al. Amphetamine and physical therapy facilitate recovery of function from stroke: correlative animal and human studies. In MR Raichle, WJ Powers (eds), Cerebrovascular Disorders. New York: Raven Press, 1987;297–305.

Dettmers C, Stephan KM, Lemon RN, Frackowiak RSJ. Reorganization of the executive motor system after stroke. Cerebrovasc Dis 1997;7:187–200.

Dobkin BH. Neurologic Rehabilitation. Philadelphia: F.A. Davis Company, 1996;Chapter 7.

Elbert T, Pantev C, Wienbruch C et al. Increased cortical representation of the fingers of the left hand in string players. Science 1995;270:305–307.

Enderby P, Broeckx J, Hospers W et al. Effect of piracetam on recovery and rehabilitation after stroke: a double-blind, placebo-controlled study. Clin Neuropharm 1994;17: 320–331.

Ferro JM, Mariano G, Madureira S. Recovery from aphasia and neglect. Cerebrovasc Dis 1999;9(Suppl. 5):6–22.

Galski T, Bruno R, Zorowitz R et al. Predicting length of stay, functional outcome, and aftercare in the rehabilitation of stroke patients. Stroke 1993;24:1794–1800.

Garraway WM, Akhtar AM, Prescott RJ, Hockey L. Management of acute stroke in the elderly: preliminary results of a controlled trial. Br Med J 1980;280:1040–1043.

Ghika-Schmid F, Bogousslavsky J. Affective disorders following stroke. Eur Neurol 1997;38:75–81.

Goldstein LB, and The Sygen in Acute Stroke Study Investigators. Common drugs may influence motor recovery after stroke. Neurology 1995;45:865–871.

Goldstein I, Lue TF, Padma-Nathan H *et al.* Oral sildenafil in the treatment of erectile dysfunction. New Engl J Med 1998;338:1397–1404.

Gompertz P, Pound P, Ebrahim S. Predicting stroke outcome: Guy's prognostic score in practice. J Neurol Neurosurg Psychiat 1994;57:932–935.

Gresham GE, Fitzpatrick TE, Wolf PA *et al.* Residual disability in survivors of stroke – the Framingham study. New Engl J Med 1975;293:954–956.

Gresham GE, Duncan P, Stason W *et al.* Post–Stroke Rehabilitation: Assessment, Referral, and Patient Management: Clinical Practice Guideline No. 16. Rockville, MD: 1995, Agency for Health Care Policy and Research Pub No. 95–0663.

Gualtieri T, Chandler M, Coons TB, Brown LT. Amantadine: a new clinical profile for traumatic brain injury. Clin Neuropharm 1989;12:258–270.

Gupta SR, Mlcoch AG, Scolaro C, Mortiz T. Bromocriptine treatment of non-fluent aphasia. Neurology 1995;45:865–871.

Hartman J, Landau WM. Comparison of formal language therapy with supportive counseling for aphasia due to acute vascular accident. Arch Neurol 1987;44:646–649.

Heiss W-D, Karbe H, Weber-Luxenburger G *et al.* Speech-induced cerebral metabolic activation reflects recovery from aphasia. J Neurol Sci 1997;145:213–217.

Heiss W-D, Kessler J, Thiel A *et al.* Differential capacity of left and right hemispheric areas for compensation of post-stroke aphasia. Ann Neurol 1999;45:430–438; see also Heiss W-D, Kessler J, Karbe H *et al.* Cerebral glucose metabolism as a predictor of recovery from aphasia in ischemic stroke. Arch Neurol 1993;50:958–964.

Hillis AE, Barker P, Beauchamp N *et al.* MR perfusion imaging reveals regions of hypoperfusion associated with aphasia and neglect. Neurology 2000;55:782–788.

Hillis AE, Wityk RJ, Tuffiash E *et al.* Hypoperfusion of Wernicke's area predicts severity of semantic deficit in acute stroke. Ann Neurol 2001; in press.

Hoenig H, Horner RD, Duncan PW *et al.* New horizons in stroke rehabilitation research. J Rehab Res Dev 1999;36:19–31.

Huber W, Willmes K, Poeck K *et al.* Piracetam as an adjuvant to language therapy for aphasia: a randomized double-blind placebo-controlled study. Arch Phys Med Rehabil 1997;78:245–250.

Illis LS, Sedgwick EM, Glanville HJ. Rehabilitation of the Neurological Patient. Oxford: Blackwell Scientific Publications, 1982;1.

Indredavik B, Bakke F, Solberg R *et al.* Benefit of a stroke unit: a randomized controlled trial. Stroke 1991;22:1026–1031.

Johnston KC, Li JY, Lyden PD *et al.* Medical and neurological complications of ischemic stroke. Experience from the RANTTAS trial. Stroke 1998;29:447–453.

Jongbloed L. Prediction of function after stroke: a critical review. Stroke 1986;17:765–776.

Kalra L, Yu G, Wilson K, Roots P. Medical complications during stroke rehabilitation. Stroke 1995;26:990–994.

Kalra L, Eade J, Wittink M. Stroke rehabilitation units: randomized trials and mainstream practice. Cerebrovasc Dis 1996;6:266–271.

Katz RC, Wertz RT. The efficacy of computer-provided reading treatment for chronic aphasic adults. J Speech Hear Res 1997;40:493–507.

Keith RA, Wilson DB, Gutierrez P. Acute and subacute rehabilitation for stroke: a comparison. Arch Phys Med Rehabil 1995;76:495–500.

Kim JS, Choi-Kwon S. Post-stroke depression and emotional incontinence. Correlation with lesion location. Neurology 2000;54:1805–1810.

Kirshner HS. Stroke rehabilitation, 1997. Tenn Med 1997;90:147–149.

Kirshner HS. Behavioral neurology in the emergency room: Language testing, brain imaging, and acute stroke therapy. Ann Neurol 2001; in press.

Kirshner HS, Alexander M, Lorch MP, Wertz RT. Disorders of speech and language. Continuum 1999;5:171–187.

Kondziolka D, Wechsler L, Goldstein S et al. Transplantation of cultured human neuronal cells for patients with stroke. Neurology 2000;55:565–569.

Korpelainen JT, Nieminen P, Myllyla VV. Sexual functioning among stroke patients and their spouses. Stroke 1999;30:715–719.

Kramer AM, Steiner JF, Schlenker RE et al. Outcomes and costs after hip fracture and stroke. A comparison of rehabilitation settings. JAMA 1997;277:396–404.

Krane RJ, Goldstein I, Tejada IS. Impotence. New Engl J Med 1989;321:1648–1659.

Kwakkel G, Wagenaar RC, Koelman TW et al. Effects of intensity of rehabilitation after stroke. A research synthesis. Stroke 1997;28:1550–1556.

Liepert J, Bauder H, Miltner WHR et al. Treatment-induced cortical reorganization after stroke in humans. Stroke 2000;31:1210–1216.

Mongra T, Lawson J, Inglis J. Sexual dysfunction in stroke patients. Arch Phys Med Rehabil 1986;67:19–22.

Mottaghy FM, Hungs M, Brugmann M et al. Facilitation of picture naming after repetitive transcranial magnetic stimulation. Neurology 1999;53:1806–1812.

Murray FT, Geisser M, Murphy TC. Evaluation and treatment of erectile dysfunction. Am J Med Sci 1995;309:99–109.

Nelles G, Spiekermann G, Jueptner M et al. Evolution of functional reorganization in hemiplegic stroke: A serial positron emission tomographic activation study. Ann Neurol 1999;46:901–909.

Nickels JL, Schneider WN, Dombovy ML, Wong TM. Clinical use of amantadine in brain injury rehabilitation. Brain Injury 1994;8:709–718.

Nighoghossian N, Trouillas P. Hyperbaric oxygen in the treatment of acute ischemic stroke: an unsettled issue. J Neurol Sci 1997;150:27–31.

Nighoghossian N, Trouillas P, Adeleine P, Salord F. Hyperbaric oxygen in the treatment of acute ischemic stroke. A double-blind pilot study. Stroke 1995;26:1369–1372.

Novack T, Haban G, Graham K et al. Prediction of stroke rehabilitation outcome from psychological screening. Arch Phys Med Rehabil 1987;68:729–734.

Nudo RJ, Milliken GW. Reorganization of movement representations in primary motor cortex following focal ischemic infarcts in adult squirrel monkeys. J Neurophysiol 1996;75:2144–2149.

Nudo RJ, Wise B, SiFuentes, Milliken GW. Neural substrates for the effects of rehabilitative training on motor recovery after ischemic infarct. Science 1996;272:1791–1794.

Ottenbacher K, Jannell S. The results of clinical trials in stroke rehabilitation research. Arch Neurol 1993;50:37–44.

Pascual-Leone A, Wassermann EM, Sadato N, Hallet M. The role of reading activity on the modulation of motor cortical outputs to the reading hand in Braille readers. Ann Neurol 1995;38:910–915.

Perani D, Vallar G, Paulesu E et al. Left and right hemisphere contributions to recovery from neglect after right hemisphere damage – An {18F}FDG PET study of two cases. Neuropsychologia 1993;31:115–125.

Pizzamiglio L, Antonucci G, Judica A et al. Cognitive rehabilitation of the hemineglect disorder in chrionic patients with unilateral right brain damage. J Clin Exp Neuropsychol 1992;14:901–923.

Reding MJ, Potes E. Rehabilitation outcome following initial unilateral hemispheric stroke: life table analysis approach. Stroke 1988;19:1354–1358.

Robertson IH, Tegner R, Tham K et al. Sustained attention training for unilateral neglect: theoretical and rehabilitation implications. J Clin Exp Neuropsychol 1995;17:416–430.

Robey RR. A meta-analysis of clinical outcomes in the treatment of aphasia. J Speech Lang Hear Res 1998;41:172–187.

Robinson RG. Neuropsychiatric consequences of stroke. Ann Rev Med 1997;48:217–229.

Robinson RG. An 82-year-old woman with mood changes following a stroke. Clinical Crossroads. JAMA 2000;283:1607–1614.

Robinson RG, Parikh RM, Lipsey JR *et al.* Pathological laughing and crying following stroke: validation of a measurement scale and a double-blind treatment study. Am J Psychiatry 1993;150:286–293.

Robinson RG, Schultz SK, Castillo C *et al.* Nortriptyline vs. fluoxetine in the treatment of depression and short-term recovery following stroke: a placebo controlled double-blind study. Am J Psychiatry 2000;157:351–359.

Rossetti Y, Rode G, Pisella L *et al.* Prismadaptation to a rightward optical deviation rehabilitates left hemispatial neglect. Nature 1998;395:166–169.

Sarno M, Levita E. Natural course of recovery in severe aphasia. Arch Phys Med Rehabil 1971;52:175–178.

Sinyor D, Jacques P, Kaloupek DG *et al.* Post-stroke depression and lesion localization: an attempted replication. Brain 1986;109:537–546.

Starkstein SE, Kubos KL, Starr LB *et al.* Mood disorders in stroke patients: importance of lesion localization Brain 1984;107:81–93.

Starkstein SF, Pearlson GD, Boston J, Robinson RG. Mania after brain injury. A controlled study of causative factors. Arch Neurol 1987;44:1069–1073.

Starkstein SE, Boston JD, Robinson RG. Mechanisms of mania after brain injury. 12 case reports and review of the literature. J Nerv Ment Dis 1988;176:87–100.

Staskin SR. Intracranial lesions that affect lower urinary tract function. In RJ Krane, MB Siroky (eds), Clinical Neuro-urology (2nd edn). Boston: Little, Brown, 1991;345–353.

Sterr A, Muller MM, Elbert T *et al.* Changed perceptions in Braille readers. Nature 1998;391:134–135.

Strand T, Asplund K, Eriksson S *et al.* A non-intensive stroke unit reduces functional disability and the need for long-term hospitalization. Stroke 1985;17:377–381.

Taub E, Miller NE, Novack TA *et al.* Technique to improve chronic motor deficit after stroke. Arch Phys Med Rehabil 1993;74:347–354.

Taub E, Crago JE, Uswatte G. Constraint-induced movement therapy, a new approach to treatment in physical rehabilitation. Rehab Psychol 1998;43:152–170.

Taub N, Wolfe C, Richardson E *et al.* Predicting the disability of first-time stroke sufferers at 1 year. Stroke 1994;25:352–357.

Triggs WJ, Kirshner HS. Improving brain function with transcranial magnetic stimulation? Neurology 2001;56:429–430.

Van der Worp HB, Kappelle LJ. Complications of acute ischaemic stroke. Cerebrovasc Dis 1998;8:124–132.

Wade DT, Hewer RL. Outlook after an acute stroke: urinary incontinence and loss of consciousness compared in 532 patients. Q J Med 1985;56:601–608.

Walker-Batson D. Use of pharmacotherapy in the treatment of aphasia. Brain Lang 2000;71:252–254.

Walker-Batson D, Smith P, Curtis S *et al.* Amphetamine paired with physical therapy accelerates motor recovery after stroke. Further evidence. Stroke 1995;26:2254–2259.

Weiller C, Isensee C, Rijintes M *et al.* Recovery from Wernicke's aphasia: a positron emission tomographic study. Ann Neurol 1995;37:723–732.

Weinberg J, Diller L, Gordon WA *et al.* Visual scanning training effect on reading-related tasks in acquired right brain damage. Arch Phys Med Rehabil 1977;58:479–486.

Wertz RT. Efficacy. In C Code, D Muller (eds), The Treatment of Aphasia: From Theory to Practice. London: Whurr Publishers Ltd, 1995;303–339.

Wertz RT, Weiss DG, Aten J *et al.* Comparison of clinic, home, and deferred language treatment for aphasia: a Veterans Administration cooperative study. Arch Neurol 1986;43:653–658.

Whurr R, Lorch MP, Nye C. A meta-analysis of studies carried out between 1946 and 1988 concerned with the efficacy of speech and language therapy treatment for aphasic patients. Eur J Dis Commun 1992;27:1–17.

Wiart L, Saintcome AB, Debelleix X *et al.* Unilateral neglect syndrome rehabilitation by trunk rotation and scanning training. Arch Phys Med Rehabil 1997;78:424–429.

Index

Page numbers printed in **bold** type refer to figures; those in *italic* to tables

Ablative surgery, in epilepsy, 388, 404
Abstract reasoning:
    in multiple sclerosis, 379
    testing, 38
Abstraction:
    in delirium, 313
    in frontal lobe dysfunction, *181*, 186
Abulia, 20, 171
    causes, 182, 194
    in frontal lobe dysfunction, 182, 184,
        191, 193, 194
    in traumatic brain injury, 417
Acalculia, 99–101, *102*
Accident neurosis, 421
N-Acetyl aspartate (NAA),
    in schizophrenia, 331
Acetylcholinesterase inhibitors,
    in Alzheimer's disease, 282
Achromatopsia, 141
Acute brain syndrome, *see* Delirium
Acute confusional state, *see* Delirium
Acute psychotic break, 327
Addison's disease, causing delirium, 316
Affect, assessment of, 30–1, 37–8
Affective agnosia, 173
Affective disorders, 332–6
    see also Bipolar affective disorder;
        Depression; Mania
Afferent agraphia, 117–18
Age associated memory impairment,
    see Mild cognitive impairment
Aggression, in epilepsy, 401–4
    ictal violence, 402–4

interictal *v.* ictal/postictal, 404
    treatment, 403
Aging:
    and Alzheimer's disease, 284
    and cognition, 248–9
    and dementia, 247–8
    intellectual functions deteriorating, 248
    intellectual functions preserved, 248
Agnosia(s), 137–58
    affective, 173
    auditory, *see* Auditory agnosia(s)
    color agnosia, 104, 141
    definition, 137
    diagnostic criteria, 137–8
    finger agnosia, 70, 101–2, *102*
    lesions, 138
    in multiple sclerosis, 379
    tactile, 36, 151–2
    types of, 137–8
    visual, *see* Visual agnosia(s)
Agoraphobia, 367
Agrammatism, 113–14
Agranular cortex, 12
Agraphesthesia, 151
Agraphia(s), 97–8, 99, *102,* 112–19
    afferent, 117–18
    allographic, 117
    aphasic, 113–14, 115
    apraxic, 115, 117
    of Broca's aphasia, 54–5
    callosal, 115–16
    central, 113–14
    classification, 113, 114

Agraphia(s) – *continued*
  constructional, 117–18
  deep agraphia, 115
  definition, 112
  graphemic buffer agraphia, 116–17
  ideational, 117
  isolated, 118, 119
  lexical, 114
  non-aphasic, 116
  orthographic, 114
  peripheral, 116–18
  phonological, 114–15
  physical-letter-code agraphia, 117
  pure agraphia, *see* Pure agraphia
  semantic, 115
  spatial, 117–18
  spelling in, 114, 115, 116–17
  surface, 114
  transitional, *see* Apraxic agraphia
  unilateral, 115–16
  visuospatial, 117–18
  see also Alexia with agraphia
AIDS dementia complex, 259, 270
Akinesia, *see* Hemiakinesia
Akinetic mutism, 20, 22, 171
  causes, 182, 194
  in frontal lobe dysfunction, 182, 184,
      191, 194
  in traumatic brain injury, 417
Akinetopsia, 141
Alcohol:
  blackouts, 224, 226, 403
  withdrawal, and delirium, 317
Alcoholic dementia, 258
Alcoholic hallucinosis, and delirium, 317
Alertness, assessment of level of, 30
Alexia(s), 97–8, 98–109, *102*
  with agraphia, *see* Alexia with agraphia
  without agraphia, *see* Alexia without
      agraphia
  angular, *see* Alexia with agraphia
  aphasic (anterior/frontal), 98, 107–9
  categories, 98
  central, *see* Alexia with agraphia
  deep alexia, 110–11
  letter-by-letter reading, 109–10
      see also Alexia without agraphia
  literal alexia, 108
  meaning, 97

  occipital, *see* Alexia without agraphia
  parietal-temporal, *see* Alexia with
      agraphia
  phonological, 111
  posterior, *see* Alexia without agraphia
  psycholinguistic syndromes of, 109–11
  pure, *see* Alexia without agraphia
  semantic, *see* Alexia with agraphia
  subangular, 105
  surface alexia, 111
  third alexia, *see* Aphasic alexia
Alexia with agraphia, 98–103
  v. alexia without agraphia, tests, 107
  anatomy, 99
  associated signs, *98, 99*
  brain imaging, **100–1**
  characteristics, *98, 99*
  localization, *98*
  stroke cases, 99
Alexia without agraphia, 103–7
  v. alexia with agraphia, tests, 107
  associated signs/symptoms, *103,* 104
  causes, 106–7
  characteristics, 103–4, *103*
  disconnection model, **106**
  disconnection syndrome, 104
  lesions, 104, **105**
  localization, *103*
Alexithymia, 369
Alfrey's syndrome, 256
Alice in Wonderland syndrome, 141
Alien hand syndrome, 23, 240–1
Allesthesia, 165
  visual, 141
Allocortex, 16
Allographic agraphia, 117
Allographic variation, 117
Alpha adrenergic antihypertensive
      agents, in stroke patients, 433
Alpha blockers, in stroke patients, 433
Alpha-methyldopa:
  causing delirium, 317
  causing mental changes, 257
Alternating sequence test, **38**
Aluminium:
  deposition in Alzheimer's disease, 282
  and dialysis dementia, 256
Alzheimer's disease, 274–84
  aging and, 284

aluminium deposition in, 282
amyloid deposition in, 281–2
brain imaging, **276**, 276–8, **277**
causing dementia, 262, 271
depression and, 365
diagnosis, 275–8, 292
electroencephalography (EEG) in,
     292–3
etiology, 280–2
genetic factors, 280–1
granulovacuolar degeneration in, 280
incidence, 247
v. Lewy body dementia, 345–6
mood and, 364–5
neuropathology, 278–80, **279**
NINCDS/ADRDA criteria, 275, *275*
'presumed Alzheimer's disease', 293
prevalence, 247
risk factors, 280
tests for, 275–6, 278
treatment, 282–4
see also Senile dementia of the
     Alzheimer type
Alzheimer's Disease Assessment Scale
     (ADAS), 28
Amantadine, in traumatic brain injury,
     433
Aminoacidurias:
   and delirium, 316
   and dementia, 269
Amnesia(s), 207–32
   amnestic syndrome, *see* Amnestic
        syndrome
   anterograde amnesia, 209, 224, 226
   categories, 208
   description, 207
   functional, 208
   global, 224–5
   partial, 208
   for personal identity, 226
   post-traumatic, 422
   psychogenic, 208, 226–7, 403
   retrograde amnesia, 209, 224,
        226, 419
   secondary to medial temporal
        ablations, 219
   transient, 223–5
   for words, 222
   see also Memory loss/disorders

Amnestic aphasia, *see* Anomic aphasia
Amnestic syndrome, 208, 211–13
   diseases associated with, 218–21
   features, 211–12, *212*
   living in eternal present, 212
   memory cues, 214
   neuropsychological mechanism,
        214–15
   primacy effect, 214
   recency effect, 214
   see also Confabulation; Transient
        amnesia
Amorphosynthesis, 167
Amphetamine psychosis, 398
Amphetamines:
   in aphasia, 88
   and delirium, 317
   in hemineglect, 170
   in stroke rehabilitation, 433
Amusia(s), 150–1
Amygdalectomy, 404
Amyloid deposition, in Alzheimer's
     disease, 281–2
Amyloidosis, cerebral, 262
Amyotrophic lateral sclerosis (ALS),
     causing dysarthria, *49, 50*
Anarithmetia, 101
Angiitis:
   granulomatous angiitis, 265–6
   see also Vasculitis
Angioencephalopathy, subacute
     diencephalic, 266
Angular alexia, *see* Alexia with agraphia
Angular gyrus syndrome, 102–3, *102*
Animal naming test, 69
Anisodiaphoria, 159, 165
Anomia, *102*
   color anomia, 70, 104, 141
   disconnection anomia, 70
   semantic, 70
   types, 69
   for verbs and nouns, 70
Anomic aphasia, 68–70
   characteristics, 69, *69*
   lesions, 70
   as stage in recovery from other
        aphasias, 64, 70
Anosognosia, 159, 165, 313
   see also Hemineglect

Anoxia, causing delirium, 315
Anterior alexia, *see* Aphasic alexia
Anterior subcortical aphasia syndromes, 76–9
  brain imaging, **78**
  syndromes, 77
Anterograde amnesia, 209, 224, 226
Anticholinergics:
  causing delirium, 317
  causing mental changes, 257
  and Parkinson's disease, 344
  in stroke patients, 433
Anticholinesterase drugs, in multiple sclerosis, 381
Anticonvulsant therapy:
  in aphasia, 86
  in epilepsy, 403, 404, 405
Antidepressants, 367
  in Alzheimer's disease, 283
  associated with mania, 335, 336
  in epilepsy, 407
  in stroke patients, 436
  in treatment of bipolar affective disorder, 336
Antiepileptics, 404–5, 407
  in bipolar affective disorder, 336, 407
  impeding recovery from stroke, 433
Antihypertensives:
  causing delirium, 317
  impeding recovery from stroke, 86, 433
Antipsychotic agents, and Parkinson's disease, 344
Anton's syndrome, 138, 314
  inverse Anton's syndrome, *see* Blindsight
Anxiety disorders, 367–9
  symptoms, 368
  treatment, 369
Apathetic hyperthyroidism, 257
Apathy, 196
Aphasia(s), 52–83
  amnestic, *see* Anomic aphasia
  anomic, 64, 68–70
  anterior subcortical aphasia syndromes, 76–9
  v. apraxia of speech, 51
  Broca's, *see* Broca's aphasia

'catastrophic reaction', 64, 166, 171, 359, 362
classification, 52–3, 73, **74**
conduction aphasia, *see* Conduction aphasia
conflicting terminology, 47
crossed aphasia in dextrals, 80–1, **81**
definition, 45, 47
dynamic, 71
expressive aphasia, 53
fluent, 73, *102*, 114, 285, 289
global, 64, 79
ideomotor apraxia relationship, 130–1
in left-handers, 76, 79–80
meaning, 97
mixed aphasia, 64
in multiple sclerosis, 379
neuroanatomy, 73
non-fluent, 73, 285, **286–7**, 289
optic, 70, 145–6
pharmacotherapy, 86
in polyglots, 82–3
primary progressive aphasia, *see* Primary progressive aphasia
v. psychosis, 48
recovery of, 88
research, future areas of, 86–8
subcortical, 75–9
tactile, 152
thalamic, 75–6
total aphasia, 64
transcortical, 71–3
  in traumatic brain injury, 417
treatment, efficacy studies, 84–6
Wernicke's, *see* Wernicke's aphasia
see also Agraphia; Alexia(s)
Aphasic agraphia, 113–14, 115
Aphasic alexia, 98, 107–9
Aphemia, 53, 58, 114
Apolipoproteins, 281, 290, 292
Apperceptive prosopagnosia, 146
Apperceptive visual agnosia, 143–4
  and pure word deafness, 148–9
Apraxia(s), 125–36
  buccofacial (oral), *126*, 126, 128, 131
  callosal, 129–30
  conceptual, 132, 133
  constructional, 70, *102*, 126, 126, 159–60

definition, 36, 125
dressing apraxia, *126,* 126, 162–3
of eyelid opening, *126,* 126
in frontal lobe dysfunction, 195
gait apraxia, *126,* 126–7, 271
ideational, *126,* 132–3, 188
ideomotor apraxia, *see* Ideomotor
    apraxia
limb apraxia, 131
limb-kinetic apraxia, *126,* 133–4
neuroanatomic model, 128, **128**
oculomotor apraxia, *126,* 126, 142
oral (buccofacial), *126,* 126,
    129, 131
of speech, *see* Apraxia of speech
tool-use apraxia, 133
traditional apraxias, *126*
types of, 125–6, *126*
verbal, *see* Apraxia of speech
Apraxia of speech, 50–2, *126,* 126
    v. aphasia, 51
    auditory features, *51,* 51
    definition, 50–1
    v. dysarthria, 51, 126
    etiology, 52
    isolated, 58
    localization, 51
Apraxic agraphia, 115, 117
Aprosodias, 173
Archicortex, 16
'Area of concepts', 71, 73
Arteriovenous malformations, 266
Arteritis, giant cell (temporal)
    arteritis, 265
Artificial grammar learning, 211
Asemantic writing, 115
Assessment of mental status, *see* Mental
    status examination
Association cortex, 11
    heteromodal, 14–15, 103
    increasing size of, 11
    right hemisphere reorganization
        after stroke, 431–2
    supramodal, 183
    unimodal, 14
Associative prosopagnosia, 146
Associative tactile agnosia, 151
Associative visual agnosia, 144–5
Astereognosis, 151

Ataxia:
    optic, 142
    sporadic, 351
Ataxia-telangiectasia, 126
Athletes, concussion in, 423
Atrophy, *see* Multisystem atrophy
Attention:
    attention span, in Alzheimer's
        disease, 40
    in delirium, 310–11
    in frontal lobe dysfunction, *181,*
        189, 196
    in multiple sclerosis, 379
    and neglect, 167–8
    requirements of, 310
Attention-arousal hypothesis, 167–8
Atypical presenile dementia, 290–1
Auditory agnosia(s), 36, 148–51
    amusias, 150
    categories of, 148
    cortical deafness, 63, 148
    non-verbal, 150
    pure word deafness, 63, 148–50, **149**
Auditory comprehension:
    in alexia with agraphia, *98,* 99
    in alexia without agraphia,
        103, *103*
    in anomic aphasia, *69,* 69
    in Broca's aphasia, *54,* 54
    in conduction aphasia, *65,* 65
    in global aphasia, *64*
    testing, 35, *35*
    in transcortical aphasias, 71, *71,* 72
    in Wernicke's aphasia, *59,* 60, 63
Auditory cortex, 13
Auditory non-verbal agnosia, 150
    discriminative, 150
    semantic-associative, 150
Automatisms, 390, 402
Awareness, *see* Self-awareness

Baclofen, withdrawal from, causing
    mania, 335
Bacterial endocarditis, causing
    delirium, 317
Bacterial meningitis, causing
    dementia, 259
Balint's syndrome, 141–2
    partial deficits, 142

Barbiturates:
  in epilepsy, 401, 404, 405
  withdrawal, and delirium, 317
Basal temporal language area, 406–7
Behavior:
  in alexia without agraphia, 104
  in anomic aphasia, 69
  in Broca's aphasia, 54
  in conduction aphasia, 65
  in dementia, 251
  in global aphasia, 64
  in Wernicke's aphasia, 59
Behavioral impairments, in right
    hemisphere disorders, 159
Behavioral neurology:
  bedside observation, 4, 7
  contemporary period, 6
  definition, 3
  history, 5–6
  overview, 3–7
Benign senescent forgetfulness, see Mild
    cognitive impairment
Benzodiazepines:
  in Alzheimer's disease, 283
  in anxiety, 368
  in aphasia, 86
  causing transient amnesia, 224
  in delirium tremens, 321
  impeding recovery from stroke, 433
  in panic disorder, 369
  in seizures, 368
  withdrawal from:
    and delirium, 317
    and mania, 335
Benztropine, and Parkinson's
    disease, 344
Bethanechol, 282
Bilingualism, 82
Binswanger's disease, 264
Biological psychiatry, 5
Bipolar affective disorder (BAD), 333–5
  causes, 334
  diagnostic criteria, 333
  hereditary factor, 334
  incidence, 333–4
  late onset, 334–5
  and multiple sclerosis, 382
  pharmacotherapy, 335–6, 407
  prevalence, 333–4

v. schizophrenia, 327–8
  secondary mania, 334
Blessed rating scales, 28
Blindness:
  cortical, see Cortical blindness
  letter blindness, 98, 108
  psychic blindness, 147
  pure word blindness, see Alexia
    without agraphia
  word blindness, 108
Blindsight, 21, 23, 139–40
Blue toes, 265
Bonnet's syndrome, 140
Boston Diagnostic Aphasia Examination
    (BDAE), 52
Bovine spongiform encephalopathy
    (BSE), 261
Boxing injuries, 422–3
Bradykinesia, in Parkinson's disease,
    341, 343
Bradyphrenia, 343
Brain, lateral/medial surfaces, 12
Brain-behavior relationships, 6, 10
Brain damage, hypoxic, and
    amnesia, 220
Brain imaging, 5
  in epilepsy, 388
  in future research, 86–8
  techniques, 6, 46
  see also under specific disorders
Brain injury:
  hypoxic brain damage, and
    amnesia, 220
  traumatic, see Traumatic brain injury
Brain mapping, see
    Electroencephalography
Brain–mind relationships, 3, 4, 19
Brain networks, 6
  consciousness and, 23
  cortical, 16–17
  cortical–subcortical, 16–17
  frontal-subcortical circuits, 181–2, 182
  neurocognitive, 16–17
Brain plasticity, reorganization after
    stroke, 428
  language cortex, 430–1
  motor cortex, 428–30
  right hemisphere association cortex,
    431–2

Brain stimulation:
  causing mood changes, 359, 363
  coma stimulation, 417–18
  in depression, 359, 363, 367
  magnetic, 432–3
  see also Vagus nerve stimulation
Brain trauma, *see* Traumatic brain injury
Brain tumors, *see* Neoplasms; Tumors
Broca's aphasia, 53–8, 107–8, 129
  agraphia of, 54–5
  and apraxia of speech, 51
  apraxic deficits, 132
  associated signs, *54*, 55–6
  auditory comprehension in, *54*, 54
  Baby Broca syndrome, 58
  behavior in, *54*
  Big Broca syndrome, 58
  brain imaging in, *57*
  features, 53–5, *54*
  lesions, *56*
  naming in, *54*, 54
  prognosis, 58
  reading in, *54*, 54
  repetition in, *54*, 54
  spontaneous speech in, 53, *54*
  v. Wernicke's aphasia, 58–9, *60*
  writing in, *54*, 54–5, 116
Broca's area, 17, 53, **55**, 56, **56, 68**
  in epilepsy, 406, 407, **408**
Brodmann areas, **12**, 13
Bromide toxicity, 317
Bromocriptine:
  in aphasia, 72, 86, 88
  associated with mania, 335
  in non-fluent aphasia, 433
  and Parkinson's disease, 344
Brucellosis, and dementia, 259
Buccofacial (oral) apraxia, *126*, 126,
  129, 131
Buproprion, in depression, 367
Buspirone:
  in Alzheimer's disease, 283
  in panic disorder, 369

CADASIL (cerebral autosomal dominant
  arteriopathy with subcortical
  infarcts and leukoencephalopathy),
  263–4
Calcarine sulcus, **11**

Calculations:
  in alexia with agraphia, 107
  in delirium, 312
  in dementia, 251
  testing, 36–7
  see also Numbers
Callosal agraphia, 115–16
Callosal apraxia, 129–30
Callosotomy surgery, 70
Cancer therapy, causing delirium and
  dementia, 268, 317
Capgras syndrome, 213, 311, 314
Carbamazepine:
  in aphasia, 86
  in epilepsy, 403, 404–5, 405, 407
  impeding recovery from stroke, 433
  in treatment of mania/bipolar
    affective disorder, 335, 336
'Catastrophic reaction', 64, 166, 171,
  359, 362
Catatonia, 328
Catecholamines, in depression,
  366, 367
Categories Test (Halstead–Reitan
  Battery), 187
Central agraphias, 113–14
Central alexia, *see* Alexia with agraphia
Cerebral amyloidosis, 262
Cerebral cortex, 9–16
  neuroanatomy, **10**, 11–12
  white matter bundles, 13, **13**
Cerebral emboli, causing delirium, 318
Cerebral lipofuscinosis, and
  dementia, 269
Cerebral tumors, *see* Neoplasms; Tumors
Cerebral vasculitis, causing delirium, 318
Cerebrovascular disease, diagnosis, 292
Chemicals, 317
Chemotherapeutic agents, and
  dementia, 268
Chlorpromazine:
  in epilepsy, 407
  and Parkinson's disease, 344–5
  in schizophrenia, 331
Cholesterol, multiple cholesterol
  emboli, 264–5
Cholesterol-lowering drugs, and
  dementia, 262
Churg–Strauss vasculitis, 265

Cimetidine:
  associated with mania, 335
  causing delirium, 317
  causing mental changes, 257
Citalopram:
  in depression, 367
  in stroke patients, 436
Clang associations:
  in bipolar affective disorder, 47
  in schizophrenia, 329
Clonidine, impeding recovery from
    stroke, 433
Clozapine:
  in Alzheimer's disease, 283–4
  in Parkinson's disease, 345
  in schizophrenia, 332
Cocaine:
  associated with mania, 335
  and delirium, 317
Cognition:
  and aging, 248–9
  in frontal lobe disorders, 185–6
  mild cognitive impairment (MCI), 249
Cognitive changes, in epilepsy, 388
Cognitive deficits/impairment:
  in depression, 366–7
  in multiple sclerosis, 378–81, 382–3
  in Parkinson's disease, 342–3, 344
  in schizophrenia, 328–9
Cognitive fatigue, in multiple sclerosis
    (MS), 379
Cognitive functioning, Rancho Los
    Amigos Scale of Cognitive
    Functioning, 418
Cognitive neuroscience, 5
Collagen vascular diseases, causing
    dementia, 265–6
Color:
  disorders of color vision, 141
  loss of perception of, see
      Achromatopsia
  visual system in monkeys, 21
Color agnosia, 104, 141
Color anomia, 70, 104, 141
Coma stimulation, 417–18
Coma vigile, 20
Commissurotomy:
  split-brain research, 235, 241
  see also Corpus callosotomy entries

Commissurotomy patients, 23, 235
  memory in, 238
  praxis in, 238
Communicating hydrocephalus, 272
Communication:
  in dementia, 251
  right hemisphere functions, 172–3
  see also Language; Speech
Comprehension, see Auditory
    comprehension
Computerized tomography (CT), 46
Computers, therapy programs, 88
Conceptual apraxia, 132, 133
Concussion, 318
  in athletes, 423
  boxing injuries, 422–3
  second impact syndrome, 423
  see also Head injuries; Traumatic
      brain injury
Conduction aphasia, 65–8, 129, 222
  brain imaging, 66, 67
  characteristics, 65, 65
  disconnection theory/syndrome,
      65–6, 68
  lesions, 65–8
  theories of, 68
Confabulation, 199, 212, 213–14
  in Anton's syndrome, 138
Confusion:
  brain imaging, 61
  definition, 31, 307
  global, 166
  in Parkinson's disease, 344–5
Connective tissue disease, 265
Consciousness, 16, 19–24
  in corpus callosotomy patients, 239
  depressed, 20
  diagnostic terminology, 23
  frontal lobes in, 22, 23
  in individual cerebral hemispheres, 236
  lesions impairing, 19–20
  non-Freudian unconscious, 22
Constraint-induced therapy, 429–30
Constructional ability, testing, 37, 37
Constructional agraphia, 117–18
Constructional apraxia, 70, 102, 126,
    126, 159–60
Constructional impairment, 159–62, 161
  CT scan, 162

in dementia, 251
localization, 160
tests of, 160
Contrecoup injuries, 416
Conversion symptoms, in multiple
    sclerosis, 382
Copper deposition, in Wilson's disease,
    349
Corollary discharge, 194
Corpus callosotomy patients:
    consciousness in, 239
    language in, 236
    spatial functions in, 238–9
    see also Commissurotomy patients
Corpus callosotomy syndrome, 235–9
Corpus callosum, **234**
    alien hand syndrome, 240–1
    corpus callosotomy syndrome,
        235–9
    history of investigation of, 233–5
    lesions, 70
    section:
        in epilepsy, 234–5, 406, 407
        partial, 239–40
    syndromes of, 233–43
    see also Commissurotomy patients;
        Corpus callosotomy patients
Cortical-basal ganglionic degeneration,
    see Corticobasal degeneration
Cortical blindness, 138–40, 314
    causes, 140
    CT scan, **139**
    diagnostic criteria, 140
Cortical deafness, 63, 148
Cortical dementias, *v.* subcortical
    dementias, 352
Cortical networks, 16–17
Cortical–subcortical networks, 16–17
Cortical visual distortions, 140–1
Cortical visual disturbances, 138–41
Corticobasal degeneration, 270, 346
Corticosteroids, associated with
    mania, 335
Creutzfeldt–Jakob disease, 260–1, 274
Crossed aphasia in dextrals, 80–1, **81**
Crossed dominance, 127, 133, 172
Crystallized intelligence, 248
CT (computerized tomography), 46
Cushing's disease, 257

Cushing's syndrome, causing
    delirium, 316
Cysticercosis, 260

Deaf hearing, 149
Deafness:
    cortical deafness, 63, 148
    pure word deafness, 63, 148–50, **149**
Declarative memory, *see* Short-term
    (recent) memory
Deep agraphia, 115
Deep alexia/dyslexia, 110–11, 112
Deinstitutionalization, 327, 332
Delirium, 307–24
    abstraction, 313
    anatomic substrates of, 313–15
    attention in, 310–11
    calculations, 312
    clinical features, 309–13, *310*
    definition, 307
    v. dementia, 253, 309
    differential diagnosis, 308–9
    disorientation, 311–12
    endocrine disorders causing, *316,* 316
    etiology, 315–20, *316*
    v. focal brain lesions, 309
    focal syndromes causing, 314
    infectious diseases causing, *316,* 317
    insight, 313
    judgment, 313
    laboratory testing, *320*
    language, 312
    management of, 320–1
    memory in, 221, 311
    metabolic disorders causing, 315, *316*
    mood, 313
    mortality, 308
    neoplasms causing, *316,* 317
    nutritional disorders causing,
        315–16, *316*
    perception in, 312–13
    personality, 313
    postoperative, 318–20
    prognosis, hypoactive *v.*
        hyperactive, 307
    v. psychosis, 308–9, 326
    risk factors, 308
    stroke and, 166
    toxic disorders causing, *316,* 317

Delirium – *continued*
  vascular diseases causing, *316*, 318
  visuospatial functions, 312–13
  see also Encephalopathy
Delirium tremens, 312, 317
Delusions, in dementia, 251
Dementia(s), 250–2
  and aging, 247–8
  alcoholic dementia, 258
  atypical presenile dementia, 290–1
  causes, treatable/non-treatable, 254,
     292, 293
  communication in, 251
  cortical *v.* subcortical, 352
  definitions, 250
  v. delirium, 253, 309
  v. depression, 252–3, 366–7
  diagnosis, 291–3
  dialysis dementia, 256
  differential diagnosis, 252–4, 254
  diseases associated primarily
     with, 274–91
  endocrine disorders causing,
     255, 256–7
  final stages, 251
  v. focal brain lesion, 253–4
  frontal lobe disease and, 188–9
  frontotemporal, *see* Frontotemporal
     dementia
  hereditary dysphasic dementia, 290
  infectious diseases causing, *255,*
     258–61
  laboratory tests, 291, *291*
  lacking specific histological features,
     290–1
  language in, 251
  life expectancy decrease, 248
  medical diseases associated with,
     254–69, *255*
  memory loss in, 221
  metabolic disorders causing, *255,* 256
  and multiple sclerosis, 269
  neoplasms causing, *255,* 268–9
  neurological diseases associated with,
     269–73, *270*
  non-specific, 290–1
  nutritional disorders causing,
     255, 256
  paraneoplastic syndrome, 268

  progression of, 250–1
  v. pseudodementia, 252–3
  v. psychosis, 326
  screening tests, 28–9
  semantic dementia, 285, 286
  stages, 251–2
  subcortical, *see* Subcortical dementia(s)
  symptoms, 250–1
    variability of, 252
  toxic disorders causing, *255,* 257–8
  vascular diseases causing, *255,* 261–8
  visual agnosia in, 147–8
  white matter dementia, 379
  see also Lewy body dementia; *and*
     individual dementing disorders
Dementia praecox, 328, 329
Dementia pugilistica, 318, 423
Depression, 332, 360–1
  and Alzheimer's disease, 365
  brain imaging, 365–6
  brain stimulation in, 359, 363
  after closed head injuries, 422
  cognitive deficits in, 366–7
  v. dementia, 252–3, 366–7
  in epilepsy, 400–1
  genetic factors, 365
  v. grief reaction, 361
  hormonal changes in, 365
  incidence, 332, 360
  major, diagnostic criteria, 360, *361*
  minor (dysthymic disorder), 360
  in multiple sclerosis, 381–2, 382–3
  in Parkinson's disease, 344, 365
  in post-concussive syndrome, 364
  post-stroke depression, 171
    treatment, 363
  in post-traumatic stress disorder, 364
  prevalence, 332
  primary, 365–7
  and pseudodementia, 252–3
  in stroke patients, 362, 436
  stroke *v.* epilepsy, 400
  suicide risk, 360
  symptoms, 332–3
  in traumatic brain injury, 363–4
  treatment, 367
  tripartite model, 366
  vagus nerve stimulation, 363, 367
  see also Mood

Depression-induced organic mental disorder, *see* Pseudodementia
Depressive cognitive impairment, clinical features, 252
Depressive pseudodementia, 364, 366
Desipramine, depression in multiple sclerosis, 382
Developmental language disorders, 47
Dexamethasone suppression tests, 171
Diabetes, and Alzheimer's disease, 280
Diabetic ketoacidosis, 315
Diagnostic dyspraxia, *see* Alien hand syndrome
Dialysis dementia, 256
Diazepam, in epilepsy, 391
Diffuse axonal injury, 416
Diffuse Lewy body disease, *see* Lewy body dementia
Diplopia, 141
Disconnection:
    in alexia without agraphia, 104, **106**
    in associative visual agnosia, 144–5
    in ideomotor apraxia, 128, 131
    in optic aphasia, 145–6
    in prosopagnosia, 147
    in tactile agnosia, 152
Disconnection anomia, 70
Disconnection theory of conduction aphasia, 65–6, **68**
Discourse:
    in frontal lobe dysfunction, 192
    in Huntington's disease, 347–8
    in traumatic brain injury, 417
'Disorders of attention', 310
Disorientation:
    in the amnestic syndrome, 212
    in delirium, 311–12
    to personal identity, 311–12
    to place and time, 212, 311, 312
    right–left disorientation, 99, *102*
    spatial, 163–4
    topographical, 163–4
Diuretics, in stroke patients, 433
Donepizil:
    in Alzheimer's disease, 282
    in multiple sclerosis, 381
    in vascular dementia, 268
Dopamine, in depression, 366

Dopamine agonists, and Parkinson's disease, 342, 344, 345
Dopamine-blocking drugs, 331
Dopamine excess, in Parkinson's disease, 343
Dopaminergic drugs:
    associated with mania, 335
    and Parkinson's disease, 344
    in progressive supranuclear palsy, 351
Dopaminergic function:
    in Huntington's disease, 348
    in schizophrenia, 330–1
Down's syndrome, 280
Dress, assessment of, 30
Dressing apraxia/impairment, *126*, 126, 162–3
    localization, 162–3
Drive, frontal lobe function, 184
Drug intoxications, causing transient amnesia, 224
Drugs, *see* Medication; Polypharmacy; *and individual drugs*
Dual personalities, 227
Dynamic aphasia, 71
Dysarthria(s), 48–50
    v. apraxia of speech, 51, 126
    ataxic, *49*, 49–50
    auditory signs, *49*
    classification, 48–50, *49*
    definition, 48
    flaccid, 48–9, *49*
    in Huntington's disease, 347
    hyperkinetic, *49*, 50
    hypokinetic, *49*, 50
    localization, *49*
    mixed, 50
    multiple sclerosis causing, *49*, 50
    spastic, *49*, 49
    spastic–flaccid, *49*, 50
    unilateral upper motor neuron (UUMN), *49*, 49
Dysgraphia, neglect dysgraphia, 118
Dyslexia:
    deep dyslexia, 110–11, 112
    letter-by-letter, 109–10
    meaning, 97
    phonological, 111, 112
    surface dyslexia, 111
    visual word-form dyslexia, 110

Dysphasia:
   conflicting terminology, 47
   definition, 47
Dyspraxia, diagnostic, see Alien
      hand syndrome
Dysthymic disorder (minor
      depression), 360
Dystonia, causing dysarthria, 49, 50
Dystonia musculorum deformans, 50

Echolalia, 71
EEG, see Electroencephalography
Electroconvulsive therapy,
      in depression, 367
Electroencephalography (EEG):
   in Alzheimer's disease diagnosis,
      292–3
   in dementia diagnosis, 292
   depth electrodes, 388
   in epilepsy, 388, 389, 391, 392,
      397, 401
   forced normalization, 397, 399
Electrolyte disturbances:
   causing delirium, 315
   causing dementia, 256
Emotion(s), 359–73
   definition, 359
   see also Mood
Emotional changes:
   in frontal lobe dysfunction, 181,
      195–8
   after stroke, 436–7
Emotional incontinence, 362–3
Emotional indifference, 170–2
Emotional lability, 362–3, 436
Encephalitis:
   and dementia:
      limbic, 268–9
      viral, 260
   herpes simplex encephalitis, 200,
      219–20, 260, 315
Encephalopathy:
   acute, see Delirium
   behavioral techniques in prevention
      of, 321
   definition, 307
   hypertensive, 318
   lead encephalopathy, 317
   patient numbers, 308

subcortical arteriosclerotic,
      see Binswanger's disease
   temporal/frontal lobe seizures
      causing, 315
   see also Delirium
Endocarditis, bacterial, and delirium, 317
Endocrine disorders:
   causing delirium, 316, 316
   causing dementia, 255, 256–7
Entacapone, in Parkinson's disease, 342
Environmental dependency syndrome,
      38, 195
Epilepsy, 387–414
   ablative surgery, 388, 404
   aggression and violence in, 401–4
      ictal violence, 402–4
      interictal v. ictal/postictal, 404
      treatment, 403
   anticonvulsant therapy, 403,
      404, 405
   behavioral effects, long-term,
      392–404
   behavioral manifestations, 388
   brain imaging, 388
   brain mapping, 46, 388, 389
   cognitive changes, 388
   cortical maps, 406, 408–9
   definition, 387–8
   depression in, 400–1
   episodic dyscontrol, 403
   hypergraphia in, 393–4, 396
   mood and, 172, 363
   personality changes, 388, 393–6,
      400, 407
   personality traits, 394–6, 394, 400
   philosophical preoccupation in,
      393, 395
   psychosis, 397–400
      complex partial seizures and, 398
      features, 398–9
      pathogenesis, 397–8
      risk factors, 398
      v. schizophrenia, 397
   religious preoccupation in, 393,
      395, 397
   v. seizures, 389
   stigma of, 388
   suicide risk, 400
   syndromes, 389

temporal lobe epilepsy, 226, 390
treatment, 404–9
   emotional and behavioral
      disorders, 407
   ictal violence, 403
   medication, 404–5
   monotherapy *v.* polytherapy, 405
   surgical, 406–7
   vagus nerve stimulation, 363, 406
   see also Seizures
Episodic dyscontrol, in epilepsy, 403
Episodic memory:
   v. semantic memory, 221
   see also Short-term (recent) memory
Estrogen therapy, in Alzheimer's
   disease, 283
Euphoria:
   in frontal lobe disorders, 196
   in multiple sclerosis, 199,
      381, 382
Examination, of mental status, *see*
   Mental status examination
Executive function, 15, 22–3
   of frontal lobe, 184
   in multiple sclerosis, 379, 380
   in Parkinson's disease, 342
Executive function network, 17
Exner's area, 118
Expressive aphasia, 53
Eye movements, in progressive
   supranuclear palsy, 350
Eyelid opening, apraxia of, *126,* 126

Facetiousness:
   in delirium, 313
   in frontal lobe disorders, 196
Facial expression, perception of, 172
Facial identification network, 17
Facial recognition:
   in Huntington's disease, 348
   in Parkinson's disease, 342
   see also Prosopagnosia
False memories, 227
Fetal cell transplantation, in Parkinson's
   disease, 343
Finger agnosia, 70, 101–2, *102*
Fluid intelligence, 248
Fluoxetine:
   in depression, 367

   in post-stroke depression, 363
   in stroke patients, 436
fMRI (functional magnetic resonance
   imaging), 46
Focal brain lesions:
   and anxiety, 368
   v. delirium, 309
   v. dementia, 253–4
   and mood, 361–5
   v. psychosis, 326
Focal stroke syndromes, causing
   delirium, 318
Focal syndromes (lesions), causing
   delirium, 314
Foix–Chavany–Marie syndrome, 198
Football injuries, 423
Forgetfulness:
   as symptom of dementia, 250
   see also Memory loss/disorders; Mild
      cognitive impairment
Fortification spectra, 141
Free will, 15
Frontal alexia, *see* Aphasic alexia
Frontal assessment battery (FAB),
   38, 195
Frontal functions, in Huntington's
   disease, 347
Frontal gait disorder, 127
   see also Gait apraxia
Frontal lobe disorders, 179–205, *181*
   abstraction in, *181,* 186
   attention and, *181,* 189, 196
   behavioral changes in, 179, 180
   behavioral effects, 183–5
   cognition in, 185–6
   dementia and, 188–9
   diagnosis, 186–7
   diseases associated with, 198–200
   emotional changes in, 179, *181,* 195–8
   environmental dependency syndrome
      in, 38, 195
   failure to respond to feedback, 188
   imitation behavior in, 182, 194–5
   judgment, lack of, 188
   language, *181,* 191–2
   memory and, *181,* 189–91
   motor changes, *181,* 193–5
   multiple sclerosis causing, 199
   penetrating injuries, 364

Frontal lobe disorders – *continued*
  personality changes in, 179, *181,*
      195–8, 422
    proverb interpretation, 186
    psychiatric disorder symptoms, 197
    spatial functions, *181,* 192–3
    utilization behavior in, 38, 182,
      194–5
    verbal understanding *v.* behavior, 186
    Wisconsin Card Sorting Test in, 186–7
Frontal lobe functions, 183–5
  corollary discharge, 194
  drive, 184
  executive control, 184
  frontal assessment battery (FAB),
      38, 195
  future memory, 184
  self-awareness, 185
  sequencing, 183–4
  testing, 37–8, 186–7
  see also Affect; Mood
'Frontal lobe syndrome', 197
Frontal lobes:
  anatomy, 180–3
  behavioral disturbances, *181*
  consciousness role, 22, 23
  see also Frontal-subcortical circuits;
      Prefrontal cortex
Frontal neglect, 193
Frontal-subcortical circuits, 181–2, *182*
Frontotemporal dementia (FTD), 287–9
  brain imaging, 288, **289**
  diagnosis, *288, 292*
  features, *288*
  molecular genetics, 290
  neuropathology, 289–90
  subsyndromes, 287
  temporal variant of, 288–9
Fugue states, 224, 226–7
  in epilepsy, 403
  organic *v.* psychogenic, 227
Functional amnesias, 208
Functional magnetic resonance imaging
    (fMRI), 46
Fungal meningitis, causing dementia, 259

GABA (gamma aminobutyric acid):
  and mania, 335
  and schizophrenia, 331

Gabapentin:
  in bipolar affective disorder, 336, 407
  in epilepsy, 405
Gage, Phineas, 179, 196
Gait abnormality, in hydrocephalus,
    271, 272
Gait apraxia, *126,* 126–7, 271
Galantamine:
  in Alzheimer's disease, 282–3
  in multiple sclerosis, 381
  in vascular dementia, 268
Galvanic skin response (GSR), 168
Gamma aminobutyric acid (GABA):
  and mania, 335
  and schizophrenia, 331
Ganser syndrome, 311, 315
Gennari, stria of, **11**, 13
Gerstmann syndrome, 70, *98,* 99–101,
    102, 407
Geschwind, Dr. Norman, 6
Gestural communication systems, 130–1
Giant cell (temporal) arteritis, 265
Gingko biloba, in Alzheimer's
    disease, 283
Glasgow Coma Scale, 415, *416*
Glatiramer, in multiple sclerosis, 381
Global aphasia, 64, 79
Global confusion, 166
Gnosis, testing, 36
Go–no go tests, 38, 187
Granular cortex, 12
Granulomatous angiitis, 265–6
Granulovacuolar degeneration,
    in Alzheimer's disease, 280
Graphemic buffer agraphia, 116–17
Grief reaction, *v.* depression, 361
Grooming:
  assessment of, 30
  in frontal lobe dysfunction, 193
Gunshot wounds, 196, 197
Gustatory cortex, 13

Hallervorden–Spatz disease, 352
  and dementia, *270*
Hallucinations:
  in delirium, 308, 312–13
  in dementia, 251
  in psychosis, 308
  visual, 140

Hallucinosis, alcoholic, and delirium, 317
Haloperidol:
  in Alzheimer's disease, 283
  in delirium, 321
  in epilepsy, 407
  in Huntington's disease, 349
  and Parkinson's disease, 344–5
Handedness:
  in ideomotor apraxia, 127, 130
  inclusion in history taking, 29–30
  see also Left-handedness; Right-
    handedness
Hashimoto's encephalopathy, 257
Head injuries:
  amnesia and, 220
  boxing injuries, 422–3
  causing frontal lobe damage, 198–9
  classification, 415
  closed:
    mania after, 364, 422
    mood and psychiatric changes
      after, 422
  features, 419–20
  headaches following, 421
  mild, 419–23
    brain imaging, 419–20
    causes, 420
    neurobehavioral effects of, 419
    pathology, 420
    post-concussive syndrome, 419,
      420–1
    treatment, 422
  severity and length of amnesia, 420
  see also Concussion; Traumatic brain
    injury
Headaches:
  effect of medication on, 421
  post-traumatic, 421
  rebound headaches, 421
Heart surgery, postoperative delirium,
  318–19
Heavy metal poisoning, 257, 317
Hematomas, as cause of dementia, 254
Hemiachromatopsia, 104, 105
Hemiakinesia, 168
Hemianopia, 105
Hemigraphia, 115–16
Hemineglect, 164
  anatomy of, 166–7

mechanisms of, 167–9
recovery, 169–70
therapy, 169–70
  see also Anosognosia; Neglect
Hemispherectomy, in refractory
  seizures, 406
Hemorrhage, intracranial, causing
  delirium, 318
Hepatic failure/dysfunction:
  and dementia, 256
  in Wilson's disease, 349
Hereditary dysphasic dementia, 290
Herpes simplex encephalitis, 200,
  219–20, 260, 315
Heteromodal association cortices,
  14–15, 103
Heteromodal frontal cortex, 22
High intensity transients (HITS), 319
History taking, mental status assessment
  during, 29–32
HIV, and dementia, 258–9
Human Genome Project, 4
Huntingtin, 348
Huntington's disease (HD), 347–9
  'anticipation' (increasing severity in
    successive generations), 348
  causing dysarthria, *49*, 50
  causing frontal lobe disturbances, 199
  course of, 347
  diagnosis, 348
  features, 347
  juvenile form, 347
  molecular genetics, 348
  pathological changes in, 348
  and subcortical dementia, 270, 271
  suicide risk, 348
  treatment, 349
Hydrocephalus, 259
  communicating hydrocephalus, 272
  and delirium, 317
  see also Normal pressure
    hydrocephalus
Hygiene:
  assessment of, 30
  in frontal lobe dysfunction, 193
Hyperactivity, 184
Hyperbaric oxygen, in stroke
  rehabilitation, 432
Hypercalcemia, and dementia, 256

Hyperglycemia, 315
Hypergraphia, in epilepsy, 393–4, 396
Hyperkinesia, 341
Hyperparathyroidism:
    causing delirium, 316
    causing dementia, 257
Hypertensive encephalopathy, 318
Hyperthyroidism, causing dementia, 257
Hypocalcemia, and dementia, 256
Hypoglycemia, 315
Hypokinesia, 341
    unilateral, 168
Hypomania, 184
Hyponatremia, and dementia, 256
Hypophonia, in Parkinson's disease,
    341–2
Hyposexuality, in epilepsy, 394
Hypothyroidism:
    causing delirium, 316
    causing dementia, 256–7
Hypoxic brain damage, and amnesia, 220

Ideation, paranoid, 328
Ideational agraphia, 117
Ideational apraxia, *126*, 132–3, 188
    definitions, 132
Ideomotor apraxia, 66, *126*, 127–32
    aphasia relationship, 130–1
    in dementing illness, 132
    diagnosis, 127
    disconnection syndrome/model,
        128, 131
    lesion sites and pathways, **128**
    lesions in, 128–9, 130, 131, 132
    phenomena of, 127–8
'Ignoring aphasic', 64
Illness, neglect of, *see* Anosognosia
Imaging, *see* Brain imaging
Imitation behavior, 182, 194–5
Implicit memory, 21, 210–11, *210*
Inattention, *see* Attention
Incontinence:
    in dementia, 251
    in normal-pressure hydrocephalus,
        271, 272
Indifference reaction, 171, 173, 362
Infectious diseases:
    causing delirium, *316*, 317
    causing dementia, *255*, 258–61

Insecticides, 317
Insight:
    assessment of, 31, 38
    in delirium, 313
Insula, 51
Intellectual functions, and aging, 248
Intelligence, crystallized/fluid, 248
Interferons, in multiple sclerosis, 381, 382
Intermanual conflict, *see* Alien
        hand syndrome
Intracranial hemorrhages, causing
        delirium, 318
Intracranial pressure, increased, and
        dementia, 268
Inverse Anton's syndrome, *see* Blindsight
Iron deposition, in Hallervorden–Spatz
        disease, 352
Irritability, 196
Ischemic vascular dementia (IVD),
        see Vascular dementia
Ischemic white matter disease, 264
Isolated agraphia, 118, 119

Jargon, 34
Jargon aphasia, 58
Joseph's disease, causing dysarthria, 50
Judgment:
    assessment of, 31, 38
    in delirium, 313
    in frontal lobe dysfunction, *181,* 188

Ketoacidosis, 315
Kluver–Bucy syndrome, 147, 219
Korsakoff's syndrome, memory in,
        212, 214
Kraepelin's disease, 290–1
Kuru, 260–1

L-DOPA-carbidopa, and Parkinson's
        disease, 344
Laboratory testing:
    Alzheimer's disease, 275–6, 278
    in delirium, *320*
    multiple sclerosis, 378
Lactate infusion, and anxiety, 368
Lacunar state, 263–4
Lamotrigine:
    in bipolar affective disorder, 336, 407
    in epilepsy, 405

Language:
  assessment of, 31–2, 34–5, *34*
  automatic sequences, testing, 34–5
  basal temporal language area, 406–7
  in corpus callosotomy patients, 236
  definition, 45
  in delirium, 312
  in dementia, 251
  developmental disorders, 47
  in frontal lobe dysfunction, *181,*
    191–2
  in Huntington's disease, 347
  inferior temporal language area, 87
  polyglots, aphasia in, 82–3
  right hemisphere functions, 172–3
  in schizophrenia, 329
  in traumatic brain injury, 417
  see also Communication; Speech; *and*
    Speech and Language *entries*
Language cortex, reorganization after
  stroke, 430–1
Language network, 17
Language syndromes, 22
Lead poisoning, 317
Left-handedness:
  agraphia and, 118
  aphasia and, 76, 79–80
  see also Handedness
Left hemisphere:
  language and praxis functions, 241
  lateral surface, 55
Letter blindness, 98, 108
Letter-by-letter reading/alexia/dyslexia,
  109–10
  see also Alexia without agraphia
Leukemia, lymphocytic, brain
  imaging, **100**
Leukoaraiosis, 264
Leukodystrophies, and dementia, 269
Leukoencephalopathies, and
  dementia, *270*
Levitiracetam, 405, 433
Levodopa:
  associated with mania, 335
  in Parkinson's disease, 342, 345
  in progressive supranuclear
    palsy, 350
Levodopa-carbidopa, in Parkinson's
  disease, 342

Lewy body dementia (LBD), 345–6
  v. Alzheimer's disease, 270, 345–6
Lexical agraphia, 114
Lhermitte's syndrome, 378
Limb apraxia, 131
Limb-kinetic apraxia, *126,* 133–4
Limbic cortex, 16
Limbic encephalitis, and dementia,
  268–9
Limbic system, 15, 16
  epilepsy and, 395, 399, 403–4
Lipid storage diseases, and dementia, 269
Lipofuscinosis, cerebral, and
  dementia, 269
Listeria monocytogenes, 259
Literal alexia, 108
Lithium, in mania treatment, 335
Lithium carbonate, in treatment of
  bipolar affective disorder, 335
Liver failure/dysfunction:
  and dementia, 256
  in Wilson's disease, 349
Lobectomy, temporal, 404
Locked-in syndrome, 20
Logorrhea, 58
Lorazepam:
  in delirium tremens, 321
  in epilepsy, 391
LSD (lysergic acid diethylamide), and
  delirium, 317
Lyme borreliosis, 259

Macropsia, 141
Mad cow disease, 261
Magnetic resonance imaging (MRI), 46
Magnetic stimulation, transcranial, in
  neurorehabilitation, 432–3
Mania:
  after closed head injuries, 364, 422
  drugs associated with, 335
  and multiple sclerosis, 382
  after stroke, 437
  treatment, 335
Manic-depressive psychosis:
  v. schizophrenia, 328
  see also Bipolar affective disorder
Mannitol, in brain injury, 417
Mapping (electrical) of brain,
  see Electroencephalography

Mapping (grammatical) therapy, 84
Marchiafava–Bignami syndrome, 258
Mattis Dementia Rating Scale, 28
Medial temporal ablations, amnesia
    secondary to, 219
Medial temporal sclerosis, 219, 391
Medication:
    effect on headaches, 421
    impeding recovery from stroke, 433
    toxic effect causing delirium, 317
    toxic effect resembling dementia, 257
    see also Polypharmacy; and individual
        medications
Megaloblastic madness, 256
Melodic intonation therapy, 151
Memory:
    artificial grammar learning, 211
    assessment of (bedside tests), 31–2,
        33, 33–4
    brain regions activated, 216–17
    classical conditioning, 21, 210, 211
    declarative, 210
        see also Short-term (recent)
            memory
    description, 207
    encoding, depth of, 217
    episodic v. semantic, 221
    explicit, 210
    immediate, 33, 208
    implicit, 21, 210–11, 210
    long-term (remote), 34, 209–10
    loss, see Memory loss/disorders
    motor, 210
    non-declarative, 210, 210, 211
    priming, 21, 210, 211
    probabilistic classification learning,
        210, 211
    procedural, 21, 210, 211
    prospective memory tests, 248
    recency tests, in frontal lobe
        disorders, 190
    recent (short-term), see Short-term
        (recent) memory
    remote (long-term), 34, 209–10
    semantic v. episodic, 221
    short-term (recent), see Short-term
        (recent) memory
    stages of, 33, 208–10
    temporal gradient, 212, 221

tests of, 33, 33–4
    types and localizations, 210
    working memory, 15, 22, 23, 208
    working-memory network, 17
    working-with memory, 190
Memory circuit, 17
Memory loss/disorders:
    in alexia without agraphia, 104, 106
    causes, 220–1
    in commissurotomy patients, 238
    cortical blindness and, 140
    in delirium, 221, 311
    in dementia, 221
    false memories, 227
    in frontal lobe dysfunction, 181,
        189–91
    future memory, frontal lobe
        function, 184
    in Huntington's disease, 347
    memory cues in, 214
    mild cognitive impairment v. normal
        loss in aging, 249
    in multiple sclerosis, 379
    in Parkinson's disease, 342
    partial, syndromes of, 221–3
    primacy effect, 214
    proactive interference, 214
    in progressive supranuclear palsy, 350
    recency effect, 214, 342
    tactile memory disorders, 223
    transient, 226
    in traumatic brain injury, 419
    verbal memory, 222
    visual memory disorder, diagnostic
        criteria, 222–3
    see also Amnesia(s); Amnestic
        syndrome
Meningeal carcinomatosis, 268
Meningiomas, as cause of
    dementia, 254
Meningitis:
    bacterial, 259
    fungal, 259
Mental competency, determination of,
    39–40, 39
Mental deterioration, in Parkinson's
    disease, 344–5
Mental impairments, in Parkinson's
    disease, 343

Mental retardation, 269
Mental status examination, 25–41
  assessment during history taking,
      29–32, 29
  bedside examination, 25–41
  dementia screening tests, 28–9
  formal, 32–8, 32
  individualized examinations, 29–32
  mental competency, 39–40, 39
  Micro Mental State examination, 27
  Mini Mental State examination
      (MMSE), 26–7, 26
  modified MMSE, 27
  necessity for, 25–6
  standardized bedside
      assessments, 26–9
Mesocortex, 16
Metabolic disorders:
  causing delirium, 315, 316
  causing dementia, 255, 256
Metachromatic leukodystrophy, and
      dementia, 269
Metamorphopsia, 141, 312
Metastases, and dementia, 268
Methylphenidate:
  in aphasia, 86
  in refractory depression, 367
Metrifonate, in Alzheimer's disease, 282
Metrizamide, causing delirium, 317
Micro Mental State examination, 27
Micropsia, 141
Midazolam, causing transient
      amnesia, 224
Middle cerebral artery, 56
Mild cognitive impairment (MCI), 249
Mind–brain relationships, 3, 4, 19
Mini Mental State examination (MMSE),
      26–7, 26
  advantages, 27
  limitations, 27
  modified MMSE (3MS), 27
Mirtazapine, in depression, 367
Mixed connective tissue disease, 265
Modified Mini Mental State examination
      (3MS), 27
Modules, 13, 14
Monoamine oxidase inhibitors,
      in refractory depression, 367
Monotherapy, 405

Mood:
  Alzheimer's disease and, 364–5
  assessment of, 30–1, 37–8
  and brain stimulation, 359, 363
  after closed head injuries, 422
  in delirium, 313
  epilepsy and, 172, 363
  focal brain lesions and, 361–5
  Parkinson's disease and, 365
  post-concussive syndrome and, 364
  post-traumatic stress disorder
      and, 364
  traumatic brain injury and, 363–4
  see also Depression; Emotion(s)
Motion, loss of perception of
      (akinetopsia), 141
Motor activity, assessment of, 30
Motor changes, in frontal lobe
      dysfunction, 181, 193–5
Motor cortex, 12
  reorganization after stroke, 428–30
Motor impersistence, 170
Motor perseveration, in frontal lobe
      dysfunction, 193–4
Motor speech disorders, 48–52
  see also individual disorders
Movement disorders, 341–57
MRI (magnetic resonance imaging), 46
Mucopolysaccharidoses, and
      dementia, 270
Multiple personalities, 227
Multiple sclerosis (MS), 377–85
  aphasia/agnosia in, 379
  benign, 377
  bipolar affective disorder and, 382
  brain imaging, 380–1
  causing dysarthria, 49, 50
  causing frontal lobe disturbances, 199
  clinical diagnosis, 377–8
  cognitive fatigue, 379
  cognitive impairment in, 378–81,
      382–3
  conversion symptoms in, 382
  course of, 377
  and dementia, 269
  depression in, 381–2, 382–3
  as disease of white matter, 379, 382
  emotional changes in, 381–2
  laboratory tests, 378

Multiple sclerosis (MS) – *continued*
  and mania, 382
  pathology, 377
  primary progressive, 377
  psychotic illness in, 382
  relapsing-remitting, 377, 381
  secondary progressive, 377
  suicide risk, 382
  temporal course of cognitive
     deficits, 381
  treatment of cognitive deficits in, 381
  treatment of depression in, 382
Multisystem atrophy (MSA), 351–2
  diagnosis, 351–2
Music:
  loss of ability and appreciation
     (amusia), 150–1
  melodic intonation therapy, 151
  musical notation in alexia with
     agraphia, 99
Muteness, 52
Mutism, akinetic, *see* Akinetic mutism
Myasthenia gravis, causing dysarthria, *49*

Naming:
  in alexia with agraphia, *98*
  in alexia without agraphia, 103, *103*
  in anomic aphasia, *69, 69*
  in Broca's aphasia, *54, 54*
  in conduction aphasia, *65, 65*
  in delirium, 312
  in dementia, 251
  in global aphasia, *64*
  in Huntington's disease, 347
  in polyglots, 82–3
  testing, 35
  in transcortical aphasias, 71, *71*, 72
  in traumatic brain injury, 417
  in Wernicke's aphasia, *59, 59*
Narcotics, in stroke patients, 433
Nefazodone, in depression, 367
Neglect, 164
  association with right hemisphere
     disease, 166
  attentional, 167–8
  of deficit itself (anosognosia), 159,
     165, 313
  delirium and, 165–6
  frontal, 193
  intentional, 168
  motor akinesia in, 168
  network approach, 169
  of sensory functions, 165
  visual, 164, 167, 170
  see also Hemineglect
Neglect dysgraphia, 118
Neglect phenomena, in frontal lobe
     disorders, 193
Neocortex, layers of, 12
Neologisms, 34
Neoplasms:
  and delirium, *316*, 317
  and dementia, *255*, 268–9
  see also Tumors
Networks, *see* Brain networks
Neural transplants, in stroke
     rehabilitation, 432
Neuroanatomy, gross/microscopic, 10
Neurocognitive networks, 16–17
Neuroleptics:
  in Alzheimer's disease, 283–4
  impeding recovery from stroke, 433
Neurological diseases, associated with
     dementia, 269–73, *270*
Neuronal thread protein, 292
Neuropsychiatric Inventory, 29
Neuropsychiatry, 5
Neuropsychology, 4
Neurosyphilis, 258–9
  causing frontal lobe disease, 200
Neurotransmitters and depression, 365
Non-aphasic misnaming, 312
Non-steroidal anti-inflammatory drugs,
     in Alzheimer's disease, 283
Norepinephrine, in depression,
     365, 366
Normal pressure hydrocephalus (NPH),
     270, 271–3
  CT scan, **273**
  diagnosis, 272–3, 292
  treatment, 273
Nortriptyline:
  in post-stroke depression, 363
  in stroke patients, 436
Nouns, anomia for, 70
Numbers:
  loss of concept of, 101
  memorizing, 208

memory testing, 33
see also Calculations
Nutritional disorders:
  causing delirium, 315–16, *316*
  causing dementia, *255, 256*

Object identification network, 17
Object recognition testing, 36
Occipital alexia, *see* Alexia
  without agraphia
Occipital cortex, **11**
Oculomotor apraxia, *126,* 126, 142
Olanzepine:
  in Alzheimer's disease, 283–4
  in delirium, 321
  in Parkinson's disease, 345
  in schizophrenia, 332
Olfactory cortex, 13, 16
Olivopontocerebellar atrophy
  (OPCA), 351
Opercular syndrome, 198
Optic agnosia, 145–6
Optic aphasia, 70, 145–6
  disconnection in, 145–6
Optic ataxia, 142
Oral (buccofacial) apraxia, *126,* 126,
  129, 131
Orbitofrontal cortex, 15, 16, 22
Organ failure syndromes
  causing delirium, 315
  and dementia, 256
Organization of information, in frontal
  lobe disorders, 187–8
Orientation, testing, 32
Orienting reflex, 189
Orthographic agraphia, 114
Oxcarbamazepine, in bipolar affective
  disorder, 336
Oxcarbazepine, in epilepsy, 405
Oxygen, hyperbaric oxygen in stroke
  rehabilitation, 432

PACE (Promoting Aphasic's
  Communicative Effectiveness), 84
Paleocortex, 16
Palinopsia, 141
Pallidotomy, in Parkinson's disease, 343
Panic disorders, 368–9
  pathophysiology, 368–9

suicide risk, 368
symptoms, 368
treatment, 369
Papez's circuit, 16, 181, 191, **216**, 216
Paralimbic cortex, 16
Paramnesia, 311, 313
  reduplicative, 163, 311
Paranoia, 313, 395
Paranoid ideation, 328
Paraphasic errors, 34, 66
Parietal cortex, 11, 15
Parietal-temporal alexia, *see* Alexia
  with agraphia
Parkinsonism:
  in boxers, 423
  with dementia, syndromes of,
    345, *346*
Parkinson's disease, 341–5
  age at onset, 341, 342
  causing dysarthria, *49, 50*
  cognitive deficits in, 342–3, 344
  with dementia, 342–3
  depression in, 344, 365
  drug therapy, 342
  effect of medications, 344–5
  features, 341–2
  memory, 342
  mental impairments in, 343, 344
  mood and, 365
  and subcortical dementia, 270, 271
  surgical treatments, 343–4
  visuoperceptual functions, 342
Paroxetine:
  in depression, 367
  in stroke patients, 436
Partial amnesias, 208
Pathological laughter and crying,
  362–3, 436
Pellagra, 256, 315
Penfield, Wilder, 6
Penicillamine, in Wilson's disease, 349
Pentoxyphilline, in vascular
  dementia, 268
Perception, in delirium, 312–13
Pergolide, and Parkinson's disease, 344
Periarteritis nodosa, 265
Perisylvian language circuit, 70, 71
Permanent vegetative state, 20
Pernicious anemia, 256

Perphenazine, in Parkinson's disease, 345
Perseveration:
  in frontal lobe disorders, 187
  motor perseveration, in frontal lobe
      dysfunction, 193–4
  in schizophrenia, 328
Persistent post-concussive syndrome,
    420–1
  predictors, 420
  symptoms, 420–1
Persistent vegetative state, 20
Personality changes:
  in delirium, 313
  in epilepsy, 388, 393–6, 400, 407
  in frontal lobe dysfunction, 179, *181*,
      195–8, 422
  in Huntington's disease, 347
Personality traits, in epilepsy, 394–6,
    394, 400
PET (positron emission tomography), 46
Phakomatoses, and dementia, 269
Phantom limb feeling, 165
Phencyclidine:
  associated with mania, 335
  and delirium, 317
Phenobarbital:
  in epilepsy, 404, 405
  impeding recovery from stroke, 433
Phenylketonuria, and dementia, 269
Phenytoin:
  in aphasia, 86
  in epilepsy, 404–5, 405
  impeding recovery from stroke, 433
Philosophical preoccupation, in epilepsy,
    393, 395
Phonological agraphia, 114–15
Phonological alexia/dyslexia, 111, 112
Physical-letter-code agraphia, 117
Pick bodies, 285
Pick complex, 290
Pick's disease, 284–5, 289
  causing frontal lobe disturbances, 200
  diagnosis, 292
Piracetam, in stroke rehabilitation, 433
Pitres' law, 82
Planning impairment, in frontal lobe
    disorders, 187
Polyglots, aphasia in, 82–3
Polyopia, 141

Polypharmacy:
  causing delirium, 317
  causing dementia, 257–8
  in epilepsy, 405
  rational, 405
Poriomania, 227, 391
Porphyria, causing delirium, 315–16
Positron emission tomography
    (PET), 46
Post-concussive syndrome, 199, 318,
    419, 420–1
  depression and, 364
  v. post-traumatic stress disorder, 421
  predictors, 420
Post-traumatic amnesia, 422
Post-traumatic headaches, 421
Post-traumatic stress disorder (PTSD)
  depression and, 364
  v. post-concussive syndrome, 421
Posterior alexia, *see* Alexia
    without agraphia
Pramipexole, and Parkinson's
    disease, 344
Praxis:
  in commissurotomy patients, 238
  in dementia, 251
  testing, 36, *36*
Prazocin, impeding recovery from
    stroke, 433
Prefrontal cortex, 181
Primary progressive aphasia (PPA),
    285–7
  brain imaging, 285–6, **286–7**
  molecular genetics, 290
  neuropathology, 289–90
Primidone, contributing to depression in
    epilepsy, 404
Priming, 21, *210,* 211
Prions, 261
Probabilistic classification learning,
    210, 211
Procedural memory, 21
  in Parkinson's disease, 342
Progressive multifocal
    leukoencephalopathy (PML), 260
Progressive supranuclear palsy (PSP),
    350–1
  differential diagnosis, 350–1
  features, 350

pathology, 351
and subcortical dementia, 270
treatment, 351
Promoting Aphasic's Communicative
Effectiveness (PACE), 84
Prosopagnosia, 146–7, 314
apperceptive, 146
associative, 146
localization, 147
Prospective memory, tests, 248
Proteins:
in Creutzfeldt–Jakob disease, 261
in dementia, 278, 292
Proverb interpretation, in frontal lobe
disorder, 186
Pseudoagnosic syndromes, 143
Pseudobulbar affect, 362–3
Pseudobulbar palsy, 49, 197–8, 362–3
Pseudodelirium, 309
Pseudodementia, 252–3
depressive, 364, 366
Pseudodepressed personality, 196
Pseudopsychopathic personality, 196
Pseudotumor cerebri, 272
Psychedelic drugs, 317
Psychiatry, biological, 5
Psychic blindness, 147
Psychogenic amnesia, 208, 226–7, 403
fugue states, 224, 226–7
transient memory loss, 226
Psychomotor retardation, 184
Psychosis, 325–39
v. aphasia, 48
v. delirium, 308–9, 326
v. dementia, 326
diagnosis, 326
epileptic, 397–400
complex partial seizures and, 398
features, 398–9
pathogenesis, 397–8
risk factors, 398
v. schizophrenia, 397
v. focal brain lesions, 326
speech and language in, 47–8
symptoms, positive/negative, 326
see also Affective disorders;
Schizophrenia
Psychotic illness, in multiple
sclerosis, 382

Psychotropic medication
in Alzheimer's disease, 283
in epilepsy, 407
Pulmonary failure, and dementia, 256
'Punch-drunk' syndrome, 318
Pure agraphia, 113, 118–19
CT scan, **119**
incidence, 118
lesions, 118
native language influencing, 118–19
Pure alexia, *see* Alexia without agraphia
Pure word blindness, *see* Alexia without
agraphia
Pure word deafness, 63, 148–50, **149**

Quetiapine:
in Alzheimer's disease, 283
in Parkinson's disease, 345
in schizophrenia, 332

Radiation therapy:
and delirium, 317
and dementia, 268
Rancho Los Amigos Scale of Cognitive
Functioning, *418*
Reading:
in alexia with agraphia, *98*
in alexia without agraphia,
103–4, *103*
in anomic aphasia, 69, *69*
in aphasic alexia, 107–9
in Broca's aphasia, 54, *54*
in conduction aphasia, 65, *65*
in dementia, 251
dissociations in, 113
in global aphasia, *64*
in Huntington's disease, 347
letter-by-letter, 109–10
lexical–phonological path to, 111
psycholinguistic model, 111–12
routes to, 108–9, **108**, 111–12
steps in, 98
testing, 35
in transcortical aphasias, 71, *71, 72*
in Wernicke's aphasia, 59, *59*
Reading disorders:
acquired, 97–8
psycholinguistic analysis of, 109–12
see also Agraphia(s); Alexia(s)

Reading disorders – *continued*
  congenital, *see* Dyslexia
  developmental, *see* Dyslexia
Reading errors, classification, *109*
Reasoning, assessment of, 31, 38
Rebound headaches, 421
Recency, *see under* Memory
Recognition, disorders of, *see* Agnosia(s)
Reduplicative paramnesia, 163, 311
Religious preoccupation, in epilepsy,
    393, 395, 397
Renal failure, and dementia, 256
Repetition:
  in alexia with agraphia, *98, 99*
  in alexia without agraphia,
      103, *103*
  in anomic aphasia, *69, 69,* 70
  in aphasia syndromes, 73
  in Broca's aphasia, *54, 54*
  in conduction aphasia, *65, 65*
  in global aphasia, *64*
  testing, 35
  in transcortical aphasias, 71, *71,* 72
  in Wernicke's aphasia, *59, 59*
Reptile brain, 15–16
Reserpine, causing depression, 365
Reticular activating system, 19, 20, 23,
    167–8, 169
Retrograde amnesia, 209, 224, 226
  in minor head injuries, 419
  shrinking, 209
Reverse digit span, 208
Ribot's Law, 82
Right-handedness:
  crossed aphasia, 80–1, **81**
  crossed dominance, 172
  see also Handedness
Right hemisphere:
  behavioral and visuospatial functions,
      159, 241
  language and communication
      functions, 172–3
  reorganization after stroke, 431–2
Right hemisphere disorders, 159–78
  anosognosia, 159, 165, 313
  aprosodias, 173
  behavioral impairments, 159
  behavioral syndromes, *160*
  communication difficulties, 172–3

constructional impairment,
    see Constructional impairment
dressing impairment, *126,* 126, 162–3
emotional indifference, 170–2
hemineglect, *see* Hemineglect
language alterations, 172–3
motor impersistence, 170
neglect, association with, 166
spatial disorientation, 163–4
topographical disorientation, 163–4
Right–left disorientation, 99, *102*
Rigidity, in Parkinson's disease, 341, 343
Risperidone:
  in Alzheimer's disease, 283–4
  in Parkinson's disease, 345
  in schizophrenia, 332
Rivastigmine:
  in Alzheimer's disease, 282
  in multiple sclerosis, 381
Ropinirole, and Parkinson's
    disease, 344

Sarcoidosis, and dementia, 259
Scanning speech, 49
Schizoaffective disorder, 328
Schizophrenia, 327–32
  in adolescents, 325, 327
  v. bipolar affective disorder, 327–8
  brain studies, 330–1
  catatonic, 328
  classification, 328
  cognitive behavioral therapies, 332
  cognitive deficits in, 328–9
  course of, 328
  diagnostic criteria, 327, *327*
  disorganized, 328
  dopaminergic function in, 330–1
  v. epileptic psychoses, 397
  etiology, 329–31
  health care cost, 327
  hebephrenic, 328
  v. manic-depressive psychosis, 328
  neurological signs, 329–30
  paranoid, 328
  prevalence, 327
  suicide risk, 325
  symptoms, 327
  treatment, 328, 331–2
Scrapie, 260

Screening tests:
  dementia, 28–9
  see also Mental status examination
Second impact syndrome, 423
Sedatives, causing delirium, 317
Seizures:
  absence (petit mal) seizures, 391–2
  alcohol withdrawal causing, 317
  clinical manifestations, 389
  definitions, 387–8, 388–9
  v. epilepsy, 389
  focal motor seizures, 390
  focal sensory seizures, 390
  forms of, 388–92, *389*
  grand mal (tonic-clonic)
    seizures, 392
  incidence, 387
  limbic seizures, 390
  partial:
    complex partial seizures, 390–1,
      392, 394, 396, 398
    with secondary generalization, 391
    simple partial seizures, 390
  petit mal (absence) seizures, 391–2
  psychomotor seizures, 390
  refractory seizures, surgical
    management, 406
  temporal lobe seizures, 390
  tonic-clonic (grand mal) seizures, 392
  see also Epilepsy
Selective serotonin reuptake
    inhibitors (SSRIs):
  in depression, 367
  in epilepsy, 407
  in multiple sclerosis, 382
  in panic disorder, 369
  in post-stroke depression, 363
  in stroke patients, 433, 436
Selegiline, in Parkinson's disease, 342
Self-analysis, *see* Self-awareness
Self-awareness:
  definition, 185
  frontal lobe function, 185
  loss of, in dementia, 250
Self-consciousness, *see* Self-awareness
Semantic agraphia, 115
Semantic alexia, *see* Alexia with
    agraphia
Semantic anomia, 70

Semantic dementia, 285, 286
Senile dementia of the Alzheimer type
    (SDAT), 274, 293
Sensorium, assessment of, 30
Sensory cortices, 12, 13
Septicemia, and delirium, 317
Sequencing, frontal lobe function, 183–4
Serial subtractions, 33
Serotonin:
  in depression, 365, 366, 367
  in schizophrenia, 331
Sertraline:
  in depression, 367
  in stroke patients, 436
7-Minute Screen for dementia, 28–9
Sexual behavior, in epilepsy, 394
Sexual dysfunction, after stroke, 435–6
Sexual function, drugs interfering
    with, 433
Shape, distortion of, 141, 312
Short-term (recent) memory,
    33–4, 208–9
  in aging, 249
  in alexia without agraphia, 106
  consolidation process, 209
  memory types functioning in
    short-term memory loss, 21
  neuroanatomy, 209, 215–17
  neurochemistry, 217–18
  processes in, 209
  recall/recognition process, 209
  recording/registration process, 209
  testing, 209
Shy–Drager syndrome, 351
Sign language, 130–1
Sildenafil, in stroke patients, 436
Silent strokes, 262, 263
Simultanagnosia, 110, 142
Singing, impaired, 151
Single photon emission computed
    tomography (SPECT), 46
Sjogren's syndrome, 265
Sneddon's syndrome, 265
Sodium hypochlorite, 261
Somatosensory cortex, 13
Spatial ability, testing, 37, *37*
Spatial agraphia, 117–18
Spatial awareness network, 17
Spatial disorientation, 163–4

Spatial functions, in corpus callosotomy
    patients, 238–9
Speaking, dissociations in, 113
SPECT (single photon emission
    computed tomography), 46
Speech:
    in alexia with agraphia, 98
    in alexia without agraphia, 103, 103
    in anomic aphasia, 69, 69
    apraxia of, see Apraxia of speech
    automatic sequences, testing, 34–5
    in Broca's aphasia, 53, 54
    in conduction aphasia, 65, 65
    definition, 45
    in dementia, 251
    dysfluency in frontal lobe
        dysfunction, 191–2
    emotional tone, 172, 173
    in global aphasia, 64, 64
    in Huntington's disease, 347
    paraphasic errors, 34, 66
    scanning speech, 49
    testing, 34
    in transcortical aphasias, 71, 71, 72
    in traumatic brain injury, 417
    in Wernicke's aphasia, 58–9, 59, 114
    word salad speech, 47, 329
    see also Communication; Language;
        Speech therapy
Speech and language disorders, 45–95
    evaluation of, 47
    history, 45–6
    see also Language; Speech; and
        individual disorders
Speech and language therapy, 431
    see also Speech therapy
Speech area, syndrome of isolation of,
    72–3
Speech therapy, 83–8
    cognitive neuropsychological
        treatment, 84
    efficacy studies, 84–6
    functional communication
        treatment, 84
    principles of, 83
    psycholinguistic treatment, 84
    stimulation–facilitation therapy, 83–4
    theories of, 83–4
    see also Speech and language therapy

Spelling:
    in agraphias, 114, 115, 116–17
    in alexia without agraphia, 103, 107
    dissociations in, 113
    in Wernicke's aphasia, 59–60, 114
Spinocerebellar atrophies, and
    dementia, 270
Split-brain research, 235, 241
Sports injuries, 422–3
Stereognosis, 15
Stimulation:
    coma stimulation, 417–18
    see also Brain stimulation; Vagus
        nerve stimulation
Stria of Gennari, 11, 13
Striatonigral degeneration, 351
    and dementia, 270
Stroke(s), 427–43
    alexia with agraphia, 99
    causing delirium, 318
    causing dysarthria, 49
    causing memory loss, 220
    constraint-induced therapy, 429–30
    emotional changes, 436–7
    lacunar strokes, 263–4
    medical complications, 435–7
    post-stroke depression, 171
        treatment, 363
    post-stroke emotional changes,
        361–3
    posterior cerebral artery (PCA)
        stroke, 314
    rehabilitation, see Stroke
        rehabilitation
    sexual dysfunction after, 435–6
    silent strokes, 262, 263
    statistics, 427
    see also Right hemisphere disorders
Stroke rehabilitation, 428–35
    association cortex reorganization,
        431–2
    economic aspects, 437–9
    efficacy of, 439
    family training, 434–5
    goals, 434–5
    hyperbaric oxygen in, 432
    inpatient admission criteria, 438
    inpatient rehabilitation, 439
    language cortex reorganization, 430–1

medications impeding recovery, 86, 433
motor cortex reorganization, 428–30
neural transplants in, 432
outcome prediction, 437–8
  G-score, 438, *438*
pharmacotherapy in, 433–4
practical aspects, 437–9
scientific basis of, 428
selection of patients for, 437–8
speech and language therapy, 431
therapies, 434
transcranial magnetic stimulation in, 432–3
Stroop test, 187
Subacute diencephalic angioencephalopathy, 266
Subacute sclerosing panencephalitis (SSPE), 260
Subangular alexia, 105
Subcortical aphasias, 75–9
Subcortical arteriosclerotic encephalopathy (Binswanger's disease), 264
Subcortical dementia(s), 269–71, 352
  v. cortical dementias, 352
  diagnosis, 292
  features, 270–1
  and multiple sclerosis, 379
Subpial transections, in refractory seizures, 406
Suicide risk:
  depression, 360
  epilepsy, 400
  Huntington's disease (HD), 348
  multiple sclerosis (MS), 382
  panic disorders, 368
  schizophrenia, 325
Sundowning, 252, 309
Supramodal association cortex, 183
Supramodal cortex, 15–16, 22
Supraspan numbers, 33, 208
Surface agraphia, 114
Surface alexia/dyslexia, 111, 112
Susac's syndrome, 265
Syphilis, 258–9
Systemic lupus erythematosus, 265

Tacrine, in Alzheimer's disease, 282
Tactile agnosia(s), 36, 151–2
  associative, 151
  mechanisms of, 152
Tactile aphasia, 152
Tactile memory disorders, 223
Tau protein, 278, 292
Tauopathies, 290
Tay–Sachs disease, and dementia, 269
Teichopsia, 141
Temporal (giant cell) arteritis, 265
Temporal lobe epilepsy, 226, 390
Temporal lobectomy, 404
Testing:
  of mental status, *see* Mental status examination
  see also Laboratory testing
Thalamic aphasia, 75–6
  brain imaging, **76**
  localization, 75
Thalamotomy, in Parkinson's disease, 343
Thiamine deficiency, 219, 256, 315
Third alexia, *see* Aphasic alexia
Thought process, assessment of, 31
Thrombotic thrombocytopenic purpura (TTP), 265
Thyrotoxicosis, causing delirium, 316
Tiagabine, in epilepsy, 405
Tip of the tongue phenomenon, 54
Todd's paralysis, 390, 392
Toes, blue toes, 265
Tool-use apraxia, 133
'Top of the basilar embolus' syndrome, 140
Topiramate:
  in bipolar affective disorder, 407
  in epilepsy, 405
Topographical disorientation, 163–4
Toxic disorders:
  causing delirium, *316*, 317
  causing dementia, *255*, 257–8
Toxic psychosis, *see* Delirium
Trailmaking test (Wechsler Adult Intelligence Scale), 187
Tranquilizers, and delirium, 317, 321
Transcortical aphasia(s), 71–3
  characteristics, *71*
  mixed, 72–3

Transcortical aphasia(s) – *continued*
  motor (TCMA), 71–2
  sensory (TCSA), 72
  in traumatic brain injury, 417
Transcranial doppler (TCD), 319
Transcranial magnetic stimulation, in
    neurorehabilitation, 432–3
Transient amnesia, 223–5
  causes, 223–4
  see also Transient global amnesia
Transient global amnesia (TGA), 224–5
  brain imaging, 225
  etiology, 225
  incidence, 225
Transitional agraphia, *see* Apraxic
    agraphia
Traumatic brain injury (TBI), 415–26
  amnesia and, 220
  brain imaging, 417, 418–19
  causing confusional state, 318
  causing frontal lobe damage, 198–9
  contrecoup injuries, 416
  depression in, 363–4
  memory loss, 419
  moderate, 418–19
    language disorders in, 417
  mood and, 363–4
  severe, 416–18
    language disorders in, 417
    management, 417
    post-injury impairments, 417
    rehabilitation, 417–18
  statistics, 415
  see also Concussion; Head injuries
Trazodone:
  in Alzheimer's disease, 283
  in post-stroke depression, 363
Tremor, in Parkinson's disease, 341, 343
Triazolam, causing transient amnesia, 224
Triethylene tetramine dihydrochloride
    (trine), in Wilson's disease, 349
Trihexyphenidyl, and Parkinson's
    disease, 344
Trine (triethylene tetramine
    dihydrochloride), in Wilson's
    disease, 349
Triune brain, 15–16
Tuberculosis, and dementia, 259
Tuberous sclerosis, and dementia, 269

Tumors:
  amnesia and, 220
  causing dementia, 188–9, 254, 268
  causing dysarthria, 49
  causing frontal lobe dysfunction, 199
  causing transient amnesia, 224
  see also Neoplasms

Uhtoff's syndrome, 377
Unawareness, *see* Self-awareness
Unconsciousness, 19
  non-Freudian unconscious, 22
  see also Consciousness
Unilateral agraphia, 115–16
Unimodal association cortex, 14
Utilization behavior, 38, 182, 194–5

Vagus nerve stimulation:
  in depression, 363, 367
  in epilepsy, 363, 406
Valproic acid:
  in Alzheimer's disease, 283
  in bipolar affective disorder, 336, 407
  in epilepsy, 405
Vascular dementia:
  diagnostic criteria, 266–7, 266, 267
  Hachinski index, 266–7, 266
  treatment, 268
Vascular disease(s):
  causing delirium, 316, 318
  causing dementia, 255, 261–8
  causing frontal lobe disturbances, 199
  multiple infarcts, 262–3
Vasculitis, 265–6:
  cerebral, causing delirium, 318
Vasodilators, in Alzheimer's disease, 283
Vegetative state, 20
Venlafaxine, in depression, 367
Verbal apraxia, *see* Apraxia of speech
Verbal memory, 222
Verbs, anomia for, 70
Violence:
  and frontal lobe damage, 197
  see also Aggression
Viral encephalitis, 260
Visual ability, testing, 37, 37
Visual agnosia(s), 138–48
  apperceptive, 143–4, 148–9
  associative, 144–5

Balint's syndrome, 141–2
    cortical visual distortions, 140–1
    cortical visual disturbances, 138–41
    in dementia, 147–8
    Kluver–Bucy syndrome, 147, 219
    optic agnosia, 145–6
    prosopagnosia, 146–7, 314
    in pure alexia, 104
    simultanagnosia, 110, 142
    visual object agnosia, 143–5
Visual allesthesia, 141
Visual awareness, 21
Visual cortex, 12–13, 13
    cell functions, 14
Visual field defects, 102
Visual memory disorder, diagnostic
        criteria, 222–3
Visual neglect, 164, 167, 170
Visual processing, 21
Visual streams, dorsal/ventral, 21
Visual word-form dyslexia, 110
'Visuokinesthetic engrams', 128
Visuoperceptual function, in Parkinson's
        disease, 342
Visuospatial agraphia, 117–18
Visuospatial dysfunction:
    in delirium, 312–13
    in dementia, 251
    in frontal lobe dysfunction, 181, 192–3
    in Huntington's disease, 347, 348
    in Parkinson's disease, 342
    in schizophrenia, 329
Vitamin B1 (thiamine) deficiency, 219,
        256, 315
Vitamin B12 deficiency, 256, 315
Vitamin E, in Alzheimer's disease, 283

Wada testing, 81
Wayward hand, see Alien hand
        syndrome
Wegener's granulomatosis, 265
Wernicke–Korsakoff syndrome, 218–19,
        317
    etiology, 218–19, 256, 258
Wernicke's aphasia, 58–63, 107
    'analogue' of, 314
    associated signs, 59, 60
    auditory comprehension in, 59,
        60, 63

behavior in, 59
brain imaging in, 60, 61–2
v. Broca's aphasia, 58–9, 60
and delirium, 314
features, 59–60, 59
'mirror image' of, 166
naming in, 59, 59
reading in, 59, 59
repetition in, 59, 59
spelling in, 59–60, 114
spontaneous speech in, 58–9, 59, 114
writing in, 59–60, 59, 114
Wernicke's area, 17, 55, 56, 63, 68
    in epilepsy, 406, 407, 408
    and ideomotor apraxia, 128–9, 128
Western Aphasia Battery (WAB), 52
Whipple's disease, 259
White matter:
    ischemic white matter disease, 264
    multiple sclerosis as disease of,
        379, 382
White matter bundles, 13, 13
    connecting Wernicke's and Broca's
        areas, 68
White matter dementia, 379
Wilson's disease, 349–50
    causing dysarthria characteristics, 50
    diagnosis, 349–50
    and subcortical dementia, 270
    symptoms, 349
    treatment, 349
Wisconsin Card Sorting Test (WCST),
        186–7
Witzelsucht, 313, 315
Word blindness, 108
    pure, see Alexia without agraphia
Word production anomia, 69
Word salad speech, 47, 329
Word selection anomia, 69
Working memory, 15, 22, 23, 208
Working-memory network, 17
Working-with memory, 190
Writing:
    in alexia with agraphia, 98, 99
    in alexia without agraphia, 103, 104
    in anomic aphasia, 69, 69
    in aphasic agraphia, 113–14
    asemantic, 115
    in Broca's aphasia, 54, 54–5, 116

Writing – *continued*
  in conduction aphasia, 65, *65*
  in delirium, 312
  in dementia, 251
  dissociations in, 113
  elements involved in, 112
  in global aphasia, *64*
  in Huntington's disease, 347
  prostheses, 116

testing, 35
in transcortical aphasias, 71, *71*
in Wernicke's aphasia, 59–60, *59*, 114
see also Agraphia

Z
Ziduvidine, causing mania, 335
Zinc, in Wilson's disease, 349
Zonisamide, in epilepsy, 405